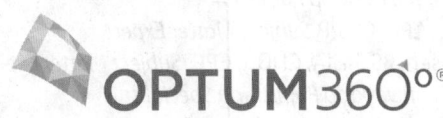

Auditors' Desk Reference

A comprehensive resource for code selection and validation

2021

optum360coding.com

Acknowledgments

Gregory A. Kemp, MA, *Product Manager*
Stacy Perry, *Manager, Desktop Publishing*
Nichole VanHorn, CPC, CCS-P, *Subject Matter Expert*
Jacqueline Petersen, BS, RHIA, CHDA, CPC, *Subject Matter Expert*
Tracy Betzler, *Senior Desktop Publishing Specialist*
Hope M. Dunn, *Senior Desktop Publishing Specialist*
Katie Russell, *Desktop Publishing Specialist*
Kimberli Turner, *Editor*

Subject Matter Experts

Nichole VanHorn, CPC, CCS-P, *Subject Matter Expert*
Ms. VanHorn has more than 20 years of experience in the health care profession. Her areas of expertise include CPT and ICD-10-CM coding in multiple specialties, auditing, and education. Most recently she served as Clinical Auditor for a multispecialty group. Ms. VanHorn was responsible for the oversight of the physician coding and education section of the Corporate Compliance Program. She has been an active member of her local American Academy of Professional Coders (AAPC) chapter for several years and has also served as an officer.

Jacqueline Petersen, BS, RHIA, CHDA, CPC, *Subject Matter Expert*
Ms. Petersen has more than 25 years of experience in the health care profession. She has served as Senior Clinical Product Research Analyst with Optum360 developing business requirements for edits to support correct coding and reimbursement for claims processing applications. Her experience includes development of data-driven and system rules for both professional and facility claims and in-depth analysis of claims data inclusive of ICD-10-CM, CPT, HCPCS, and modifiers. Her background also includes consulting work for Optum, serving as a SME, providing coding and reimbursement education to internal and external clients. Ms. Petersen is a member of the American Academy of Professional Coders (AAPC), and the American Health Information Management Association (AHIMA).

At our core, we're about coding.

Essential medical code sets are just that — essential to your revenue cycle. In our ICD-10-CM/PCS, CPT®, HCPCS and DRG coding tools, we apply our collective coding expertise to present these code sets in a way that is comprehensive, plus easy to use and apply. Print books are inexpensive and easily referenced, created with intuitive features and formats, such as visual alerts, color-coding and symbols to identify important coding notes and instructions — plus great coding tips.

Find the same content, tips and features in a variety of formats. Choose from print products, online coding tools, data files or web services, as well as from various educational opportunities.

Your coding, billing and reimbursement product team,

Ryan Nichole Greg LaJuana
Regina Ken Julie Denise Leanne
Jacqui Marianne Elizabeth Nann
Anita Debbie Karen

Put Optum360 medical coding, billing and reimbursement content at your fingertips today. Choose what works for you.

📖 Print books

🛠️ Online coding tools

📁 Data files

🖥️ Web services

Visit us at **optum360coding.com** to browse our products, or call us at **1-800-464-3649, option 1** for more information.

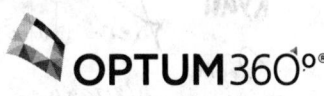

CPT is a registered trademark of the American Medical Association.

What if you could go back in time?

How much time do you think you spend researching elusive codes? Too much, probably. Time you would like to have back. We can't give time back, but we can help you save it. Our all-in-one coding solutions consolidate specialty coding processes so you can find information more easily and quickly. Each specialty-specific procedure code includes its official and lay descriptions, coding tips, cross-coding to common ICD-10-CM codes, relative value units, Medicare edit guidance, *CPT Assistant®* references, CCI edits and, when relevant, specific reimbursement and documentation tips.

With tools available for 30 specialties, we're sure you'll find the right resource to meet your organization's unique needs, even if those needs are allergy, anesthesia/pain management, behavioral health, cardiology, cardiothoracic surgery, dental, dermatology, emergency medicine, ENT, gastroenterology, general surgery, hematology, laboratory/pathology, nephrology, neurology, neurosurgery, OB/GYN, OMS, oncology, ophthalmology, orthopaedics, pediatrics, physical therapy, plastics, podiatry, primary care, pulmonology, radiology, urology or vascular surgery.

Say good-bye to time wasted digging for those elusive codes.

Your coding, billing and reimbursement product team,

Ryan   Nichole   Greg   LaJuana
        Ken   Julie
Regina   Marianne   Denise   Leanne
Jacqui   Anita   Debbie   Elizabeth   Nann
                    Karen

Put Optum360 medical coding, billing and reimbursement content at your fingertips today. Choose what works for you.

- Print books
- Online coding tools
- Data files
- Web services

Visit us at **optum360coding.com** to browse our products, or call us at **1-800-464-3649, option 1** for more information.

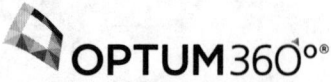

CPT is a registered trademark of the American Medical Association.

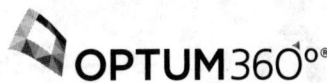

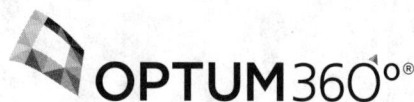

Optum360 **Learning**
LEARN. PRACTICE. APPLY.

Education suiting your specialty, learning style and schedule

Optum360® Learning is designed to address exactly what you and your learners need. We offer several delivery methods developed for various adult learning styles, general public education, and tailor-made programs specific to your organization — all created by our coding and clinical documentation education professionals.

Our strategy is simple — education must be concise, relevant and accurate. Choose the delivery method that works best for you:

eLearning

- **Web-based** courses offered at the most convenient times
- **Interactive**, task-focused and developed around practical scenarios
- **Self-paced** courses that include "try-it" functionality, knowledge checks and downloadable resources

Instructor-led training

On-site or remote courses built specifically for your organization and learners
- CDI specialists
- Coders
- Providers

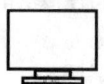

Webinars

Online courses geared toward a broad market of learners and delivered in a live setting

No matter your learning style, Optum360 is here to help you

 Visit **optum360coding.com/learning**

 Call **1-800-464-3649, option 1**

 You've worked hard for your credentials, and now you need an easy way to maintain your certification.

Contents

© 2020 Optum360, LLC

Chapter 1

Auditing Processes and Protocols

Many years ago getting reimbursed for a service was simple, requiring only a handwritten or typed claim form that included the procedure performed, the fee, and the diagnosis. CPT® and ICD-10-CM codes were not necessary. Life was easy. Now the entire process has evolved and everything is much more complicated. Processes have been streamlined, requiring a uniform process for all providers to follow. This chapter discusses some of these processes, and includes information as to why it is necessary to include audits as a part of each practice.

Claims Reimbursement

Receiving appropriate reimbursement for professional services can sometimes be difficult due to the complexity of rules involved. There are a number of things that are important to consider. The following section discusses some of the various requirements for getting a claim paid promptly and correctly.

Coverage Issues

Covered services are services payable by the insurer in accordance with the terms of the benefit-plan contract. Such services must be properly documented and medically necessary in order for payment to be made.

Medical necessity has been defined by CMS as "services or supplies that are proper and needed for the diagnosis or treatment of [a] medical condition; are provided for the diagnosis, direct care, and treatment of [a] medical condition; meet the standards of good medical practice in the local area; and aren't mainly for the convenience of [a patient] or doctor."

Section 1862 (a)(1) of the Social Security Act prohibits Medicare from covering items and services that "are not reasonable and necessary for the diagnosis or treatment of illness or injury, or to improve the function of a malformed body member."

Typically, most payers define medically necessary services or supplies as:

- Services that have been established as safe and effective
- Services that are consistent with the symptoms or diagnosis
- Services that are necessary and consistent with generally accepted medical standards
- Services that are furnished at the most appropriate, safe, and effective level

 DENIAL ALERT

Medical necessity denial decisions must be based on a detailed and thorough analysis of the patient's condition, need for care, safety and effectiveness of the service, and coverage policies.

Documentation must be provided to support the medical necessity of a service, procedure, and/or other item. Remember, payers may request the medical record documentation to determine medical necessity. This documentation should show:

- What service or procedure was rendered
- To what extent the service or procedure was rendered
- Why the service, procedure, or other item was medically warranted

Services, procedures, and/or other items that may not be considered medically necessary are:

- Services that are not typically accepted as safe and effective in the setting where they are provided
- Services that are not generally accepted as safe and effective for the condition being treated
- Services that are not proven to be safe and effective based on peer review or scientific literature
- Experimental or investigational services
- Services that are furnished at a duration, intensity, or frequency that is not medically appropriate
- Services that are not furnished in accordance with accepted standards of medical practice
- Services that are not furnished in a setting appropriate to the patient's medical needs and condition

If a service rendered is not deemed to be medically necessary, that service will be denied. For Medicare, unless the patient was previously notified of this fact and an Advance Beneficiary Notice (ABN, also referred to as a Waiver of Liability Statement) has been completed, the patient may not be billed for these services.

Code Selection

Providers must translate the services they provide and the reason for providing those services into codes. In 1983, Medicare's administrative body established the Healthcare Common Procedural Coding System (HCPCS). There are two tiers to HCPCS codes. Level I is the *Physicians' Current Procedural Terminology, Fourth Edition* (CPT), published by the American Medical Association (AMA), used primarily to report provider services and procedures. The second tier, HCPCS Level II (pronounced as "Hick Picks"), is used to report nonphysician services, durable medical equipment and supplies, and certain drugs.

The *International Statistical Classification of Diseases and Related Health Problems, Tenth Revision* (ICD-10), is published by the World Health Organization (WHO). It is the classification used in cause-of-death coding in the United States. The *International Statistical Classification of Diseases and Related Health Problems, 10th revision, Clinical Modification* (ICD-10-CM) is the United States' clinical modification of the World Health Organization's ICD-10. The term "clinical" is used to emphasize the modification's intent to serve as a useful tool in the areas of:

- Classification of morbidity data for indexing of health records
- Medical care review, including ambulatory and other healthcare programs
- Basic health statistics

DEFINITIONS

Advance Beneficiary Notice. Written communication with a Medicare beneficiary given before Part B services are rendered, informing the patient that the provider (including independent laboratories, imaging centers, physicians, practitioners, and/or suppliers) believes Medicare will not pay for some or all of the services to be rendered. Form CMS-R-131 may be used for all situations where Medicare payment is expected to be denied.

HIPAA. Health Insurance Portability and Accountability Act of 1996. Federal law that allows persons to qualify immediately for comparable health insurance coverage when they change their employment relationships. Title II, subtitle F, of HIPAA gives the Department of Health and Human Services the authority to mandate the use of standards for the electronic exchange of health care data; to specify what medical and administrative code sets should be used within those standards; to require the use of national identification systems for health care patients, providers, payers (or plans), and employers (or sponsors); and to specify the types of measures required to protect the security and privacy of personally identifiable health care information.

To describe the clinical picture of the patient, the codes must be more precise than those needed only for statistical groupings and trend analysis. Annual revisions to ICD-10-CM are made based on the established update process for ICD-10-CM (ICD-10-CM Coordination and Maintenance Committee) and the World Health Organization's ICD-10 (Update and Revision Committee).

The Health Insurance Portability and Accountability Act (HIPAA) mandated that professional services should be identified using current CPT and HCPCS Level II codes. The reason for the encounter should be reported using ICD-10-CM diagnostic codes.

Coding is often a major reason for claim delays, denials, and in some cases payer audits. Some of the most commonly reported claim denials can encompass a wide variety of errors, including but not limited to:

- Failure to code to the highest degree of specificity (ICD-10-CM)
- Transposing code numbers
- Using nonspecific codes (NEC, NOS, or unlisted)
- Unbundling services
- Improper use of modifiers
- Reporting invalid codes

A major key to successful coding and reporting of medical services involves ongoing education and training to stay current with the annual changes to the codes themselves, as well as the guidelines for proper reporting. In addition, maintaining updated code books and other reference materials, such as charge tickets and superbills, is a must to minimize the possibility of reporting invalid codes. A thorough understanding of the code sets, medical terminology, and proper use of coding books and other resources is essential to not only reducing claim denials but also to limiting liability from erroneous or fraudulent claims processing practices. It is not only detrimental to the revenue cycle process and the practice's bottom line to code improperly but it can also increase risk and liability while exposing the practice to audits and ongoing reviews of claims. These types of actions can significantly impede the processing of claims, which leads to slow reimbursement because each claim must be individually reviewed and approved.

Coding issues are one of the main areas of focus when consultants are asked to audit a medical practice for issues related to the revenue cycle process and yet, are one of the most easily remedied issues as well. Many times the errors found through an audit include simple fixes to coding errors, which can lead to significant increases in revenue, and identifying missed or underreported services, which can have a tremendous impact on a practice's bottom line.

Preauthorization and Precertification

Another simple but time consuming issue that can significantly impact claim reimbursement is preauthorization or precertification. Many payers require a preauthorization or precertification prior to a procedure or service for payment to be made.

Failure to comply with this requirement results in claim denials. Unlike coding issues, a denial for failure to preauthorize or precertify a service cannot be appealed. Instead, processes must be developed to alert staff as to which procedures and services require preauthorization or precertification and the steps necessary to do so. Many payers maintain a list of procedures that require some type of preapproval as part of the process to submit the claim for payment. When a list is not available, larger practices have a designated staff member who performs this vital service or in a single or small group practice, oftentimes the clinical or nursing staff member does it.

Preauthorization or precertification describes a process in which coverage is approved for a specific procedure, service, or even a medication based upon meeting the medical necessity criteria as defined by the particular payer. The terms are often used interchangeably but more commonly preauthorization is applied toward surgical services or procedures and precertification refers to an approval for an inpatient hospital stay. The key point being that the service, whether a hospital admission or a surgical procedure, requires a prior approval before the service can be submitted and considered for payment.

In order to secure prior authorization or approval for the service in question, the provider must demonstrate medical necessity and the appropriateness of the plan of treatment for the service being requested. This may entail providing the specific CPT and ICD-10-CM codes that represent the procedure to be performed and the diagnosis code for the condition being treated, as well as the place of service where the service will be performed, such as inpatient or at an ambulatory surgery center. Medical records, provider notes, reports from lab or other ancillary services, and/or radiology films may be required by the payer prior to issuing an authorization number.

Due to the lack of consistency and uniformity in how commercial plans and contracts are administered, it is strongly suggested that a practice contact the patient's individual payer and check whether preapproval is needed in the absence of a plan matrix that specifies this information. It is always better to be safe than sorry.

Once this process has been completed, the next step is to communicate that the procedure has been approved and a precertification or preauthorization number has been issued. This number needs to be included on the claim when it is submitted. There should be policies and procedures in place to ensure easy transfer of this information through direct entry into the practice management billing system or through an established manual process.

Claims denied for lack of a preauthorization number should be examined to see whether a number was, in fact, obtained but omitted on the claim or whether the preapproval process was not completed at all. Clearly, a remedy for the latter situation is much more difficult and would require evaluating existing work processes to try and determine how this type of oversight can happen and what steps should be implemented to avoid this happening in the future. It may be possible to contact the payer and ascertain what, if any, options are available. The good news is that in many cases when the provider office overlooks or fails to obtain the preauthorization or precertification number, the facility where the procedure is being performed serves as a "back up" and the provider can obtain the preapproval number through the facility. Still, this should be the exception and not the rule.

Role of Audits

A chart audit is a detailed review of a medical record to determine what service/procedure was performed, and to see if it was reported correctly. There

© 2020 Optum360, LLC

are a number of performance components that can be measured in a chart audit, including:

- Provider and staff compliance with documentation requirements
- Provider and staff compliance with payer guidelines
- Adherence to office protocols
- Appropriate and accurate reimbursement

An audit can be conducted on virtually any aspect of the chart, including medical and surgical care. The data should be complete, accurate, and must be available in the chart. A chart audit also involves reviewing data that may be deemed confidential; therefore, it is necessary to consult the appropriate institutional privacy guidelines prior to reviewing charts.

While most frequently performed to determine compliance with coding and billing requirements, chart audits may also be performed for clinical care quality improvement. A chart audit for quality improvement measures how often and how well something is being done (or not done). For example, a chart audit may involve reviewing a pediatric practice's charts to see how often the chicken pox vaccine is offered, administered, or declined. If the audit determines that the vaccine is not being offered or administered as recommended, then there is room for improvement.

There are a few steps that can be taken by clinical staff to help avoid mistakes, including:

- Document thoroughly all communication with the patient.
- Develop written policies and procedures and distribute them to the clinical and administrative staff.
- Create a written compliance plan and educate all employees on its content.
- Ensure adherence with internal compliance policies and procedures by all clinical and administrative staff.
- Provide coding and billing education to clinical staff on a regular basis (i.e., annual code and guideline changes).
- Provide access to current coding books and regulation manuals as references.
- Conduct periodic internal audits and document the results.
- Educate, educate, educate.

Background of Audits

Auditing is used by government and commercial payers alike to determine if payments are being made appropriately. The Office of Inspector General (OIG) audits that began in 1996 are the most extensive in terms of the size of the settlements and the implications for providers. Large and small physician offices and hospitals alike have been selected for audit with the dollar recovery amounts often being in the millions. Billing errors, failure to combine outpatient charges with inpatient stays, and misapplied codes have brought penalties of treble damages, fines, and the threat of criminal prosecution. It has been a visible attempt by the federal government to control fraud and abuse and everyone takes these audits quite seriously.

 DEFINITIONS

chargemaster. File, usually in an electronic billing system, where charge amounts are kept for all procedures, services, and supplies in a hospital for use with billing software in claims submission.

compliance committee. Individuals assigned to help the compliance officer teach and comply with all laws, regulations, and guidelines related to health care.

fraud. Intentional deception, misrepresentation, or a statement that is known to be false that could result in an unauthorized benefit to the patient, provider, or other persons.

OIG. Office of Inspector General. Agency within the Department of Health and Human Services that is ultimately responsible for investigating instances of fraud and abuse in the Medicare and Medicaid and other government health care programs. Annual OIG work plan details the areas of focus for fraud and abuse investigations.

External Audits

External audits are performed by an agency or organization other than the provider or provider group, commonly by federal or state agencies, Medicare contractors, and commercial payers. External audits and investigations can be initiated by a payer requesting the medical record documentation associated with a date of service or with a search warrant, a grand jury subpoena, or by an investigator contacting an employee at work or at home. The key is to be prepared and to have written procedures in place, including the telephone number of the provider's attorney for these different scenarios.

Internal Audits

Each practice should implement an internal auditing program. Auditing provider charges and billing practices is a large task to undertake, but the results typically lead to improved claims management processes, cash flow, and compliance with payer rules and regulations. Chart audits can serve many purposes, from compliance to research to administrative to clinical. A practice can conduct a chart audit on virtually any aspect of care that is documented in the medical record. Auditing charts allows practices to identify specific coding issues that may occur in claims submissions. There may be a high number of similar types of claim errors that can be identified and, in this case, pre-submission monitoring and review of these may safeguard against repeated errors that result in a claim denial and decreased revenue. An internal audit allows the provider and staff to identify incorrect billing patterns before claims are denied or payer audits arise and penalties are assessed.

The results of these regular and periodic internal audits can be used to develop an action plan addressing deficiencies and other findings and recommendations. Involve staff, other departments, and upper management in developing procedures to correct the problems. Some issues cross department lines (e.g., coding issues) and it may take a focused task force to resolve some of the deficiencies.

The compliance committee, or the individual responsible for compliance, should be expected to complete the following reviews and actions in a diligent search to uncover deficient or noncompliant areas:

- Review the OIG fraud alerts and major fraud cases
- Identify patterns of billing denials or focused reviews
- Review survey deficiencies, internal/external audits, agency audits, independent auditor's recommendation, and prior audits to verify if identified issues have been resolved
- Develop a compliance plan modeled after the OIG compliance guidance plan
- Perform routine internal audits
- Identify any signs of potential violations in the areas of:
    - equipment, or services given to physicians or hospitals
    - chargemasters that may not have been updated in years
    - billing insurance only and failing to balance bill patients
    - discounts to patients, physicians, or employees
    - giving or receiving gifts to induce referrals
    - contracts that have not been reviewed for years or by an attorney

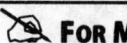
FOR MORE INFO

OIG fraud alerts and fraud cases can be found at:
http://oig.hhs.gov/fraud/enforcement/criminal/

FOR MORE INFO

The OIG compliance resource portal can be found at https://oig.hhs.gov/compliance/compliance-resource-portal/

Audit Types

There are two types of internal audits that can be performed: prospective or retrospective.

A prospective billing audit is a review of claims before they are submitted to the payer, paying special attention to coding and documentation to ensure that code assignment is correct and that payer guidelines have been adhered to.

A retrospective billing audit is a review of claims after they are paid. Coding assignment and payer guidelines are reviewed. If any overpayments or billing errors are identified, they are dealt with according to payer guidelines.

If audits reveal repeated errors, the claims should be corrected and education should be provided to staff to resolve the issue, so as not to create a pattern that will be identified by payers and result in penalties. The time frame of audits may vary from practice to practice depending on the issues found. For example, if a provider is consistently overbilling, the practice may decide to audit that provider quarterly instead of yearly.

Audit Responsibility

Many practices assign a staff member to conduct internal audits or hire a consultant that specializes in the practice's specialty. Once the audits have been performed, providers and other staff members need to be educated on the findings. This can be performed by the same staff member who conducted the audits or by the compliance officer.

Medical Record Documentation

Overview

When auditing a service, medical record documentation easily ranks among the top areas of concern or focus in any hospital, physician practice, or other health care facility or organization. The reason is simple: medical record documentation indicates what services were provided and the reason for providing them. Additionally, medical records are an essential component of providing quality patient care and serve as an important source of data. By its very nature, the medical record is the means by which providers communicate and ensure the patient's continuity of care and treatment. As a result, it is vitally important that medical record documentation standards are established and maintained for current, complete, and accurate health information necessary to provide quality care, precise coding, timely billing, and correct reimbursement. Lastly, the medical record is a *legal* document and is therefore used to support or substantiate the care and treatment provided to a patient, thereby adding to the need for up-to-date, consistent, and thorough information.

As simple as it sounds, if a practice wants to get claims paid, documentation must be accurate and speak the proper coding language. Providers use a common language of names and terms (nomenclature) to communicate with other providers and with the organizations that reimburse them for the services they perform. Specific codes serve as a type of shorthand for this nomenclature and are recognized and accepted by most insurance payers. These codes represent diagnoses (ICD-10-CM), provider services and procedures (CPT), and medical services and supplies (HCPCS). Fair and appropriate reimbursement in a timely fashion by third-party payers requires providers and billing specialists to fully understand and use these codes correctly. In order to do so, it is necessary to be familiar with and have a strong working knowledge of medical record documentation.

Any discussion of medical documentation should include defining the meaning of this term as it applies to the practice or organization. In simple terms, medical documentation is the means in which the patient's care is chronicled in order to establish and maintain a lasting record of encounters and treatment from health care providers.

As healthcare becomes increasingly more regulated and complex, documentation and other paperwork requirements have increased. In the hurried and hectic provider practice, medical documentation can seem like yet another benign task adjunct to the business of medicine rather than central to it. Rarely, in the course of human interactions, however, does so much rely upon so little. A few hurried chart entries by a provider in some anonymous late-night call room can become the focus of thousands of hours of retrospective legal and professional scrutiny with millions of dollars riding on the deliberations. The creation and maintenance of an accurate and sound patient record stands aside from most of the controversies surrounding health care today. Medical documentation is inseparable from the patient care it describes and, when performed professionally with precision, becomes the mirror into which we view the way medicine is practiced. Omissions, skewed observations, and errors serve only to distort the picture or, perhaps worse, surround it in suspicion and uncertainty.

The medical record serves a variety of purposes, all of which are important to the proper functioning of a hospital, outpatient facility, or medical or surgical practice.

The medical record should detail information pertinent to the care of the patient, document the performance and medical necessity of billable services, and serve as a legal document that describes a course of treatment. Periodic audits help ensure the record adequately meets these requirements.

The record contains information about the patient's history of illnesses and treatments in a variety of locations, including office, inpatient, and outpatient settings. It also contains opinions and consultations provided by other health care providers and findings from ancillary services such as lab and x-ray results.

A chart that is comprehensive, well-organized, and accurate enables the physician and other health care professionals to quickly access needed information and is essential in providing quality patient care.

In addition, much of what the provider documents in the medical record is translated by medical coding specialists into ICD-10-CM and CPT codes. Codes submitted for reimbursement become part of the statistics that are used for quality assurance, research, grants, studies (medical, revenue, etc.), vital statistics (births, infectious disease, morbidity, and mortality), tumor registry, utilization review, and case management. Payers expect the information submitted by the provider to be accurate, detailed, and specific.

Methodologies

Medical records are the only source of written information about patient encounters and are essential to the assignment and/or substantiation of ICD-10-CM, CPT, or HCPCS Level II codes. The primary purpose of the medical record is to document patient care, showing exactly which services were provided and why. An organized medical record allows the provider or anyone

---

 DENIAL ALERT

No documentation and insufficient documentation account for a large percentage of denials found by the Comprehensive Error Rate Testing (CERT) reviews.

---

else using the record, to retrieve information quickly, since the documents are classified chronologically and, in some cases, by content.

The necessity of complete and precise medical record documentation cannot be stressed enough, especially given the medico-legal concerns over the medical record.

Various methods exist to document the patient encounter, from handwritten to dictated and transcribed notes to sophisticated, state of the art electronic medical records. Depending on the method or technique employed to record the encounter, standards must be established to ensure the quality and integrity of the health information.

Electronic Records

Greater emphasis has been placed on the adoption of electronic health records (EHR) in the hospital and outpatient clinical settings. Some of the obvious benefits include legibility, portability within a clinic or facility, and improved quality of care. Some EHRs are so sophisticated that clinicians rarely consult hard copy patient documents. Even laboratory and radiological studies can be retrieved and viewed on screen. These systems typically feature organized patient documents that can be readily accessed and searched for pertinent information. Providers may enter encounter or procedural information by keyboard, voice recognition software, or by conventional dictation that is converted into the system. However, whenever using EHR documentation, careful attention must be paid to include only those elements that occur during the encounter. Populating a note with outdated, conflicting, incomplete, or inaccurate information can result from many of the copy functions available in an EHR. The ability to default or auto-populate checkboxes (primarily in review of systems and physical exams) to "no" or "negative" upon starting a new note or closing a note may inadvertently include conflicting information in a single note. At the present time there is much concern within the industry that providers who use an EHR tend to document notes that are repetitive, inconsistent, or identical and the use of "cloned" or "canned" notes can call into question the medical necessity of the care and result in payment denial, payer audits, or other types of investigation. Additionally, documentation that is long and cluttered with "canned" text could result in increased risk that pertinent, new, and critical information is overlooked by other providers, coding and billing staff, and payers if an audit should occur.

Each health care provider on staff has an electronic signature embedded within the system, which is applied upon approval of the notes. Once the signature is placed, the document becomes locked as "read-only" and any addenda must be entered and signed separately. Payers embrace these systems, since supporting documentation can be electronically exchanged and even attached to electronic claims billing, in some instances.

The coding staff may be limited in the way hard copy or electronic records are accessed. Electronic systems are typically protected by a password protocol that logs activity and files are "read-only." Consider all clinical files to be "locked," whether they are or not, and never introduce material into them. Many electronic systems employ an abstract template for coding purposes. Fields are presented on screen and essential elements entered. In almost all settings, billing and coding records are segregated from the clinical records form or in some fashion.

Preprinted encounter forms (e.g., checklists of diagnoses and CPT codes) are not considered documentation and should not find their way into the medical record. Checklists for claim generation should be kept on file to verify code selection and actual services billed.

In addition to the risks and benefits of an EHR described previously, there are also some areas of concern surrounding the protection of patient privacy, interoperability, and the high cost of implementation.

In an effort to address some of these concerns, legislative action and guidelines were issued by the Department of Health and Human Services (HHS). The Health Information Technology for Economic and Clinical Health Act (HITECH Act) was created to encourage the implementation of electronic health records (EHR) and supporting technology in the United States. President Obama signed HITECH into law on February 17, 2009 as part of the economic stimulus bill, the American Recovery and Reinvestment Act of 2009 (ARRA).

In the early years, ARRA contained specific incentives designed to accelerate the adoption of electronic health record (EHR) systems among providers through the Centers for Medicare and Medicaid Services (CMS) EHR Incentive Programs, also known as Meaningful Use. With this legislation there was a substantial expansion in the exchange of electronic protected health information. The HITECH Act expanded the scope of privacy and security protections available under HIPAA, and it increased the potential legal liabilities for non-compliance and allowed more enforcement.

In 2019, the U.S. Department of Health and Human Services (HHS) announced in the "Notification of Enforcement Discretion Regarding HIPAA Civil Monetary Penalties," April 30, 2019, edition of the *Federal Register* (84 Fed. Reg. 18151) that it had reduced the penalties for HIPAA violations in certain tiers after a review of the wording of the HITECH Act. There are four penalty tiers in the Act per the *Federal Register*:

- Tier 1–the person did not know (and, by exercising reasonable diligence, would not have known) that the person violated the provision;

- Tier 2–the violation was due to reasonable cause and not willful neglect;

- Tier 3–the violation was due to willful neglect that is timely corrected; and

- Tier 4–the violation was due to willful neglect that is not timely corrected.

If any of the penalty definitions were met, a penalty for each such violation may be enforced. Per the *Federal Register* the penalties are as follows:

Tier	Minimum Penalty	Maximum Penalty	Annual Limit
Tier 1	$100	$50,000	$25,000
Tier 2	$1,000	$50,000	$100,000
Tier 3	$10,000	$50,000	$250,000
Tier 4	$50,000	$50,000	$1,500,000

Dictation

Dictated and transcribed records are common today and certain standards have emerged to govern their function. The provider always reviews the transcripts for content and handwritten edits are entered. The entry should be signed and dated. This is necessary since many third-party payers, including Medicare,

 FOR MORE INFO

More information regarding the HITECH Act may be found in H.R. 1, 2009 from the Government Printing Office or at http://www.gpo.gov/fdsys/pkg/BILLS-111hr1enr/pdf/BILLS-111hr1enr.pdf.

 AUDITOR'S ALERT

The EHR Incentive Programs was renamed the Promoting Interoperability (PI) Programs in April 2018. More information may be found at http://www.cms.gov/Regulations-and-Guidance/Legislation/EHRIncentivePrograms/index.html.

 DEFINITIONS

Meaningful Use. *1)* Sets of guidelines that must be followed as part of the HITECH Act. Three main components of the Act include use of certified EHR in a meaningful manner (e.g., e-prescribing), electronic exchange of health information to improve the quality of healthcare, and submission of clinical quality and other measures. *2)* Use of certified electronic health technology in measurable ways of both quality and quantity. The Medicare EHR Incentive Program, aka Meaningful Use, ended reporting on 12/31/2016; components from this program have been included in the Quality Payment Program (QPP) mandated under the MACRA legislation.

require that the information be "authenticated." No information should ever be removed from a medical record. Errors should be corrected by including a notation and never deleted or erased. When it is necessary to amend medical record documentation, the edit should be made, initialed, and dated. Practices should establish a protocol or policy about documenting encounters in a timely manner, procedures for editing medical record documentation, the content that should be included, and the structure of the content in the practice compliance plan. Typically, a handwritten summary is available to other clinicians until the formal dictated transcript reaches the patient's chart.

Checks and balances should be initiated to make certain that each patient encounter is documented with a transcribed note. Verifying each medical record against a copy of the appointment schedule can help identify any patients whose visit note may not have been dictated or is missing when the typed notes are returned from the transcription service.

Medical Necessity

Medical necessity refers to services required to prevent harm to the patient or an adverse effect on the patient's quality of life. The term usually determines whether insurance will cover a procedure or service. It is important to remember that the most accurate method of supporting medical necessity is through good, clear, and complete documentation.

Medicare pays for services that are determined to be reasonable and necessary for the diagnosis and treatment of a specific illness or injury, or in the treatment of a malformed or missing body member.

Private payers often define medical necessity as:

- Services appropriate to prevent, diagnose, or treat the patient's condition, illness, or injury

- Consistent with standards of good medical practice in the United States

- Not primarily for personal comfort of the patient, the family, or the provider

- Not part of or associated with scholastic education or vocational training of the patient

- In the case of inpatient care, cannot be provided safely on an outpatient basis

For example, based on findings from a routine x-ray exam, a radiologist may feel additional studies are warranted. The record must clearly demonstrate the medical necessity for performing the additional studies. In such a situation, the radiologist is usually not required to check with the ordering provider before proceeding. However, the service may require prior authorization from the payer, depending upon that payer's guidelines.

Legal and Commonly Accepted Documentation Standards

Due to the variances in laws and regulations pertaining to medical record content by state and practice site, there is currently no standard definition of what constitutes a legal record. Nonetheless, there are some widely held principles that can be followed when creating a definition of content in a medical record for use in a practice or facility.

General Standards

Documentation is the recording of pertinent facts and observations about a patient's health history, including past and present illnesses, tests, treatments, and outcomes. The medical record chronologically documents the care of the patient to:

- Enable a physician or other health care professional to plan and evaluate the patient's treatment
- Enhance communication and promote continuity of care among physicians and other health care professionals involved in the patient's care
- Facilitate claims review and payment
- Assist in utilization review and quality of care evaluations
- Reduce hassles related to medical review
- Provide clinical data for research and education
- Serve as a legal document to verify the care provided (e.g., as defense in the case of a professional liability claim)

Payers want to know that their health care dollars are well spent because they have contractual obligations to their subscribers to validate that the services rendered are:

- Appropriate for treating the patient's condition
- Medically necessary for the diagnosis
- Coded correctly
- Properly reimbursed
- Compliant with any third-party payer utilization guidelines
- Follow medical record documentation principles and provide a basis for maintaining adequate medical health information

Representatives of the American Health Information Management Association (AHIMA), American Health Quality Association (AHQA), American Hospital Association (AHA), American Medical Association (AMA), Blue Cross and Blue Shield Association (BCBSA), and America's Health Insurance Plans (AHIP) have developed several principles of medical record documentation, including:

- The medical record should be complete and legible.
- The documentation of each patient encounter should include the date; reason for the encounter; appropriate history and physical exam; review of lab, x-ray data, and other ancillary services as appropriate; assessment; and plan for care (including discharge plan, as appropriate).
- Past and present diagnoses should be accessible to the treating or consulting health care professional.
- The reasons for, and results of, x-rays, lab tests, and other ancillary services should be documented or included in the medical record.
- Relevant health risk factors should be identified.
- The patient's progress, including response to treatment, change in treatment, change in diagnosis, and patient noncompliance should be documented.

- The written plan for care should include, when appropriate, treatments and medications, specifying frequency and dosage; referrals and consultations; patient and family education; and specific instructions for follow-up.

- The documentation should support the intensity of the patient evaluation and treatment, including thought processes and the complexity of medical decision making.

- All entries to the medical record should be dated and authenticated.

- The codes reported on the health insurance claim form or billing statement should reflect the documentation in the medical record.

Proper documentation practices are essential for quality patient care. A correctly documented medical record conveys critical information to other health care providers about the patient, the medical services provided, and their outcomes. In addition, good patient record keeping techniques help protect providers against an unfavorable outcome in the event of a medical malpractice lawsuit, and ensure accurate and timely reimbursement. Medicare and private payers will not reimburse an undocumented service, and a claim accompanied by incomplete documentation may be delayed and/or denied. But, what constitutes proper documentation and how much documentation is enough? The answer is not straightforward. Unfortunately, documentation is not formally taught in medical school, there are no national guidelines, and private payers' requirements differ greatly.

However, below are some basic guidelines to help ensure quality patient care, as well as support the medical necessity of the services provided:

- Create a separate medical record for each patient
- Document all handwritten entries in blue or black ink
- Write legibly or dictate
- Record all entries promptly
- Date and time all entries
- Avoid eraser or white out
- Line through incorrect entries with a single line
- Abstain from having blank spaces in patient records
- Ensure all entries are reviewed and signed off by the provider
- Make changes to the record according to defined protocols, such as an addenda
- Avoid subjective judgment and vague references
- Know how to appropriately word a patient's opinion of another provider
- Document consultations, concurrent care, or transfer of care situations carefully
- Reference only standard acronyms and abbreviations
- Utilize drawings, illustrations, and pictures whenever possible
- Employ appropriate systems of measurement for documentation

Beyond the medical documentation requirements listed above, additional steps that ensure medical records are complete and accurate should include:

- Patient health history and updates

- Copies of signed consent forms or concurrent entries documenting the discussion regarding informed consent with the patient

- Results of laboratory studies and x-ray interpretations

- Copies of all prescriptions and clear documentation of medications being taken by the patient

- Treatment summary for each office visit

- Summary of telephone conversations with the patient

- Scheduled appointments and missed appointments

- Return to care (RTC) notations

- Referral notations or consultations concerning other health care providers and consent to release records

- Admission orders

- Operative, procedure, or treatment reports or notes

Chart Authentication and Signature Requirements

Another element of the auditing process is to routinely check for provider signatures. It cannot be overemphasized that **all** documentation in the patient's medical chart *must* be signed and dated by the provider. As previously stated, many electronic medical records require the provider's unique electronic signature to close and lock the record. Dictated and handwritten documentation must also be signed and dated by the provider. In addition, dictated documentation should be read and reviewed to ensure accuracy and to validate revisions before being initialed. Some payers will not accept unsigned notes, whether electronic, dictated, or handwritten.

Remember, commonly accepted documentation standards always include a provider signature or "identifier." However, Medicare and commercial payers require a handwritten or electronic signature for all services provided or ordered.

Note that there is a possibility of misuse or abuse for providers opting to use electronic systems. Appropriate administrative procedures should be in place to protect against modifications and should correlate to recognized existing standards and laws. Keep in mind that the individual whose name is listed as the alternate signature, as well as the provider, share the responsibility for authenticity of all information being attested to. Finally, all state licensure and practice regulations continue to apply and where state law is more restrictive than Medicare, the state law standard is applied.

Complying with payers' signature guidelines is vital, especially if your practice is audited. CMS has changed signature guidelines several times over the years. These guidelines not only apply to providers, but they are a reference for medical reviewers when reviewing medical records and claim documentation.

The guidelines stress the importance of having all services rendered or ordered supported by documentation authenticated by the provider who authored it. The guidelines specifically state that authentication methods include a handwritten or electronic signature (stamped signatures are permitted only when the authenticator can provide proof to a CMS contractor of the inability to sign due to a disability). Handwritten signatures are considered any mark or sign by an individual on a document that denotes acknowledgment, approval, acceptance, or obligation.

 AUDITOR'S ALERT

According to CMS, a scribe is not required to sign/date the documentation; however, the treating provider's signature on a note indicates that the physician/NPP affirms the note adequately documents the care provided. Reviewers are only required to look for the signature (and date) of the treating provider on the note.

  © 2020 Optum360, LLC

If a signature is illegible, practices can use a signature log (a list of the typed or printed name of the author associated with initials or illegible signatures) or an attestation statement to determine the identity of the author of a medical record entry.

When a signature is missing from the medical record, an attestation statement may be completed. Following is an example of a CMS approved attestation statement:

> "I, _____ *[print full name of the physician/practitioner]*, hereby attest that the medical record entry for _____ *[date of service]* accurately reflects signatures/notations that I made in my capacity as _____ *[insert provider credentials, e.g., M.D.]* when I treated/diagnosed the above-listed Medicare beneficiary. I do hereby attest that this information is true, accurate, and complete to the best of my knowledge, and I understand that any falsification, omission, or concealment of material fact may subject me to administrative, civil, or criminal liability."

Providers should use signature attestation rather than add late signatures to the medical record (beyond the short delay that occurs during the transcription process). The signature attestation can also be used for illegible signatures.

Below are a few things to note regarding signatures if your medical records are subject to a payer audit.

- If the signature is illegible, medical reviewers (MACs, ZPICs/UPICs, SMRC, and CERT) may consider a signature log, attestation statement, or other documentation to determine the identity of the author of a medical record entry.

- If the signature is missing from an order, medical reviewers are instructed to disregard the order during the claims review. In other words, the reviewer proceeds as if the order was not received.

- If the signature is missing from any other medical documentation (other than an order), MACs, SMRC, and CERT accept a signature attestation from the author of the medical record entry.

- If the medical reviewers find reasons for denial unrelated to signature requirements, the reviewer does not need to proceed to signature authentication. When the contractor reviewer finds that the documentation contains all of the information necessary to process the claim but that it contains a missing or illegible signature, the contractor then follows the requirements for assessing the signature.

While authentication is required, there are some exceptions to this requirement for medical review purposes, which include:

Exception 1: Facsimiles of original written or electronic signatures are acceptable for the certifications of terminal illness for hospice.

Exception 2: There are some circumstances for which an order does not need to be signed. For example, orders for some clinical diagnostic tests are not required to be signed. The rules in 42 CFR 410 and Pub.100-02, chapter 15, §80.6.1, state that if the order for the clinical diagnostic test is unsigned, there must be medical documentation (e.g., a progress note) by the treating physician that he/she intended the clinical diagnostic test be performed. This documentation showing the intent that the test be performed must be authenticated by the author via a handwritten or electronic signature.

Exception 3: Other regulations and the CMS's instructions regarding conditions of payment related to signatures (such as timeliness standards for particular benefits) take precedence. For medical review purposes, if the relevant regulation, NCD, LCD, and CMS manuals are silent on whether the signature needs to be legible or present and the signature is illegible or missing, the reviewer follows the guidelines listed below to discern the identity and credentials (e.g., MD, RN, etc.) of the signator. When the relevant regulation, NCD, LCD and CMS manuals have specific signature requirements, those signature requirements take precedence.

Exception 4: CMS permits use of a rubber stamp for signature in accordance with the Rehabilitation Act of 1973 in the case of an author with a physical disability who can provide proof to a CMS contractor of his/her inability to sign their signature due to their disability. By affixing the rubber stamp, the provider is certifying that he or she has reviewed the document.

These exceptions apply to MACs, CERT, RACs, SMRC, and ZPICs/UPICs.

Note that in cases where the relevant regulation (NCD, LCD, and CMS manuals) has specific signature requirements, those requirements take precedence.

Diagnosis Coding

ICD-10-CM codes relate directly to medical diagnoses and are used to classify illnesses, injuries, and reasons for patient encounters within the health care system. Patients may have one primary and several secondary diagnoses.

Medical diagnoses are sequenced by order of severity or importance. Describing the onset of the problem and objectively documenting the patient's impairment and are essential to accurate coding. Diagnosis confirmation is based on objective measurements performed and values obtained during an assessment. The diagnostic description of the current problem for which the patient is being treated should be defined by:

- Subjective complaint described in the patient's own words
- Date of onset of the problem or condition
- Confirmation of the diagnosis by objective test values
- Treatment and prognosis

Procedure Coding

CPT and HCPCS Level II codes were developed specifically to define and describe provider services and procedures. Used by payers, in combination with ICD-10-CM codes, the codes are analyzed and reviewed to identify practice patterns related to specific diagnoses and to project costs of procedures for diagnosis groups. Correct use of procedure codes depends on the accuracy and specificity of the documentation for the evaluation and treatment provided. In order to substantiate the CPT codes reported, documentation should describe:

- Evaluation/management services and/or procedures performed
- Unusual circumstances requiring additional time and/or effort
- Reduction of normal service provided including explanation

- Responses/observations
- Time

Medical History

Health care providers should record and maintain a proper medical history for each patient. Health histories should gather information about all health problems that may impact the evaluation of the risks involved in a contemplated medical procedure or treatment plan. The completed health history in the patient's file should make the provider aware of any hazards the patient may present and any negative impact or side effects in which treatment may result. The completed health history should be discussed with the patient prior to the start of any treatment or procedure to avoid misunderstandings, inaccurate terminology, or errors in the documentation.

Responses that indicate a patient has symptoms reflecting potential underlying medical problems should prompt further follow up by the clinician who should document additional information and patient discussions within the medical record. For more information on medical history, see chapter 4.

Omissions from the Patient Record and Addenda

When auditing a medical record, it is necessary to determine if information was added appropriately. In cases where information is omitted from a patient's record, it is permissible to include an "addendum" or amendment to the record under certain guidelines. For example, if the results of a patient's lab studies are not recorded in the chart at the time they are received, they can and should be added as soon as is reasonably possible. However, it is important to record the information chronologically by the date the results are actually entered in the chart. They should not be recorded under an earlier date despite being received earlier. Another valid reason for amending a patient record is to document any step inadvertently or accidentally left out of the original dictated report of a surgery or procedure.

One acceptable method for dealing with an omission is to include an addendum to document the missing step or have the provider re-dictate the entire procedure report. In either case, the provider should date and sign the addendum and attach it in chronological order to the health record. Do not replace the original notes, though a note acknowledging the missing information and referencing the addendum should be included with the original documentation.

Chapter 2

Focusing and Performing Audits

Conducting an effective chart audit requires careful planning. A well thought out plan is essential to completing a chart audit that yields useable data.

Some questions to consider before starting the audit are:

- What is the topic/focus of the audit (e.g., evaluation and management, surgery, etc.)?
- Is the topic/focus too narrow or too broad?
- Is there a measure for the topic/focus (e.g., level for established patient visits)?
- Is the measure available in the medical record (e.g., recorded by the provider in review of systems)?
- Has the topic/focus been measured before?
  - If yes, then a benchmark or standard exists.
  - If no, then a standard for comparison may not exist.

Once the answers to the above questions have been determined, the practice must decide which steps are necessary to perform a complete and accurate audit.

Ten Steps To Audits

Step 1. Determine who will perform the audit. An internal audit is typically performed by coding staff within the practice that are proficient in coding and interpreting payer guidelines. Depending upon the size of the practice and the number of services provided annually, a compliance department with full-time auditors may be established. If not, the person performing the audit should not audit claims that he or she completed.

Step 2. Define the scope of the audit. Determine what types of services to include in the review. Utilize the most recent Office of Inspector General (OIG) work plan, Recovery Audit Contractor (RAC) issues, and third-party payer provider bulletins, which will help identify areas that can be targeted for upcoming audits. Review the OIG work plan to determine if there are issues of concern that apply to the practice. Determine specific coding issues or claim denials that are experienced by the practice. The frequency and potential effect to reimbursement or potential risk can help prioritize which areas should be reviewed. Services that are frequently performed or have complex coding and billing issues should also be reviewed, as the potential for mistakes or impact to revenue could be substantial.

Step 3. Determine the type of audit to be performed and the areas to be reviewed. Once the area of review is identified, careful consideration should be given to the type of audit performed. Reviews can be prospective or retrospective. If a service is new to the practice, or if coding and billing guidelines have recently been revised, it may be advisable to create a policy stating that a prospective review is performed on a specified number of claims as part of a compliance plan. The basic coding audit should include, at minimum, validation of CPT® code use, including the level of E/M visit assigned; undocumented or underdocumented services; correct use of modifiers; and accuracy of diagnosis codes and whether the source document supports medical necessity. Additional areas of review may include verifying that the correct place of service was billed, the correct category of service was billed, and whether there were services documented but not billed.

Step 4. Request necessary medical record, billing, and reporting documentation. To verify the accuracy of the services reported, request the patient chart to review the documentation. Also obtain copies of the superbill or charge ticket, along with a copy of the claim form. By examining these documents, problematic areas may be identified, such as data entry errors, use of outdated code sets, incorrect or missing modifier usage, or improperly sequenced surgery CPT codes, which can result in incorrect reimbursement.

Step 5. Assemble reference materials. Reference materials, such as current editions of coding manuals, NCCI edits, and CMS or other third-party policies pertinent to the services being reviewed, should be collected. When auditing evaluation and management (E/M) services, determine which set of CMS documentation guidelines (1995 or 1997) are appropriate for the review and have the corresponding E/M audit worksheet available.

Step 6. Develop customized data capture tools. Use an audit worksheet. Audit worksheets (available in the appendix of this book) can aid in the audit process. They help verify that signatures were obtained, that patient identifying information (such as complete name, date of birth) is correct, that the practice is in compliance with "incident-to" guidelines, and that time-based codes are documented and reported appropriately.

Step 7. Develop a reporting mechanism for findings. Once the audit is complete, written recommendations should be made. The recommendations can include conducting a more frequent focused audit, implementing improved documentation templates, or conducting targeted education on CPT or ICD-10-CM coding. Each practice should have benchmarks set up that all providers must meet. For example, if 10 charts are reviewed, 90 percent must be correct. It is also important to identify claims that may need to be corrected or payments that need to be refunded to the payer.

Step 8. Determine recommendations and corrective actions. The next step is to schedule meetings with the providers to provide feedback, recommendations, and education. Typically it works best to meet with a provider on an individual basis and have his or her audit results and charts available as examples so that they can be reviewed and discussed. The provider should be given the opportunity to explain the rationale behind his or her coding, and perhaps even provide additional information to help the coder further understand the code selected. Allowing the provider to give feedback also helps build a better auditor-provider relationship. This relationship may make the provider feel comfortable enough with the auditor to ask questions about future coding issues, instead of reporting incorrect codes to payers. A word to the wise, when discussing a

 AUDITOR'S ALERT

Keep current with weekly CMS updates by signing up for CMS e-news at https://www.cms.gov/ Outreach-and-Education/Outreach/ FFSProvPartProg/Provider-Partnership -Email-Archive. These notifications are published every Thursday and include Medicare updates and information about CMS national provider calls.

coding error with a provider, it is a good idea to have a copy of the source document supporting discussion of the error.

Step 9. Implement quality improvement initiatives. After addressing the identified issues, set up a process to monitor these areas. Formal training programs, one-on-one coaching, and regularly scheduled audits can be beneficial. After an audit process is in place, it may be necessary to update practice policies and procedures that need to be monitored on a regular basis. Lastly, designate an individual who is responsible for each area of compliance and document the follow-through so that providers stay on the right track with billing practices.

Step 10. Determine if corrective actions have resolved issues. Once the corrective actions have been in place for a reasonable time, the practice may wish to perform a second review to determine if the desired results have been achieved. This could be done through a comprehensive audit or a "mini" review. Staff should also be interviewed to determine if additional modifications to the corrective actions are necessary.

Identifying Potential Problem Areas

Key elements to a successful claims processing cycle include monitoring claims, responding to correspondence, and carefully reviewing the remittance advice notices, all of which require diligence and follow through. The task of ensuring that the claim has reached its destination and is processed correctly may seem mundane and tedious and yet is vitally important to the financial well being of the practice. Likewise, responding to requests for additional information or reviewing a remittance advice (RA) notice to determine how a claim was processed may not initially appear to impact the bottom line but it certainly can and does. For example, claims pending receipt of requests for documentation that are not responded to can be worth hundreds or even thousands of dollars. Or, the remittance notice not carefully reviewed can represent noncovered service amounts that could be balance billed to the patient, generating additional revenue for the practice.

Clean Claims

One reason to audit claims is to ensure that "clean claims" are sent to payers on the first attempt. Ideally, every claim submitted to a payer would be a "clean claim," processed timely and paid correctly. Unfortunately, the reality is quite different. Payers define a clean claim as one that does not require the payer to investigate or develop on a prepayment basis. Clean claims must be filed within the timely filing limit as outlined in the provider contract.

Most payers consider clean claims to be:

- Claims that pass all edits
- Claims that do not require external development (i.e., investigated within the claims, medical review, or payment office even if the investigator does not need to contact the provider, the beneficiary, or other outside source)

 AUDITOR'S ALERT

The Medicare Learning Network has free online training on a variety of compliance issues. CMS' Quarterly Compliance Newsletter is another valuable resource to educate providers on common billing issues and how to avoid them. This information is found at https://www.cms.gov/Outreach-and-Education/Medicare-Learning-Network-MLN/MLNProducts/ProviderCompliance.html.

📖 **DEFINITIONS**

common working file. System of local databases containing total beneficiary histories developed by CMS to improve Medicare claims processing. Medicare fiscal intermediaries, and/or carriers, interact with these databases to obtain data on eligibility, utilization, Medicare secondary payer (MSP), and other detailed claims information.

remittance advice. Statement, voucher, or notice received by the service provider from a payer reflecting the status of adjudicated claims, either paid or denied.

- Claims not approved for payment by the common working file (CWF) within seven days of the original claim submittal for reasons beyond the carrier's or provider's control (e.g., CWF system/communication difficulties) (Medicare only)

- Claims where the beneficiary is not on the CWF host and CWF has to locate and identify where the beneficiary record resides (CWF out-of-service area [OSA] claims) (Medicare only)

- Claims subject to medical review but complete medical evidence is attached by the provider

- Claims pending additional requests for information developed on a postpayment basis

- Claims that have all basic information necessary to adjudicate the claim, and all required supporting documentation is attached

Claims that do not meet the aforementioned definition are considered "other." Other claims require additional investigation or external development by the payer prior to payment. Examples of claims that may be considered "other" include:

- Claims that require additional information from the provider or another external source by the payer (e.g., routine data omitted from the bill, medical information, or information needed to resolve discrepancies)

- Claims where information or assistance must be requested from another payer (e.g., requests for charge data from Medicare or any other request for information from the Medicare contractor)

- Requests for information that is necessary for a coverage determination by the payer

- Claims that require sequential processing when an earlier claim is in development

- Claims that require the contractor to perform outside development as a result of a CWF edit (Medicare only)

Claims defined as "unprocessable" are those with incomplete or missing information or any claim that contains complete but invalid information.

Returning an unprocessable claim to the provider (RTP) does not mean the payer physically returns the claim it received. Rather, payers use some of the techniques shown below as a means of considering the claim "returned:"

- Incomplete or invalid information is detected at the front end of the payer claims processing system. The claim is returned to the provider electronically or in a hardcopy/checklist type form explaining the error and how to correct the error prior to resubmission. Claim data is not usually retained in the payer's system for returned as unprocessable claims. In these cases, the payer does not issue a remittance advice (RA).

- Incomplete or invalid information is detected at the front end of the claims processing system and the claim is suspended for development. If requested corrections and/or medical documentation are submitted within a predefined period, the claim is processed. Otherwise, the suspended portion is returned and the supplier or provider of service is notified by the RA.

 SPECIAL ALERT

Medicare defines incomplete information as missing required or conditional information on a claim (i.e., no national provider identifier [NPI]).

- Incomplete or invalid information is detected within the claims processing system and the claim is rejected through the remittance process. Suppliers or providers of service are notified of any error and how to correct the error prior to resubmission through the RA.

A claim that is returned to the provider as unprocessable due to incomplete or invalid information does not meet the criteria to be considered an adjudicated claim, is not denied, and, as such, cannot be appealed. Instead, the provider should determine what information is missing, correct the errors, and resubmit the corrected claim following the payer's established guidelines.

Medical Reviews

In an effort to identify provider billing errors and fraudulent billing many payers have implemented a medical review process. In this process, an analysis of claims data is performed by a third-party payer to identify areas of overutilization and areas at risk for incorrect coding and payment. The statutory authority for the majority of medical review policies can be found in section 1862 (a)(1)(A) of the Social Security Act, which prohibits Medicare payment for "items or services that are not considered to be reasonable and necessary for the diagnosis or treatment of illness or injury or to improve the functioning of a malformed body member." Medicare and other third-party payers routinely monitor claims, which means that many claims submitted undergo some type of prepayment review without a provider being notified or aware of it. Paid claims may also be subject to review.

Circumstances that appear suspicious and warrant a review may include, but are not limited to:

- Sudden billing changes
- Spike billing
- Billing a service not usually performed by a specific specialty
- Billing of inappropriate questionable diagnoses
- Increased complaints from beneficiaries
- Compromised beneficiary and provider identities
- Geographical billing changes
- High CERT rate
- Identity theft (provider and/or beneficiary)
- Beneficiary recruitment (capping)
- High utilization accounting for a disproportionate share of "ordered" services for a provider or group
- Submitting claims for deceased patients with dates of service *after* the date of death
- Billing for Part B services during an inpatient, Part A, institutional stay
- Billing for ordered services (e.g., IDTF, clinical laboratory, DME, etc.) when the ordering physician has no billing relationship for the patient (implying lack of clinical relationship for the ordering physician and beneficiary)
- Billing on behalf, or using the NPI of a deceased physician or clinical practitioner to submit "ordered" services

Medicare Medical Reviews

CMS contracts with various types of contractors in its effort to fight improper payments and promote provider compliance in the Medicare fee-for-service (FFS) program. These may include:

- Comprehensive Error Rate Testing (CERT) contractors
- Medicare Administrative Contractors (MAC)
- Program Integrity Contractors (ZPIC)
- Recovery Auditors (RA)
- Supplemental Medical Review Contractors (SMRC)
- Unified Program Integrity Contractors (UPIC)

CERT contractors are used in the CERT program CMS implemented, which establishes error rates and estimates of improper payments. The CERT review contractor is responsible for reviewing claims randomly selected by the CERT statistical contractor.

Recovery Auditors are outside auditors that are used to assist CMS by conducting additional claim reviews. They are responsible for reviewing claims where improper payments have been made or there is a high probability that improper payments were made. Due to the amount of claims CMS processes each year (more than 1 billion), CMS uses the Recovery Audit Program to detect and correct improper payments in the Medicare FFS program and provide information to CMS and review contractors that could help prevent future improper payments.

The Supplemental Medical Review Contractors' main tasks are to perform and/or provide support for a variety of tasks aimed at lowering the improper payment rates and increasing efficiencies of the medical review functions of the Medicare and Medicaid programs. Having a centralized medical review resource that can perform a large volume of medical reviews nationally allows for a timely and consistent execution of medical review, activities, and decisions. The focus of the reviews may include but are not limited to issues identified by CMS internal data analysis, the CERT program, professional organizations, and other Federal agencies, such as the OIG/Government Accountability Office (GAO) and comparative billing reports.

The primary goal of UPICs is to investigate instances of suspected fraud, waste, and abuse in Medicare or Medicaid claims. They develop investigations early, and in a timely manner, and take immediate action to ensure Medicare Trust Fund monies are not inappropriately paid. They also identify any improper payments that are to be recouped by the Medicare Administrative Contractors (MAC). Actions UPICs take to detect and deter fraud, waste, and abuse in the Medicare or Medicaid programs include:

- Investigate potential fraud and abuse for CMS administrative action or referral to law enforcement
- Conduct investigations in accordance with the priorities established by the Center for Program Integrity (CPI) Fraud Prevention System
- Perform medical reviews, as appropriate
- Perform data analysis in coordination with CPI's Fraud Prevention System, IDR, and OnePI

 © 2020 Optum360, LLC

- Identify the need for administrative actions, such as payment suspensions, prepayment or auto-denial edits, revocations, postpay overpayment determination

- Share information (e.g., leads, vulnerabilities, concepts, approaches) with other UPICs/ZPICs to promote the goals of the program and the efficiency of operations at other contracts

- Refer cases to law enforcement to consider civil or criminal prosecution

MACs review billed services that have significant potential to be noncovered or incorrectly coded. Medical reviewers may evaluate problem areas that demonstrate a significant risk to the Medicare program as a result of inappropriate billing or improper payments. MACs also have a program in place to perform an ongoing analysis of claims and data from Recovery Auditors and CERT, among other sources, in order to focus intervention efforts on the most significant errors.

MACs have the discretion to select target areas with:

- High volume of services

- High cost

- Dramatic change in frequency of use

- High-risk, problem-prone areas

- Recovery Auditor, CERT, Office of Inspector General (OIG), or Government Accounting Office (GAO) data demonstrating vulnerability

There are three types of Medicare medical reviews: Medical Record Review, Nonmedical Record Review, and Automated Review. The following chart indicates which contractors perform each type of review:

Contractor Type	Prepayment			Postpayment	
	Medical Record Review	Nonmedical Record Review	Automated Reviews	Medical Record Review	Nonmedical Record Review
MACs	Yes	Yes	Yes	Yes	Yes
CERT	No	No	No	Yes	No
RACs	No	No	No	Yes	No
SMRC	No	No	No	Yes	Yes
ZPIC/UPIC	Yes	No	No	Yes	Yes

A medical record review involves requesting, receiving, and reviewing medical documentation associated with a claim. The purpose is to determine the medical necessity of the service reported and requires a licensed medical professional to use clinical review judgment to evaluate the medical record documentation.

Per CMS, clinical review judgment involves two steps:

1. The combination of all submitted medical record information (e.g., progress notes, diagnostic findings, medications, nursing notes, etc.) to create a clinical picture of the patient.

2. The resulting clinical picture identified above is reviewed, using standard review criteria and relevant policies, by the MAC, CERT, RAC, and/or ZPIC/UPIC to determine that all necessary requirements are met.

Note: CMS stresses that clinical review judgment does not replace poor or inadequate medical records. Clinical review judgment by definition is not a process that MACs, CERT, RACs, and ZPICs/UPICs can use to override, supersede, or disregard a policy requirement.

The MACs, CERTs, and ZPICs/UPICs employ licensed medical professionals to perform their medical record reviews. For the purpose of making coverage determinations, the reviews are performed by licensed nurses (RNs and LPNs) or physicians, unless this task is delegated to other licensed health care professionals. For ZPICs/UPICs, RACs, and the SMRC, they ensure that the credentials of their reviewers are consistent with the requirements in their respective statements of work (SOW).

Nonmedical record reviews use manual intervention, but only to the extent that a reviewer can make a determination based on claim information. It does not require clinical judgment in review of medical record documentation. Contractors only perform a nonmedical record review for denials of related claims and/or no receipt of additional documentation requests (ADR) where such denials cannot be automated.

Automated review is a medical review where a payment decision is made at the system level, using available electronic information, with no manual intervention. The automated prepayment and postpayment denials are based on clear policy that serves as the basis for denial—or a Medically Unlikely Edit (MUE)—or occurs when no timely response is received to an ADR. When a clear policy exists (or in the case of a MUE), MACs, RACs, SMRC, and ZPICs/UPICs have the discretion to automatically deny the services without stopping the claim for manual review, even if documentation is attached or simultaneously submitted.

The term "clear policy" means a statute, regulation, NCD, coverage provision in an interpretive manual, coding guideline, LCD, or MAC article that specifies the circumstances under which a service will always be considered noncovered, incorrectly coded, or improperly billed.

Prepayment Reviews

Prepayment reviews are performed before a claim is paid. The payer may request the medical record documentation when performing prepayment reviews. There are different types of prepayment reviews. For example, an automated prepayment review is done at the system level, using electronic information. The system selects claims containing specific services for review, such as comparing diagnosis to procedure code.

Postpayment reviews

Postpayment reviews are performed after the claim is paid. During a postpayment review, medical record documentation is requested and subsequently compared to the claim.

Probe Reviews

CMS utilzes a Targeted Probe and Educate (TPE) review process. The purpose of TPE is to reduce appeals, decrease provider burden, and improve the medical review/education process. This is a required process for providers targeted by medical review. TPE reviews can be prepayment or postpayment and involve MACs focusing on specific providers/suppliers that bill a particular item or service. A round of TPE typically involves the review of 20 to 40 claims, per provider/supplier, per service/item, and corresponding education. The TPE

AUDITOR'S ALERT

CERT refers to all reviews where no documentation was requested as "T-claim review" and are a claim category reviewed by CERT. T-claims were automatically denied by the MAC. The RACs refer to all reviews where no documentation was requested as "automated review."

review process includes three rounds of a prepayment probe review with education. However a MAC may discontinue the process if/when providers/suppliers become compliant. If there are continued high denials after the first three rounds, the MAC will refer the provider and results to CMS. CMS determines additional action, which may include extrapolation, referral to the Zone Program Integrity Contractor (ZPIC/UPIC), referral to Recovery Auditor (RA) contractor, etc.

Statistical Sample Reviews and Estimation of Overpayments

CMS has given very specific guidance to contractors on when this type of review may be used. The contractor should use statistical sampling when it has been determined that a sustained or high level of payment error exists. The use of statistical sampling may be used after documented educational intervention has failed to correct the payment error. For purposes of extrapolation, a sustained or high level of payment error should be determined to exist through a variety of means, including, but not limited to:

- Allegations of wrongdoing by current or former employees of a provider/supplier

- Audits or evaluations conducted by the OIG

- CMS approval provided in connection to a payment suspension

- High-error rate determinations by the contractor or by other medical reviews (i.e., greater than or equal to 50 percent from a previous pre- or postpayment review)

- Information from law enforcement investigations

- Provider/supplier history (i.e., prior history of noncompliance for the same or similar billing issues, or historical pattern of noncompliant billing practices)

If the contractor believes that statistical sampling and/or extrapolation should be used for purposes of estimation, and it does not meet any of the criteria listed above, the contractor should consult with a Contracting Officer's Representative (COR)/Business Function Lead (BFL) prior to creating a statistical sample and issuing a request for medical records from the provider/supplier. Examples of this may include, but are not limited to, billing for noncovered services, billing for services not rendered, etc.

Comprehensive Error Rate Testing Program

The Comprehensive Error Rate Testing (CERT) program is one of the programs that CMS established to monitor and report the accuracy of Medicare fee-for-service payments.

Under this program, independent reviewers review random samples of claims as they are accepted into contractor and intermediary claims processing systems and follow them through the system. CERT medical reviewers strictly follow documentation standards as outlined in Medicare regulation, statute, and policy, including local coverage determinations (LCD), rather than allowing for clinical review judgment based on billing history and other available information.

The decisions of the independent reviewer are then entered into a tracking database, which allows CMS to identify trends as they arise. CERT is also used to identify where corrective action may be needed and to monitor and direct the performance of contractors. In addition, the large volume of claims in the database that have undergone independent review can be utilized to test new software.

As a result of the CERT program and its strict adherence to policy requirements, a significant number of errors have been identified, including:

- Missing/no documentation for the services provided
- Missing signature or not legible signature
- Medical record does not support medical necessity
- Medical record documentation received from a provider is insufficient to substantiate a claim
- Incorrect coding

The CERT contractor requests medical records and supporting documentation from the provider. Once they are received, the contractor's medical review staff (i.e., nurses, physicians, and other qualified health care practitioners) perform a complete review, comparing the claims data to the medical record to verify the services billed were rendered and medically necessary. If the documentation supports the service and medical necessity, no further action is required. However, if the documentation fails to support the service billed, an error is determined and a refund requested.

The 2019 fiscal year (FY) CERT report (the most recent information available at printing) indicates that the Medicare FFS program improper payment for Part B services, which includes physicians, is 8.6 percent of improper payments. The report projects that for physician services, the following improper payments by type of error in billions of dollars have been made:

No Documentation	$0.3
Insufficient Documentation	$3.9
Medical Necessity	$0.1
Incorrect Coding	$2.4
Other	$0.1
Total	**$6.7**

Evaluation and management services continue to be problematic, often resulting in the E/M service being downcoded one level. The following tables illustrate the projected improper payments for E/M services.

E/M Service	Claims Reviewed	Projected Improper Payment
Emergency room visit	538	$290,076,940
Hospital, initial	962	$663,196,743
Hospital, subsequent	1,559	$755,207,786
Hospital, critical care	266	$189,815,652
Nursing home visit	665	$257,492,434
Office, new	708	$383,093,483
Office, established	1,451	$1,017,331,298

Type of Service	Improper Payment Rate	Type of Error				
		No Documentation	Insufficient Documentation	Medical Necessity	Incorrect Coding	Other
Subsequent Hospital Visits	12.9%	12.1%	36.1%	0.0%	51.8%	0.0%
Established Patient E/M	6.6%	2.8%	24.1%	0.0%	73.1%	0.0%
Initial Hospital Visits	22.2%	2.0%	28.0%	0.0%	70.0%	0.0%
New Patient E/M	12.7%	0.7%	8.1%	0.0%	90.0%	1.1%
Emergency Room	11.7%	3.8%	13.2%	0.0%	83.0%	0.0%

 DENIAL ALERT

Insufficient documentation is responsible for a high percentage of improper payments. When auditing records internally, carefully determine medical record documentation errors and perform internal education to resolve the issue.

E/M claims have a number of basic components that substantiate the service and are expected to be included on the claim or in the medical record:

- Complete and legible medical record
- Reason for, and date of, the visit, appropriate and relevant beneficiary history, physical exam and medical decision making that includes findings, results of diagnostic tests, diagnosis, plan of care, and the identity of the provider
- Documented or easily inferred rationale for ordering diagnostic and other ancillary services
- Past, present, and revised diagnoses
- Health risk factors
- Progress notes/treatment plans

E/M coding continues to be an ongoing issue for providers. The majority of incorrect payments for E/M services were due to lack of documentation in the medical record that failed to support the service reported or missing and inadequate documentation to substantiate the level of E/M service reported.

In terms of insufficient documentation, there were a number of claims denoted as being in error because the provider's intent for ordering services was missing or inadequate, or the records did not contain the appropriate physician authentication.

Due to CMS's stringent adherence to documentation policies, the CERT program processes have been revised many times. The process for measuring the improper payment rate and the sampling methodology continue to be improved to provide additional improper payment information on high-risk areas. In addition, CMS continually reviews data gathered from the CERT program and improves areas that show programmatic weakness. CERT results are also used to provide feedback to Medicare contractors on ways to enhance their medical review efforts, develop education and outreach efforts, and improve their overall operations. A number of corrective actions are in place or being developed that minimize the number of improper payments arising from inadequate insufficient documentation and medical necessity errors. Finally, CMS intends to implement some programmatic changes that are expected to reduce improper payments and safeguard the legitimacy of the services providers and suppliers bill.

Recovery Audit Contractor

The RAC program is mandated by the Medicare Prescription Drug, Improvement and Modernization Act of 2003 (MIPAA) to find and correct improper Medicare payments erroneously paid to health care providers. In general, CMS contracts with RACs to review claims and recover improper payments. A three-year demonstration program showed tremendous success collecting more than $1.03 billion in improper payments and became the driving force behind establishing a permanent program.

The program was extended to include Medicaid claims. Each was required to establish a Medicaid RAC program per the Affordable Care Act (ACA). As with Medicare RACs, Medicaid RAC contractors are tasked with finding and recovering over- and underpayments made by state Medicaid programs.

Goals of the Medicare Medical Review Program

Medical reviews are a strategic part of CMS's efforts to prevent inappropriate, abusive, or fraudulent billings. The goal of the medical review program is to reduce payment errors by preventing the initial payment of claims that do not comply with Medicare's coverage, coding, payment, and billing policies.

MACs and SMRCs help ensure that the goals of the medical review program are met.

MACS:

- Identify provider noncompliance with coverage, coding, billing, and payment policies through analysis of data (e.g., profiling of providers, services, or utilization of services) and evaluation of other information (e.g., complaints, enrollment, and/or cost report data).

- Act to prevent and/or address the identified improper payment.

- Emphasize reducing the paid claims error rate by notifying individual billing entities (e.g., providers, suppliers, or other approved clinician) of review findings identified by contractors and making appropriate referrals to provider outreach and education (POE), Program Safeguard Contractor (PSC), and Zone Program Integrity Contractors (ZPIC).

SMRCs:

- Identify provider noncompliance with coverage, coding, billing, and payment policies through the research and analysis of data related to assigned tasks (e.g., profiling of providers, services, or beneficiary utilization)

- Perform medical reviews

- Perform extrapolations

- Notify the individual billing entities (i.e., providers, suppliers, or other approved clinicians) of review findings identified and make appropriate recommendations for provider outreach education (POE) and ZPIC referrals

© 2020 Optum360, LLC

Electronic Submission of Medical Documentation

As a result of the increase in documentation requests due to contractor reviews, CMS developed an electronic method for the submission of medical documentation. Electronic Submission of Medical Documentation (esMD) is a system that allows providers or health information handlers (HIH) to submit medical documentation over secure electronic means.

The primary intent of esMD is to reduce provider costs and cycle time by minimizing paper processing and mailing of medical documentation to review contractors.

CMS uses "gateways" to securely exchange electronic private health information. The gateways are built on the sender and receiver ends. Gateways built for the esMD project follow the set of health information exchange standards, services, and policies that the Office of the National Coordinator for Health IT (ONC) has adopted. CMS esMD Gateway is built using the open source CONNECT software. This solution enables secure exchange of electronic health information adhering to various Health Information Technology (HIT) interoperability standards. Currently the gateway securely receives the electronic medical documents submitted by various HIHs on behalf of providers.

There are two options providers may use to access a CONNECT-compatible gateway:

- Larger providers, such as hospital chains or large group practices, may choose to build their own gateway.

- Providers may choose to obtain gateway services by entering into a contract or other arrangement with an approved Health Information Handler (HIH) that offers esMD gateway services.

A list of HIHs that offer esMD services can be found at https://www.cms.gov/Research-Statistics-Data-and-Systems/Computer-Data-and-Systems/ESMD/Information_for_HIHs.html.

Medicare administrative contractors (MAC) and comprehensive error rate testing (CERT) contractors that accept esMD are encouraged to state in their additional documentation request (ADR) how providers can get more information about using this system. CMS encourages all MACs, CERT contractors, and recovery auditors to post a statement on their websites indicating whether they do or do not accept esMD transactions along with a link to an instructional website about how a provider HIH can submit medical documentation via the esMD. Information about the esMD system can be found at http://www.cms.gov/Research-Statistics-Data-and-Systems/Computer-Data-and-Systems/ESMD/index.html?redirect=/esMD.

In addition to medical documentation requests, esMD also allows providers to obtain prior authorization requests. Suppliers, providers, and Health Information Handlers (HIH) can electronically submit prior authorization requests to review contractors and also receive electronically prior authorization request response.

Advanced Determination of Medical Coverage may also be obtained through esMD. Suppliers and beneficiaries can request prior approval and determine, in advance of delivery, if the purchase of a DME item is likely to be covered.

CMS expanded the esMD system to enable providers to submit first- and second-level appeal requests electronically in PDF format to review contractors who participate in this functionality on a voluntary basis. The system also accepts Recovery Auditor Discussion Requests (RADR) electronically in PDF format to recovery auditors.

Prior Authorization of Durable Medical Equipment, Prosthetics, Orthotics, and Supplies Through the esMD

Effective July 2017, CMS implemented a prior authorization model for Durable Medical Equipment, Prosthetics, Orthotics, and Supplies (DMEPOS) in seven states (California, Florida, Illinois, Michigan, New York, North Carolina, and Texas), and will focus on select codes related to the provision of power wheelchairs.

Participation in this program is voluntary; however, many health care providers find that it reduces costs, increases efficiency, and shortens processing times. Providers may continue to mail or fax documentation to review contractors.

For a complete listing of contractors accepting the above requests, visit https://www.cms.gov/Research-Statistics-Data-and-Systems/Computer-Data-and-Systems/ESMD/Which_Review_Contractors_Accept_esMD_Transactions.html.

The Appeals Process

There are times when, for a number of reasons, claims are paid inappropriately or inaccurately. In these instances, it is often worth the time and effort to appeal these claims. In fact, studies have shown that initial decisions are reversed in whole or in part for more than 50 percent of reviewed claims. Below is the process Medicare uses. Each payer may have a different process so it is wise to contact the payer or look at the payer's website for details.

Appealing Medicare Claims

When appealing Medicare claims, there is a well-defined five-level process:

- Redetermination
- Reconsideration
- Administrative law judge (ALJ) hearing
- Departmental Appeals Board (DAB) Review/Appeals Council
- Federal court review

The following is a flow chart to help you understand the Medicare appeals process.

Medicare Appeals Process

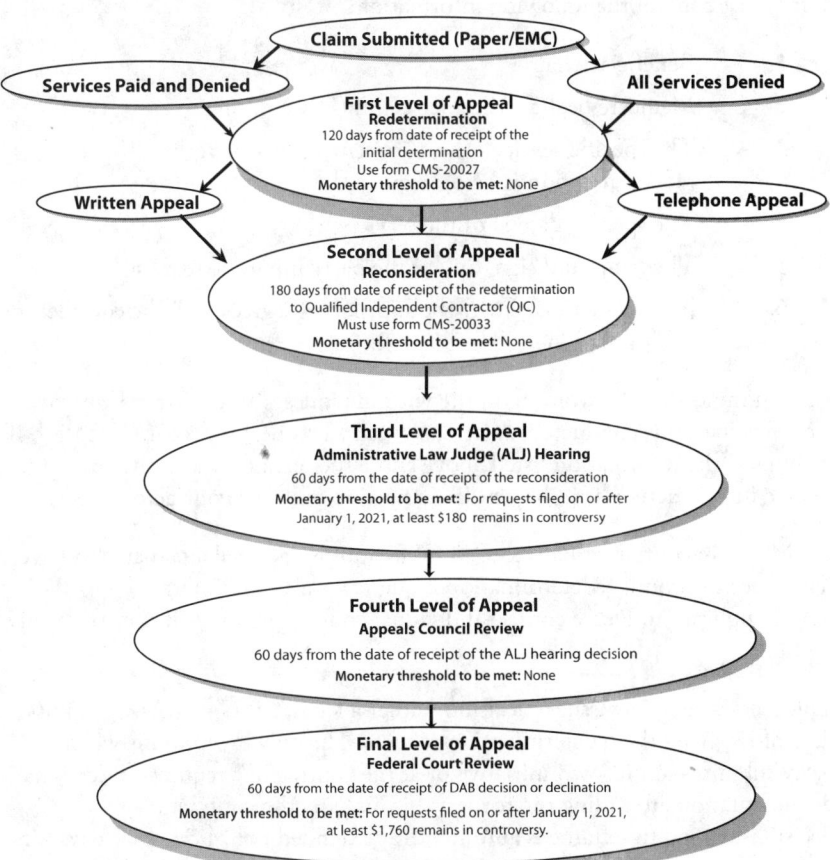

Redetermination

The First Level of Appeal—Redetermination

If a provider is dissatisfied with the outcome of the initial appeal determination, it may request, in writing, to have a different contractor review the determination. This step is considered the first level of appeal for Part A and Part B claims. Essentially, this is a "second look" at the claim and supporting documentation.

The individual filing the appeal must file the request for redetermination with the contractor as noted on the Medicare summary notice (MSN) or remittance advice (RA) within 120 days from the date of receipt of the initial determination. A minimum monetary threshold is not required to request a redetermination.

When the filing deadline for a redetermination ends on a Saturday, Sunday, legal holiday, or any other nonwork day, the contractor applies a rollover period that extends the filing deadline to the first work day after the nonwork day.

As mentioned, all appeals for redetermination must be made in writing. Appeal requests submitted electronically via a facsimile or secure internet portal/application shall be considered to have been received in writing. There are two ways of submitting a written appeal: a completed form CMS-20027 or a written request or letter. The CMS-20027, which can be found on the CMS website, is considered "completed" when all applicable spaces are filled out and all necessary attachments are included with the request. A written request or letter must contain the following information:

1. Beneficiary name
2. Medicare health insurance claim (HIC) number
3. The specific service(s) and/or item(s) for which the redetermination is being requested
4. The specific date(s) of the service
5. The name and signature of the party filing the request
6. An explanation of why the appellant disagrees with the contractor's determination

Keep in mind that the wording in the written request can determine whether a redetermination is conducted. A letter serves as a request for redetermination if it contains the information listed above and either explicitly asks the contractor to take further action or indicates dissatisfaction with the contractor's decision.

If a Medicare contractor has received CMS approval, appellants may also have the choice to submit redetermination requests via a secure Internet portal/application. Please contact individual contractors to see if they offer this option.

Contractors generally issue a decision (either a letter, MSN or RA) within 60 days of receiving the redetermination request. The only exception is when a party submits—on its own initiative or at the contractor's request—additional documentation after filing the request. In this case, the contractor's 60-day decision-making timeframe is automatically extended for 14 calendar days for each submission. This extension should not be applied routinely unless extra time is needed to consider additional documentation.

Note: It is important that the request for redetermination be filed with the proper contractor based on the claims processing jurisdiction rules Medicare established. Contractors are expected to have standard operational procedures in place, including maintaining a record of these cases, to ensure that misdirected requests are forwarded to the proper contractor jurisdiction within 60 calendar days of receipt.

The Second Level of Appeal—Reconsideration

When a party that participated in the redetermination is still dissatisfied with the outcome of the redetermination, a reconsideration may be requested. The qualified independent contractor (QIC) reconsideration process allows for an independent review of an initial determination, including the redetermination, which may include review of medical necessity issues by a panel of physicians or other health care professionals.

A request for reconsideration must be submitted, in writing, on the CMS-20033 form or, if not on the 20033 form, it should contain all of the same information identified above for the redetermination process, as well as the name of the contractor who made the redetermination. The request for reconsideration should clearly explain the reason for disputing the redetermination decision. Also include a copy of the RA or Medicare Redetermination Notice (MRN), and any other useful documentation.

Requests for reconsideration must be filed with a QIC who is specified in the redetermination notice and who has the jurisdiction within 180 days of receipt of the redetermination. A minimum monetary threshold is not required to request a reconsideration.

The QIC processes reconsideration requests within 60 days of receiving the required information and notifies the requester of the action to be taken. In many cases, the QIC's decision requires the contractor to issue a payment. If the QIC's decision is favorable to the appellant and gives a specific amount to be paid, the contractor issues payment within 30 calendar days of receiving the notice from the QIC.

The Third Level of Appeal—Administrative Law Judge Hearing

A party can request an administrative law judge hearing or a review of the administrative record by an attorney adjudicator within the Office of Medicare Hearings and Appeals (OMHA). An appellant has the opportunity to escalate to an ALJ or attorney adjudicator if the adjudication period for the QIC to complete its reconsideration has elapsed and the QIC is unable to complete the reconsideration by the deadline. The request is submitted within 60 days after receipt of the QIC's reconsideration and the dollar requirement is met. The amount in question must be at least $180 for all ALJ hearings made on or after January 1, 2021.

A provision of the Medicare Prescription Drug, Improvement, and Modernization Act (MMA) of 2003 mandates that the AIC threshold must be adjusted annually based on the increase in the medical care component of the consumer price index. If this adjusted amount is not a multiple of $10, the amount is rounded to the nearest multiple of $10. The adjusted amount is published in the *Federal Register*.

The request for an ALJ hearing must be made in writing and contain the following information:

- Name, address, and Medicare health insurance claim number of the beneficiary whose claim is being appealed, and the beneficiary's telephone number if the beneficiary is the appealing party and not represented

- Name, address, and telephone number of the appellant, when the appellant is not the beneficiary

- Name, address, and telephone number of the authorized or appointed representative, if any

- Medicare appeal number or document control number, if any, assigned to the QIC reconsideration or dismissal notice being appealed

- Dates of service

- Reasons the appellant disagrees with the decision made by the QIC during reconsideration or other determination being appealed

For the convenience of parties, forms may be used to request a Medicare ALJ hearing. These can be found on the CMS website. The contractor provides copies of the form to parties upon request. It is not necessary, however, that this form be used to make a written request. Form OMHA-100 is the hearing request form used when the request follows a QIC reconsideration. When multiple beneficiaries are associated with a single request for an ALJ hearing or a review of dismissal, form OMHA 100A is used. These forms may be found at (OMHA-100) https://www.hhs.gov/sites/default/files/OMHA-100.pdf and (OMHA 100A) https://www.hhs.gov/sites/default/files/OMHA-100A-Multiple-Claim-Attachment.pdf

KEY POINT

As part of the effort to reduce the outstanding number of ALJ hearing requests, the Office of Medicare Hearings and Appeals (OMHA) implemented two programs: Settlement Conference Facilitation (SCF) and Statistical Sampling Initiative. SCF is an alternative dispute resolution process that uses mediation principles. Statistical Sampling Initiative applies to appellants with a large volume of claim disputes.

ALJ hearing requests should be filed with the entity specified in the reconsideration notice from the QIC.

In most cases, OMHA will: 1) issues a decision based on the request for an ALJ hearing; 2) issues an order of dismissal of the appellant's request for ALJ hearing; or 3) remands the case to the QIC. In most cases, when OMHA's decision is partially or wholly favorable to the appellant, the contractor is given a specific amount to be paid and issues payment within 30 calendar days of receiving the notice from the administrative AdQIC. If OMHA decides that an overpayment was made, the money is recouped.

The Fourth Level of Appeal—Appeals Council Review

This level is available to appellants after the ALJ hearing decision, OMHA attorney adjudicator review, or dismissal order has been issued. The request for a review by the appeals council must be submitted within 60 days of the receipt of the notice of the ALJ's hearing decision or dismissal. A minimum monetary threshold is not required to request appeals council review.

The request for an Appeals Council may be in writing by following OMHA instructions. The request should include:

- The beneficiary's name
- The beneficiary's Medicare number
- The specific service(s) or item(s) for which the review is requested
- The specific date(s) of service
- The date of the ALJ's decision or dismissal order
- The name of the party or the representative of the party

A Council review request can be made by completing form DAB-101 found at: https://www.hhs.gov/sites/default/files/dab101.pdf.

The appeals council may receive the decision and adopt, modify, or reverse the ALJ's or attorney adjudicator's decision, or remand the case back to an ALJ for further proceedings. In the event of a dismissal from the ALJ or attorney adjudicator's decision, the council may deny review or remand the case back to an ALJ or attorney adjudicator for further proceedings. It may also dismiss a request for a hearing for any reason the ALJ or attorney adjudicator could have used to dismiss the request for hearing. The appeals council may also decide on its own motion to review a decision or dismissal issued by an ALJ or attorney adjudicator within 60 days after the date of the hearing decision or dismissal.

The Fifth Level of Appeal—U.S. District Court Review

In limited circumstances (outlined in 42 CFR 405.1136), an appeal or escalation to the U.S. District Court level of review is permitted. A contractor is not permitted to accept requests for judicial review. A request may be made to have a judicial review after the appeals council issues a decision. The appellant must file a complaint with the U.S. District Court within 60 days. The amount in dispute must be at least $1,760 for requests made on or after January 1, 2021.

The address to file with the U.S. District Court is:

> Department of Health and Human Services
> General Counsel
> 200 Independence Avenue, S.W.
> Washington, D.C. 20201

Waste, Fraud, and Abuse

Determining Waste, Fraud, and Abuse

Compliance is generally defined as "adherence to official requirements." Compliance in the physician practice means acting in accordance with the principles of ethical medical and business practices, as well as state and federal regulations. This involves ensuring that all activities follow the standards, laws, and regulations governing medical practice, as well as the internal policies and procedures established by the practice. Third parties, such as government agencies, enforce compliance by reviewing medical claims, contractual agreements, medical record documentation, or other forms of documentation to ensure adherence to these standards, laws, and regulations.

Compliance has become a major concern for physicians and other health care providers due to increasing regulatory requirements. There are currently thousands of health care regulations, both state and federal, and federal health care fraud criminal statutes, as well as additional voluntary standards, and the risks associated with noncompliance continue to grow significantly. With total health care expenditures in the trillions and Medicare and Medicaid alone in the billions, it is no surprise that health care is one of the most heavily regulated industries. Compliance goes beyond coding and billing; providers must comply with federal regulations covering licensing and clinical practice guidelines, investment and compensation arrangements, professional liability, controlled substances, informed consent, patient abuse or neglect, medical record documentation, and retention, storage, and release of information to name a few.

With the passage of the False Claim Act, Medicare and other payers have the means necessary to protect themselves from waste, fraud, and abuse.

What is waste?

CMS defines waste as overutilization of services or other practices that, directly or indirectly, result in unnecessary costs to the Medicare program. Waste is generally not considered to be caused by criminally negligent actions but rather the misuse of resources.

What is fraud?

Generally, health care fraud involves a provider's intentional use of false statements or schemes, such as kickbacks, to obtain payment for or to cause someone else to obtain payment for items or services payable under a federal health care program. CMS identifies some of the following as examples of fraud:

- Billing for services not furnished
- Soliciting, offering, or receiving a kickback, bribe, or rebate
- Billing based on "gang visits," an example of this would be when a physician visits a nursing home and bills for multiple nursing home visits without furnishing any specific service to individual patients.
- Billing noncovered or nonchargeable services as covered items.
- Misrepresentations of dates and descriptions of services furnished or the identity of the beneficiary or the individual who furnished the services.
- Repeatedly violating the participation agreement, assignment agreement, and the limitation amount.
- Giving false information about provider ownership in a clinical laboratory.

- Using another person's Medicare card to obtain medical care.
- Consistently using procedure codes that describe more extensive services than those actually performed (upcoding)

There are a number of federal statutes under which a practice can be indicted for fraud.

What is Abuse?

Abuse involves inappropriate payment for items or services when the provider has not knowingly or intentionally misrepresented facts to obtain payment. Abusive practices may directly or indirectly result in improper payment for services that fail to meet the recognized standards of care, or that are medically unnecessary. Inappropriate or abusive billing or coding practices that have been identified but not remedied may be considered fraudulent by payers. For example, when a provider ignores the payer's guidance, education, warnings, and/or advice and continues to bill for a service inappropriately, the action may then be interpreted as fraudulent.

Examples of abuse include:

- Billing for services/items in excess of those needed by the patient
- Charging in excess for services or supplies (lack of medical necessity documentation)
- Routinely filing duplicate claims (even if it does not result in duplicate payment)
- Collecting in excess of the deductible or coinsurance amounts due from a patient

Administrative sanctions may be imposed if fraudulent or abusive behavior is noted, including suspension of provider payments and Corporate Integrity Agreements (CIA) requiring the provider to satisfy a corrective action plan and be subject to periodic audits by federal agencies.

The OIG imposes CIAs on providers that settle civil fraud cases in exchange for not excluding the provider from participating in the federal health care programs. CIAs usually last five years and require the provider to put a variety of compliance measures in place.

The federal government continues to investigate physicians and other health care providers for violations using these and other enforcement tools. Funded through the Health Care Fraud and Abuse Control (HCFAC) program, a variety of investigations are performed. Since its inception in 1997, HCFAC has returned more than $43 billion through audit and investigative recoveries.

The False Claims Act (FCA) is a primary enforcement tool used to prosecute fraudulent billing practices under Medicare and Medicaid. Under FCA, any individual who knowingly makes a false claim to the government is liable for mandatory civil penalties and fines. The FCA authorized civil penalties which may include recovery of up to three times the amount of damages sustained by the Government as a result of the false claims, plus penalties up to $22,927 (in 2019) per false claim filed. Under this Act, each item or a service on a claim form is counted as a claim, so the fines can add up quickly. Many payers are now aggressively pursuing providers that are suspected of fraudulent activity. CERT is one of the programs that CMS established to monitor and report the accuracy of Medicare fee-for-service payments. Private organizations are contracted under

DEFINITIONS

corporate integrity agreement. Agreement between the government and a provider who has entered into a settlement with the government due to a health care fraud and abuse investigation. Providers must agree to follow the corporate integrity agreement, which is essentially a government-mandated compliance program.

fee for service. Payment for services, usually physician services, on a service-by-service basis rather than an alternative payment system like capitation. Fee-for-service arrangements may be discounted or undiscounted rates.

the Medicare Integrity Program to review health care professional's activities, such as utilization and fraud. CMS also has the national Recovery Audit Contractor (RAC) program, which is an aggressive program to find and prevent Medicare waste, fraud, and abuse. Enforcement options range from claim denials, audits, and overpayment recoveries to civil actions and even criminal prosecution.

Anti-Kickback Statute

The Anti-Kickback statute prohibits physicians from knowingly and willfully paying or receiving remuneration in exchange for the referral of a patient, and violations can result in civil and criminal penalties including fines, imprisonment, and health care program exclusion. Remuneration includes anything of value and can take many forms besides cash, such as excessive compensation for medical directorships or consulting, expensive hotel stays and meals, and free rent. The criminal statute applies to any individual who accepts or solicits payment for referring patients to a facility, physician, or any other health care provider that provides items or services paid for by Medicare or Medicaid. Anyone convicted under these felony provisions may be fined up to $100,000 per kickback plus three times the amount of the remuneration, imprisoned up to 10 years, or both.

Anti-Physician Self-Referral (Stark) Law

The Anti-Physician Self-Referral (Stark) Law prohibits a provider from referring a patient for certain designated health care services if the provider or a family member has a financial relationship with the entity providing the service. Stark designated health care services include:

- Clinical laboratory services
- Durable medical equipment (DME) and supplies
- Home health services
- Inpatient and outpatient hospital services
- Outpatient prescription drugs
- Outpatient speech-language pathology services
- Parenteral and enteral nutrients, equipment, and supplies
- Physical and occupational therapy
- Prosthetics, orthotics, and prosthetic devices and supplies
- Radiology and certain other imaging services
- Radiation therapy services and supplies

Penalties for physicians who violate the Stark Law may include fines, Civil Monetary Penalties (CMPs) up to $25,372 (in 2019) for each service, repayment of claims, and potential exclusion from participation in the federal health care programs.

Regulatory Agencies

Efforts to identify and eliminate health care waste, fraud, and abuse involve contractors, beneficiaries, and federal agencies such as CMS, OIG, Department of Justice (DOJ), and the Department of Health and Human Services (HHS).

The Health Insurance Portability and Accountability Act of 1996 (HIPAA) established a comprehensive program to combat health care fraud: the national Health Care Fraud and Abuse Control program. The program coordinates federal, state, and local law enforcement efforts in health care fraud and abuse. The DOJ and HHS have overseen the HCFAC program enforcement efforts since 1997. HIPAA also gave the OIG and the DOJ funding to increase penalties for health care fraud and abuse violations of the False Claims Act and other federal laws. In addition to significant financial penalties, under HIPAA health care fraud became a federal crime carrying a federal prison term of up to 10 years. Therefore it is vital that physicians understand who the investigating agencies are, what they do, and the physician's legal rights and obligations.

Federal program enforcers include:

- Office of Inspector General (OIG)
- Department of Justice (DOJ)
- Federal Bureau of Investigation (FBI)
- Medicare Administrative Contractors (MAC)
- Recovery Audit Contractors (RAC)
- Quality Improvement Organizations (QIO)
- Program Safeguard Contractors (PSC)
- Medicare Zone Program Integrity Contractors (ZPIC)
- Supplemental Medical Review Contractors (SMRC)
- Medicaid Fraud Control Units (MFCU)
- State Attorney Generals
- Unified Program Integrity Contractor (UPIC)

Remittance Advice Review

Another tool that can be utilized when auditing is the payer remittance advice (RA) review. An RA is a notification of how the claim was adjudicated, including payments and adjustments. Adjustments refer to any change about why the claim was paid differently from the original billing. The RA contains many details that can be crucial in identifying common denials.

Once third-party payers have acknowledged receipt of the claim, the next step usually involves some type of notification from the payer to the physician practice in the form of a payment or an explanation of how the claim was processed (deductible, noncovered, etc.), a request for additional information, or an outright denial of that claim via the RA.

CMS lists seven general types of adjustments:

- Denied claim
- Zero payment
- Partial payment
- Reduced payment
- Penalty applied
- Additional payment
- Supplemental payment

A remittance advice document provides detailed information related to how the health care claim was processed. It is used by providers to post payments and adjustments, as well as to understand the reasoning behind the claim adjudication process. When a claim does not meet coverage, medical necessity, or policy requirements, the provider may be afforded appeal rights with additional information for redetermination based on guidance contained in the RA.

In the case of Medicare, this document has historically been referred to by a number of names including RA, remittance notice, explanation of Medicare benefits (EOMB), and the Medicare summary voucher. Providers typically use the term RA or explanation of benefits interchangeably, for Medicare and non-Medicare payers. An RA can cover single or multiple patients.

Each RA should be carefully reviewed to determine if billing, coding, or reimbursement errors have occurred and, if so, what steps are necessary to make corrections. This review should also determine if this was a simple, one-time oversight or if policies and procedures should be developed to prevent repetitive errors from occurring in the future. Payers make mistakes, too. Carefully look over the RA to make sure the payer has not made any errors when processing the claim.

 DEFINITIONS

downcode. Reduction in the value and code on a claim when documentation does not support the level of service billed by a provider.

When reviewing the RA, first crosscheck the patient's health insurance claim number (HICN) with the office record for that patient to ensure payment is posted to the correct account. Next, verify that the date of service matches the date of service in the record. This allows staff to determine what services and/or procedures should have been processed for that date.

Compare the HCPCS Level II and/or CPT codes on the RA with those shown on the claim. This determines whether the payer has downcoded the claim or requires services be identified with a different code. Downcoded claims are paid at a reduced amount. Many providers identify that a procedure code has been changed by the inclusion of HCPCS Level II modifier CC.

Take note of whether a service or procedure identified by multiple codes was bundled into a single code. This can occur when component procedure codes are combined into a single, more comprehensive code. (The correct coding initiative will be discussed in detail later in this chapter.) If the individual codes were more appropriately identified by the single, more comprehensive code, be sure to share this information with the coding and billing staff in order to avoid repeating the same error. In addition, always ensure the appropriate place of service was used for the type of service provided. For example, a provider reports an initial nursing facility care code 99304 with a nail debridement service 11721 using POS code 32 for the visit and POS code 11 for the debridement. The payer classifies the claim as "fractured" and payment is made for the nursing facility visit only while the nail debridement is denied due to the incorrect place of service. The payer's thought process is that if the patient was able to come into the office for a nail debridement, why was there a need for the nursing facility visit? Of course, the patient did not come into the office and thus the nail procedure was denied. The claim could be reconsidered once the POS code was amended to reflect the proper location. Always verify the information submitted on the claim against the remittance advice and flag any changes, omissions, reduced payment items, or denials for follow up.

Note that there may be a message on the RA that indicates an interest payment by Medicare. The secretary of the treasury certifies an interest rate quarterly. The

Department of the Treasury uses the most comprehensive data available on consumer interest rates to determine the certified rate. Medicare regulations provide the assessment of interest for Medicare over and underpayments. For 2021, the interest rate is 9.375 percent.

Non-medical Code Sets

HIPAA code sets used to describe a general administrative situation rather than a medical condition or service are referred to as non-medical code sets. A few examples of these code sets are listed below.

Claim Adjustment Reason Codes

Claim adjustment reason codes (CARC) provide the financial information about claim processing decisions, such as an adjustment or why a claim or line item was paid differently than it was billed. When no adjustment is made to the claim or line item, no CARC is used. CARCs were designed to replace proprietary coding systems used by each payer prior to HIPAA and to alleviate the burden of interpreting different systems faced by providers. Examples of this type of code include:

1	Deductible amount
2	Co-insurance amount
3	Co-payment amount
4	The procedure code is inconsistent with the modifier used. Usage: Refer to the 835 Healthcare Policy Identification Segment (loop 2110 Service Payment Information REF), if present.
5	The procedure code/type of bill is inconsistent with the place of service. Usage: Refer to the 835 Healthcare Policy Identification Segment (loop 2110 Service Payment Information REF), if present.
40	Charges do not meet qualifications for emergent/urgent care. Usage: Refer to the 835 Healthcare Policy Identification Segment (loop 2110 Service Payment Information REF), if present.
96	Non-covered charge(s). At least one Remark Code must be provided (may be comprised of either the NCPDP Reject Reason Code, or Remittance Advice Remark Code that is not an ALERT.) Usage: Refer to the 835 Healthcare Policy Identification Segment (loop 2110 Service Payment Information REF), if present.

Remittance Advice Remark Codes

Remittance advice remark codes (RARC) are used in conjunction with CARCs to provide additional detail on an adjustment. Some of these code types start with descriptors such as "ALERT," which are used to provide general claim processing information for things such as appeal rights. This type of RARC can be used without an associated CARC or when no adjustment has been made. CMS maintains the remittance advice remark codes but any other health care payer may use them when appropriate. Examples of this code type include:

M2	Not paid separately when the patient is an inpatient
M13	Only one initial visit is covered per specialty per medical group

 © 2020 Optum360, LLC

M125   Missing/incomplete/invalid information on the period of time for which the service/supply/equipment will be needed

N1   Alert: You may appeal this decision in writing within the required time limits following receipt of this notice by following the instructions included in your contract, plan benefit documents, or jurisdiction statutes. Refer to the URL provided in the ERA for the payer website to access the appeals process guidelines.

N24   Missing/incomplete/invalid electronic funds transfer (EFT) banking information

Claim adjustment reason codes and remittance advice remark codes are updated three times each year. A list of the latest codes is available at https://x12.org/codes.

Common Reasons for Denial for Medicare

The following section discusses the types of errors that may result in denial of services and/or procedures. Also included are steps a practice can take to prevent recurrence of these errors.

Medical Necessity Denials

As stated earlier, CMS defines medical necessity as "services or supplies that are proper and needed for the diagnosis or treatment of a medical condition; are provided for the diagnosis, direct care, and treatment of [a] medical condition; meet the standards of good medical practice in the local area; and are not simply for the convenience of [a patient] or doctor." Many commercial payers also follow this guideline or one similar.

Medical record documentation is key to avoiding this type of denial and should include not only the service or procedure rendered, but also *why* the service or procedure was medically warranted.

In the event the claim is denied due to medical necessity, first determine that the correct ICD-10-CM diagnosis code was submitted. Check to make certain that the digits were not transposed, that the condition was coded to the highest level of specificity, and that all conditions documented in the medical record were included on the claim at the time of submission.

Note that some services or procedures have coverage limitations that permit payment only after specific criteria are met. For example, coverage may only be provided for a specific diagnosis after other less invasive or costly services have been attempted and are unsuccessful in treating the condition or when the patient is over a certain age.

Specific Coverage Criteria

Many payers, including Medicare, only offer coverage on services when a specific medical condition is present.

National Coverage Determinations

For Medicare services, when a coverage decision has been made on a national basis, a national coverage determination (NCD) is created. NCDs can be found in the Medicare IOM, Pub. 100-03, the *Medicare National Coverage Determinations Manual.* Examples of coverage indications in this manual include those for electrocardiograms, ambulatory blood pressure monitoring,

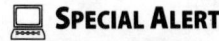

SPECIAL ALERT

A revised Advance Beneficiary Notice of Noncoverage (ABN), Form CMS-R-131, has been approved. Use will be mandatory starting 8/31/20. More information can be found at: https://www.cms.gov/Medicare/Medicare-General-Information/BNI/ABN

neuromuscular electrical stimulation (NMES), magnetic resonance angiography, and many others.

It is strongly suggested and recommended that providers review the table of contents for this online manual periodically. Determine what procedures the providers are likely to perform or refer patients for. Print these specific decisions and include them in the compliance manual once all clinical and administrative staff have reviewed them. Refer to them frequently before providing or referring patients for procedures to ensure coverage and that all necessary requirements have been met. If not, ask the patient to sign an advance beneficiary notice (ABN) or notice of exclusion from Medicare benefits (NEMB), whichever is appropriate.

Local Coverage Determinations

Individual Medicare contractors also develop policies that apply to local coverage. These policies are called local coverage determinations (LCD). Like NCDs, these coverage decisions often indicate a specific reason a service or procedure may be covered. LCDs can be found on the contractor website or on the Medicare website at http://www.cms.gov/medicare/coverage/determinationprocess/LCDs.html.

Usually, the remittance advice notifies the provider of a denial to a local coverage issue by the following remittance advice remark:

> The decision was based on a local coverage determination (LCD). An LCD provides a guide to assist in determining whether a particular item or service is covered. A copy of this policy is available at http://www.cms.gov/mcd, or the contractor may be contacted to request a copy of the LCD.

It is recommended that providers frequently review contractor bulletins and websites for local coverage decisions. Print these decisions and include them in the coding compliance manual after clinical staff have been educated.

Claims Submission Errors

Claim errors account for a large percentage of denied claims. Many Medicare contractors release the top claim submission errors on a monthly basis. Below are a few of the errors that are frequently seen on the monthly reports.

- **Patient not identified as insured.** Always enter the patient's name and HICN or policy number as it is shown on the insurance or benefit card. Verify that all numbers are entered correctly and that no numbers have been transposed; also make sure the letter at the end of the Medicare number is correct. Check eligibility and benefits prior to the visit.

- **Missing, incomplete, or invalid NPI of ordering or referring physician.** Ensure that staff are knowledgeable and educated as to what services and circumstances require the referring/ordering physician's NPI number. Failure to provide this information results in an "unprocessable" claim denial.

- **Claim/service lacks information that is needed for adjudication.** Make sure that there is a formal process in place so that staff is aware of how this should be dealt with. If this type of denial continues to occur it should be investigated to see if there are missing steps in the process. Whether it is omitted demographics, authorization numbers, or secondary payer information, the problem should be able to be resolved.

- **Claim not covered by this payer/contractor. Claims must be sent to the correct payer/contractor.** Staff should be asking patients at every visit for a copy of their current insurance card. It is also important for staff to identify whether a patient's claims should be covered by other insurance before, or in addition to, Medicare. This information helps determine who to bill and how to file claims with Medicare.

- **Duplicate claim/service.** Allow 30 days from the date a claim was received to process the claim for payment. Prior to resubmitting a claim, check the claim status using the payers' online inquiry system or inquire by telephone.

- **These are noncovered services because this is not deemed a medical necessity by the payer.** Reviewing national and local medical policies regularly for procedures and services performed in the practice helps keep staff familiar with the requirements needed to report them.

Commercial Payers

Commercial payers also have specific coverage indications for procedures and services. Providers are most frequently notified of these requirements by the provider manual or provider bulletins.

As with Medicare coverage issues, it is suggested that providers review these publications and determine any services likely to be provided or ordered by the practice. Print this information and include it in the coding compliance manual. Be certain the clinical staff is aware of any specific requirements.

It may also be helpful to create a spreadsheet that staff can refer to for a quick reference. An example follows:

Service	Requirements			
	Medicare	Payer 1	Payer 2	Payer 3
Thermography	NCD. Excluded from Medicare Coverage. Get NEMB	Covered for breast lesions	Noncovered	Noncovered
Percutaneous image guided breast biopsy	NCD. Nonpalpable and graded as BIRADS III, IV, or V	No special coverage requirements	See Medicare coverage	See Coding Compliance Manual

Common Claim Denial Reasons for Commercial Payers

In today's economy it is crucial that provider practices earn their potential. This means there needs to be an ongoing effort within the practices to track denials and resolve them in order to receive the revenue that the practice justly deserves. Each practice should determine the denial codes that have the most impact on their revenue and concentrate on those.

The following pages outline many of the common denials encountered by provider practices. Each of these denials are discussed in detail and include guidance on evaluating the impact on claims, how to determine the root cause of the denial, and, finally, how to prevent future denials.

Duplicate Claim/Service

As indicated in the table above, "duplicate claim/service" is the reason noted by payers for most claim denials. This error is responsible for a significant loss of revenue.

Code Type: Claim Adjustment Reason Codes

18	Exact duplicate claim/service (Use only with Group Code OA except where state workers' compensation regulations require CO) *Start: 01/01/1995	Last Modified: 06/02/2013*
97	The benefit for this service is included in the payment/allowance for another service/procedure that has already been adjudicated. Usage: Refer to the 835 Healthcare Policy Identification Segment (loop 2110 Service Payment Information REF), if present. *Start: 01/01/1995	Last Modified: 07/01/2017*

Code Type: Remittance Advice Remark Codes

M80	Not covered when performed during the same session/date as a previously processed service for the patient. *Start: 01/01/1997	Last Modified: 10/31/2002* *Notes: (Modified 10/31/02)*
M86	Service denied because payment already made for same/similar procedure within set time frame. *Start: 01/01/1997	Last Modified: 06/30/2003* *Notes: (Modified 6/30/03)*
N111	No appeal right except duplicate claim/service issue. This service was included in a claim that has been previously billed and adjudicated. *Start: 02/28/2002*
N522	Duplicate of a claim processed, or to be processed, as a crossover claim. *Start: 11/01/2009	Last Modified: 03/01/2010*

Code Type: Claim Status Codes

54	Duplicate of a previously processed claim/line. *Start: 01/01/1995*
78	Duplicate of an existing claim/line, awaiting processing. *Start: 01/01/1995*

A denial of this type may indicate that more than one claim was submitted for the same service. Additionally, this denial may occur because the same service (frequently evaluation and management services) was provided by different providers on the same date of service.

Provider offices should not simply resubmit outstanding claims that have not been processed in what may be considered a normal time frame by a practice. Unnecessary duplicate filing of claims costs the provider's office valuable time and resources. Additionally, duplicate claims submissions can be viewed as potentially abusive or fraudulent.

Corrective Actions

To reduce duplicate claim filings, providers are encouraged to adopt the following processes:

- Allow 30 days from the date a claim was received to process the claim for payment. (Medicare contractors generally process electronic claims within 14 days and paper claims within 29 days.)

- Check claim status through an online inquiry system or by telephone before resubmitting.

© 2020 Optum360, LLC

- Payment staff should pay special attention to remittance advice noting zero-pay claims to determine if the claim should be resubmitted. Often these claims are not paid because the allowed amount was applied to the patient's deductible.

- Procedures performed multiple times on the same day require that modifier 76 be appended to the procedure listed on the claim.

- When billing consultations to Medicare using the initial hospital care code (99221–99223) or initial nursing facility care code (99304–99306), modifier AI should be appended to the procedure code reported by the attending physician. Failure to do so could result in one or more providers having their claim denied as a duplicate service.

- Duplicate services denied because the same service was provided by a different provider, such as in the case of an E/M service, requires staff to validate appropriate ICD-10-CM code assignment for the condition treated by the respective providers and then resubmit the claim.

Additional Information Needed

This claim adjustment reason code is one of the most significant sources of denied services and may indicate some type of failure within the practice's procedures.

Code Type: Claim Adjustment Reason Codes

16	Claim/service lacks information or has submission/billing error(s). Usage: Do not use this code for claims attachment(s)/other documentation. At least one Remark Code must be provided (may be comprised of either the NCPDP Reject Reason Code, or Remittance Advice Remark Code that is not an ALERT.) Refer to the 835 Healthcare Policy Identification Segment (loop 2110 Service Payment Information REF), if present. *Start: 01/01/1995	Last Modified: 03/01/2018*
197	Precertification/authorization/notification/pre-treatment absent. *Start: 10/31/2006	Last Modified: 05/01/2018*
206	National Provider Identifier - missing. *Start: 07/09/2007	Last Modified: 09/30/2007*
207	National Provider identifier - Invalid format *Start: 07/09/2007	Last Modified: 06/01/2008*
208	National Provider Identifier - Not matched. *Start: 07/09/2007	Last Modified: 09/30/2007*

Remittance Advice Remark Codes

M127	Missing patient medical record for this service. *Start: 01/01/1997	Last Modified: 02/28/2003* *Notes: (Modified 2/28/03)*
N257	Missing/incomplete/invalid billing provider/supplier primary identifier. *Start: 12/02/2004*
N479	Missing Explanation of Benefits (Coordination of Benefits or Medicare Secondary Payer). *Start: 07/01/2008*
N516	Records indicate a mismatch between the submitted NPI and EIN. *Start: 03/01/2009*

The CARC is accompanied by an additional CARC or a remittance advice remark code (RARC) that provides more detail as to the nature of the information that is missing, including patient demographic information, provider information, other payer explanation of benefits needed for coordination of benefits, or information regarding the service or procedure.

When determining the root cause of the denial, the additional remark code must be established. Providers should then determine if there is a pattern. For example, if 60 claims with CARC denial code 16 are examined and 45 of those denials have the additional remarks code of M127, then further investigation as to why medical record requests were not replied to would be necessary.

Corrective Actions

A common root cause could be that a formal process for responding to these requests has not been defined. In this instance, identify a staff member who is responsible for fulfilling these requests and a method of tracking requests (i.e., the nature of the missing information and responses to these requests), such as a log. The log should be reviewed periodically to determine the number of requests and whether the requests are being handled in a timely fashion. If there are a large number of requests for additional information, the type of information missing should be tracked and investigated.

Benefit Included in the Payment/Allowance for Another Service/Procedure

This type of denial includes inappropriate billing of a procedure or service that is considered an integral part of a more comprehensive service or procedure. In other words, this includes unbundling or exploding services.

Code Type: Claim Adjustment Reason Codes

97	The benefit for this service is included in the payment/allowance for another service/procedure that has already been adjudicated. Usage: Refer to the 835 Healthcare Policy Identification Segment (loop 2110 Service Payment Information REF), if present. *Start: 01/01/1995	Last Modified: 07/01/2017*

Code Type: Remittance Advice Remark Codes

M15	Separately billed services/tests have been bundled as they are considered components of the same procedure. Separate payment is not allowed. *Start: 01/01/1997*
M80	Not covered when performed during the same session/date as a previously processed service for the patient. *Start: 01/01/1997	Last Modified: 10/31/2002* *Notes: (Modified 10/31/02)*
M86	Service denied because payment already made for same/similar procedure within set time frame. *Start: 01/01/1997	Last Modified: 06/30/2003* *Notes: (Modified 6/30/03)*
M144	Pre-/postoperative care payment is included in the allowance for the surgery/procedure. *Start: 01/01/1997*
N111	No appeal right except duplicate claim/service issue. This service was included in a claim that has been previously billed and adjudicated. *Start: 02/28/2002*

Code Type: Claim Status Codes

735	This service/claim is included in the allowance for another service or claim. *Start: 06/06/2010*

This type of denial may be caused by reporting a service/procedure that is included in the CPT global surgical package. CPT has identified procedures that are typically included when performing a surgical procedure, although they may vary by patient.

In defining the specific services included in a given CPT surgical code, the following services are always included in addition to the surgical procedure itself by the American Medical Association (AMA):

- Local infiltration; metacarpal, metatarsal, or digit block; or topical anesthesia

- Subsequent to the decision for surgery, one related E/M encounter on the date immediately prior to or on the date of procedure (including history and physical)

- Immediate postoperative care, including dictating operative notes, talking with the family, and other physicians

- Writing orders

- Evaluating the patient in the postanesthesia recovery area

- Typical postoperative follow-up care

Another reason for this denial is that components of a surgical procedure may be bundled into a more comprehensive procedure under the National Correct Coding Initiative (NCCI). Under the NCCI there is an official list of codes from CMS's National Correct Coding Policy Manual for Part B Medicare Carriers that identifies services considered an integral part of a comprehensive code or mutually exclusive of it.

Corrective Actions:
Before reporting a group of procedures it is wise to consult the NCCI to verify that one or more of the procedures is not a component of a more comprehensive procedure. The most comprehensive procedure should be the one that is reported. (The NCCI will be discussed in further detail later in this chapter.)

Coordination of Benefits or Incorrect payer/contractor
This type of error is often due to the failure to determine if the patient has additional coverage or if a condition is related to an accident or injury that would result in another payer, such as auto insurance or worker's compensation, being the primary payer.

 DEFINITIONS

bundled services. Items or services grouped together for reporting and reimbursement purposes. The items or services may be related or unrelated, but all defined elements must be present to constitute a specific bundle.

Code Type: Claim Adjustment Reason Codes

19	This is a work-related injury/illness and thus the liability of the Worker's Compensation Carrier. *Start: 01/01/1995 | Last Modified: 09/30/2007*
20	This injury/illness is covered by the liability carrier. *Start: 01/01/1995 | Last Modified: 09/30/2007*
21	This injury/illness is the liability of the no-fault carrier. *Start: 01/01/1995 | Last Modified: 09/30/2007*
22	This care may be covered by another payer per coordination of benefits. *Start: 01/01/1995 | Last Modified: 09/30/2007*
109	Claim/service not covered by this payer/contractor. You must send the claim/service to the correct payer/contractor. *Start: 01/01/1995 | Last Modified: 01/29/2012*
B11	The claim/service has been transferred to the proper payer/processor for processing. Claim/service not covered by this payer/processor. *Start: 01/01/1995*

Code Type: Remittance Advice Remark Codes

MA16	The patient is covered by the Black Lung Program. Send this claim to the Department of Labor, Federal Black Lung Program, P.O. Box 828, Lanham-Seabrook MD 20703. *Start: 01/01/1997*
MA18	Alert: The claim information is also being forwarded to the patient's supplemental insurer. Send any questions regarding supplemental benefits to them. *Start: 01/01/1997 | Last Modified: 04/01/2007* *Notes: (Modified 4/1/07)*
MA19	Alert: Information was not sent to the Medigap insurer due to incorrect/invalid information you submitted concerning that insurer. Please verify your information and submit your secondary claim directly to that insurer. *Start: 01/01/1997 | Last Modified: 04/01/2007* *Notes: (Modified 4/1/07)*
N4	Missing/incomplete/invalid prior insurance carrier(s) EOB. *Start: 01/01/2000 | Last Modified: 03/06/2012* *Notes: (Modified 2/28/03, 3/6/2012)*
N5	EOB received from previous payer. Claim not on file. *Start: 01/01/2000*
N155	Alert: Our records do not indicate that other insurance is on file. Please submit other insurance information for our records. *Start: 10/31/2002 | Last Modified: 04/01/2007* *Notes: (Modified 4/1/07)*
N196	Alert: Patient eligible to apply for other coverage which may be primary. *Start: 02/25/2003 | Last Modified: 04/01/2007* *Notes: (Modified 4/1/07)*
N479	Missing explanation of benefits (Coordination of Benefits or Medicare Secondary Payer). *Start: 07/01/2008*
M480	Incomplete/invalid explanation of benefits (Coordination of Benefits or Medicare Secondary Payer). *Start: 07/01/2008*

Code Type: Claim Status Codes

52	Investigating existence of other insurance coverage. *Start: 01/01/1995*

This type of denial may be caused by submitting a claim to an incorrect payer, whether it is the initial submission or for coordination of benefits. When a patient has more than one insurance plan, there are coordination of benefits (COB) rules that determine which plan will process claims first. Under COB, the benefits of the primary plan are applied to the cost of care. After considering what has been covered by the primary plan, the secondary plan may cover the remainder of the cost of service according to the plan's payment guidelines.

Most payers use guidelines implemented by the National Association of Insurance Commissioners (NAIC) for determining primary and secondary benefit plans. The most common guidelines are listed below:

- Active/inactive rule: The plan that covers an active employee (not as a laid-off employee or retiree) is primary over the plan that covers a laid-off employee or retiree.

- Birthday rule: This is a method used to determine when a plan is primary or secondary for a dependent child when covered by both parents' benefit plan. The plan covering the parent whose birthday falls earlier in the year is the primary carrier. If both parents have the same birthday, the plan that has provided coverage longest is the primary carrier.

Dependent Children of Separated or Divorced Parents

If a child is covered by more than one group plan and the parents are separated or divorced, the plans must pay in the following order:

- The plan of the parent with custody of the child
- The plan of the spouse of the parent with custody of the child
- The plan of the parent not having custody of the child
- The plan of the parent's spouse not having custody of the child

However, if terms of a court decree state that one parent is responsible for a child's health care expenses and the insurance company has been informed of the responsibility, that plan is the primary carrier over the plan of the other parent.

Dependent Children of Parents with Joint Custody

The birthday rule applies in this situation.

If a patient is covered by Medicare and has another group insurance as well, the COB rules are set by CMS.

Corrective Action

As a rule of thumb, always verify a patient's insurance coverage prior to performing a service/procedure. Additionally, if a patient is seen due to an accident or injury, it is advisable to determine the cause of the accident or injury and if some personal injury protection insurer (automobile, homeowners) or worker's compensation should be the primary payer.

It should also be noted that some payers have edits that automatically request additional information from the patient when an injury diagnosis code is indicated on a claim. Stress the importance of completing this information in a timely manner to the patient and when acceptable to the payer, indicate the appropriate V codes on the claim describing the circumstances of the injury.

Noncovered Services Due To Medical Necessity

This type of error is responsible for a large amount of claim denials and, therefore, there is the potential of significant revenue loss.

Code Type: Claim Adjustment Reason Codes

50	These are non-covered services because this is not deemed a "medical necessity" by the payer. Usage: Refer to the 835 Healthcare Policy Identification Segment (loop 2110 Service Payment Information REF), if present. *Start: 01/01/1995	Last Modified: 07/01/2017*
150	Payer deems the information submitted does not support this level of service. *Start: 10/31/2002	Last Modified: 09/30/2007*
186	Level of care change adjustment. *Start: 06/30/2005	Last Modified: 09/30/2007*
B12	Services not documented in patient's medical records. *Start: 01/01/1995	Last Modified: 03/01/2018*

Code Type: Remittance Advice Remark Codes

M25	The information furnished does not substantiate the need for this level of service. If you believe the service should have been fully covered as billed, or if you did not know and could not reasonably have been expected to know that we would not pay for this level of service, or if you notified the patient in writing in advance that we would not pay for this level of service and he/she agreed in writing to pay, ask us to review your claim within 120 days of the date of this notice. If you do not request an appeal, we will, upon application from the patient, reimburse him/her for the amount you have collected from him/her in excess of any deductible and coinsurance amounts. We will recover the reimbursement from you as an overpayment. *Start: 01/01/1997	Last Modified: 11/01/2010* *Notes: (Modified 10/1/02, 6/30/03, 8/1/05, 11/5/07, 11/01/10)*
M26	The information furnished does not substantiate the need for this level of service. If you have collected any amount from the patient for this level of service, any amount that exceeds the limiting charge for the less extensive service, the law requires you to refund that amount to the patient within 30 days of receiving this notice. The requirements for refund are in 1824(l) of the Social Security Act and 42CFR411.408. The section specifies that physicians who knowingly and willfully fail to make appropriate refunds may be subject to civil monetary penalties and/or exclusion from the program. If you have any questions about this notice, please contact this office. *Start: 01/01/1997	Last Modified: 11/05/2007* *Notes: (Modified 10/1/02, 6/30/03, 8/1/05, 11/5/07. Also refer to N356)*
N115	This decision was based on a Local Coverage Determination (LCD). An LCD provides a guide to assist in determining whether a particular item or service is covered. A copy of this policy is available at http://www.cms.gov/mcd, or if you do not have web access, you may contact the contractor to request a copy of the LCD. *Start: 05/30/2002	Last Modified: 07/01/2010* *Notes: (Modified 4/1/04, 07/01/10)*
N124	Payment has been denied for the/made only for a less extensive service/item because the information furnished does not substantiate the need for the (more extensive) service/item. The patient is liable for the charges for this service/item as you informed the patient in writing before the service/item was furnished that we would not pay for it, and the patient agreed to pay. *Start: 09/26/2002*

© 2020 Optum360, LLC

N125	Payment has been (denied for the/made only for a less extensive) service/item because the information furnished does not substantiate the need for the (more extensive) service/item. If you have collected any amount from the patient, you must refund that amount to the patient within 30 days of receiving this notice.
	The requirements for a refund are in §1834(a)(18) of the Social Security Act (and in §§1834(j)(4) and 1879(h) by cross-reference to §1834(a)(18)). Section 1834(a)(18)(B) specifies that suppliers which knowingly and willfully fail to make appropriate refunds may be subject to civil money penalties and/or exclusion from the Medicare program. If you have any questions about this notice, please contact this office. *Start: 09/26/2002	Last Modified: 08/01/2005* *Notes: (Modified 08/01/2005. Also refer to N356)*
N163	Medical record does not support code billed per the code definition. *Start: 02/28/2003*
N206	The supporting documentation does not match the information sent on the claim. *Start: 06/30/2003	Last Modified: 03/06/2012* *Notes: (Modified 03/06/2012)*
N356	Not covered when performed with, or subsequent to, a non-covered service. *Start: 08/01/2005	Last Modified: 03/08/2011* *Notes: (Modified 03/08/2011)*
N386	This decision was based on a National Coverage Determination (NCD). An NCD provides a coverage determination as to whether a particular item or service is covered. A copy of this policy is available at www.cms.gov/mcd/search.asp. If you do not have web access, you may contact the contractor to request a copy of the NCD. *Start: 04/01/2007	Last Modified: 07/01/2010* *Notes: (Modified 07/01/2010)*

This type of denial occurs when third-party payers will not provide coverage for services deemed as not medically necessary.

Medicare defines a covered service as:

- Services that are considered medically reasonable and necessary to the overall diagnosis and treatment of the patient's condition.

Services or supplies are considered medically necessary when they meet one or more of the following requirements:

- Proper and needed for the diagnosis or treatment of the patient's medical condition
- Furnished for the diagnosis, direct care, and treatment of the patient's medical condition
- Meet standards of good medical practice
- Not provided mainly for the convenience of the patient, provider, or supplier

In this type of denial, it is essential to have medical record documentation that includes not only the service or procedure rendered, but also an explanation of why the service or procedure was medically warranted.

In the event the claim is denied due to medical necessity, first determine that the correct ICD-10-CM diagnosis code was submitted. Check to make sure that the digits were not transposed, that the condition was coded to the highest level of specificity, and that all conditions documented in the medical record were included on the claim.

Note that some services or procedures have coverage limitations that permit payment only after specific criteria are met. For example, coverage may only be provided for a specific diagnosis after other less invasive or costly services have been attempted and are unsuccessful in treating the condition, or when the patient is over a certain age.

Corrective Actions

- Providers should familiarize themselves with NCDs and LCDs. It is recommended that providers review these periodically and determine which procedures the providers are likely to perform or refer patients. Print these specific decisions and include them in the coding compliance manual. Refer to them frequently before providing or referring patients for procedures to ensure coverage and that all necessary requirements have been met. If not, ask the patient to sign an ABN or NEMB, whichever is appropriate.

- Commercial payers also have specific coverage indications for procedures and services. It is suggested that providers review their provider manual or provider bulletins and determine any services likely to be provided or ordered by the practice. A copy of these citations should be included in the coding compliance manual. Clinical staff should be made aware of any specific requirements.

- Confirm that the patient's medical documentation and records are complete prior to submitting a claim. Ensure that diagnosis codes reported on the claim correspond with the documentation.

- Diagnosis and/or symptoms responsible for the reason the procedure or service is performed should be coded to the highest degree of specificity available using official ICD-10-CM coding guidelines.

- A valid Advance Beneficiary Notice (ABN) may be necessary when billing a service that falls under an NCD or LCD. An ABN is a written notice completed by the provider and given to a Medicare beneficiary informing them that the service or procedure to be provided will likely not be paid for by Medicare. The purpose of the ABN is to inform the Medicare patient *before* the item or service is provided; therefore, it is important that the ABN be processed *prior to the service being rendered*. Clinical staff should be educated regarding coverage guidelines for services commonly performed. Additionally, clinical staff should be trained to consider coverage of procedures and, if questionable, request coverage guidance from administrative staff. Blanket ABNs should not be executed. The ABN must specify the service and a genuine reason that denial by Medicare is expected. ABN standards are not satisfied by generic statements signed by the beneficiary indicating that, should Medicare deny payment for anything, the patient agrees to pay for the service.

💻 SPECIAL ALERT

A revised Advance Beneficiary Notice of Noncoverage (ABN), Form CMS-R-131, has been approved. Use will be mandatory starting 8/31/20. More information can be found at: https://www.cms.gov/Medicare/Medicare-General-Information/BNI/ABN

Timely Filing Deadline Exceeded

Code Type: Claim Adjustment Reason Code

29	The time limit for filing has expired. *Start: 01/01/1995*
164	Attachment/other documentation referenced on the claim was not received in a timely fashion. *Start: 06/30/2004 | Last Modified: 06/02/2013*
226	Information requested from the Billing/Rendering Provider was not provided or not provided timely or was insufficient/incomplete. At least one Remark Code must be provided (may be comprised of either the NCPDP Reject Reason Code, or Remittance Advice Remark Code that is not an ALERT.) *Start: 09/21/2008 | Last Modified: 07/01/2013*

Code Type: Claim Status Code

718	Claim/service not submitted within the required timeframe (timely filing). *Start: 01/24/2010*

Most health plans have a defined time period in which a health insurance claim can be submitted. If the claim arrives beyond this date, the claim will be denied.

The time period for filing Medicare fee-for-service (FFS) claims was amended to reduce the maximum time period for submission of all Medicare FFS claims to one calendar year after the date of service.

Corrective Actions

- Providers should identify unprocessed or unpaid patient claims and submit to the payer within the period specified in the contract.
- Reports should be used to track outstanding claims that may have been denied or are not on file with the payer in order to correct and resubmit.

Category: Patient Coverage

This category includes services denied due to exclusions in the patient's insurance plan or the patient was not eligible for benefits on the date services were performed.

Code Type: Claim Adjustment Reason Codes

26	Expenses incurred prior to coverage. *Start: 01/01/1995*
27	Expenses incurred after coverage terminated. *Start: 01/01/1995*
33	Insured has no dependent coverage. *Start: 01/01/1995 | Last Modified: 09/30/2007*
34	Insured has no coverage for newborns. *Start: 01/01/1995 | Last Modified: 09/30/2007*
49	This is a noncovered service because it is a routine/preventive exam or a diagnostic/screening procedure done in conjunction with a routine/preventive exam. Usage: Refer to the 835 Healthcare Policy Identification Segment (loop 2110 Service Payment Information REF), if present. *Start: 01/01/1995 | Last Modified: 07/01/2017*

51	These are non-covered services because this is a pre-existing condition. Usage: Refer to the 835 Healthcare Policy Identification Segment (loop 2110 Service Payment Information REF), if present. *Start: 01/01/1995	Last Modified: 07/01/2017*
96	Non-covered charge(s). At least one Remark Code must be provided (may be comprised of either the NCPDP Reject Reason Code, or Remittance Advice Remark Code that is not an ALERT.) Usage: Refer to the 835 Healthcare Policy Identification Segment (loop 2110 Service Payment Information REF), if present. *Start: 01/01/1995	Last Modified: 07/01/2017*
200	Expenses incurred during lapse in coverage. *Start: 10/31/2006*
B1	Non-covered visits. *Start: 01/01/1995*

Code Type: Remittance Advice Remark Codes

N216	We do not offer coverage for this type of service or the patient is not enrolled in this portion of our benefit package. *Start: 04/01/2004	Last Modified: 03/14/2014* *Notes: (modified 03/01/2010, 03/14/2014)*
N356	Not covered when performed with, or subsequent to, a non-covered service. *Start: 08/01/2005| Last Modified: 03/08/2011* *Notes: (Modified 03/08/2011)*

Code Type: Claim Status Codes

81	Contract/plan does not cover pre-existing conditions. *Start: 01/01/1995*
83	No coverage for newborns. *Start: 01/01/1995*
585	Denied Charge or Non-covered Charge. *Start: 10/31/2004	Last Modified: 07/09/2007*

Many denials result from claims submitted for members who have no coverage on the date of service or who do not have coverage for the services provided. Such denials can be avoided by implementing insurance verification processes.

Insurance plans renew and change throughout the year, not just in January. A patient's employment status can change or the insurance plan may change with the current employer. The patient may not remember to inform the practice of any changes, so it is very important to ask if any changes have occurred and make a copy of any new insurance cards. Be sure to update the patient's account in the practice management software system with any new information prior to submitting any claims.

Many payers have a list of excluded services that are never covered. Again, it is of utmost importance to verify the patient's coverage *before* performing services to ensure payment.

Medicare has established a list of noncovered services. Although a waiver is not needed for these services, it is suggested that providers inform beneficiaries of the likelihood of a claim denial as a courtesy and to prevent future animosity and/or failure for the patient to pay for these services. The patient's EOMB automatically reflects the beneficiary as liable for excluded services; therefore, no modifier is required. Even though it is not required to bill Medicare for services not payable due to statutory exclusion, if the beneficiary requests the provider to do so (e.g., for supplemental insurance purposes), then the claim should be submitted to Medicare.

The following are examples of some of the services that do not require an advance written notice as they are specifically excluded from the limitation of liability provision:

- Cosmetic surgery
- Custodial care
- Dental services
- Personal comfort items
- Routine eye care, most eyeglasses, and examinations
- Hearing aids and hearing examinations
- Routine physical checkups and certain immunizations
- Orthopaedic shoes or other supportive devices for the feet
- Routine foot care and flat foot care
- Investigational devices
- Services required as a result of war
- Physicians' services performed by a physician assistant, midwife, psychologist, or nurse anesthetist, when furnished to an inpatient, unless they are furnished under arrangement with the hospital
- Items and services furnished by the beneficiary's immediate relatives and members of the beneficiary's household

Corrective Actions

- Obtain a current insurance ID card on every visit.
- Verify effective dates of coverage for each member. Benefits cannot be paid for services prior to the patient's effective date.
- It is imperative to always verify benefits prior to rendering services. This can be done by telephone or an online inquiry system.
- Providers should familiarize themselves with NCDs and LCDs.
- A valid Advance Beneficiary Notice (ABN) may be necessary when billing a service that falls under an LCD. An ABN is a written notice that a provider completes and gives to a Medicare patient indicating that the service or procedure that is about to be provided will probably not be paid by Medicare. Since the purpose of the ABN is to inform the Medicare patient *before* the item or service is provided, it is important that the ABN be processed *prior to the service being rendered*. Therefore, clinical staff should be educated regarding coverage guidelines for services commonly performed. Clinical staff should be trained to consider coverage of procedures and, if questionable, then request coverage guidance from administrative staff. Blanket ABNs should not be executed. The ABN must specify the service and a genuine reason that denial by Medicare is expected. ABN standards are not satisfied by generic statements signed by the beneficiary indicating that, should Medicare deny payment for anything, the patient agrees to pay for the service.

General Coding Principles That Influence Payment

This section addresses general coding principles, issues, and policies that should be applied when reporting services or procedures performed. They should also be used as a guide when auditing services and procedures to make sure that they have been adhered to. This principles in this section are strictly enforced by Medicare, but as always other payers tend to follow suit. Examples within the text are often utilized to clarify principles, issues, or policies and do not represent the only codes to which the principles, issues, or policies apply.

Correct Coding Initiative

The Health Insurance Portability and Accountability Act established standard code sets that must be used for reporting procedures and services. The regulation identifies the HCPCS/CPT coding systems as the required code sets. Providers utilize these code sets to report medical services and procedures to most third-party payers.

HCPCS (Healthcare Common Procedure Coding System) consists of Level I CPT (Current Procedural Terminology) codes and Level II codes. CPT codes are defined in the American Medical Association's (AMA) CPT book, which is updated and published annually. HCPCS Level II codes are defined by CMS and are updated throughout the year as necessary. Changes in CPT codes are approved by the AMA CPT Edi7torial Panel, which meets three times per year.

CPT and HCPCS Level II codes define medical and surgical procedures performed on patients. Some procedure codes are very specific defining a single service (e.g., code 93000 Electrocardiogram) while other codes define procedures consisting of many services (e.g., code 58263 Vaginal hysterectomy with removal of tube(s) and/or ovary(s); with repair of enterocele). Because many procedures can be performed by different approaches, different methods, or in combination with other procedures, there are often multiple HCPCS/CPT codes defining similar or related procedures. CPT and HCPCS Level II code descriptors usually do not define all services included in a procedure. There are often services inherent in a procedure or group of procedures. For example, anesthesia services include certain preparation and monitoring services.

CMS developed the NCCI program to prevent inappropriate payment of services. Prior to April 1, 2012, there were two tables, NCCI "Column One/Column Two Correct Coding Edit Table" or the "Mutually Exclusive Edit Table." However, on April 1, 2012, the edits in the "Mutually Exclusive Edit Table" were moved to the "Column One/Column Two Correct Coding Edit Table" to simplify researching NCCI edits. The NCCI table contains edits that are pairs of HCPCS/CPT codes that, in general, should not be reported together. Each edit has a column one and column two HCPCS/CPT code. If a provider reports the two codes of an edit pair, the column two code is denied, and the column one code is eligible for payment. However, if it is clinically appropriate to utilize an NCCI-associated modifier, both the column one and column two codes are eligible for payment.

When the NCCI was established and during its early years, the "Column One/Column Two Correct Coding Edit Table" was termed the "Comprehensive/Component Edit Table." This latter terminology was a misnomer. Although the column two code is often a component of a more comprehensive column one code, this relationship is not true for many edits. In the latter type of edit, the code pair edit simply represents two codes that should not be reported together. For example, a provider should not report a vaginal hysterectomy code and total abdominal hysterectomy code together.

Use of the term "physician" does not restrict the policies to physicians only, but applies to all providers eligible to bill the relevant HCPCS/CPT codes pursuant to applicable portions of the Social Security Act (SSA) of 1965, the Code of Federal Regulations (CFR), and Medicare rules.

Beginning in 2010, the CPT book modified the numbering of codes so that the sequence of codes as they appear in the CPT book does not necessarily correspond to a sequential numbering of codes. In the *National Correct Coding Initiative Policy Manual for Medicare Services,* use of a numerical range of codes reflects all codes that numerically fall within the range regardless of their sequential order in the CPT book.

Coding Based on Standards of Medical/Surgical Practice

Most HCPCS/CPT procedure codes include services that are integral to them. Some of these integral services have specific CPT codes for reporting the service when not performed as an integral part of another procedure. For example, CPT code 36000 Introduction of needle or intracatheter into a vein, is integral to all nuclear medicine procedures requiring injection of a radiopharmaceutical into a vein.

Code 36000 is not reported individually with these types of nuclear medicine procedures. However, code 36000 may be reported alone if the only service provided is the introduction of a needle into a vein. Other integral services do not have specific CPT codes. For example, wound irrigation is integral to the treatment of all wounds and does not have a HCPCS/CPT code. Services integral to HCPCS/CPT procedure codes are included in those procedures based on the standards of medical/surgical practice. It is inappropriate to separately report services that are integral to another procedure with that procedure.

Many NCCI edits are based on the standards of medical/surgical practice. Services that are integral to another service are component parts of the more comprehensive service. When integral component services have their own HCPCS/CPT codes, NCCI edits place the comprehensive service in column one and the component service in column two. Since a component service integral to a comprehensive service is not reported individually, the column two code is not reported individually with the column one code.

Often, services are integral to large numbers of procedures. Other services are integral to a more limited number of procedures. Examples of services integral to a large number of procedures include:

- Cleansing, shaving, and prepping of skin
- Draping and positioning of patient
- Insertion of intravenous access for medication administration
- Insertion of urinary catheter
- Sedative administration by the physician performing a procedure
- Local, topical, or regional anesthesia administered by the physician performing the procedure

- Surgical approach including identification of anatomical landmarks, incision, evaluation of the surgical field, debridement of traumatized tissue, lysis of adhesions, and isolation of structures limiting access to the surgical field such as bone, blood vessels, nerve, and muscles including stimulation for identification or monitoring

- Surgical cultures

- Wound irrigation

- Insertion and removal of drains, suction devices, and pumps into same site

- Surgical closure and dressings

- Application, management, and removal of postoperative dressings and analgesic devices (peri-incisional)

- TENS unit

- Institution of patient controlled anesthesia

- Imaging and/or ultrasound guidance

- Preoperative, intraoperative, and postoperative documentation, including photographs, drawings, dictation, or transcription as necessary to document the services provided

- Surgical supplies, except for specific situations where CMS policy permits separate payment

Note: It is not possible to discuss all NCCI edits based on the principle of the standards of medical/surgical practice because of space limitations. However, there are several general principles that can be applied to the edits as follows:

- The component service is an accepted standard of care when performing the comprehensive service.

- The component service is usually necessary to complete the comprehensive service.

- The component service is not a separately distinguishable procedure when performed with the comprehensive service.

Specific examples of services that are not separately reportable because they are components of more comprehensive services follow.

Medical
- Since interpretation of cardiac rhythm is an integral component of the interpretation of an electrocardiogram, a rhythm strip is not reported separately.

- Since determination of ankle/brachial indices requires both upper and lower extremity Doppler studies, an upper extremity Doppler study is not reported separately.

- Since a cardiac stress test includes multiple electrocardiograms, an electrocardiogram is not reported separately.

Surgical
- Since a myringotomy requires access to the tympanic membrane through the external auditory canal, removal of impacted cerumen from the external auditory canal is not reported separately.

- A "scout" bronchoscopy to assess the surgical field, anatomic landmarks, extent of disease, etc., is not reported individually with an open pulmonary procedure such as a pulmonary lobectomy. By contrast, an initial diagnostic bronchoscopy is reported individually. If the diagnostic bronchoscopy is performed at the same patient encounter as the open pulmonary procedure and does not duplicate an earlier diagnostic bronchoscopy by the same or another physician, the diagnostic bronchoscopy may be reported with modifier 58 appended to the open pulmonary procedure code to indicate a staged procedure. A cursory examination of the upper airway during a bronchoscopy with the bronchoscope should not be reported individually as a laryngoscopy. However, separate endoscopies of anatomically distinct areas with different endoscopes may be reported individually (e.g., thoracoscopy and mediastinoscopy).

- If an endoscopic procedure is performed at the same patient encounter as a non-endoscopic procedure to ensure no intraoperative injury occurred or verify the procedure was performed correctly, the endoscopic procedure is not reported separately with the non-endoscopic procedure.

- Since a colectomy requires exposure of the colon, the laparotomy and adhesiolysis to expose the colon are not reported individually.

Medical/Surgical Package

Most medical and surgical procedures include preprocedure, intraprocedure, and postprocedure work. When multiple procedures are performed at the same patient encounter, there is often overlap of the preprocedure and postprocedure work. Payment methodologies for surgical procedures account for the overlap of the preprocedure and postprocedure work.

The component elements of the preprocedure and postprocedure work for each procedure are included component services of that procedure as a standard of medical/surgical practice.

Some general guidelines follow:

- Many invasive procedures require vascular and/or airway access. The work associated with obtaining the required access is included in the preprocedure or intraprocedure work. The work associated with returning a patient to the appropriate postprocedure state is included in the postprocedure work.

  For example, airway access is necessary for general anesthesia and is not separately reportable. There is no CPT code for elective endotracheal intubation. Code 31500 describes an emergency endotracheal intubation and should not be reported for elective endotracheal intubation.

  Likewise, visualization of the airway is a component part of an endotracheal intubation, and CPT codes describing procedures that visualize the airway (e.g., nasal endoscopy, laryngoscopy, bronchoscopy) should not be reported with an endotracheal intubation. These CPT codes describe diagnostic and therapeutic endoscopies, and it is a misuse of these codes to report visualization of the airway for endotracheal intubation.

- Intravenous access (e.g., codes 36000, 36400, 36410) is not reported separately when performed with many types of procedures (e.g., surgical procedures, anesthesia procedures, radiological procedures requiring intravenous contrast, nuclear medicine procedures requiring intravenous radiopharmaceutical). After vascular access is achieved, the access must be maintained by a slow infusion (e.g., saline) or injection of heparin or saline into a "lock." Since these services are necessary for maintenance of the vascular access, they are not reported individually with the vascular access CPT codes or procedures requiring vascular access as a standard of medical/surgical practice. Codes 37211–37214 Transcatheter therapy, infusion for thrombolysis, should not be reported for use of an anticoagulant to maintain vascular access. The global surgical package includes the administration of fluids and drugs during the operative procedure. Codes 96360–96377 should not be reported individually for that operative procedure.

  When a procedure requires more invasive vascular access services (e.g., central venous access, pulmonary artery access), the more invasive vascular service is reported separately if it is not typical of the procedure and the work of the more invasive vascular service has not been included in the valuation of the procedure. Insertion of a central venous access device (e.g., central venous catheter, pulmonary artery catheter) requires passage of a catheter through central venous vessels and, in the case of a pulmonary artery catheter, through the right atrium and ventricle. These services often require the use of fluoroscopic guidance. Separate reporting of CPT codes for right heart catheterization, selective venous catheterization, or pulmonary artery catheterization is not appropriate when reporting a CPT code for insertion of a central venous access device. Since code 77001 describes fluoroscopic guidance for central venous access device procedures, codes for more general fluoroscopy (e.g., 76000, 77002) should not be reported individually.

- Medicare anesthesia rules prevent separate payment for anesthesia services by the same physician performing a surgical or medical procedure. The physician performing a surgical or medical procedure should not report codes 96360–96377 for the administration of anesthetic agents during the procedure. If it is medically reasonable and necessary that a separate provider (anesthesia practitioner) perform anesthesia services (e.g., monitored anesthesia care) for a surgical or medical procedure, a separate anesthesia service may be reported by the second provider. When anesthesia services are not reported separately, physicians and facilities should not unbundle components of anesthesia and report them in lieu of an anesthesia code.

- If an endoscopic procedure is performed at the same patient encounter as a non-endoscopic procedure to ensure that no intraoperative injury occurred or to verify that the procedure was performed correctly, the endoscopic procedure is not reported separately with the non-endoscopic procedure.

- Many procedures require cardiopulmonary monitoring by the physician performing the procedure or an anesthesia practitioner. Since these services are integral to the procedure, they are not separately reportable. Examples of these services include cardiac monitoring, pulse oximetry, and ventilation management (e.g., 93000–93010, 93040–93042, 94760, 94761).

- A biopsy performed at the time of another more extensive procedure (e.g., excision, destruction, removal) is separately reportable under specific circumstances. If the biopsy is performed on a separate lesion, it is separately reportable. This situation may be reported with anatomic modifiers or modifier 59 or XS. If the biopsy is performed on the same lesion on which a more extensive procedure is performed, it is separately reportable only if the biopsy is utilized for immediate pathologic diagnosis prior to the more extensive procedure, and the decision to proceed with the more extensive procedure is based on the diagnosis established by the pathologic examination. The biopsy is not separately reportable if the pathologic examination at the time of surgery is for the purpose of assessing margins of resection or verifying resectability. When separately reportable, modifier 58 may be reported to indicate that the biopsy and the more extensive procedure were planned or staged procedures.

  If a biopsy is performed and submitted for pathologic evaluation that will be completed after the more extensive procedure is performed, the biopsy is not separately reportable with the more extensive procedure. If a single lesion is biopsied multiple times, only one biopsy code may be reported with a single unit of service. If multiple lesions are non-endoscopically biopsied, a biopsy code may be reported for each lesion appending a modifier indicating that each biopsy was performed on a separate lesion.

  For endoscopic biopsies, multiple biopsies of a single or multiple lesions are reported with one unit of service of the biopsy code. If it is medically reasonable and necessary to submit multiple biopsies of the same or different lesions for separate pathologic examination, the medical record must identify the precise location and separate nature of each biopsy.

- Exposure and exploration of the surgical field is integral to an operative procedure and is not reported separately. For example, an exploratory laparotomy (code 49000) is not reported separately with an intra-abdominal procedure. If exploration of the surgical field results in additional procedures other than the primary procedure, the additional procedures may generally be reported individually. However, a procedure designated by the CPT code descriptor as a "separate procedure" is not reported separately if performed in a region anatomically related to the other procedure(s) through the same skin incision, orifice, or surgical approach.

- If a definitive surgical procedure requires access through diseased tissue (e.g., necrotic skin, abscess, hematoma, seroma), a separate service for this access (e.g., debridement, incision and drainage) is not reported separately. Types of procedures to which this principle applies include, but are not limited to, -ectomy, -otomy, excision, resection, -plasty, insertion, revision, replacement, relocation, removal, and closure. For example, debridement of skin and subcutaneous tissue at the site of an abdominal incision made to perform an intraabdominal procedure to repair a fracture is not reported separately.

- If removal, destruction, or other form of elimination of a lesion requires coincidental elimination of other pathology, only the primary procedure may be reported. For example, if an area of pilonidal disease contains an abscess, incision and drainage of the abscess during the procedure to excise the area of pilonidal disease is not reported separately.

- An excision and removal (-ectomy) includes the incision and opening (-otomy) of the organ. A HCPCS/CPT code for anatomy procedure should not be reported with an -ectomy code for the same organ.

- Multiple approaches to the same procedure are mutually exclusive of one another and should not be reported individually. For example, both a vaginal hysterectomy and abdominal hysterectomy should not be reported individually.

- If a procedure utilizing one approach fails and is converted to a procedure utilizing a different approach, only the completed procedure may be reported. For example, if a laparoscopic hysterectomy is converted to an open hysterectomy, only the open hysterectomy procedure code may be reported.

- If a laparoscopic procedure fails and is converted to an open procedure, the physician should not report a diagnostic laparoscopy in lieu of the failed laparoscopic procedure. For example, if a laparoscopic cholecystectomy is converted to an open cholecystectomy, the physician should not report the failed laparoscopic cholecystectomy or a diagnostic laparoscopy.

- If a diagnostic endoscopy is the basis for and precedes an open procedure, the diagnostic endoscopy may be reported with modifier 58 appended to the open procedure code. However, the medical record must document the medical reasonableness and necessity for the diagnostic endoscopy. A scout endoscopy to assess anatomic landmarks and extent of disease is not reported separately with an open procedure. When an endoscopic procedure fails and is converted to another surgical procedure, only the completed surgical procedure may be reported. The endoscopic procedure is not reported separately with the completed surgical procedure.

- Treatment of complications of primary surgical procedures is separately reportable with some limitations. The global surgical package for an operative procedure includes all intraoperative services that are normally a usual and necessary part of the procedure. Additionally, the global surgical package includes all medical and surgical services required of the surgeon during the postoperative period of the surgery to treat complications that do not require return to the operating room. Thus, treatment of a complication of a primary surgical procedure is not separately reportable if: 1) it represents usual and necessary care in the operating room during the procedure or 2) it occurs postoperatively and does not require return to the operating room. For example, control of hemorrhage is a usual and necessary component of a surgical procedure in the operating room and is not separately reportable. Control of postoperative hemorrhage is also not separately reportable unless the patient must be returned to the operating room for treatment. In the latter case, the control of hemorrhage may be reported individually with modifier 78.

Evaluation and Management Services

Medicare global surgery rules define the rules for reporting E/M services with procedures covered by these rules. This section summarizes some of the rules. All procedures on the Medicare Physician Fee Schedule are assigned a global period of 000, 010, 090, MMM, XXX, YYY, or ZZZ. The global concept does not apply to XXX procedures. The global period for YYY procedures is defined by the Medicare contractor. All procedures with a global period of ZZZ are related to another procedure, and the applicable global period for the ZZZ code is determined by the related procedure. Procedures with a global period of MMM are maternity procedures.

Since NCCI edits are applied to same day services by the same provider to the same beneficiary, certain global surgery rules are applicable to NCCI. An E/M service is separately reportable on the same date of service as a procedure with a global period of 000, 010, or 090 under limited circumstances.

If a procedure has a global period of 090 days, it is defined as a major surgical procedure. If an E/M service is performed on the same date of service as a major surgical procedure for the purpose of deciding whether to perform this surgical procedure, the E/M service is separately reportable with modifier 57. Other preoperative E/M services on the same date of service as a major surgical procedure are included in the global payment for the procedure and are not reported individually. NCCI does not contain edits based on this rule because Medicare contractors have separate edits for this rule.

If a procedure has a global period of 000 or 010 days, it is defined as a minor surgical procedure. In general, E/M services on the same date of service as the minor surgical procedure are included in the payment for the procedure. The decision to perform a minor surgical procedure is included in the payment for the minor surgical procedure and should not be reported separately as an E/M service. However, a significant and separately identifiable E/M service unrelated to the decision to perform the minor surgical procedure is separately reportable with modifier 25. The E/M service and minor surgical procedure do not require different diagnoses. If a minor surgical procedure is performed on a new patient, the same rules for reporting E/M services apply. The fact that the patient is "new" to the provider is not sufficient alone to justify reporting an E/M service on the same date of service as a minor surgical procedure.

NCCI does contain some edits based on these principles, but the Medicare contractors have separate edits. Neither the NCCI nor Medicare contractors have all possible edits based on these principles.

Example
If a physician determines that a new patient with head trauma requires sutures, confirms the allergy and immunization status, obtains informed consent, and performs the repair, an E/M service is not separately reportable. However, if the physician also performs a medically reasonable and necessary full neurological examination, an E/M service may be reported separately.

For major and minor surgical procedures, postoperative E/M services related to recovery from the surgical procedure during the postoperative period are included in the global surgery package as are E/M services related to complications of the surgery that do not require additional trips to the operating room. Postoperative visits unrelated to the diagnosis for which the surgical procedure was performed unless related to a complication of surgery may be reported separately on the same day as a surgical procedure with modifier 24 Unrelated Evaluation and Management Service by the Same Physician or Other Qualified Health Care Professional During a Postoperative Period.

Procedures with a global surgery indicator of "XXX" are not covered by these rules. Many of these "XXX" procedures are performed by physicians and have inherent preprocedure, intraprocedure, and postprocedure work usually performed each time the procedure is completed. This work should never be reported as a separate E/M code.

Other "XXX" procedures are not usually performed by a physician and have no physician work relative value units associated with them. A physician should never report a separate E/M code with these procedures for the supervision of others performing the procedure or for the interpretation of the procedure.

With most "XXX" procedures, the physician may, however, perform a significant and separately identifiable E/M service on the same date of service, which may be reported by appending modifier 25 to the E/M code. This E/M service may be related to the same diagnosis necessitating performance of the "XXX" procedure but cannot include any work inherent in the "XXX" procedure, supervision of others performing the "XXX" procedure, or time for interpreting the result of the "XXX" procedure. Appending modifier 25 to a significant, separately identifiable E/M service when performed on the same date of service as an "XXX" procedure is correct coding.

Modifiers and Modifier Indicators
NCCI edits also affect modifiers. Please see a detailed explanation in chapter 3.

Standard Preparation/Monitoring Services for Anesthesia
With few exceptions, anesthesia HCPCS/CPT codes do not specify the mode of anesthesia for a particular procedure. Regardless of the mode of anesthesia, preparation and monitoring services are not separately reportable with anesthesia service HCPCS/CPT codes when performed in association with the anesthesia service. However, if the provider of the anesthesia service performs one or more of these services prior to and unrelated to the anticipated anesthesia service or after the patient is released from the anesthesia practitioner's postoperative care, the service may be separately reportable with modifier 59 or -X{EU}.

Anesthesia Service Included in the Surgical Procedure
Under the CMS Anesthesia Rules, with limited exceptions, Medicare does not allow separate payment for anesthesia services performed by the physician who also furnishes the medical or surgical service. In this case, payment for the anesthesia service is included in the payment for the medical or surgical procedure. For example, separate payment is not allowed for the physician's performance of local, regional, or most other anesthesia including nerve blocks if the physician also performs the medical or surgical procedure. However, Medicare allows separate reporting for moderate conscious sedation services (codes 99151–99153) when provided by the same physician performing a medical or surgical procedure except for those procedures listed in appendix G of the CPT book. CPT codes describing anesthesia services (00100–01999) or services that are bundled into anesthesia should not be reported in addition to the surgical or medical procedure requiring the anesthesia services if performed by the same physician. Examples of improperly reported services that are bundled into the anesthesia service when anesthesia is provided by the physician performing the medical or surgical procedure include introduction of needle or intracatheter into a vein (code 36000), venipuncture (code 36410), intravenous infusion/injection (codes 96360–96368, 96374–96377), or cardiac assessment (e.g., codes 93000–93010, 93040–93042).

However, if these services are not related to the delivery of an anesthetic agent, or are not an inherent component of the procedure or global service, they may be reported individually.

The physician performing a surgical or medical procedure should not report an epidural/subarachnoid injection (codes 62320–62327) or nerve block (codes 64400–64530) for anesthesia for that procedure.

HCPCS/CPT Procedure Code Definition

The HCPCS/CPT code descriptors of two codes are often the basis of an NCCI edit. If two HCPCS/CPT codes describe redundant services, they should not be reported individually. Several general principles follow:

- A family of CPT codes may include a code followed by one or more indented codes. The first CPT code descriptor includes a semicolon. The portion of the descriptor of the first code in the family preceding the semicolon is a common part of the descriptor for each subsequent code of the family.

  For example, code 70120 Radiologic examination, mastoids; less than three views per side, and code 70130 complete, minimum of three views per side. The portion of the descriptor preceding the semicolon ("Radiologic examination, mastoids") is common to both codes 70120 and 70130. The difference between the two codes is the portion of the descriptors following the semicolon. Often, as in this case, two codes from a family may not be reported individually. A physician cannot report codes 70120 and 70130 for a procedure performed on ipsilateral mastoids at the same patient encounter.

  It is important to recognize, however, that there are numerous circumstances when it may be appropriate to report more than one code from a family of codes. For example, codes 70120 and 70130 may be reported individually if the two procedures are performed on contralateral mastoids or at two separate patient encounters on the same date of service.

- If a HCPCS/CPT code is reported, it includes all components of the procedure defined by the descriptor. For example, code 58291 includes a vaginal hysterectomy with "removal of tube(s) and/or ovary(s)." A physician cannot report a salpingooophorectomy (code 58720) separately with code 58291.

- CPT code descriptors often define correct coding relationships where two codes may not be reported individually with one another at the same anatomic site and/or same patient encounter. A few examples follow:

  - a "partial" procedure is not separately reportable with a "complete" procedure
  - a "partial" procedure is not separately reportable with a "total" procedure
  - a "unilateral" procedure is not separately reportable with a "bilateral" procedure
  - a "single" procedure is not separately reportable with a "multiple" procedure
  - a "with" procedure is not separately reportable with a "without" procedure
  - an "initial" procedure is not separately reportable with a "subsequent" procedure

CPT Book and CMS Coding Manual Instructions

CMS often publishes coding instructions in its rules, manuals, and notices. Physicians must utilize these instructions when reporting services rendered to Medicare patients. The CPT book also includes coding instructions in the introduction, individual chapters, and appendices. In individual chapters, the instructions may appear at the beginning of a chapter, at the beginning of a subsection of the chapter, or after specific CPT codes. Physicians should follow CPT book instructions unless CMS has provided different coding or reporting instructions. The American Medical Association publishes *CPT Assistant,* which contains coding guidelines. CMS does not review nor approve the information in this publication. In the development of NCCI edits, CMS occasionally disagrees with the information in this publication. If a physician utilizes information from *CPT Assistant* to report services rendered to Medicare patients, it is possible that Medicare contractors may utilize different criteria to process claims.

CPT Separate Procedure Definition

If a CPT code descriptor includes the term "separate procedure," the CPT code may not be reported individually with a related procedure. CMS interprets this designation to prohibit the reporting of a separate procedure when performed with another procedure in an anatomically related region often through the same skin incision, orifice, or surgical approach. A CPT code with the separate procedure designation may be reported with another procedure if it is performed at a separate patient encounter on the same date of service or at the same patient encounter in an anatomically unrelated area often through a separate skin incision, orifice, or surgical approach. Modifier 59 or -X{ES}, (or a more specific modifier, e.g., anatomic modifier) may be appended to the separate procedure CPT code to indicate that it qualifies as a separately reportable service.

Family of Codes

The CPT book often contains a group of codes that describe related procedures that may be performed in various combinations. Some codes describe limited component services, and other codes describe various combinations of component services. Physicians must utilize several principles in selecting the correct code to report:

- A HCPCS/CPT code may be reported if and only if all services described by the code are performed.

- The HCPCS/CPT code describing the services performed should be reported. A physician should not report multiple codes corresponding to component services if a single comprehensive code describes the services performed. There are limited exceptions to this rule that are specifically identified in the NCCI manual.

- HCPCS/CPT codes corresponding to component services of other more comprehensive HCPCS/CPT codes should not be reported individually with the more comprehensive HCPCS/CPT codes that include the component services.

- If the HCPCS/CPT codes do not correctly describe the procedure performed, the physician should report a "not otherwise specified" CPT code rather than a HCPCS/CPT code that most closely describes the procedure performed.

More Extensive Procedure

The CPT book often describes groups of similar codes differing in the complexity of the service. Unless services are performed at separate patient encounters or at separate anatomic sites, the less complex service is included in the more complex service and is not separately reportable.

Several examples of this principle follow:

- If two procedures only differ in that one is described as a "simple" procedure and the other as a "complex" procedure, the "simple" procedure is included in the "complex" procedure and is not reported separately unless the two procedures are performed at separate patient encounters or at separate anatomic sites.

- If two procedures only differ in that one is described as a "simple" procedure and the other as a "complicated" procedure, the "simple" procedure is included in the "complicated" procedure and is not reported separately unless the two procedures are performed at separate patient encounters or at separate anatomic sites.

- If two procedures only differ in that one is described as a "limited" procedure and the other as a "complete" procedure, the "limited" procedure is included in the "complete" procedure and is not reported separately unless the two procedures are performed at separate patient encounters or at separate anatomic sites.

- If two procedures only differ in that one is described as an "intermediate" procedure and the other as a "comprehensive" procedure, the "intermediate" procedure is included in the "comprehensive" procedure and is not reported separately unless the two procedures are performed at separate patient encounters or at separate anatomic sites.

- If two procedures only differ in that one is described as a "superficial" procedure and the other as a "deep" procedure, the "superficial" procedure is included in the "deep" procedure and is not reported separately unless the two procedures are performed at separate patient encounters or at separate anatomic sites.

- If two procedures only differ in that one is described as an "incomplete" procedure and the other as a "complete" procedure, the "incomplete" procedure is included in the "complete" procedure and is not reported separately unless the two procedures are performed at separate patient encounters or at separate anatomic sites.

- If two procedures only differ in that one is described as an "external" procedure and the other as an "internal" procedure, the "external" procedure is included in the "internal" procedure and is not reported separately unless the two procedures are performed at separate patient encounters or at separate anatomic sites.

Sequential Procedure

Some surgical procedures may be performed by different surgical approaches. If an initial surgical approach to a procedure fails and a second surgical approach is utilized at the same patient encounter, only the HCPCS/CPT code corresponding to the second surgical approach may be reported. If there are different HCPCS/CPT codes for the two different surgical approaches, the two procedures are considered "sequential," and only the HCPCS/CPT code corresponding to the second surgical approach may be reported. For example, a physician may begin a cholecystectomy procedure utilizing a laparoscopic approach and have to convert the procedure to an open abdominal approach. Only the CPT code for the open cholecystectomy may be reported. The CPT code for the failed laparoscopic cholecystectomy is not reported separately.

Laboratory Panel

The CPT book defines organ and disease specific panels of laboratory tests. If a laboratory performs all tests included in one of these panels, the laboratory may report the CPT code for the panel or the CPT codes for the individual tests. If the laboratory repeats one of these component tests as a medically reasonable and necessary service on the same date of service, the CPT code corresponding to the repeat laboratory test may be reported with modifier 91 appended.

Misuse of Column Two Code with Column One Code

CMS manuals and instructions often describe groups of HCPCS/CPT codes that should not be reported together for the Medicare program. Edits based on these instructions are often included as a misuse of a column two code with a column one code. A HCPCS/CPT code descriptor does not include exhaustive information about the code. Physicians who are not familiar with a HCPCS/CPT code may incorrectly report the code in a context different than intended. The NCCI has identified HCPCS/CPT codes that are incorrectly reported with other HCPCS/CPT codes as a result of the misuse of the column two code with the column one code. If these edits allow use of NCCI-associated modifiers (modifier indicator of "1"), there are limited circumstances when the column two code may be reported on the same date of service as the column one code. Two examples follow:

- Three or more HCPCS/CPT codes may be reported on the same date of service. Although the column two code is misused if reported as a service associated with the column one code, the column two code may be appropriately reported with a third HCPCS/CPT code reported on the same date of service. For example, CMS limits separate payment for use of the operating microscope for microsurgical techniques (CPT code 69990) to a group of procedures listed in the online *Claims Processing Manual* (Chapter 12, Section 20.4.5 [Allowable Adjustments]). The NCCI has edits with column one codes of surgical procedures not listed in this section of the manual and column two code of 69990. Some of these edits allow use of NCCI-associated modifiers because the two services listed in the edit may be performed at the same patient encounter as a third procedure for which code 69990 is reported separately.

- There may be limited circumstances when the column two code is separately reportable with the column one code. For example, the NCCI has an edit with column one code of 80061 (lipid profile) and column two code of 83721 (LDL cholesterol by direct measurement). If the triglyceride level is less than 400 mg/dl, the LDL is a calculated value utilizing the results from the lipid profile for the calculation, and code 83721 is not separately reportable. However, if the triglyceride level is greater than 400 mg/dl, the LDL may be measured directly and may be reported separately with code 83721 utilizing an NCCI-associated modifier to bypass the edit.

Misuse of a code as an edit rationale may be applied to procedure-to-procedure edits where the column two code is not reported separately with the column one code based on the nature of the column one procedure. This edit rationale may also be applied to code pairs where use of the column two code with the column one code is deemed to be a coding error.

Mutually Exclusive Procedures

Many procedure codes cannot be reported together because they are mutually exclusive of each other. Mutually exclusive procedures cannot reasonably be performed at the same anatomic site or same patient encounter. An example of a mutually exclusive situation is the repair of an organ that can be performed by two different methods. Only one method can be chosen to repair the organ.

A second example is a service that can be reported as an "initial" service or a "subsequent" service. With the exception of drug administration services, the initial service and subsequent service cannot be reported at the same patient encounter.

Gender-Specific Procedures

The descriptor of some HCPCS/CPT codes includes a gender-specific restriction on the use of the code. HCPCS/CPT codes specific for one gender should not be reported with HCPCS/CPT codes for the opposite gender. For example, CPT code 53210 describes a total urethrectomy including cystostomy in a female, and CPT code 53215 describes the same procedure in a male. Since the patient cannot have both the male and female procedures performed, the two CPT codes cannot be reported together. Edits based on this principle are included in the mutually exclusive edit table since the two procedures of a code pair edit cannot be performed on the same patient.

Add-on Codes

Certain codes in the CPT book are identified as "add-on" codes. These codes describe a service or procedure that can be reported only in addition to a primary (usually more comprehensive) procedure. CPT book instructions indicate the primary procedure code(s) related to most add-on codes; however, in some instances the primary procedure code(s) is (are) not specified. When the CPT book identifies a specific primary code, the add-on code should not be reported as an additional service for other HCPCS/CPT codes not identified as a primary code.

Add-on codes permit the reporting of significant supplemental services commonly performed during the same encounter as the primary procedure. Add-on procedures should not be confused with incidental services that are required to accomplish the primary procedure (e.g., lysis of adhesions in the course of an open cholecystectomy). Incidental services and procedures are not reported separately. Similarly, complications inherent in an invasive procedure such as the control of bleeding occurring during the procedure are not reported separately.

In general, NCCI procedure-to-procedure edits do not include edits with most add-on codes because edits related to the primary procedure(s) apply. However, NCCI does contain additional edits for selected add-on codes when coding edits related to the primary procedures must be augmented. Examples include edits with add-on HCPCS/CPT codes 69990 (Microsurgical techniques requiring use of operating microscope) and 95940/95941/G0453.

HCPCS/CPT codes that are not designated as add-on codes should not be misused as an add-on code to report a supplemental service. A HCPCS/CPT code may be reported if and only if all services described by the CPT code are performed. A HCPCS/CPT code should not be reported with another service because a portion of the service described by the HCPCS/CPT code was performed with the other procedure. For example, if an ejection fraction is estimated from an echocardiogram study, it would be inappropriate to additionally report code 78472 Cardiac blood pool imaging with ejection fraction with the echocardiography (code 93307). Although the procedure described by code 78472 includes an ejection fraction, it is measured by gated equilibrium with a radionuclide that is not utilized in echocardiography.

Excluded Service
The NCCI does not address issues related to HCPCS/CPT codes describing services that are excluded from Medicare coverage or are not otherwise recognized for payment under the Medicare program.

Unlisted Procedure Codes
The CPT book includes codes to identify services or procedures not described by other HCPCS/CPT codes. These unlisted procedure codes are identified as XXX99 or XXXX9 codes and are located at the end of each section or subsection of the manual. If a physician provides a service that is not accurately described by other HCPCS/CPT codes, the service should be reported utilizing an unlisted procedure code. A physician should not report a CPT code for a specific procedure if it does not accurately describe the service performed. It is inappropriate to report the best fit HCPCS/CPT code unless it accurately describes the service performed, and all components of the HCPCS/CPT code were performed. Since unlisted procedure codes may be reported for a very diverse group of services, the NCCI generally does not include edits with these codes.

Modified, Deleted, and Added Code Pairs/Edits
NCCI edits are adopted after due consideration of Medicare policies including the principles described in the *National Correct Coding Initiative Policy Manual for Medicare Services,* HCPCS and CPT code descriptors, CPT book coding guidelines, coding guidelines of national societies, standards of medical and surgical practice, current coding practice, and provider billing patterns. Since the NCCI is developed by CMS for the Medicare program, the most important consideration is CMS policy. Prior to initial implementation of the NCCI in 1996, the proposed edits were evaluated by Medicare Part B Carrier Medical Directors, representatives of the American Medical Association's CPT Advisory Committee, and representatives of other national medical and surgical societies.

The NCCI undergoes continuous refinement with revised edit tables published quarterly. There is a process to address annual changes (additions, deletions, and modifications) of HCPCS/CPT codes and CPT book coding guidelines. Other sources of refinement are initiatives by the CMS central office and comments from the CMS regional offices, AMA, national medical, surgical, and other health care societies/organizations and Medicare contractor medical directors, providers, consultants, other third-party payers, and other interested parties. Prior to implementing new edits, CMS generally provides a review and comment period to representative national organizations that may be impacted by the edits. However, there are situations when CMS thinks that it is prudent to implement edits prior to completion of the review and comment period. CMS Central Office evaluates the input from all sources and decides which edits are modified, deleted, or added each quarter.

Medically Unlikely Edits
To lower the error rate for Medicare fee-for-service paid claims, CMS established units of service edits referred to as medically unlikely edits (MUE). An MUE is defined as an edit that tests individual claim lines for the same beneficiary,

HCPCS code, date of service, and billing provider against a criteria number of units of service.

An MUE for a HCPCS/CPT code is the maximum number of units of service (UOS) under most circumstances allowable by the same provider for the same beneficiary on the same date of service. The ideal MUE value for a HCPCS/CPT code is the unit of service that allows the vast majority of appropriately coded claims to pass the MUE.

On April 1, 2013, CMS introduced date of service (DOS) MUEs. If the MUE is adjudicated as a claim line edit, the units of service (UOS) on each claim line are compared to the MUE value for the HCPCS/CPT code on that claim line. If the UOS exceed the MUE value, all UOS on that claim line are denied. If the MUE is adjudicated as a DOS MUE, all UOS on each claim line for the same date of service for the same HCPCS/CPT code are summed, and the sum is compared to the MUE value. If the summed UOS exceeds the MUE value, all UOS for the HCPCS/CPT code for that date of service are denied. Denials due to claim line MUEs or DOS MUEs may be appealed to the local claims processing contractor. DOS MUEs are utilized for HCPCS/CPT codes where it would be extremely unlikely that more UOS than the MUE value would ever be performed on the same date of service for the same patient. Over time CMS will convert many, but not all, MUEs to DOS MUEs. Since April 1, 2013, MUEs are adjudicated as claim line edits or DOS edits. The MUE files on the CMS NCCI website display an "MUE Adjudication Indicator" (MAI) for each HCPCS/CPT code.

There are three MUE adjudicator indicator types:

MAI	Type
1	Line Edit
2	Date of Service Edit, Policy
3	Date of Service, Clinical

The MUE also indicates a rationale for the edit. An example of the MUE table is shown below.

HCPCS/CPT Code	Practitioner Services MUE Values	MUE Adjudication Indicator	MUE Rationale
11641	2	3 Date of Service Edit: Clinical	Clinical: Data
11642	3	3 Date of Service Edit: Clinical	Clinical: Data
11643	2	3 Date of Service Edit: Clinical	Clinical: Data
11644	2	3 Date of Service Edit: Clinical	Clinical: Data
11646	2	3 Date of Service Edit: Clinical	Clinical: Data
11719	1	2 Date of Service Edit: Policy	Anatomic Consideration
11720	1	2 Date of Service Edit: Policy	Anatomic Consideration
11721	1	2 Date of Service Edit: Policy	Anatomic Consideration
11730	1	2 Date of Service Edit: Policy	Anatomic Consideration
11732	4	3 Date of Service Edit: Clinical	Clinical: Data

Both the MAI and MUE values for each HCPCS/CPT code are based on one or more of the following considerations:

- Anatomic considerations may limit units of service based on anatomic structures. For example:
  - The MUE value for an appendectomy is "1" since there is only one appendix.
  - The MUE for a knee brace is "2" because there are two knees and Medicare policy does not cover back-up equipment.
  - The MUE value for a lumbar spine procedure reported per lumbar vertebra or per lumbar interspace cannot exceed "5" since there are only five lumbar vertebrae or interspaces.
  - The MUE value for a procedure reported per lung lobe cannot exceed "5" since there are only five lung lobes (three in right lung and two in left lung).
- CPT code descriptors/CPT coding instructions in the CPT book may limit units of service. For example:
  - A procedure described as the "initial 30 minutes" would have an MUE value of "1" because of the use of the term "initial." A different code may be reported for additional time.
  - If a code descriptor uses the plural form of the procedure, it must not be reported with multiple units of service. For example, if the code descriptor states "biopsies," the code is reported with "1" unit of service regardless of the number of biopsies performed.
  - The MUE value for a procedure with "per day," "per week," or "per month" in its code descriptor is "1" because MUEs are based on number of services per day of service.
  - The MUE value of a code for a procedure described as "unilateral" is "1" if there is a different code for the procedure described as "bilateral."
  - The code descriptors of a family of codes may define different levels of service, each having an MUE of "1." For example, CPT codes 78102–78104 describe bone marrow imaging. CPT code 78102 is reported for imaging a "limited area," CPT code 78103 is reported for imaging "multiple areas." CPT code 78104 is reported for imaging the "whole body."
  - The MUE value for CPT code 86021 Antibody identification; leukocyte antibodies, is "1" because the code descriptor is plural including testing for any and all leukocyte antibodies. On a single date of service only one specimen from a patient would be tested for leukocyte antibodies.
- Edits based on established CMS policies may limit units of service (UOS). For example:
  - The MUE value for a surgical or diagnostic procedure may be based on the bilateral surgery indicator on the Medicare Physician Fee Schedule Database (MPFSDB).
    - If the bilateral surgery indicator is "0," a bilateral procedure must be reported with "1" unit of service (UOS). There is no additional payment for the code if reported as a unilateral or bilateral procedure because of anatomy or physiology. Alternatively, the code descriptor may specifically state that the procedure is a

© 2020 Optum360, LLC

unilateral procedure, and there is a separate code for a bilateral procedure.

- If the bilateral surgery indicator is "1," a bilateral surgical procedure must be reported with "1" UOS and modifier 50 Bilateral Procedure. A bilateral diagnostic procedure may be reported with "2" UOS on one claim line, "1" UOS and modifier 50 on one claim line, or "1" UOS with modifier RT on one claim line plus "1" UOS and modifier LT on a second claim line.

- If the bilateral surgery indicator is "2," a bilateral procedure must be reported with "1" UOS. The procedure is priced as a bilateral procedure because (1) the code descriptor defines the procedure as bilateral; (2) the code descriptor states that the procedure is performed unilaterally or bilaterally; or (3) the procedure is usually performed as a bilateral procedure.

- If the bilateral surgery indicator is "3," a bilateral surgical procedure must be reported with "1" UOS and modifier 50 Bilateral Procedure. A bilateral diagnostic procedure may be reported with "2" UOS on one claim line, "1" UOS and modifier 50 on one claim line, or 1 UOS with modifier RT on one claim line plus "1" UOS and modifier LT on a second claim line.

– The MUE value for a code may be "1" where the code descriptor does not specify a UOS and CMS considers the default UOS to be "per day."

– The MUE value for a code may be "0" because the code is listed as invalid, not covered, bundled, not separately payable, statutorily excluded, not reasonable and necessary, etc. based on:

- The Medicare Physician Fee Schedule Database
- Outpatient Prospective Payment System Addendum B
- Alpha-Numeric HCPCS Code File
- DMEPOS Jurisdiction List
- Medicare Internet-Only Manual

• The nature of an analyte may limit units of service and is, in general, determined by one of two considerations:

– The nature of the specimen may limit the units of service. For example, CPT code 82575 describes a creatinine clearance test and has an MUE of "1" because the test requires a 24-hour urine collection, OR

– The physiology, pathophysiology, or clinical application of the analyte is such that a maximum unit of service for a single date of service can be determined. For example, the MUE for CPT code 82747 Folic acid; RBC, is "1" because the test result would not be expected to change during a single day, and thus it is not necessary to perform the test more than once on a single date of service.

• The nature of a procedure/service may limit units of service and is, in general, determined by the amount of time required to perform a procedure/service (e.g., overnight sleep studies) or clinical application of a procedure/service (e.g., motion analysis tests).

– The MUE for many surgical or medical procedures is "1" because the procedure is rarely, if ever, performed more than one time per day (e.g., colonoscopy, motion analysis tests).

– The MUE value for a procedure is "1" because of the amount of time required to perform the procedure (e.g., overnight sleep study).

- The nature of equipment may limit units of service and is, in general, determined by the number of items of equipment that would be utilized. For example, the MUE value for a wheelchair code is "1" because only one wheelchair is used at one time, and Medicare policy does not cover back-up equipment.

- Although clinical judgment considerations and determinations based on input from numerous physicians and certified coders are sometimes initially utilized to establish some MUE values, these values are subsequently validated or changed based on submitted and/or paid claims data.

- Prescribing information is based on FDA labeling as well as off-label information published in CMS-approved drug compendia. See below for additional information about how prescribing information is utilized in determining MUE values.

- Submitted and paid claims data (100%) from a six-month period is utilized to ascertain the distribution pattern of UOS typically reported for a given HCPCS/CPT code.

- Published policies of the Durable Medical Equipment (DME) Medicare Administrative Contractors (MACs) may limit units of service for some durable medical equipment, prosthetics, orthotics, and supplies (DMEPOS). For example:

  - The MUE values for many ostomy and urological supply codes, nebulizer codes, and CPAP accessory codes are typically based on a three-month supply of items.

  - The MUE values for surgical dressings, parenteral and enteral nutrition, immunosuppressive drugs, and oral anti-cancer drugs are typically based on a one month supply.

  - The MUE values take into account the requirement for reporting certain codes with date spans.

  - The MUE value of a code may be "0" if the item is noncovered, not medically necessary, or not separately payable.

  - The MUE value of a code may be "0" if the code is invalid for claim submission to the DME MAC.

HCPCS J code and drug related C and Q code MUEs are based on prescribing information and 100 percent claims data for a six month period of time. Utilizing the prescribing information, the highest total daily dose for each drug is determined. This dose and its corresponding units of service are evaluated against paid and submitted claims data. Some of the guiding principles utilized in developing these edits are as follows:

- If the prescribing information defined a maximum daily dose, this value is used to determine the MUE value. For some drugs there is an absolute maximum daily dose. For others there is a maximum "recommended" or "usual" dose. In the latter two cases, the daily dose calculation is evaluated against claims data.

- If the maximum daily dose calculation is based on actual body weight, a dose based on a weight range of 110-150 kg is evaluated against the claims data. If the maximum daily dose calculation is based on ideal body weight, a dose based on a weight range of 90-110 kg is evaluated against claims data. If the maximum daily dose calculation is based on body surface area (BSA), a dose based on a BSA range of 2.4-3.0 square meters is evaluated against claims data.

- For "as needed" (PRN) drugs and drugs where maximum daily dose is based on patient response, prescribing information and claims data are utilized to establish MUE values.

- Published off label usage of a drug is considered for the maximum daily dose calculation.

- The MUE values for some drug codes are set to 0. The rationale for such values include but are not limited to discontinued manufacture of drug, non-FDA-approved compounded drug, practitioner MUE values for oral antineoplastic, oral antiemetic, and oral immune suppressive drugs that should be billed to the DME MACs, and outpatient hospital MUE values for inhalation drugs that should be billed to the DME MACs, MACs, and practitioner/ASC MUE values for HCPCS C codes describing medications that would not be related to a procedure performed in an ASC.

The MUE files on the CMS NCCI website display an "Edit Rationale" for each HCPCS/CPT code. Although an MUE may be based on several rationales, only one is displayed on the website. One of the listed rationales is "Data." This rationale indicates that 100 percent of claims data from a six-month period of time was the major factor in determining the MUE value. If a physician appeals an MUE denial for a HCPCS/CPT code where the MUE is based on "Data," the reviewer usually confirms that (1) the correct code is reported; (2) the correct UOS is utilized; (3) the number of reported UOS were performed; and (4) all UOS were medically reasonable and necessary.

Some contractors allow providers to report repetitive services performed over a range of dates on a single line of a claim with multiple units of service. If a provider reports services in this fashion, the provider should report the "from date" and "to date" on the claim line. Contractors are instructed to divide the units of service reported on the claim line by the number of days in the date span and round to the nearest whole number. This number is compared to the MUE value for the code on the claim line.

A denial of services due to an MUE is a coding denial, not a medical necessity denial. A provider/supplier may not issue an advanced beneficiary notice (ABN) of noncoverage in connection with services denied due to an MUE and cannot bill the beneficiary for units of service denied based on an MUE. Most MUE values are set so that a provider or supplier would only very occasionally have a claim line denied or a claim returned to the provider. If a provider encounters code with frequent denials due to the MUE, frequent returns to the provi'' due to the MUE, or frequent use of a CPT modifier to bypass the M'' provider or supplier should consider the following:

- Is the HCPCS/CPT code being used correctly?

- Is the unit of service being counted correctly?

- Are all reported services medically reasor

- Why does the provider's or supplier's pract. patterns?

A provider or supplier may choose to discuss these ques Medicare contractor or a national health care organizatio frequently perform the procedure. Most MUE values are pt. MUE webpage http://www.cms.gov/Medicare/Coding/ NationalCorrectCodInitEd/MUE.html.

However, some MUE values are not published and are confidential. These values should not be published in oral or written form by any party that acquires one or more of them. MUEs are not utilization edits. Although the MUE value for some codes may represent the commonly reported units of service (e.g., MUE of "1" for appendectomy), the usual units of service for many HCPCS/CPT codes is less than the MUE value. Claims reporting units of service less than the MUE value may be subject to review by claims processing contractors, Unified Program Integrity Contractor (UPICs), Recovery Audit Contractors (RAC), and the Department of Justice (DOJ). Since MUEs are coding edits rather than medical necessity edits, claims processing contractors may have units of service edits that are more restrictive than MUEs. In such cases, the more restrictive claims processing contractor edit would be applied to the claim. Similarly, if the MUE is more restrictive than a claims processing contractor edit, the more restrictive MUE would apply. A national health care organization, provider/supplier, or other interested third party may request a reconsideration of an MUE value for a HCPCS/CPT code by submitting a written request to: NCCIPTPMUE@cms.hhs. The written request should include a rationale for reconsideration, as well as a suggested remedy.

Add-on Code Edit Tables

CMS publishes a list of add-on codes and their primary codes annually prior to January 1. The list is updated quarterly based on the AMA's "CPT Errata" documents or implementation of new HCPCS/CPT add-on codes. CMS identifies add-on codes and their primary codes based on CPT book instructions, CMS interpretation of HCPCS/CPT codes, and CMS coding instructions.

The NCCI program includes three add-on code edit tables, one table for each of three "types" of add-on codes. Each table lists the add-on code with its primary codes. An add-on code, with one exception, is eligible for payment if and only if one of its primary codes is also eligible for payment.

The "Type I Add-on Code Edit Table" lists add-on codes for which the CPT book or HCPCS tables define all acceptable primary codes. Claims processing contractors should not allow other primary codes with type I add-on codes. Code 99292 (Critical care, evaluation and management of the critically ill or critically injured patient; each additional 30 minutes [List separately in addition to code for primary service]) is included as a type I add-on code since its only primary code is 99291 (Critical care, evaluation and management of the critically ill or critically injured patient; first 30-74 minutes). For Medicare purposes, code 99292 may be eligible for payment to a physician without code 99291 if another physician of the same specialty and physician group reports and is paid for code 99291.

The "Type II Add-on Code Edit Table" lists add-on codes for which the CPT book and HCPCS tables do not define any primary codes. Claims processing contractors should develop their own lists of acceptable primary codes.

The "Type III Add-on Code Edit Table" lists add-on codes for which the CPT book or HCPCS tables define some, but not all, acceptable primary codes. Claims processing contractors should allow the listed primary codes for these add-on codes but may develop their own lists of additional acceptable primary codes.

Although the add-on code and primary code are normally reported for the same date of service, the two services may be reported for different dates of service (e.g., codes 99291 and 99292) under some unusual circumstances.

The first Add-On Code edit tables were implemented April 1, 2013. For subsequent years, new Add-On Code edit tables will be published to be effective for January 1 of the new year based on changes in the new year's CPT book. CMS also issues quarterly updates to the Add-On Code edit tables as required due to publication of new HCPCS/CPT codes or changes in add-on codes or their primary codes. The changes in the quarterly update files (April 1, July 1, or October 1) are retroactive to the implementation date of that year's annual Add-On Code edit files unless the files specify a different effective date for a change. Since the first Add-On Code edit files were implemented on April 1, 2013, changes in the July 1 and October 1 quarterly updates for 2013 were retroactive to April 1, 2013 unless the files specified a different effective date for a change.

Claims denied due to a CCI or MUE edit should be carefully reviewed to ensure appropriate coding and reporting of the services provided to ensure that the coding was correct and did not involve unbundling of services or submission of codes that would not be performed together. In addition, attention should be paid to verify the correct number of units was reported. Finally, review the CCI and/or MUE edits against the denied claim to determine whether there is a legitimate issue on the provider end or if the payer has made an error in the processing of the claim.

Correspondence

When a claim is submitted to the insurance carrier electronically, staff should review the generated report each time claims are transmitted. By doing so, several issues can be immediately addressed and corrected, such as making sure the claim transmitted correctly. Claims that did transmit but contain errors can often be corrected, resubmitted, and even paid before correspondence from the payer related to the errors is ever generated and arrives in the office.

Resubmission

When a claim is denied, one of the first thoughts is to resubmit, an option that is both fast and easy. However, claims may be resubmitted only when the entire claim is denied. This most typically occurs when information on the claim is missing or when the payer requests additional information. Routine resubmission of a claim can create a number of problems for accounts receivable and CMS can consider routine resubmissions fraudulent activity. According to CMS, some of the most common scenarios in which a claim can be resubmitted include:

- Incorrect patient name, health insurance claim number (HICN), or sex
- Missing billing provider information
- Missing diagnosis
- Missing performing provider number
- Missing place of service code
- Missing or incorrect quantity of service billed
- Missing/incorrect provider identification number (PIN)

Chapter 3. **Modifiers**

Over the last 20 years, physicians and hospitals have learned that coding and billing are closely connected processes. Coding provides the universal language through which providers and hospitals can communicate—or bill—their services to third-party payers, including managed care organizations, the federal Medicare program, and state Medicaid programs.

The use of modifiers is an important part of coding and billing for health care services. Modifier use has increased as various commercial payers, who in the past did not incorporate modifiers into their reimbursement protocol, recognize and accept HCPCS codes appended with these specialized billing flags.

Correct modifier use is also an important part of avoiding fraud and abuse or noncompliance issues, especially in coding and billing processes involving the federal and state governments. One of the top 10 billing errors determined by federal, state, and private payers involves the incorrect use of modifiers. With that being said, modifier use should also be incorporated into a practice's audit plan.

What is a modifier?

A modifier is a two-digit numeric alpha or alphanumeric code appended to a CPT® or HCPCS code to indicate that a service or procedure has been altered by some special circumstance, but for which the basic code description itself has not changed. A modifier can also indicate that an administrative requirement, such as completion of a waiver of liability statement, has been performed. Both the CPT and HCPCS Level II coding systems contain modifiers.

The CPT code book, *CPT 2021,* lists the following examples of when a modifier may be appropriate (this list does not include all of the applications for modifiers).

- A service or procedure has both a professional and technical component, but both components are not applicable
- A service or procedure was performed by more than one physician or other health care professional and/or in more than one location
- A service or procedure has been increased or reduced
- Only part of a service was performed
- An adjunctive service was performed
- A bilateral procedure was performed
- A service or procedure was performed more than once
- Unusual events occurred
- The physical status of a patient for the administration of anesthesia must be defined

Modifiers from either level may be applied to a procedure code. In other words, a CPT or HCPCS Level II modifier may be applied to a CPT or HCPCS Level II code.

Types of Modifiers

There are basically two types of modifiers: informational modifiers (those that do not affect payment) and payment modifiers (modifiers that affect reimbursement)

Informational Modifiers

Although informational modifiers may not have a direct impact on reimbursement, it should be noted that the improper use of an informational modifier may affect coverage of a service or procedure. Failure to use or to apply informational modifiers correctly may result in claim denial or can affect balance billing.

For example, a patient receives a service that is unlikely to be covered by Medicare. The office fails to complete an advance beneficiary notice (ABN); however, the claim is submitted with modifier GA Waiver of liability statement on file, appended to the procedure code. The Medicare contractor contacts the office and requests that the completed waiver be faxed as proof that it was obtained.

Since the office cannot comply, the service is denied and the Medicare remittance advice (RA) indicates that the patient cannot be billed for the noncovered service.

Payment Modifiers

Other modifiers have a direct impact on the amount a provider may be paid for a service or procedure. For example, a physician provides only the postoperative care following a laparoscopic cholecystectomy. In this instance, CPT code 47562 Laparoscopy, surgical; cholecystectomy, is submitted with modifier 55 Postoperative management only, appended to the code. The payer reimburses the physician the postoperative care portion of the procedure fee only.

Using Modifiers

There are two levels of modifiers within the HCPCS coding system. Level I (CPT) and Level II (HCPCS Level II) modifiers are applicable nationally for many third-party payers and all Medicare Part B claims. Level I or CPT modifiers are developed by the American Medical Association (AMA). HCPCS Level II modifiers are developed by the Centers for Medicare and Medicaid Services (CMS).

The Health Insurance Portability and Accountability Act (HIPAA) guidelines indicate that all codes and modifiers are to be standardized. Some coding and modifier information issued by CMS differs from the AMA's coding advice in the CPT book; a clear understanding of each payer's rules is necessary to assign such modifiers correctly.

Generally speaking, modifiers are specific to certain sections of the CPT book. The following table contains a list of CPT modifiers and the CPT section to which they can be applied.

CPT Modifiers and Applicable Sections

Table 1

Modifier	Brief Description	Applicable Sections
22	Increased procedural services	Anesthesia, Surgery, Radiology, Pathology and Laboratory, Medicine
23	Unusual anesthesia	Anesthesia
24	Unrelated evaluation and management service by the same physician or other qualified health care professional during a postoperative period	E/M
25	Significant, separately identifiable evaluation and management service by the same physician or other qualified health care professional on the same day of the procedure or other service	E/M
26	Professional component	Surgery, Radiology, Pathology and Laboratory, Medicine
32	Mandated services	E/M, Anesthesia, Surgery, Radiology, Pathology and Laboratory, Medicine
33	Preventive service	E/M, Surgery, Radiology, Pathology & Laboratory, Medicine (Services rated "A" or "B" by the USPSTF, Preventive care and screenings)
47	Anesthesia by surgeon	Surgery
50	Bilateral procedure	Surgery, Radiology, Medicine
51	Multiple procedures	Anesthesia, Surgery, Radiology, Medicine
52	Reduced services	Surgery, Radiology, Pathology and Laboratory, Medicine
53	Discontinued procedure	Anesthesia, Surgery, Radiology, Pathology and Laboratory, Medicine
54	Surgical care only	Surgery
55	Postoperative management only	Surgery, Medicine
56	Preoperative management only	Surgery, Medicine
57	Decision for surgery	E/M, Medicine
58	Staged or related procedure or service by the same physician or other qualified health care professional during the postoperative period	Surgery, Radiology, Medicine
59	Distinct procedural service	Anesthesia, Surgery, Radiology, Pathology and Laboratory, Medicine
62	Two surgeons	Surgery
63	Procedure performed on infants less than 4kg	Surgery
66	Surgical team	Surgery

Modifier	Brief Description	Applicable Sections
76	Repeat procedure or service by same physician or other qualified health care professional	Surgery, Radiology, Medicine
77	Repeat procedure by another physician or other qualified health care professional	Surgery, Radiology, Medicine
78	Unplanned return to the operating/procedure room by the same physician or other qualified health care professional following initial procedure for a related procedure during the postoperative period	Surgery, Medicine
79	Unrelated procedure or service by the same physician or other qualified health care professional during the postoperative period	Surgery, Medicine
80	Assistant surgeon	Surgery
81	Minimum assistant surgeon	Surgery
82	Assistant surgeon (when qualified resident surgeon not available)	Surgery
90	Reference (outside) laboratory	Pathology and Laboratory
91	Repeat clinical diagnostic laboratory test	Pathology and Laboratory
92	Alternative laboratory platform testing	Pathology and Laboratory
96	Habilitative Services	Medicine
97	Rehabilitative Services	Medicine
99	Multiple modifiers	Surgery, Radiology, Medicine

OIG Reports and Payer Review of Modifiers

One of the top 10 billing errors, as determined by federal, state, and private payers, involves the incorrect use of modifiers. Additionally, incorrect modifier assignment is often responsible for overpayments. For these reasons, third-party payers including Medicare often review claims containing modifiers.

An automated claim processing system usually contains edits that look for combinations of certain modifiers being reported with specific CPT codes. If the claim does not contain a modifier with the code, the claim may be suspended for manual review.

Other payers may periodically perform manual reviews of claims containing a modifier that they consider to have been billed incorrectly or inappropriately in the past. For example, if the payer finds that there is a high error rate on claims using modifier 22 Increased procedural services, they may select to manually review every 10th claim received that contains that modifier.

Payers may also elect to place a particular provider's claim containing specific procedure or modifier combinations under review. For example, a payer determined that Dr. Smith incorrectly appends modifier 59 Distinct procedural service, to procedure codes.

Every month the Office of Inspector General (OIG) issues an update to the work plan, identifying areas of concern. These are areas that Medicare contractors will most likely focus their reviews. The OIG Work Plan monthly updates can be found at: https://oig.hhs.gov/reports-and-publications/workplan/index.asp

The agency's work plan is released monthly and is a useful tool in determining what, if any, modifier inconsistencies have been discovered and what contractors will be monitoring. Each practice should monitor these areas.

Another tool that can be used to identify provider's commonly made errors and areas where providers should monitor and audit is the comprehensive error rate testing (CERT) reports. CERT reports can be located at https://www.cms.gov/Research-Statistics-Data-and-Systems/Monitoring-Programs/Medicare-FFS-Compliance-Programs/CERT/CERT-Reports.html.

Modifiers and Modifier Indicators

The AMA CPT book and CMS define modifiers that may be appended to HCPCS/CPT codes to provide additional information about the services rendered. Modifiers may be appended to HCPCS/CPT codes only if the clinical circumstances justify the use of the modifier. A modifier should not be appended to a HCPCS/CPT code solely to bypass a National Correct Coding Initiative (NCCI) edit if the clinical circumstances do not justify its use. If the Medicare program imposes restrictions on the use of a modifier, the modifier may only be used to bypass an NCCI edit if the Medicare restrictions are fulfilled.

Modifiers that may be used under appropriate clinical circumstances to bypass an NCCI edit include:

- **Anatomic modifiers:** E1-E4, FA, F1-F9, TA, T1-T9, LT, RT, LC, LD, LM, RC, RI
- **Global surgery modifiers:** 24, 25, 57, 58, 78, 79
- **Other modifiers:** 27, 59, 91, XE, XS, XP, XU

It is very important that NCCI-associated modifiers only be used when appropriate. In general, these circumstances relate to separate patient encounters, separate anatomic sites, or separate specimens. Most edits involving paired organs or structures (e.g., eyes, ears, extremities, lungs, kidneys) have NCCI modifier indicators of "1" because the two codes of the code pair edit may be reported if performed on the contralateral organs or structures. Most of these code pairs should not be reported with NCCI-associated modifiers when performed on the ipsilateral organ or structure unless there is a specific coding rationale to bypass the edit. The existence of the NCCI edit indicates that the two codes generally cannot be reported together unless the two corresponding procedures are performed at two separate patient encounters or two separate anatomic locations. However, if the two corresponding procedures are performed at the same patient encounter and in contiguous structures in the same organ or anatomic region, NCCI-associated modifiers generally should not be utilized.

The appropriate use of most of these modifiers is straight-forward. However, further explanation is provided regarding modifiers 25, 58, and 59. Although

 DEFINITIONS

NCCI. National correct coding initiative. Official list of codes from the Centers for Medicare and Medicaid Services' (CMS) National Correct Coding Policy Manual for Part B Medicare Carriers that identifies services considered an integral part of a comprehensive code or mutually exclusive of it.

modifier 22 is not a modifier that bypasses an NCCI edit, its use is occasionally relevant to an NCCI edit and is discussed below.

Modifier 22: Modifier 22 is defined by the CPT book as "increased procedural services." This modifier should not be reported routinely unless the service performed is substantially more extensive than the usual service included in the procedure described by the HCPCS/CPT code reported. Occasionally a provider may perform two procedures that should not be reported together based on an NCCI edit. If the edit allows use of NCCI-associated modifiers to bypass it and the clinical circumstances justify use of one of these modifiers, both services may be reported with the NCCI-associated modifier. However, if the NCCI edit does not allow use of NCCI-associated modifiers to bypass it and the procedure qualifies as an unusual procedural service, the physician may report the column one HCPCS/CPT code of the NCCI edit with modifier 22. The Medicare contractor may then evaluate the unusual procedural service to determine whether additional payment is justified. For example, CMS limits payment for CPT code 69990 Microsurgical techniques, requiring use of operating microscope, to procedures listed in the *Internet-Only Manual* (IOM) (*Claims Processing Manual*, Pub. 100-4, 12- §20.4.5).

If a physician reports CPT code 69990 with two other CPT codes and one of the codes is not on this list, an NCCI edit with the code not on the list will prevent payment for CPT code 69990. Claims processing systems do not determine which procedure is linked with CPT code 69990. In situations such as this, the physician may submit his claim to the local Medicare contractor for re-adjudication appending modifier 22 to the CPT code. Although the Medicare contractor cannot override an NCCI edit that does not allow use of NCCI-associated modifiers, the Medicare contractor has discretion to adjust payment to include use of the operating microscope based on modifier 22.

Modifier 25: The CPT book defines modifier 25 as a "significant, separately identifiable evaluation and management service by the same physician or other qualified health care professional on the same day of the procedure or other service." Modifier 25 may be appended to an evaluation and management (E/M) CPT code to indicate that the E/M service is significant and separately identifiable from other services reported on the same date of service. The E/M service may be related to the same or different diagnosis as the other procedure.

Modifier 25 may be appended to E/M services reported with minor surgical procedures (global periods of 000 or 010 days) or procedures not covered by global surgery rules (global indicator of XXX). Since minor surgical procedures and XXX procedures include preprocedure, intraprocedure, and postprocedure work inherent in the procedure, the provider should not report an E/M service for this work. Furthermore, Medicare global surgery rules prevent the reporting of a separate E/M service for the work associated with the decision to perform a minor surgical procedure whether the patient is a new or established patient.

Modifier 58: Modifier 58 is defined by the CPT book as a "staged or related procedure or service by the same physician or other qualified health care professional during the postoperative period." It may be used to indicate that a procedure was followed by a second procedure during the postoperative period of the first procedure. This situation may occur because the second procedure was planned prospectively, was more extensive than the first procedure, or was therapy after a diagnostic surgical service. Use of modifier 58 will bypass NCCI edits that allow use of NCCI-associated modifiers.

If a diagnostic endoscopic procedure results in the decision to perform an open procedure, both procedures may be reported with modifier 58 appended to the HCPCS/CPT code for the open procedure. However, if the endoscopic procedure preceding an open procedure is a "scout" procedure to assess anatomic landmarks and/or extent of disease, it is not reported individually. Diagnostic endoscopy is never reported separately with another endoscopic procedure in the same organ(s) or anatomic region when performed at the same patient encounter. Similarly, diagnostic laparoscopy is never reported separately with a surgical laparoscopic procedure of the same body cavity when performed at the same patient encounter. If a planned laparoscopic procedure fails and is converted to an open procedure, only the open procedure may be reported. The failed laparoscopic procedure is not reported separately. The NCCI contains many, but not all, edits bundling laparoscopic procedures into open procedures. Since the number of possible code combinations bundling a laparoscopic procedure into an open procedure is much greater than the number of such edits in NCCI, the principle stated in this paragraph is applicable regardless of whether the selected code pair combination is included in the NCCI tables. A provider should not select laparoscopic and open HCPCS/CPT codes to report because the combination is not included in the NCCI tables.

Modifier 59: Modifier 59 is an important NCCI-associated modifier that is often used incorrectly. For NCCI, its primary purpose is to indicate that two or more procedures are performed at different anatomic sites or different patient encounters. One function of NCCI edits is to prevent payment for codes that report overlapping services except when the services are "separate and distinct." Modifier 59 should be used only if no other modifier more appropriately describes the relationships of the two or more procedure codes.

The CPT book defines modifier 59 as follows: "Modifier 59: Distinct Procedural Service: Under certain circumstances, it may be necessary to indicate that a procedure or service was distinct or independent from other non-E/M services performed on the same day. Modifier 59 is used to identify procedures/services, other than E/M services, that are not normally reported together, but are appropriate under the circumstances. Documentation must support a different session, different procedure or surgery, different site or organ system, separate incision/excision, separate lesion, or separate injury (or area of injury in extensive injuries) not ordinarily encountered or performed on the same day by the same individual. However, when another already established modifier is appropriate, it should be used rather than modifier 59. Only if no more descriptive modifier is available, and the use of modifier 59 best explains the circumstances, should modifier 59 be used. Note: Modifier 59 should not be appended to an E/M service. To report a separate and distinct E/M service with a non-E/M service performed on the same date, see modifier 25."

One of the common misuses of modifier 59 is related to the portion of the definition used to describe "different procedure or surgery." The code descriptors of the two codes of a code pair edit usually represent different procedures or surgeries. The edit indicates that the two procedures/surgeries cannot be reported together if performed at the same anatomic site and same patient encounter. The provider cannot use modifier 59 for such an edit based on the two codes being different procedures/surgeries. However, if the two procedures/surgeries are performed at separate anatomic sites or at separate patient encounters on the same date of service, modifier 59 may be appended to indicate that they are different procedures/surgeries on that date of service.

Modifier 59 or XS is used appropriately for different anatomic sites during the same encounter only when procedures which are not ordinarily performed or encountered on the same day are performed on different organs, different anatomic regions, or in limited situations on different, non-contiguous lesions in different anatomic regions of the same organ.

There are several exceptions to this general principle:

- When a diagnostic procedure precedes a surgical or nonsurgical therapeutic procedure and is why the decision to perform the surgical or nonsurgical therapeutic procedure is made, that diagnostic procedure may be considered a separate and distinct procedure as long as:

  - it occurs before the therapeutic procedure and is not combined with services that are required for the therapeutic intervention
  - it clearly provides the information needed to decide whether to proceed with the therapeutic procedure
  - it does not constitute a service that would have otherwise been required during the therapeutic intervention. If the diagnostic procedure is an inherent component of the surgical or non-surgical therapeutic procedure, it should not be reported separately.

- When a diagnostic procedure follows a surgical procedure or nonsurgical therapeutic procedure, that diagnostic procedure may be considered a separate and distinct procedure as long as:

  - it occurs after the completion of the therapeutic procedure and is not interspersed with or otherwise commingled with services that are only required for the therapeutic intervention
  - it does not constitute a service that would have otherwise been required during the therapeutic intervention. If the postprocedure diagnostic procedure is an inherent component or otherwise included (or not separately payable) postprocedure service of the surgical procedure or nonsurgical therapeutic procedure, it should not be reported separately

- There is an appropriate use for modifier 59 that is applicable only to codes for which the unit of service is a measure of time (e.g., per 15 minutes, per hour). If two separate and distinct timed services are provided in separate and distinct time blocks, modifier 59 may be used to identify the services. The separate and distinct time blocks for the two services may be sequential to one another or split. When the two services are split, the time block for one service may be followed by a time block for the second service followed by another time block for the first service. All Medicare rules for reporting timed services are applicable. For example, the total time is calculated for all related timed services performed. The number of reportable units of service is based on the total time, and these units of service are allocated between the HCPCS/CPT codes for the individual services performed. The physician is not permitted to perform multiple services, each for the minimal reportable time, and report each of these as separate units of service (e.g., a physician or therapist performs eight minutes of neuromuscular reeducation [97112] and eight minutes of therapeutic exercises [97110]. Since the physician or therapist performed 16 minutes of related timed services, only one unit of service may be reported for one, not each, of these codes.)

Use of modifier 59 to indicate different procedures/surgeries does not require a different diagnosis for each HCPCS/CPT coded procedure/surgery. Additionally, different diagnoses are not adequate criteria for use of modifier 59.

The HCPCS/CPT codes remain bundled unless the procedures/surgeries are performed at different anatomic sites or separate patient encounters.

From an NCCI perspective, the definition of different anatomic sites includes different organs, different anatomic regions, or different lesions in the same organ. It does not include treatment of contiguous structures in the same organ or anatomic region. For example, treatment of the nail, nail bed, and adjacent soft tissue constitutes treatment of a single anatomic site. Treatment of posterior segment structures in the ipsilateral eye constitutes treatment of a single anatomic site. Arthroscopic treatment of a shoulder injury in adjoining areas of the ipsilateral shoulder constitutes treatment of a single anatomic site.

If the same procedure is performed at different anatomic sites, it does not necessarily imply that a HCPCS/CPT code may be reported with more than one unit of service (UOS). Determining whether additional UOS may be reported depends in part upon the HCPCS/CPT code descriptor, including the definition of the code's unit of service, when present.

Example:
The column one/column two code edit with column one CPT code 38221 Diagnostic bone marrow; biopsy, and column two CPT code 38220 Diagnostic bone marrow, aspiration, includes two distinct procedures when performed at separate anatomic sites (e.g., contralateral iliac bones) or separate patient encounters. In these circumstances, it would be acceptable to use modifier 59. However, if both 38221 and 38220 are performed on the same iliac bone at the same patient encounter which is the usual practice, modifier 59 would NOT be used. Although CMS does not allow separate payment for code 38220 with code 38221 when bone marrow aspiration and biopsy are performed on the same iliac bone at a single patient encounter, a physician may report code 38222 Diagnostic bone marrow; biopsy(ies) and aspiration(s).

Example:
The procedure-to-procedure edit with column one code 11055 (paring or cutting of benign hyperkeratotic lesion...) and column two code 11720 (debridement of nail[s] by any method; 1 to 5) may be bypassed with modifier 59 only if the paring/cutting of a benign hyperkeratotic lesion is performed on a different digit (e.g., toe) than one that has nail debridement. Modifier 59 should not be used to bypass the edit if the two procedures are performed on the same digit.

However, CMS recognized that the use of modifier 59 resulted in inappropriate payment under certain circumstances because the modifier lacks specificity and providers sometimes use it to bypass the NCCI edits.

Modifiers XE, XP, XS, XU: These modifiers, effective January 1, 2015, were developed to provide greater reporting specificity in situations where modifier 59 was previously reported and may be utilized in lieu of modifier 59 whenever possible. Modifier 59 should only be utilized if no other more specific modifier is appropriate. Although NCCI will eventually require use of these modifiers rather than modifier 59 with certain edits, physicians may begin using them for claims with dates of service on or after January 1, 2015. The modifiers are defined as follows:

- XE Separate encounter, a service that is distinct because it occurred during a separate encounter

- XS Separate structure, a service that is distinct because it was performed on a separate organ/structure
- XP Separate practitioner, a service that is distinct because it was performed by a different practitioner
- XU Unusual non-overlapping service, the use of a service that is distinct because it does not overlap usual components of the main service

Modifiers 76 Repeat procedure or service by same physician or other qualified health care professional, and 77 Repeat procedure by another physician or other qualified health care professional, are not NCCI associated modifiers. Use of either of these modifiers does not bypass an NCCI edit.

Auditing Modifiers

There are a significant number of modifiers and determining which modifiers to review is very important. When making this decision, identify the most commonly used modifiers within the practice. The next step is to determine which, if any, of these modifiers are known to have a high incidence of incorrect use or payer review. Also identify those modifiers that have the highest impact to revenue. Finally, establish a protocol and develop a worksheet that will be used. A sample worksheet can be found in appendix 1.

When auditing medical records to determine appropriate modifier assignment, a number of factors must be reviewed. These factors are discussed in the following paragraphs.

Medical Record Documentation

Does the medical record documentation indicate a modifier is necessary?
For example, does the operative report reveal that a procedure was performed bilaterally? If yes, does the CPT code description indicate that the procedure is a unilateral procedure only? If so, was modifier 50 Bilateral procedure, assigned?

Does the medical record documentation provide sufficient detail to support the modifier assignment?
For example, modifier 22 Increased procedural services, was appended to a procedure code. The medical record documentation should paint a picture of how the service was unusual, the amount of time and effort that the service was increased by, and any conditions that complicated care.

Is the medical record documentation authenticated?
Many third-party payers will not recognize the validity of documentation if the provider does not authenticate it. In most instances, this means the provider's signature or initials.

Modifier Assignment

Was the modifier appended to the correct procedure code?
As previously shown in Table 1, some modifiers can only be assigned to specific codes. Review a claim to verify that the modifier was correctly appended to the procedure code. For example, modifier 25 Significant separately identifiable evaluation and management service, must be appended to the E/M code, not the procedure code, when performed during the same encounter.

Is the modifier valid for the procedure per payer guidelines?

Many payers, including Medicare, developed edits that screen for appropriateness of modifier to procedure relationships. For example, Medicare indicates that modifier 80 Assistant surgeon, is not valid with CPT code 38210 T cell depletion within harvest. This information can also be verified in the MPFSDB.

Does the payer have specific guidelines for the modifier indicated? If so, were they followed?

As mentioned previously, while the AMA creates many of the modifier guidelines, payers also develop their own guidelines. These guidelines sometimes conflict with the AMA. When this occurs, the payer-specific guidelines must be followed. For example, the AMA states that modifier 78 Unplanned return to the operating/procedure room by the same physician or other qualified health care professional following initial procedure for a related procedure during the postoperative period, can include a treatment room; however, many payers, including Medicare, consider only an operating room the appropriate setting.

Is there a specific procedure code that accurately reflects the alteration of the service?

For example, the physician performs an interpretation of an electrocardiogram. The office assigns code 93000-26. However, CPT code 93010 reflects the interpretation and report component of the more comprehensive service without the use of a modifier. Correct code assignment for this service, therefore, should have been 93010.

Reimbursement Issues

Were any necessary fee revisions made?

Since some modifiers affect payment, it may be necessary to adjust the fee for the service. For example, modifier 52 Reduced service, often indicates a lesser fee. Was the fee submitted on the claim reduced and, if so, was the reduction amount appropriate?

Some offices elect not to reduce the fee, allowing the payer to determine what the payment for the affected procedure should be. If this is the practice's policy, was it adhered to on the claim?

Payer Issues

Did the payer process the modifier?

Most payers will indicate that a modifier has been processed by including it on the remittance advice (RA).

Did the modifier prevent a claim denial as it should have?

Some services, when billed together, trigger a denial unless a modifier, indicating a special circumstance (such as modifier 59 Distinct procedural service), is appended. The RA should be reviewed to determine that the modifier did, in fact, override edits as appropriate.

Did the payer make the appropriate payment adjustment?

Certain modifiers, such as modifier 51 Multiple procedures, result in payment reductions. The RA should be reviewed to determine that the appropriate payment adjustments were applied.

Claim Issues

Was the modifier indicated correctly on the claim?
Most payers require that the modifier be indicated on the same line as the procedure code; however, some payers may require that the modifier be indicated on the line below the procedure code. Examine the claim to make certain that any payer-specific guidelines were followed.

Were necessary claim attachments submitted with the claim?
Some modifiers, such as modifier 22 Increased procedural services, require supporting documentation be submitted with the claim to substantiate modifier use and permit the payer to compute payment.

Were requests for additional information acknowledged?
There are times when a payer may request additional information before the claim may be processed, particularly when a modifier is assigned. If a request has been made by the payer, determine that it was responded to in a timely fashion. The payer should confirm receipt of the requested information and verify that the claim has been released for processing.

Modifier Tips and Traps
The following is a detailed discussion of modifiers that are often used incorrectly. Each modifier is described along with a discussion of when the modifier is to be used, correct usage of the modifier, and incorrect usage of the modifier. Again, note that not all modifiers are included, only those that are frequently used inappropriately.

CPT Modifiers

22   Increased Procedural Services
When the work required to provide a service is substantially greater than typically required, it may be identified by adding modifier 22 to the usual procedure code. Documentation must support the substantial additional work and the reason for the additional work (i.e., increased intensity, time, technical difficulty of procedure, severity of patient's condition, physical and mental effort required). **Note:** This modifier should not be appended to an E/M service.

When to use this modifier:
Modifier 22 is appended to the procedure or service code that warranted the increased effort and should typically be submitted with a narrative detailing the specific increased work and complexity that necessitated the use of this modifier.

Correct usage of this modifier:
- Modifier 22 is appended to the basic CPT procedure code when the service provided is greater than usually required for the listed procedure. Use of modifier 22 allows the claim to undergo individual consideration.

- Modifier 22 is used to identify an increment of work that is infrequently encountered with a particular procedure and is not described by another code.

- Surgical procedures that require additional physician work due to complications or medical emergencies may warrant the use of modifier 22 after the surgical procedure code.

- Modifier 22 is applied to any code of a multiple procedure claim, whether or not that code is the primary or secondary procedure. In these instances, the Medicare contractor first applies the multiple surgery reduction rules

---

🖥 SPECIAL ALERT

A claim with modifier 22 will be processed on a by-report basis.

The frequent reporting of modifier 22 has prompted many payers to simply ignore it. When using modifier 22, the claim must be accompanied by documentation and a cover letter explaining the unusual circumstances.

Language that indicates unusual circumstances would be difficulty, increased risk, extended, hemorrhage, blood loss over 600cc, unusual findings, etc. If slight extension of the procedure was necessary (a procedure extended by 15 to 20 minutes) or, for example, routine lysis of adhesions was performed, these scenarios do not validate the use of modifier 22.

(e.g., 100 percent, 50 percent, 50 percent, 50 percent, 50 percent). Then, a decision is made as to whether modifier 22 should be paid. For example, if the fee schedule amounts for procedures A, B, and C are $1,000, $500, and $250 respectively, and modifier 22 is submitted with procedure B, the contractor would apply the multiple surgery payment reduction rule first (major procedure 100 percent of the Medicare fee schedule) and reduce the procedure B (second surgical procedure) fee schedule amount from $500 to $250. The contractor would then decide whether or not to pay an additional amount above the $250 based on the documentation submitted with the claim for increased procedural services, as designated by modifier 22.

- Modifier 22 should be appended only to procedure codes that have a global period of 0, 10, or 90 days.

Incorrect usage of this modifier:

- Appending modifier 22 to a surgical code without documentation in the medical record of an unusual occurrence.

- Using modifier 22 on a routine basis to do so would most certainly cause scrutiny of submitted claims and may result in an audit.

- Using modifier 22 to indicate that the procedure was performed by a specialist; specialty designation does not warrant use of modifier 22.

- Reporting increased E/M service time, skill, or service with modifier 22.

Regulatory and coding guidance:

- Overuse of modifier 22 could trigger a payer audit, as payers monitor the use of this modifier very carefully. Make sure that modifier 22 is used only when sufficient documentation is present in the medical record.

- A claim submitted with modifier 22 is generally forwarded to the medical review staff for review and pricing. With sufficient documentation of medical necessity, increased payment may be allowed.

- Do not bombard third-party payers with unnecessary documentation. All attachments to the claim for justification of the increased procedural services should explain the special circumstances in a concise, clear manner. This information should be easy to locate within the attached documentation. Highlight this information, if necessary, to facilitate the medical reviewer's access to the pertinent supporting data.

- CPT codes for use with modifier 22 are 00100–01999, 10004–69990, 70010–79999, 80047–89398, 90281–99199, and 99500–99607 unless limited by the payer.

The following flow chart can aid in an audit by helping determine if modifier 22 is being used correctly and whether additional documentation might be required.

Modifier 22

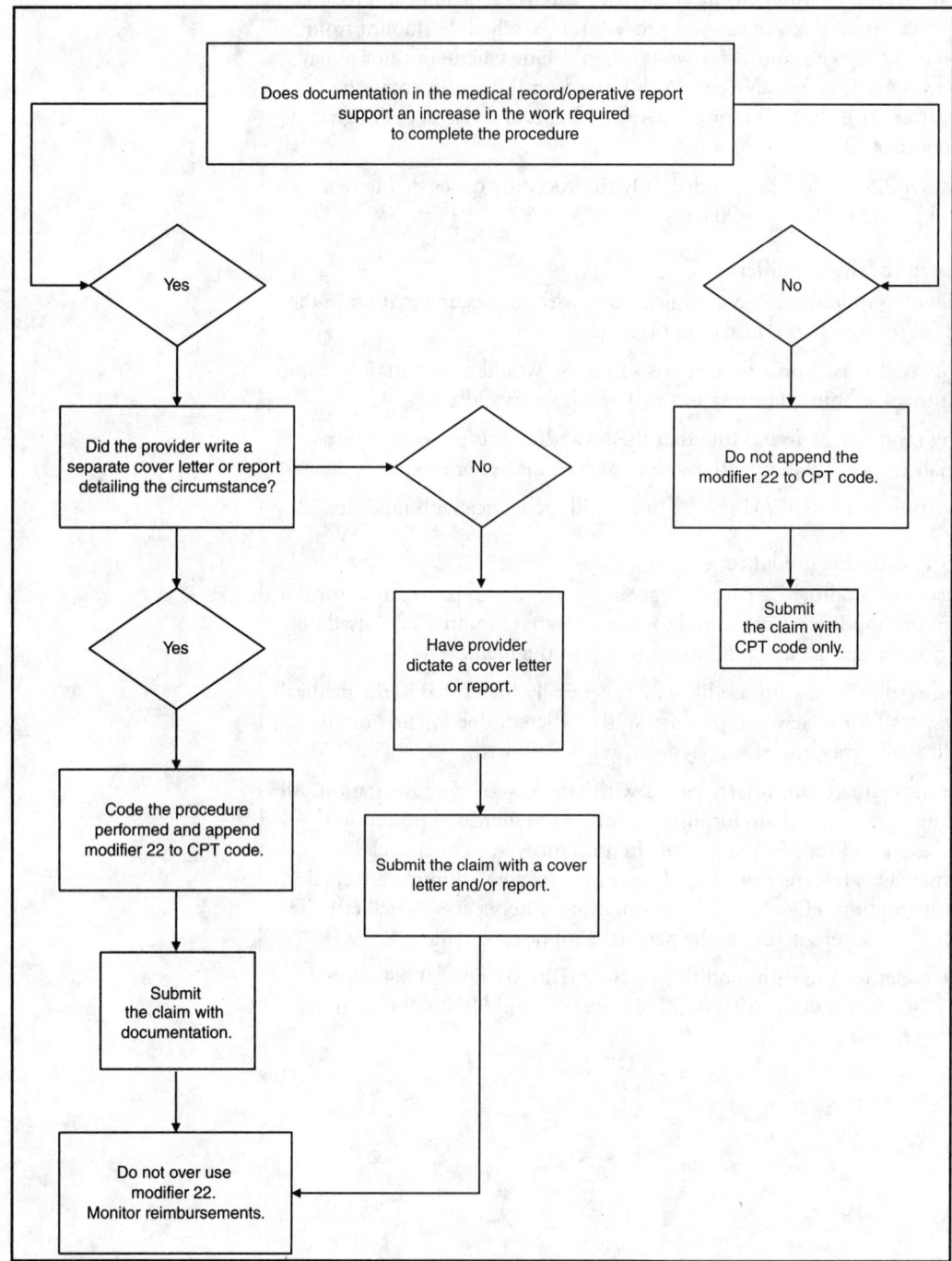

23   Unusual Anesthesia

Occasionally, a procedure, which usually requires either no anesthesia or local anesthesia, because of unusual circumstances must be done under general anesthesia. This circumstance may be reported by adding modifier 23 to the procedure code of the basic service.

When to use this modifier:

Modifier 23 is appended to anesthesia service codes to identify circumstances in which additional work is required over and beyond the usual service.

Correct usage of this modifier:

- Use this modifier when general anesthesia is administered in situations that typically would not require this level of anesthesia, or in situations in which local anesthesia might have been required, but would not be sufficient under the circumstances.

- Modifier 23 should be used on basic service procedure codes (00100–01999).

Incorrect usage of this modifier:

- Using modifier 23 for local anesthesia.

- Using modifier 23 to report anesthesia provided by the surgeon.

- It is inappropriate to report modifier 23 with the administration of moderate sedation by the surgeon or another provider. This modifier should be used only when general or monitored anesthesia is administered.

Example

A 2-year-old child is brought to the emergency room with a severe leg laceration covered in gravel and dirt that resulted from falling off his tricycle and onto asphalt and dirt. The patient is extremely agitated, scared, crying, and uncontrollable. Due to the patient's age and the significant stress being placed on the child, the emergency physician advises the parents that the use of a general anesthesia is necessary to adequately debride and suture the complex wound. The anesthesiologist is consulted and the procedure performed. The anesthesiologist should append modifier 23 to the appropriate anesthesia code to indicate the unusual circumstances necessitating the use of general anesthesia. The surgeon should also report the correct debridement and/or repair codes.

🖥 SPECIAL ALERT

When using modifier 23, the claim must be accompanied by documentation and a cover letter from the provider explaining the need for the unusual anesthesia.

The following flow chart can aid in an audit by helping determine if modifier 23 is being used correctly and whether additional documentation might be required.

Modifier 23

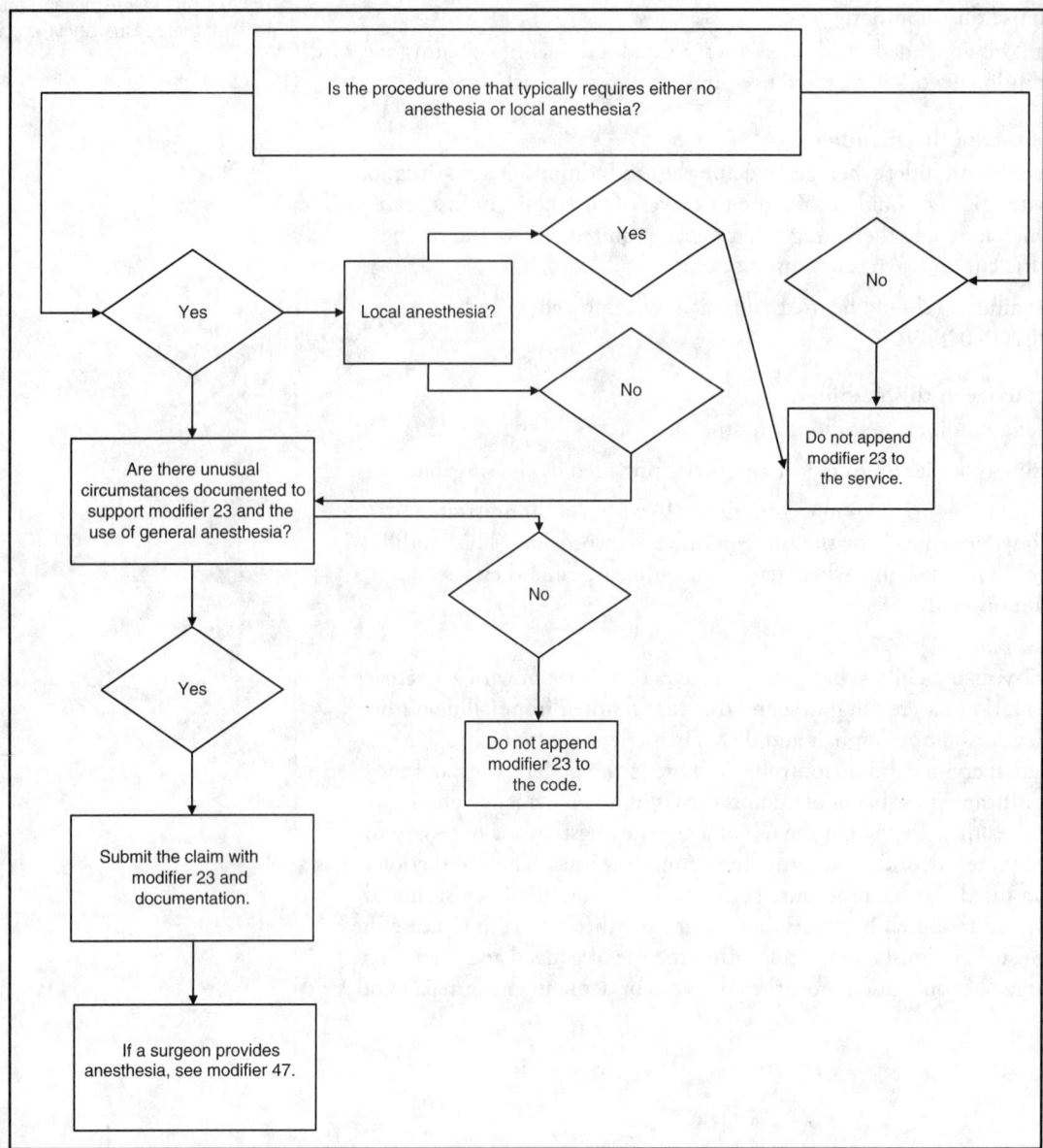

24 Unrelated Evaluation and Management Service by the Same Physician or Other Qualified Health Care Professional During a Postoperative Period

The physician or other qualified health care professional may need to indicate that an evaluation and management service was performed during a postoperative period for a reason(s) unrelated to the original procedure. This circumstance may be reported by adding modifier 24 to the appropriate level of E/M service.

When to use this modifier:
Modifier 24 is appended to an E/M code when an E/M service is performed during a postoperative period for a reason unrelated to the original procedure.

Correct usage of this modifier:
- Append modifier 24 to the E/M code for an unrelated service, for major or minor surgical procedures.

- Append modifier 24 when the same physician or other qualified health care professional provides unrelated critical care to the patient during the postoperative period.

- Append modifier 24 to an unrelated E/M service beginning the day after a procedure, when the E/M is performed by the surgeon during the 10- or 90-day postoperative period.

- Append modifier 24 to an E/M code when the surgeon is managing immunosuppressant therapy during the postoperative period of a transplant.

- Append modifier 24 to an E/M code when the surgeon is managing chemotherapy during the postoperative period of a procedure.

- When a patient is admitted to a skilled nursing facility (SNF) for an unrelated condition in a global period, report modifier 24 with the appropriate SNF admission code.

- A provider who is responsible for postoperative care (i.e., one who has reported modifier 55) may also use modifier 24 to report any unrelated visits.

Incorrect usage of this modifier:
- Using modifier 24 with the SNF admission code when a surgeon admits a patient to a SNF and the patient's admission is related to the surgery. This service is included in the global package and is not paid separately. Follow individual third-party payer guidelines, as some commercial health insurance plans may pay separately for these services.

- Reporting modifier 24 with subsequent hospital care codes (99231–99233). These services performed by the surgeon during the same hospitalization as the surgery are normally related to the surgery. Separate payment for such visits is not allowed even when billed with modifier 24 unless a different diagnosis is reported with the E/M code identifying the service as unrelated to the original procedure. Follow individual third-party payer guidelines, as some commercial health insurance plans pay separately for these services.

- Reporting modifier 24 when the E/M service is for a surgical complication or injection, which is included in the surgical package.

> **SPECIAL ALERT**
>
> Medicare rules state to report modifier 24 with E/M services provided in the postoperative period of a major or minor procedure (i.e., those with a 10 or 90-day follow-up, respectively) only if the E/M service is not related to the surgical procedure. A diagnosis code that clearly identifies the reason for the E/M service as unrelated to the procedure is necessary.

The following flow chart can aid in an audit by helping determine if modifier 24 is being used correctly and whether additional documentation might be required.

Modifier 24

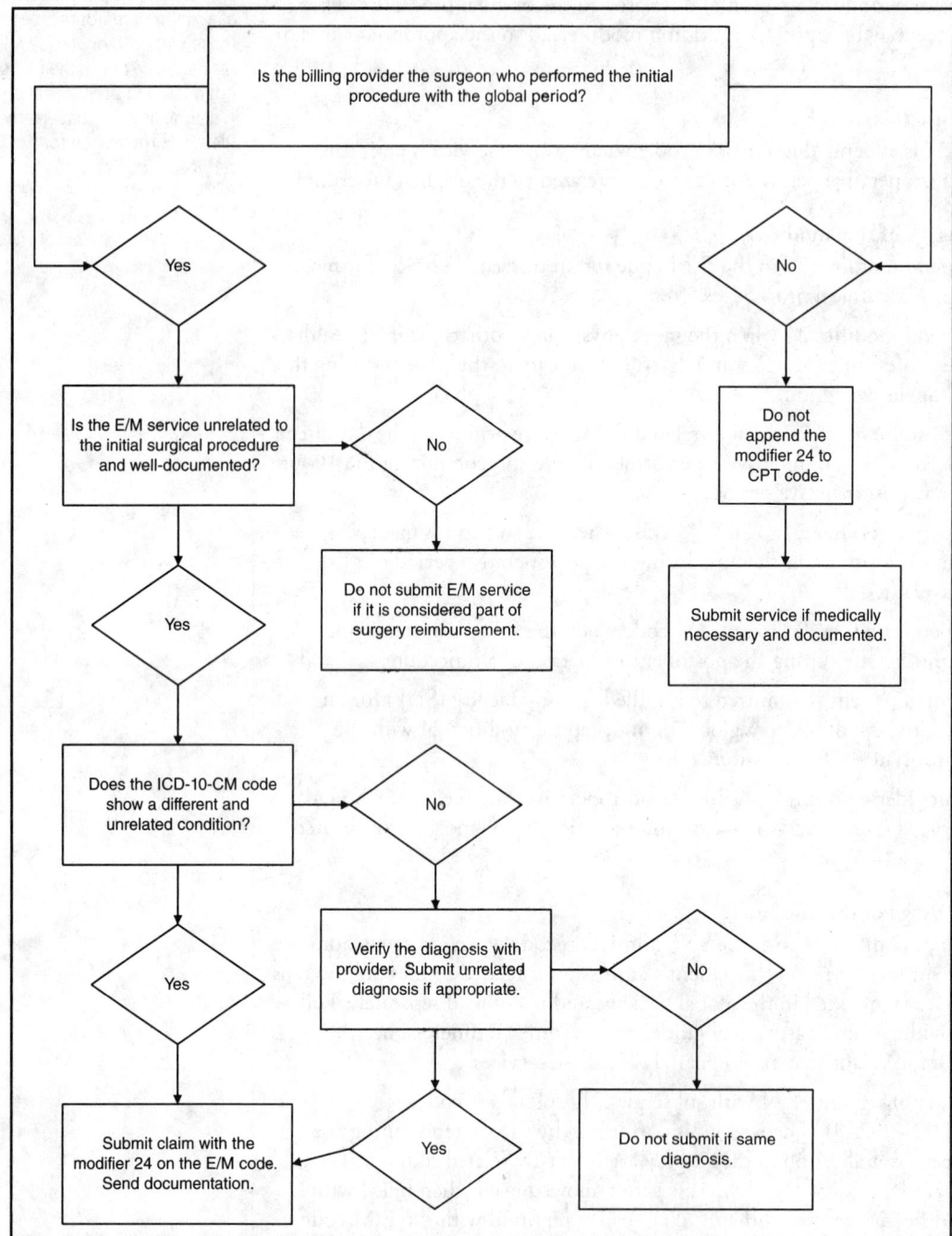

25 Significant Separately Identifiable Evaluation and Management Service by the Same Physician or Other Qualified Health Care Professional on the Same Day of the Procedure or Other Service

It may be necessary to indicate that on the day a procedure or service identified by a CPT code was performed, the patient's condition required a significant, separately identifiable E/M service above and beyond the other service provided or beyond the usual preoperative and postoperative care associated with the procedure that was performed. A significant, separately identifiable E/M service is defined or substantiated by documentation that satisfies the relevant criteria for the respective E/M service to be reported (see Evaluation and Management Services Guidelines for instructions on determining level of E/M service). The E/M service may be prompted by the symptom or condition for which the procedure and/or service was provided. As such, different diagnoses are not required for reporting of the E/M services on the same date. This circumstance may be reported by adding modifier 25 to the appropriate level of E/M service.

Note: This modifier is not used to report an E/M service that resulted in a decision to perform surgery, see modifier 57. For significant, separately identifiable non-E/M services, see modifier 59.

When to use this modifier:
Append modifier 25 to indicate that on the day of a procedure or service, the patient's condition required a significant, separately identifiable E/M service above and beyond the other service provided.

Correct usage of this modifier:
- Modifier 25 is used when the E/M service is separate from that required for the procedure and a clearly documented, distinct, and significantly identifiable service was rendered. Although the CPT book does not limit modifier 25 to use only with a specific type of procedure or service, many third-party payers will not accept modifier 25 on an E/M service when billed with a minor procedure on the same day.

- It is appropriate to use modifier 25 when preoperative critical care codes are billed within a global surgical period. Reporting these E/M services with modifier 25 indicates that they are significant and separately identifiable services. The diagnosis must support that the service was unrelated to the performance of critical care.

- Modifier 25 should be indicated for an E/M service performed at the same session as a preventive care visit when a significant, separately identifiable E/M service is performed in addition to the preventive care. The E/M service must be carried out for a nonpreventive clinical reason, and the ICD-10-CM code(s) for the E/M service should clearly indicate the nonpreventive nature of the E/M service.

- Modifier 25 may be appended to the E/M code representing a significant, separately identifiable service performed on the same day as routine foot care. The visit must be medically necessary.

- Using modifier 25 on an unrelated E/M service when billed on the same date as a dialysis service.

Incorrect usage of this modifier:
- Using modifier 25 to report an E/M service that resulted in the decision to perform major surgery (see modifier 57).

- Using modifier 25 on an E/M service performed on a different day than the procedure. For example, a surgeon sees a patient in his office to follow

SPECIAL ALERT

Medicare allows separate payment for two office visits provided on the same date, by the same provider, when each visit is rendered for an unrelated problem. Both visits must occur at different times of the day and both visits must be medically necessary. This particular circumstance is considered rare, and requires modifier 25 to be appended to the second visit, not modifier 59. Medicare contractors have been instructed by CMS to conduct claim reviews to detect high use of modifier 25 by individual providers or groups. When an individual or group has been identified, a case-by-case review of all claims and supporting documentation will be performed on subsequent submissions containing modifier 25.

up an abnormal mammogram. After discussing the findings with the patient, he schedules and performs a breast biopsy the next day. It would be incorrect to add modifier 25 to the E/M code.

- Using modifier 25 on a surgical code (10004–69990) since this modifier is used to explain the special circumstance of providing the E/M service on the same day as a procedure.

- Using modifier 25 on the office visit E/M level of service code when on the same day a minor procedure was performed, when the patient's trip to the office was explicitly for the minor procedure.

The following flow chart can aid in an audit by helping determine if modifier 25 is being used correctly and whether additional documentation might be required.

Modifier 25

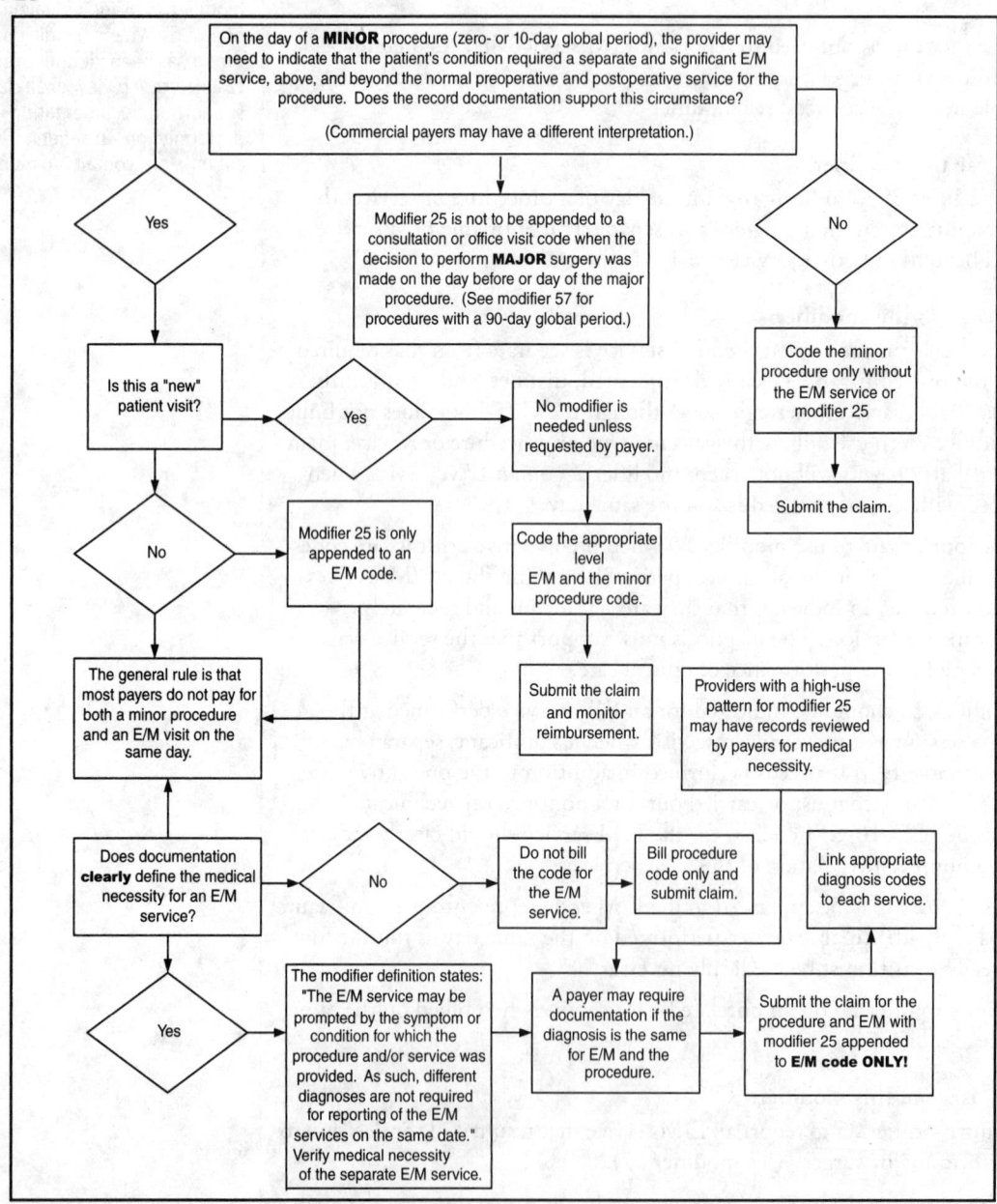

26   Professional Component

Certain procedures are a combination of a physician or other qualified health care professional component and a technical component. When the physician or other qualified health care professional component is reported separately, the service may be identified by adding modifier 26 to the usual procedure number.

When to use this modifier:

Modifier 26 should be used when the provider is rendering only the professional component of a global procedure or service code. This modifier is never reported on evaluation and management service codes.

> *Example*
> Complex dynamic pharyngeal and speech evaluation by cine or video recording is performed in an outpatient hospital setting. Report code 70371 with modifier 26.

Correct usage of this modifier:

Modifier 26 is used in those instances in which a physician is providing the interpretation of the diagnostic test/study performed. The interpretation of the diagnostic test or study is a patient-specific service that is separate, distinct, written, and signed.

- Modifier 26 is appended to procedures that have a "1" in the PC/TC field on the MPFSDB

Incorrect usage of this modifier:

- Using modifiers 26 and TC for a technical component (except for purchased diagnostic tests) when a diagnostic test or radiology service is performed globally (both components are performed by the same provider). When a global service is performed, the code representing the complete service should be reported without modifiers. The payment for the global service reflects the allowances for both components.

- Using modifier 26 for a re-read of results of an interpretation initially provided by another physician.

- Reporting modifier 26, indicating that only the professional portion of the service was provided, and modifier 52, for reduced services together. It is not necessary to use modifier 52 because the professional component modifier already indicates that only a portion of the complete service was performed.

🖥 **SPECIAL ALERT**

In order to use the professional component modifier 26, the provider must prepare a written report that includes findings, relevant clinical issues, and, if appropriate, comparative data. If a postpayment review of the medical record reveals that no separate written interpretive report exists, overpayment recoveries may be sought.

The following flow chart can aid in an audit by helping determine if modifier 26 is being used correctly and whether additional documentation might be required.

Modifier 26

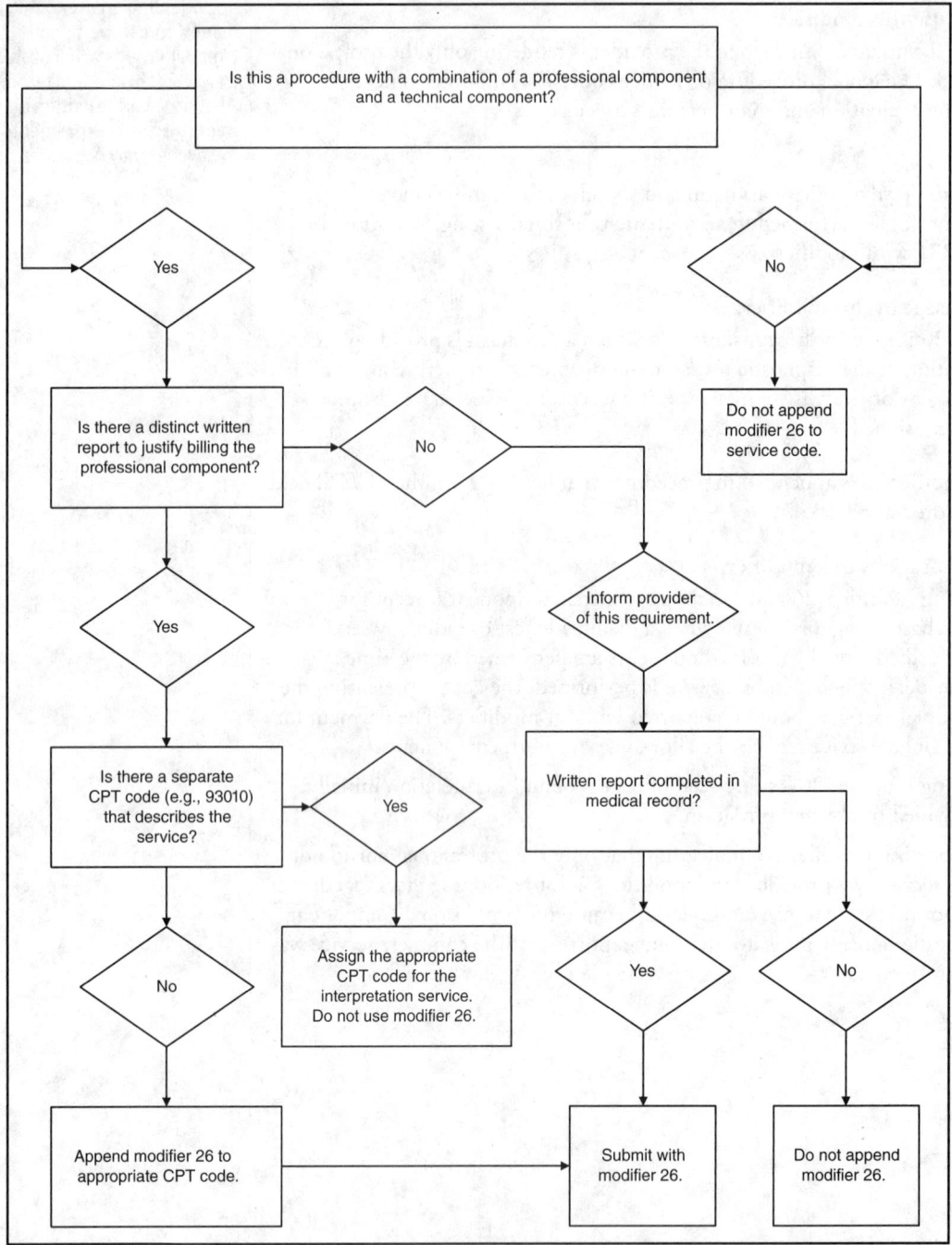

© 2020 Optum360, LLC

32   Mandated Services

Services related to *mandated* consultation and/or related service (e.g., third-party payer, governmental, legislative, or regulatory requirement) may be identified by adding modifier 32 to the basic procedure.

When to use this modifier:

This modifier is used to report that the service provided was at the request of an appropriate source, such as a third-party payer, governmental, legislative, or regulatory requirement. Append modifier 32 to the basic procedure.

> #### Example
> The unmarried parents of a 3-month-old female infant are ordered by the court to undergo DNA testing to determine paternity and establish court-ordered visitation and child support as appropriate. The laboratory performing the testing would report the service and append modifier 32 to indicate that the testing is being conducted at the judge's request.

Correct usage of this modifier:

- Modifier 32 should be used when the provider is aware of third-party involvement regarding mandated services.

- Modifier 32 may be appended to all sections of CPT.

Incorrect usage of this modifier:

- This modifier should not be used when a patient or family member requests a second opinion from another provider.

- Reporting modifier 32 for second opinions or confirmatory consultations requested by the patient or the patient's family.

- Reporting modifier 32 when another physician evaluates a patient for medical clearance prior to a procedure.

🖥 SPECIAL ALERT

A common example of using modifier 32 appropriately is when a third-party payer requests that the patient see a different provider for another opinion. The provider rendering the opinion would append modifier 32 to the E/M service code to indicate that a third-party requested this service.

The following flow chart can aid in an audit by helping determine if modifier 32 is being used correctly and whether additional documentation might be required.

Modifier 32

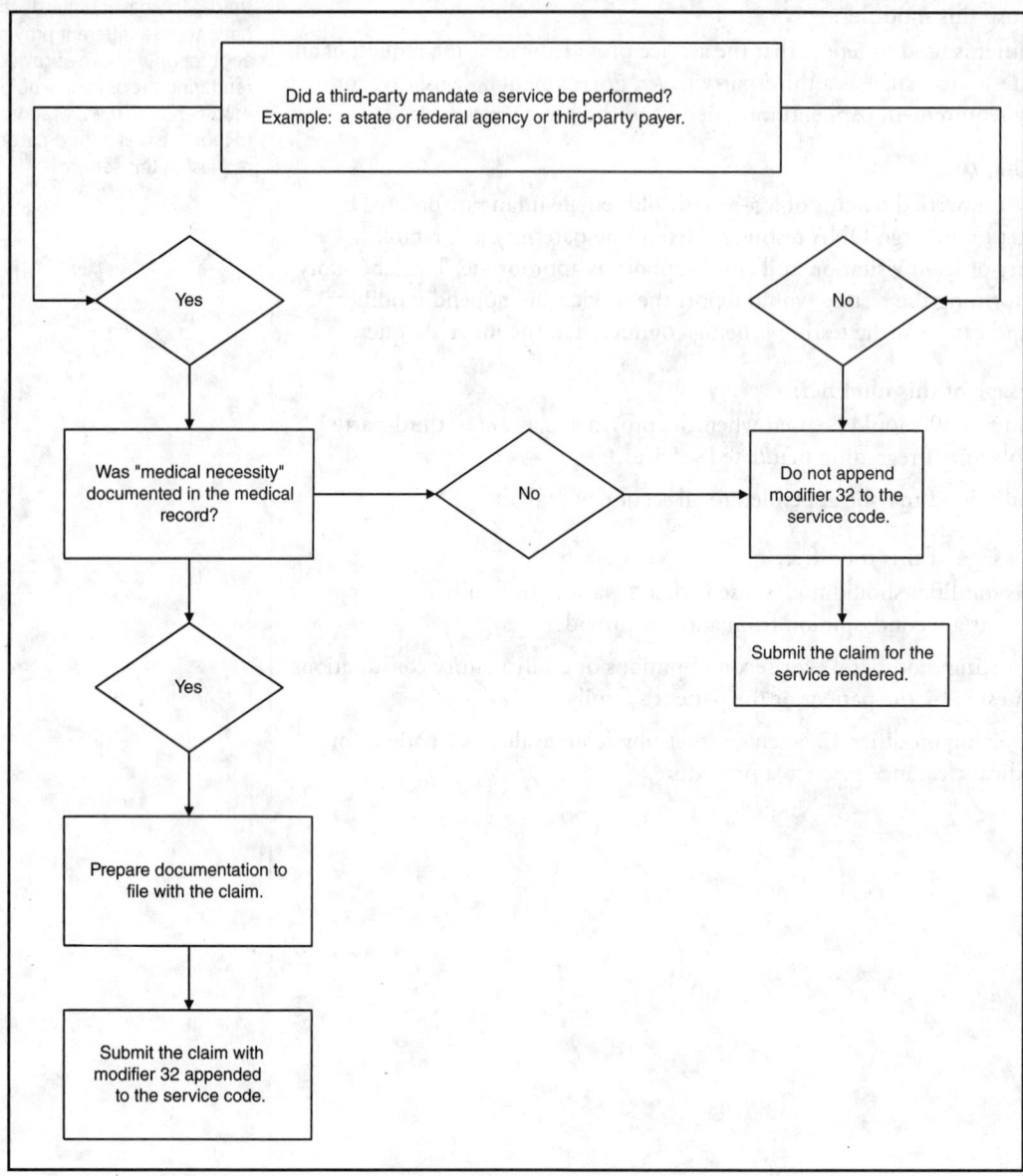

33   Preventive Service

When the primary purpose of the service is the delivery of an evidence-based service in accordance with a US Preventive Services Task Force A or B rating in effect and other preventive services identified in preventive services mandates (legislative or regulatory), the service may be identified by adding 33 to the procedure code. For separately reported services specifically identified as preventive, the modifier should not be used.

When to use this modifier:

This modifier should be reported with codes that represent preventive services with the exception of those codes that are inherently preventive, such as a screening mammography or an immunization recognized by the Advisory Committee on Immunization Practices (ACIP).

Correct usage of this modifier:

- This modifier should be used when the service is listed with an A or B rating per US Preventive Services Task Force.

- Modifier 33 is applicable for identifying preventive services without an associated cost share in the following four categories:

  1. Services rated "A" or "B" by the USPSTF (see table on the following page) as posted annually on the Agency for Healthcare Research and Quality's website: https://www.uspreventiveservicestaskforce.org/uspstf/recommendation-topics/uspstf-and-b-recommendations

  2. Immunizations for routine use in children, adolescents, and adults, as recommended by the Advisory Committee on Immunization Practices of the Centers for Disease Control and Prevention.

  3. Preventive care and screenings for children as recommended by Bright Futures (American Academy of Pediatrics) and Newborn Testing (American College of Medical Genetics) as supported by the Health Resources and Services Administration.

  4. Preventive care and screenings provided for women (not included in the task force recommendations) in the comprehensive guidelines supported by the Health Resources and Services Administration.

- A and B rated services are those recommended by the USPSTF to be offered or provided.

- When multiple preventive medicine services are performed on the same day, modifier 33 should be appended to each of the individual codes representing the specific services.

- Modifier 33 is also useful in helping to identify services that began as preventive but were subsequently converted to a therapeutic procedure. For example, a patient having a screening colonoscopy undergoes a polypectomy via snare technique due to the presence of a colon polyp.

Incorrect usage of this modifier:

- Modifier 33 should not be used for separately reported services specifically identified as preventive (99381-99429).

> 🖥 **SPECIAL ALERT**
>
> Modifier 33 should not be appended to codes for any services that are inherently preventive.

The following is a list of preventive services that have a rating of A or B from the U.S. Preventive Services Task Force that are relevant for implementing the Affordable Care Act.

USPSTF A and B Recommendations by Date

Topic	Description	Grade	Release Date of Current Recommendation
Abdominal Aortic Aneurysm: Screening: men aged 65 to 75 years who have ever smoked	The USPSTF recommends 1-time screening for abdominal aortic aneurysm (AAA) with ultrasonography in men aged 65 to 75 years who have ever smoked.	B	December 2019*
Abnormal Blood Glucose and Type 2 Diabetes Mellitus: Screening: adults aged 40 to 70 years who are overweight or obese	The USPSTF recommends screening for abnormal blood glucose as part of cardiovascular risk assessment in adults aged 40 to 70 years who are overweight or obese. Clinicians should offer or refer patients with abnormal blood glucose to intensive behavioral counseling interventions to promote a healthful diet and physical activity.	B	October 2015*
Aspirin Use to Prevent Cardiovascular Disease and Colorectal Cancer: Preventive Medication: adults aged 50 to 59 years with a ≥10% 10-year cvd risk	The USPSTF recommends initiating low-dose aspirin use for the primary prevention of cardiovascular disease (CVD) and colorectal cancer (CRC) in adults aged 50 to 59 years who have a 10% or greater 10-year CVD risk, are not at increased risk for bleeding, have a life expectancy of at least 10 years, and are willing to take low-dose aspirin daily for at least 10 years.	B	April 2016*
Asymptomatic Bacteriuria in Adults: Screening: pregnant persons	The USPSTF recommends screening for asymptomatic bacteriuria using urine culture in pregnant persons.	B	September 2019*
BRCA-Related Cancer: Risk Assessment, Genetic Counseling, and Genetic Testing: women with a personal or family history of breast, ovarian, tubal, or peritoneal cancer or an ancestry associated with brca1/2 gene mutation	The USPSTF recommends that primary care clinicians assess women with a personal or family history of breast, ovarian, tubal, or peritoneal cancer or who have an ancestry associated with breast cancer susceptibility 1 and 2 (BRCA1/2) gene mutations with an appropriate brief familial risk assessment tool. Women with a positive result on the risk assessment tool should receive genetic counseling and, if indicated after counseling, genetic testing.	B	August 2019*
Breast Cancer: Medication Use to Reduce Risk: women at increased risk for breast cancer	The USPSTF recommends that clinicians offer to prescribe risk-reducing medications, such as tamoxifen, raloxifene, or aromatase inhibitors, to women who are at increased risk for breast cancer and at low risk for adverse medication effects.	B	September 2019*
Breast Cancer: Screening: women aged 50 to 74 years	The USPSTF recommends biennial screening mammography for women aged 50 to 74 years. †	B	January 2016*
Breastfeeding: Primary Care Interventions: pregnant women, new mothers, and their children	The USPSTF recommends providing interventions during pregnancy and after birth to support breastfeeding.	B	October 2016*
Cervical Cancer: Screening: women aged 21 to 65 years	The USPSTF recommends screening for cervical cancer every 3 years with cervical cytology alone in women aged 21 to 29 years. For women aged 30 to 65 years, the USPSTF recommends screening every 3 years with cervical cytology alone, every 5 years with high-risk human papillomavirus (hrHPV) testing alone, or every 5 years with hrHPV testing in combination with cytology (cotesting). See the Clinical Considerations section for the relative benefits and harms of alternative screening strategies for women 21 years or older.	A	August 2018*

† The Department of Health and Human Services, under the standards set out in revised Section 2713(a)(5) of the Public Health Service Act and Section 9(h)(v)(229) of the 2015 Consolidated Appropriations Act, utilizes the 2002 recommendation on breast cancer screening of the U.S. Preventive Services Task Force. To see the USPSTF 2016 recommendation on breast cancer screening, go to http://www.uspreventiveservicestaskforce.org/uspstf/recommendation/breast-cancer-screening1.

* Previous recommendation was an "A" or "B."

 © 2020 Optum360, LLC

Topic	Description	Grade	Release Date of Current Recommendation
Colorectal Cancer: Screening: adults aged 50 to 75 years	The USPSTF recommends screening for colorectal cancer starting at age 50 years and continuing until age 75 years. The risks and benefits of different screening methods vary. See the Clinical Considerations section and the Table for details about screening strategies.	A	June 2016*
Dental Caries in Children from Birth Through Age 5 Years: Screening: children from birth through age 5 years	The USPSTF recommends that primary care clinicians prescribe oral fluoride supplementation starting at age 6 months for children whose water supply is deficient in fluoride.	B	September 2014*
Dental Caries in Children from Birth Through Age 5 Years: Screening: children from birth through age 5 years	The USPSTF recommends that primary care clinicians apply fluoride varnish to the primary teeth of all infants and children starting at the age of primary tooth eruption.	B	September 2014*
Depression in Adults: Screening: general adult population, including pregnant and postpartum women	The USPSTF recommends screening for depression in the general adult population, including pregnant and postpartum women. Screening should be implemented with adequate systems in place to ensure accurate diagnosis, effective treatment, and appropriate follow-up.	B	January 2016*
Depression in Children and Adolescents: Screening: adolescents aged 12 to 18 years	The USPSTF recommends screening for major depressive disorder (MDD) in adolescents aged 12 to 18 years. Screening should be implemented with adequate systems in place to ensure accurate diagnosis, effective treatment, and appropriate follow-up.	B	February 2016*
Falls Prevention in Community-Dwelling Older Adults: Interventions: adults 65 years or older	The USPSTF recommends exercise interventions to prevent falls in community-dwelling adults 65 years or older who are at increased risk for falls.	B	April 2018*
Folic Acid for the Prevention of Neural Tube Defects: Preventive Medication: women who are planning or capable of pregnancy	The USPSTF recommends that all women who are planning or capable of pregnancy take a daily supplement containing 0.4 to 0.8 mg (400 to 800 µg) of folic acid.	A	January 2017*
Gestational Diabetes Mellitus, Screening: asymptomatic pregnant women, after 24 weeks of gestation	The USPSTF recommends screening for gestational diabetes mellitus (GDM) in asymptomatic pregnant women after 24 weeks of gestation.	B	September 2014
Chlamydia and Gonorrhea: Screening: sexually active women	The USPSTF recommends screening for gonorrhea in sexually active women age 24 years and younger and in older women who are at increased risk for infection.	B	September 2014*
Chlamydia and Gonorrhea: Screening: sexually active women	The USPSTF recommends screening for chlamydia in sexually active women age 24 years and younger and in older women who are at increased risk for infection.	B	September 2014*
Healthful Diet and Physical Activity for Cardiovascular Disease Prevention in Adults With Cardiovascular Risk Factors: Behavioral Counseling: adults who are overweight or obese and have additional cvd risk factors	The USPSTF recommends offering or referring adults who are overweight or obese and have additional cardiovascular disease (CVD) risk factors to intensive behavioral counseling interventions to promote a healthful diet and physical activity for CVD prevention.	B	September 2014

† The Department of Health and Human Services, under the standards set out in revised Section 2713(a)(5) of the Public Health Service Act and Section 9(h)(v)(229) of the 2015 Consolidated Appropriations Act, utilizes the 2002 recommendation on breast cancer screening of the U.S. Preventive Services Task Force. To see the USPSTF 2016 recommendation on breast cancer screening, go to http://www.uspreventiveservicestaskforce.org/uspstf/recommendation/breast-cancer-screening1.

* Previous recommendation was an "A" or "B."

Topic	Description	Grade	Release Date of Current Recommendation
Hepatitis B Virus Infection in Pregnant Women: Screening: pregnant women	The USPSTF recommends screening for hepatitis B virus (HBV) infection in pregnant women at their first prenatal visit	A	July 2019*
Hepatitis B Virus Infection: Screening, 2014: persons at high risk for infection	The USPSTF recommends screening for hepatitis B virus (HBV) infection in persons at high risk for infection.	B	September 2014
Hepatitis C Virus Infection in Adolescents and Adults: Screening: adults aged 18 to 79 years	The USPSTF recommends screening for hepatitis C virus (HCV) infection in adults aged 18 to 79 years.	B	March 2020*
Human Immunodeficiency Virus (HIV) Infection: Screening: pregnant persons	The USPSTF recommends that clinicians screen for HIV infection in all pregnant persons, including those who present in labor or at delivery whose HIV status is unknown.	A	June 2019*
Human Immunodeficiency Virus (HIV) Infection: Screening: adolescents and adults aged 15 to 65 years	The USPSTF recommends that clinicians screen for HIV infection in adolescents and adults aged 15 to 65 years. Younger adolescents and older adults who are at increased risk of infection should also be screened. See the Clinical Considerations section for more information about assessment of risk, screening intervals, and rescreening in pregnancy.	A	June 2019*
High Blood Pressure in Adults: Screening: adults aged 18 years or older	The USPSTF recommends screening for high blood pressure in adults aged 18 years or older. The USPSTF recommends obtaining measurements outside of the clinical setting for diagnostic confirmation before starting treatment (see the Clinical Considerations section).	A	October 2015*
Intimate Partner Violence, Elder Abuse, and Abuse of Vulnerable Adults: Screening: women of reproductive age	The USPSTF recommends that clinicians screen for intimate partner violence (IPV) in women of reproductive age and provide or refer women who screen positive to ongoing support services. See the Clinical Considerations section for more information on effective ongoing support services for IPV and for information on IPV in men.	B	October 2018*
Latent Tuberculosis Infection: Screening: asymptomatic adults at increased risk for infection	The USPSTF recommends screening for latent tuberculosis infection (LTBI) in populations at increased risk.	B	September 2016*
Low-Dose Aspirin Use for the Prevention of Morbidity and Mortality From Preeclampsia: Preventive Medication : pregnant women who are at high risk for preeclampsia	The USPSTF recommends the use of low-dose aspirin (81 mg/d) as preventive medication after 12 weeks of gestation in women who are at high risk for preeclampsia.	B	September 2014
Lung Cancer: Screening: adults aged 55-80, with a history of smoking	The USPSTF recommends annual screening for lung cancer with low-dose computed tomography (LDCT) in adults aged 55 to 80 years who have a 30 pack-year smoking history and currently smoke or have quit within the past 15 years. Screening should be discontinued once a person has not smoked for 15 years or develops a health problem that substantially limits life expectancy or the ability or willingness to have curative lung surgery.	B	September 2014
Obesity in Children and Adolescents: Screening: children and adolescents 6 years and older	The USPSTF recommends that clinicians screen for obesity in children and adolescents 6 years and older and offer or refer them to comprehensive, intensive behavioral interventions to promote improvements in weight status.	B	June 2017*

† The Department of Health and Human Services, under the standards set out in revised Section 2713(a)(5) of the Public Health Service Act and Section 9(h)(v)(229) of the 2015 Consolidated Appropriations Act, utilizes the 2002 recommendation on breast cancer screening of the U.S. Preventive Services Task Force. To see the USPSTF 2016 recommendation on breast cancer screening, go to http://www.uspreventiveservicestaskforce.org/uspstf/recommendation/breast-cancer-screening1.

* Previous recommendation was an "A" or "B."

Topic	Description	Grade	Release Date of Current Recommendation
Ocular Prophylaxis for Gonococcal Ophthalmia Neonatorum: Preventive Medication: newborns	The USPSTF recommends prophylactic ocular topical medication for all newborns to prevent gonococcal ophthalmia neonatorum.	A	January 2019*
Osteoporosis to Prevent Fractures: Screening: postmenopausal women younger than 65 years at increased risk of osteoporosis	The USPSTF recommends screening for osteoporosis with bone measurement testing to prevent osteoporotic fractures in postmenopausal women younger than 65 years who are at increased risk of osteoporosis, as determined by a formal clinical risk assessment tool. See the Clinical Considerations section for information on risk assessment.	B	June 2018*
Osteoporosis to Prevent Fractures: Screening: women 65 years and older	The USPSTF recommends screening for osteoporosis with bone measurement testing to prevent osteoporotic fractures in women 65 years and older.	B	June 2018*
Perinatal Depression: Preventive Interventions: pregnant and postpartum persons	The USPSTF recommends that clinicians provide or refer pregnant and postpartum persons who are at increased risk of perinatal depression to counseling interventions.	B	February 2019
Preeclampsia: Screening: pregnant woman	The USPSTF recommends screening for preeclampsia in pregnant women with blood pressure measurements throughout pregnancy.	B	April 2017*
Prevention of Human Immunodeficiency Virus (HIV) Infection: Preexposure Prophylaxis: persons at high risk of hiv acquisition	The USPSTF recommends that clinicians offer preexposure prophylaxis (PrEP) with effective antiretroviral therapy to persons who are at high risk of HIV acquisition. See the Clinical Considerations section for information about identification of persons at high risk and selection of effective antiretroviral therapy.	A	June 2019
Prevention and Cessation of Tobacco Use in Children and Adolescents: Primary Care Interventions: school-aged children and adolescents who have not started to use tobacco	The USPSTF recommends that primary care clinicians provide interventions, including education or brief counseling, to prevent initiation of tobacco use among school-aged children and adolescents.	B	April 2020*
Rh(D) Incompatibility: Screening: unsensitized rh(d)-negative pregnant women	The USPSTF recommends repeated Rh(D) antibody testing for all unsensitized Rh(D)-negative women at 24 to 28 weeks' gestation, unless the biological father is known to be Rh(D)-negative.	B	February 2004*
Rh(D) Incompatibility: Screening: pregnant women, during the first pregnancy-related care visit	The USPSTF strongly recommends Rh(D) blood typing and antibody testing for all pregnant women during their first visit for pregnancy-related care.	A	February 2004*
Sexually Transmitted Infections: Behavioral Counseling: sexually active adolescents and adults at increased risk	The USPSTF recommends behavioral counseling for all sexually active adolescents and for adults who are at increased risk for sexually transmitted infections (STIs). See the Practice Considerations section for more information on populations at increased risk for acquiring STIs.	B	August 2020*
Skin Cancer Prevention: Behavioral Counseling: young adults, adolescents, children, and parents of young children	The USPSTF recommends counseling young adults, adolescents, children, and parents of young children about minimizing exposure to ultraviolet (UV) radiation for persons aged 6 months to 24 years with fair skin types to reduce their risk of skin cancer.	B	March 2018*

† The Department of Health and Human Services, under the standards set out in revised Section 2713(a)(5) of the Public Health Service Act and Section 9(h)(v)(229) of the 2015 Consolidated Appropriations Act, utilizes the 2002 recommendation on breast cancer screening of the U.S. Preventive Services Task Force. To see the USPSTF 2016 recommendation on breast cancer screening, go to http://www.uspreventiveservicestaskforce.org/uspstf/recommendation/breast-cancer-screening1.

* Previous recommendation was an "A" or "B."

Topic	Description	Grade	Release Date of Current Recommendation
Statin Use for the Primary Prevention of Cardiovascular Disease in Adults: Preventive Medication: adults aged 40 to 75 years with no history of cvd, 1 or more cvd risk factors, and a calculated 10-year cvd event risk of 10% or greater	The USPSTF recommends that adults without a history of cardiovascular disease (CVD) (ie, symptomatic coronary artery disease or ischemic stroke) use a low- to moderate-dose statin for the prevention of CVD events and mortality when all of the following criteria are met: 1) they are aged 40 to 75 years; 2) they have 1 or more CVD risk factors (ie, dyslipidemia, diabetes, hypertension, or smoking); and 3) they have a calculated 10-year risk of a cardiovascular event of 10% or greater. Identification of dyslipidemia and calculation of 10-year CVD event risk requires universal lipids screening in adults aged 40 to 75 years. See the "Clinical Considerations" section for more information on lipids screening and the assessment of cardiovascular risk.	B	November 2016*
Syphilis Infection in Nonpregnant Adults and Adolescents: Screening : asymptomatic, nonpregnant adults and adolescents who are at increased risk for syphilis infection	The USPSTF recommends screening for syphilis infection in persons who are at increased risk for infection.	A	June 2016*
Syphilis Infection in Pregnant Women: Screening: pregnant women	The USPSTF recommends early screening for syphilis infection in all pregnant women.	A	September 2018*
Tobacco Smoking Cessation in Adults, Including Pregnant Women: Behavioral and Pharmacotherapy Interventions: pregnant women	The USPSTF recommends that clinicians ask all pregnant women about tobacco use, advise them to stop using tobacco, and provide behavioral interventions for cessation to pregnant women who use tobacco.	A	September 2015*
Tobacco Smoking Cessation in Adults, Including Pregnant Women: Behavioral and Pharmacotherapy Interventions: adults who are not pregnant	The USPSTF recommends that clinicians ask all adults about tobacco use, advise them to stop using tobacco, and provide behavioral interventions and U.S. Food and Drug Administration (FDA)-approved pharmacotherapy for cessation to adults who use tobacco.	A	September 2015*
Unhealthy Alcohol Use in Adolescents and Adults: Screening and Behavioral Counseling Interventions: adults 18 years or older, including pregnant women	The USPSTF recommends screening for unhealthy alcohol use in primary care settings in adults 18 years or older, including pregnant women, and providing persons engaged in risky or hazardous drinking with brief behavioral counseling interventions to reduce unhealthy alcohol use.	B	November 2018*
Unhealthy Drug Use: Screening: adults age 18 years or older	The USPSTF recommends screening by asking questions about unhealthy drug use in adults age 18 years or older. Screening should be implemented when services for accurate diagnosis, effective treatment, and appropriate care can be offered or referred. (Screening refers to asking questions about unhealthy drug use, not testing biological specimens.)	B	June 2020
Vision in Children Ages 6 Months to 5 Years: Screening: children aged 3 to 5 years	The USPSTF recommends vision screening at least once in all children aged 3 to 5 years to detect amblyopia or its risk factors.	B	September 2017*
Weight Loss to Prevent Obesity-Related Morbidity and Mortality in Adults: Behavioral Interventions: adults	The USPSTF recommends that clinicians offer or refer adults with a body mass index (BMI) of 30 or higher (calculated as weight in kilograms divided by height in meters squared) to intensive, multicomponent behavioral interventions.	B	September 2018*

† The Department of Health and Human Services, under the standards set out in revised Section 2713(a)(5) of the Public Health Service Act and Section 9(h)(v)(229) of the 2015 Consolidated Appropriations Act, utilizes the 2002 recommendation on breast cancer screening of the U.S. Preventive Services Task Force. To see the USPSTF 2016 recommendation on breast cancer screening, go to http://www.uspreventiveservicestaskforce.org/uspstf/recommendation/breast-cancer-screening1.

* Previous recommendation was an "A" or "B."

The following flow chart can aid in an audit by helping determine if modifier 33 is being used correctly and whether additional documentation might be required.

Modifier 33

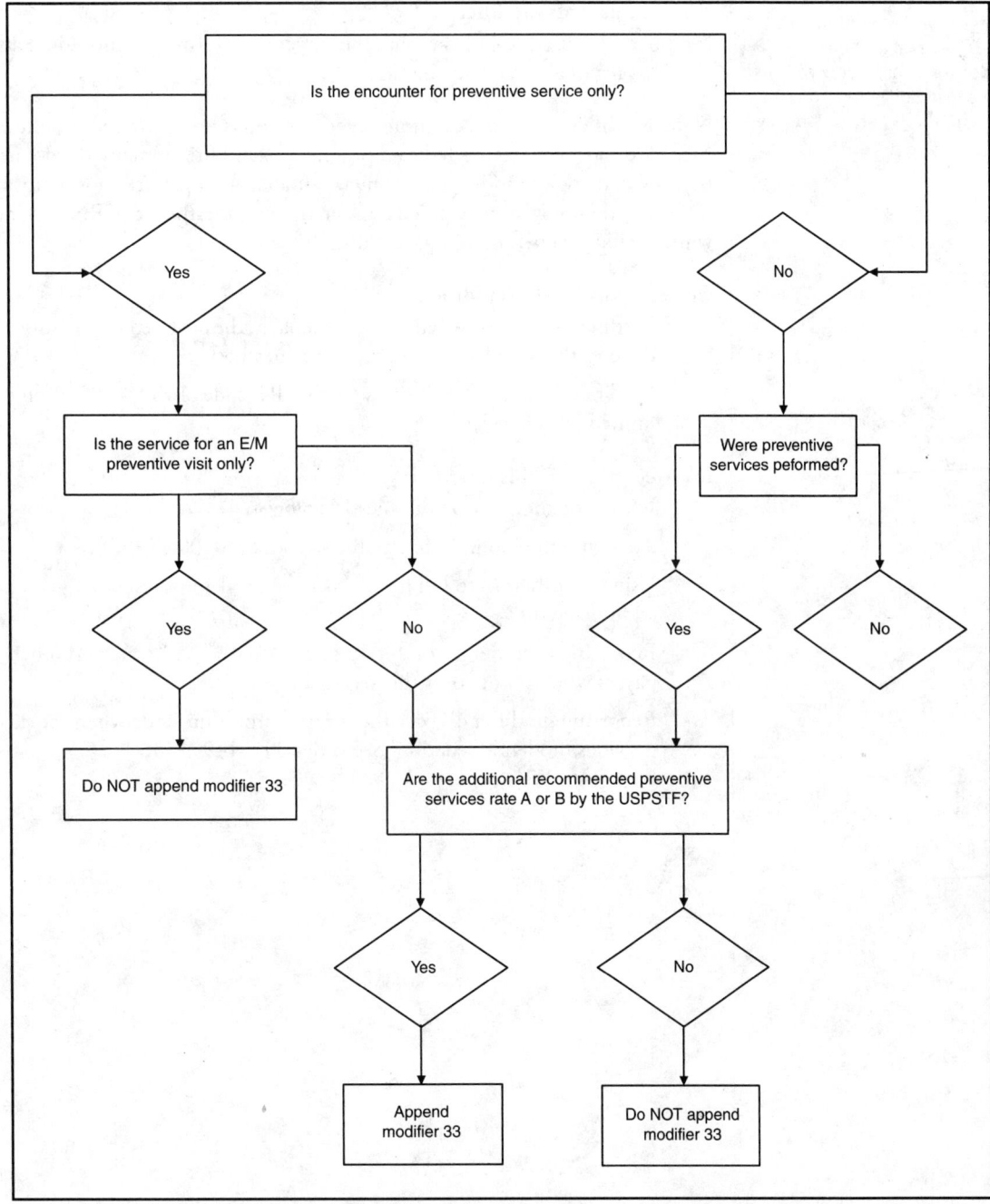

47 Anesthesia by Surgeon

Regional or general anesthesia provided by the surgeon may be reported by adding modifier 47 to the basic service. (This does not include local anesthesia.) **Note:** Modifier 47 would not be used as a modifier for the anesthesia procedures.

When to use this modifier:

Modifier 47 is used to indicate that the surgeon performing a procedure also provided regional or general anesthesia.

Note: Modifier 47 is not commonly reported and is not a covered benefit under Medicare and many state Medicaid programs. In addition, many third-party payers will deny any additional payment for anesthesia services not performed by an anesthesiologist or certified registered nurse anesthetist (CRNA). Check with specific payers for coverage details.

Correct usage of this modifier:

- Modifier 47 is used when the anesthesia is administered by the surgeon. It denotes the use of regional or general anesthesia.

- Modifier 47 is approved for use with CPT codes 10004–69990 unless limited by the payer.

Incorrect usage of this modifier:

- Use of the modifier by the anesthesiologist.

- Attaching the modifier to anesthesia codes (00100–01999).

- Using modifier 47 to bill for payment of local anesthesia a surgeon has administered.

- Reporting modifier 47 on services submitted to Medicare and other payers who do not cover this service.

- Reporting modifier 47 with the surgical procedure code when the surgeon provides moderate sedation. See codes 99151–99153.

The following flow chart can aid in an audit by helping determine if modifier 47 is being used correctly and whether additional documentation might be required.

Modifier 47

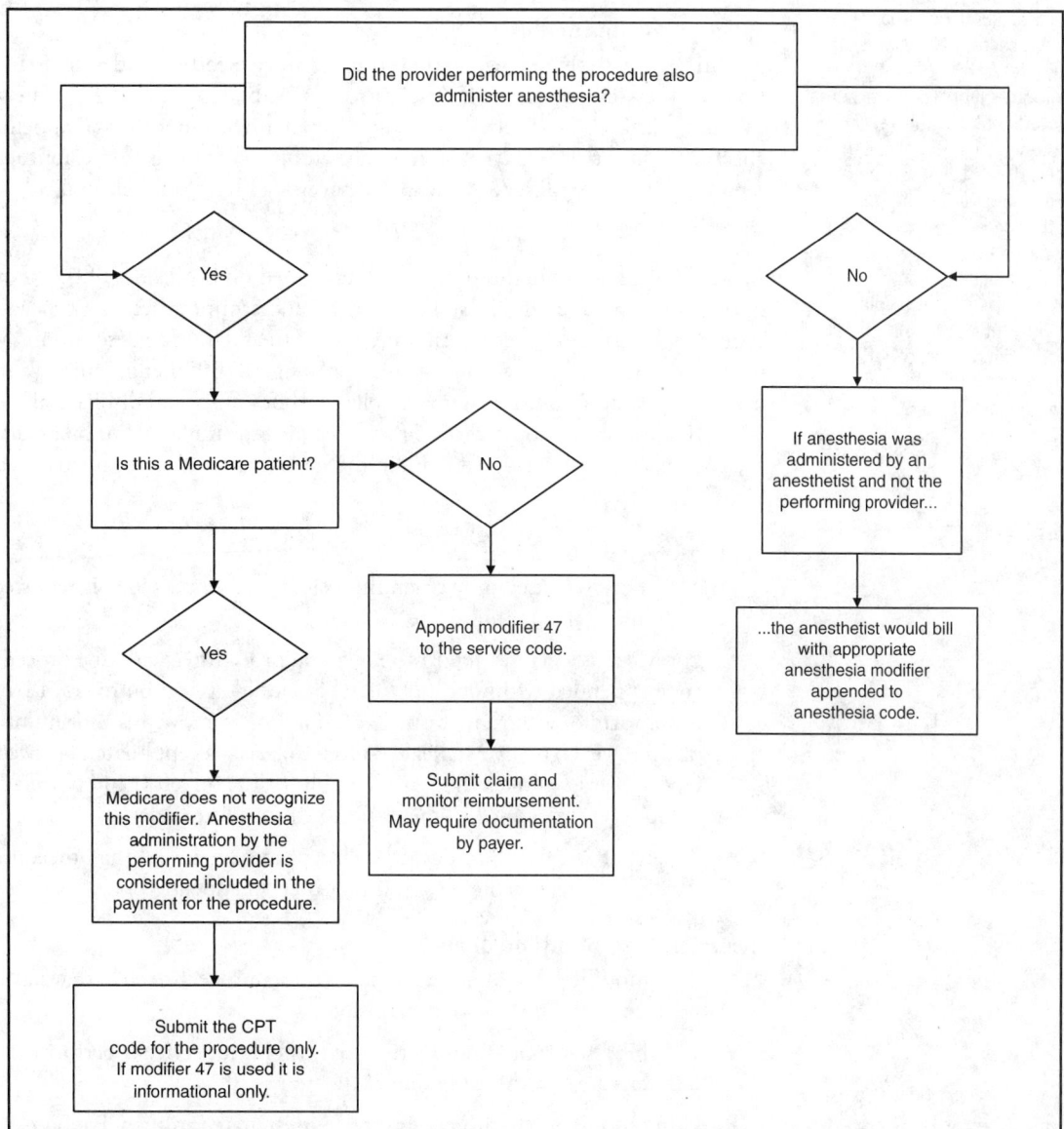

🖥️ **SPECIAL ALERT**

Medicare guidelines for the use of modifier 50 differ among many third-party payers. The CMS *Internet Only Manual* (IOM), Pub.100-04, chapter 12, section 40.7 states, "If a procedure is not identified by its terminology as a bilateral procedure (or unilateral or bilateral), report the procedure with modifier 50. Report such procedures as a single line item." For example, if a bilateral otoplasty procedure was performed on a Medicare patient, the procedure would be reported as follows: 69300-50 Otoplasty, protruding ear, with or without size reduction. The second, or bilateral, procedure is made inherent in the one line-item by appending modifier 50 to the procedure code.

50   Bilateral Procedure

Unless otherwise identified in the listings, bilateral procedures that are performed at the same session should be identified by adding modifier 50 to the appropriate 5 digit code. **Note:** This modifier should not be appended to designated "add-on" codes (see Appendix D).

When to use this modifier:

Modifier 50 is appended to the procedure or service code that describes a unilateral service performed on the mirror image body part or organ. The code should typically be submitted as a single line item with modifier 50 appended; check with the specific payer for guidance and instruction as to the appropriate reporting of this modifier as third-party payers can have different policies concerning its use.

Bilateral procedures are those surgeries performed on both sides of the body during the same operative session. In order to determine whether a procedure should be billed as "bilateral," carefully review the CPT code description. Many procedure codes include the term "bilateral" (e.g., 27395 Lengthening of the hamstring tendon; multiple tendons, bilateral) or "unilateral or bilateral" (e.g., 52290 Cystourethroscopy; with ureteral meatotomy, unilateral or bilateral) in the code narrative. Codes that contain these terms should never be reported as bilateral services.

Correct usage of this modifier:

- Modifier 50 is used only when the exact same service/code is reported for each bilateral anatomical site.

- For Medicare claims, report the bilateral procedures with one procedure code appended with modifier 50. This should appear on the CMS-1500 claim form or electronic format as a one-line item, with a unit number of one. However, many Medicare contractors also accept bilateral procedures reported as two-line items with the right (RT) and left (LT) HCPCS Level II modifiers appended to the respective procedure codes.

- When the MPFSDB indicator for the procedure is "1," the procedure code can be reported once, with modifier 50 appended.

Incorrect usage of this modifier:

- This modifier should not be appended to a procedure code that has the word bilateral in its CPT description.

- This modifier should not be reported when the service is performed on a different area on the same side of the body.

- Using modifier 51 with codes that are designated in the CPT book as add-on codes. These services are identified by a plus (+) sign next to the code. These codes are listed in Appendix D.

The following flow chart can aid in an audit by helping determine if modifier 50 is being used correctly and whether additional documentation might be required.

Modifier 50

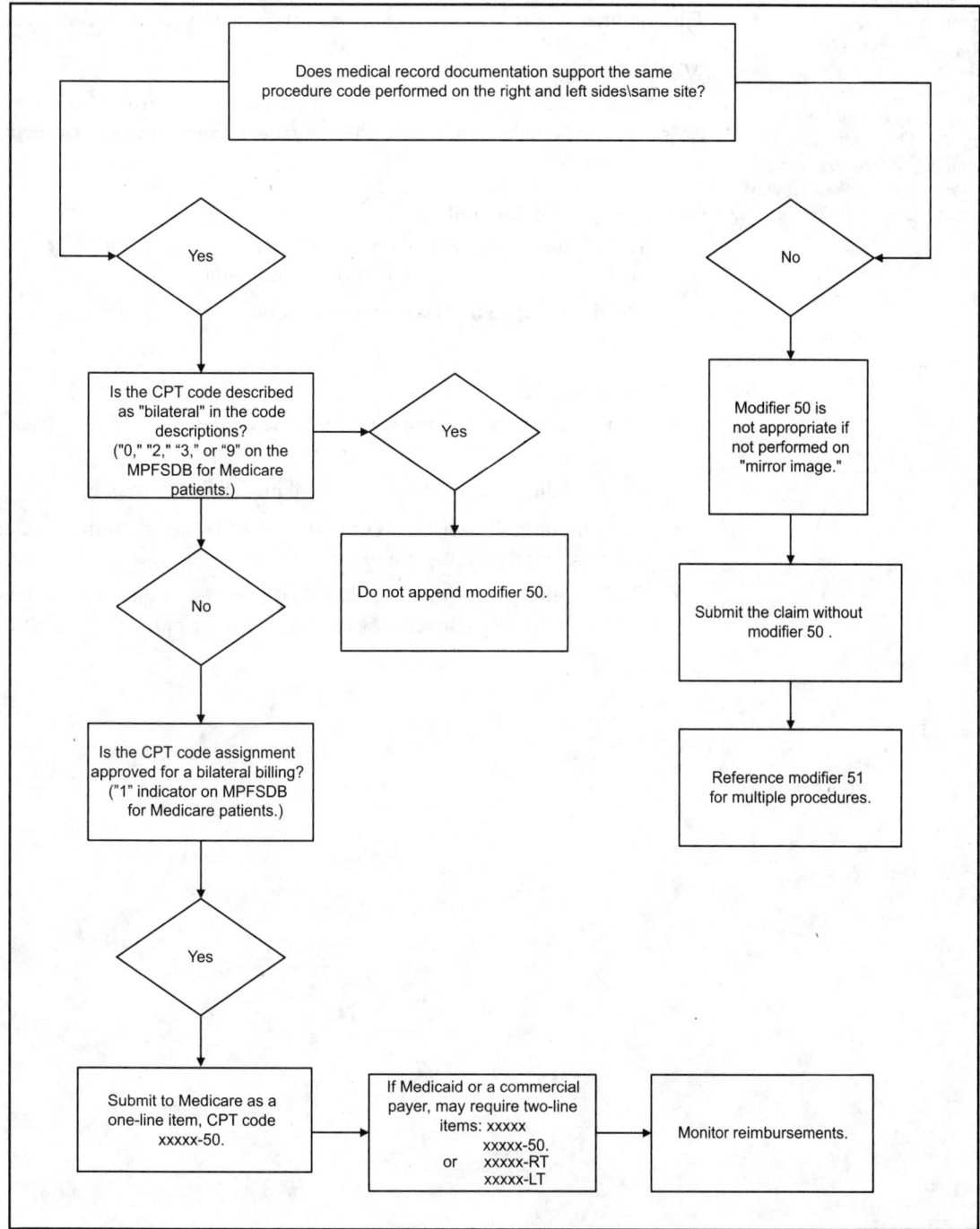

51 Multiple Procedures

When multiple procedures, other than E/M services, Physical Medicine and Rehabilitation services, or provision of supplies (e.g., vaccines), are performed at the same session by the same individual, the primary procedure or service may be reported as listed. The additional procedure(s) or service(s) may be identified by appending modifier 51 to the additional procedure or service code(s). **Note:** This modifier should not be appended to designated "add-on" codes.

When to use this modifier:

Modifier 51 is used to identify subsequent procedures performed on the same day at the same operative session as the primary or main procedure or service by the same provider.

Correct usage of this modifier:

- To indicate that more than one surgical service was performed by the same provider on the same patient at the same session.

- When more than one classification of wound repairs is performed, use modifier 51.

Incorrect usage of this modifier:

- Using modifier 51 on procedures that are considered components of a primary procedure.

- Using modifier 51 to report incidental procedures separately.

- Using modifier 51 when two or more providers each perform distinctly different, unrelated surgeries on the same day.

- Using modifier 51 with codes that are designated in the CPT book as "add-on" codes. These services are identified by a plus (+) sign next to the code.

© 2020 Optum360, LLC

The following flow chart can aid in an audit by helping determine if modifier 51 is being used correctly and whether additional documentation might be required.

Modifier 51

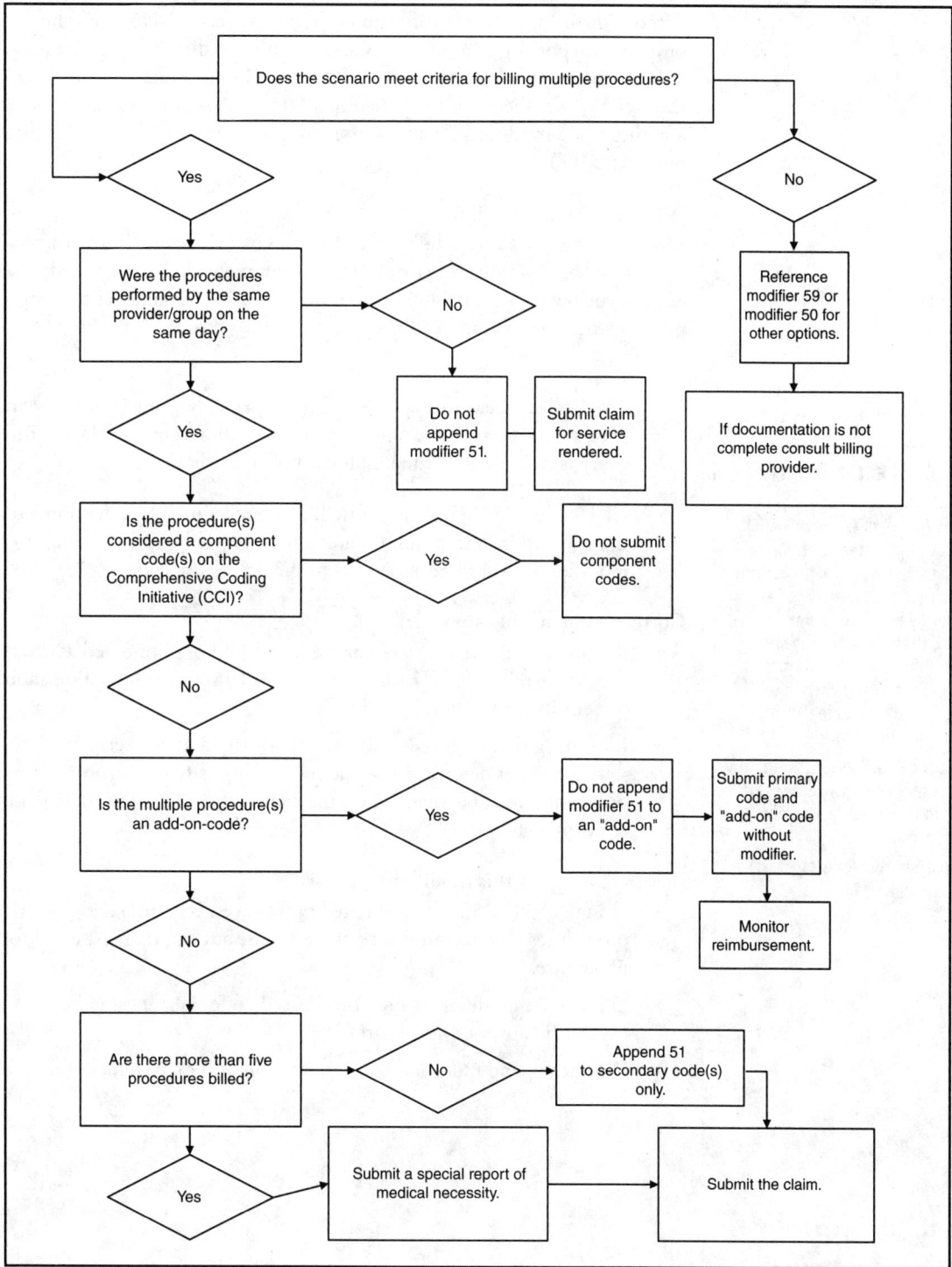

52   Reduced Services

Under certain circumstances a service or procedure is partially reduced or eliminated at the discretion of the physician or other qualified health care professional. Under these circumstances the service provided can be identified by its usual procedure number and the addition of modifier 52, signifying that the service is reduced. This provides a means of reporting reduced services without disturbing the identification of the basic service. **Note:** For hospital outpatient reporting of a previously scheduled procedure/service that is partially reduced or cancelled as a result of extenuating circumstances or those that threaten the well-being of the patient prior to or after administration of anesthesia, see modifiers 73 and 74 (see modifiers approved for ASC hospital outpatient use).

When to use this modifier:

Modifier 52 is used when the provider decides to reduce or eliminate a service or procedure based on his or her professional judgment as demonstrated in the example below in which a procedure is described as bilateral, yet the surgeon performs the service unilaterally.

> *Example*
> A radical trachelectomy, with unilateral pelvic lymphadenectomy and para-aortic lymph node sampling biopsy, with removal of the left tube and ovary is performed for metastatic cervical cancer.
>
> CPT code 57531-52 is submitted. The procedure was not completed per the CPT code description (bilateral total pelvic lymphadenectomy) so modifier 52 would be appended to the procedure code.

Correct usage of this modifier:

- Reporting services that were partially reduced or eliminated at the provider's discretion. Documentation explaining the reduction should be present in the medical record.

- Indicating that a procedure is being performed at a lesser level. A concise statement that describes how the service differs from the normal procedure must be included on the claim or in the appropriate field for electronic claims.

Incorrect usage of this modifier:

- Using modifier 52 for terminated procedures. It is intended for procedures that accomplished some result, but less than expected for the procedure.

- Do not use modifier 52 on a time-based code (i.e., anesthesia, psychotherapy, or critical care).

- Do not append modifier 52 on evaluation and management services.

The following flow chart can aid in an audit by helping determine if modifier 52 is being used correctly and whether additional documentation might be required.

Modifier 52

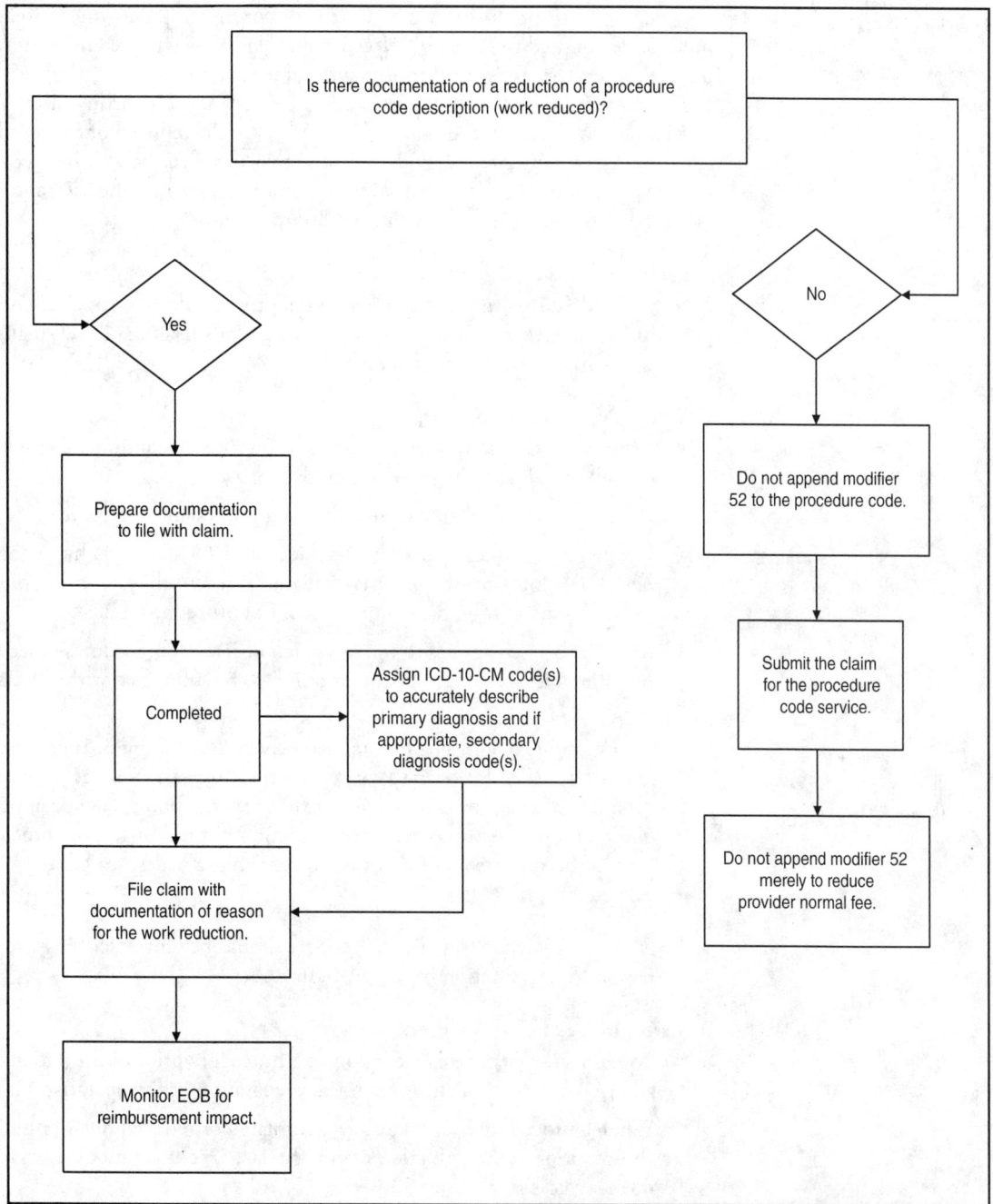

53   Discontinued Procedure

Under certain circumstances, the physician or other qualified health care professional may elect to terminate a surgical or diagnostic procedure. Due to extenuating circumstances or those that threaten the well-being of the patient, it may be necessary to indicate that a surgical or diagnostic procedure was started but discontinued. This circumstance may be reported by adding modifier 53 to the code reported by the individual for the discontinued procedure. **Note:** This modifier is not used to report the elective cancellation of a procedure prior to the patient's anesthesia induction and/or surgical preparation in the operating suite. For outpatient hospital/ambulatory surgery center (ASC) reporting of a previously scheduled procedure/service that is partially reduced or cancelled as a result of extenuating circumstances or those that threaten the well-being of the patient prior to or after administration of anesthesia, see modifiers 73 and 74 (see modifiers approved for ASC hospital outpatient use).

When to use this modifier:

Modifier 53 describes situations in which the provider decides to terminate a procedure or service due to concern over the patient's health and well-being or perhaps due to an extenuating circumstance.

Correct usage of this modifier:

- When a procedure was actually started, but was discontinued before completion due to the patient's condition.

- If the procedure was discontinued after anesthesia was induced.

- If a surgery is discontinued due to uncontrollable bleeding, hypotension, neurologic impairment, or situations that threaten the well-being of the patient, append modifier 53 to the surgical procedure code.

- Modifier 53 also applies to the physician office. All procedures billed with modifier 53 may require documentation to be submitted with the claim.

  Example
  A surgical oncologist begins a radical pelvic exenteration on a patient that had been treated for ovarian cancer in previous years. She has once again been diagnosed with cancer that is extensive and requires a radical pelvic exenteration. The surgeon begins dissection but terminates the procedure when it becomes evident that the cancer is more widespread than expected.

  Submit CPT code 51597-53. A report should be sent describing the reason for termination of the procedure.

Incorrect usage of this modifier:

- To report the elective cancellation of a procedure prior to the patient's anesthesia induction and/or surgical preparation in the operative suite.

- When a procedure is prematurely terminated or reduced due to physician choice, prior to the induction of anesthesia. The correct modifier to report these services is modifier 52.

- Use of modifier 53 on an E/M code.

- Use of modifier 53 with time-based procedure codes (e.g., critical care and psychotherapy).

The following flow chart can aid in an audit by helping determine if modifier 53 is being used correctly and whether additional documentation might be required.

Modifier 53

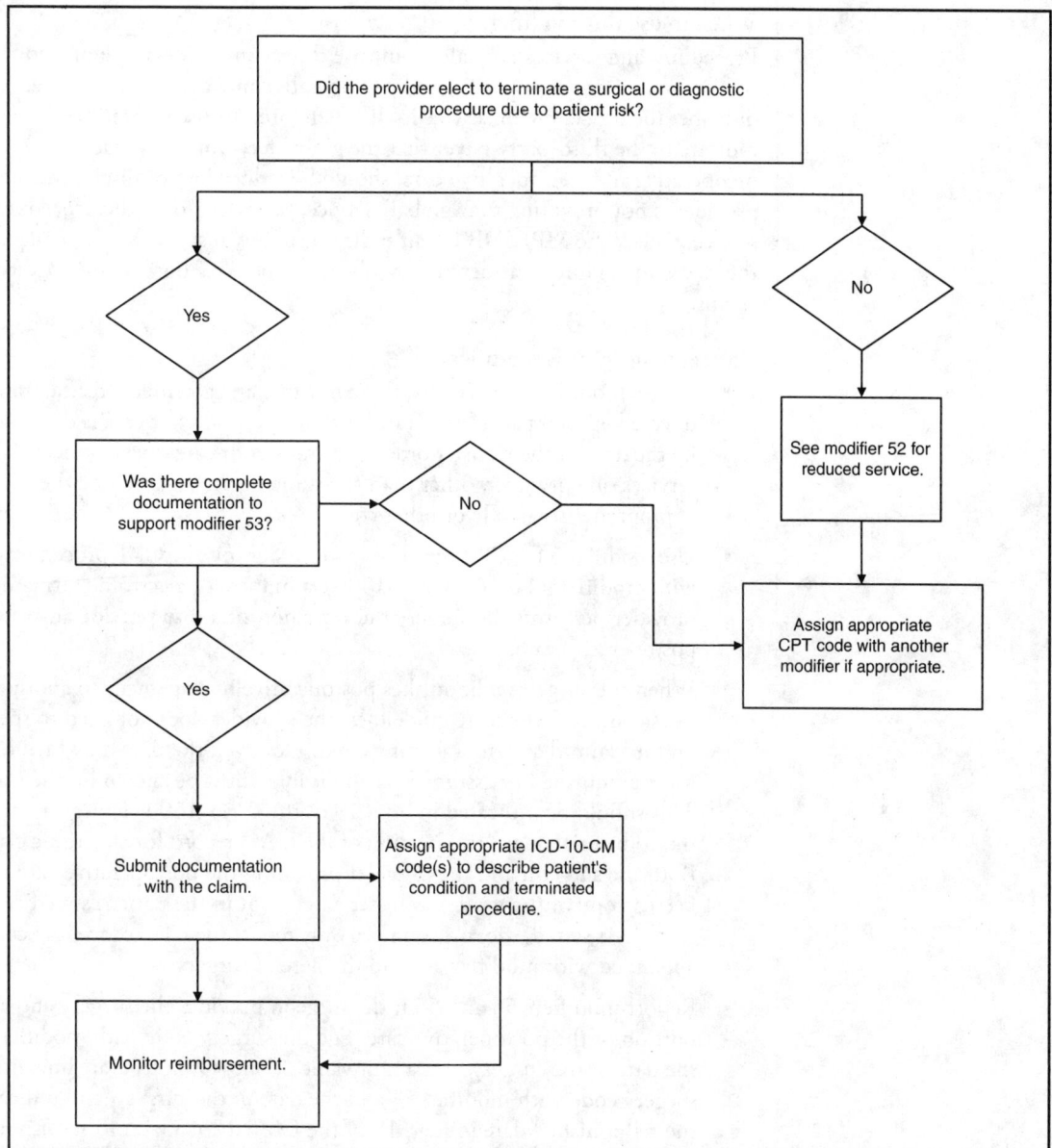

54   Surgical Care Only

When one physician or other qualified health care professional performs a surgical procedure and another provides preoperative and/or postoperative management, surgical services may be identified by adding modifier 54 to the usual procedure number.

When to use this modifier:

Procedures and services typically comprise three components: the procedure or service itself, preoperative care, and postoperative management. Modifier 54 describes the procedure or service itself. Therefore, the use of modifier 54 would indicate to the third-party payer that the global fee, which includes the preoperative and postoperative care, should be reduced accordingly since the provider is not providing the "global" service, but rather only the procedure or service. Check the MPFSDB for an indicator that will show the percentage of the global procedure considered to be the intraoperative portion for Medicare claims.

Correct usage of this modifier:

- To use modifier 54 correctly, there must be an agreement for the transfer of care between providers. Transfer of responsibility of care is determined by the date of the transfer order. If a transfer of care does not occur, the services of a provider, other than the surgeon, are reported by the appropriate E/M code or other code.

- Use modifier 54 with surgical codes only. Submit the CPT procedure code with modifier 54 on the CMS-1500 claim form or electronic format if the provider performs the surgery but does not intend to provide any of the postoperative care.

- When the surgeon relinquishes postoperative management to another physician, per Medicare guidelines, the provider does not need to specify on the claim that care was transferred. However, the date on which care was relinquished or assumed, as applicable, must be shown on the claim. This should be indicated in item 19 of the CMS-1500 claim form or in the appropriate narrative portion of the HAO record for electronic claims. Both the surgeon and the provider providing the postoperative care must keep a copy of the written transfer agreement in the patient's medical record. As stated, the surgeon need only report the CPT procedure code(s) appended with modifier 54, and the date of surgery.

- Report modifiers 54 and 55 if the surgeon provides the surgery and a portion of the postoperative care. File the surgery code with modifier 54, the date of the surgery, and a unit value of one. On a separate line, list the surgery code with modifier 55 and the date of the surgery, and indicate the relinquished date in item 19 of the CMS-1500 claim form or in the appropriate narrative portion of the HAO record for electronic claims.

- For each surgical CPT code, third-party payers have established a certain percentage for each of the three components (i.e., preoperative, intraoperative, and postoperative). If the split care modifiers (54, 55, 56) are used, these percentages help determine payment.

Incorrect usage of this modifier:

- Appending modifier 54 to a surgical procedure without a global surgery period (e.g., global surgery period equal to zero days).

- Using modifier 54 for a minor surgical service (global period zero or 10 days) performed in the ED for a patient who is referred back to his or her primary care physician or other non-ED provider for follow-up care.

- Using modifier 54 for an assistant-at-surgery service.
- Using modifier 54 when the individual is the covering provider (i.e., locum tenens) or part of the same group as the surgeon who performed the procedure and provided most of the postoperative care.

The following flow chart can aid in an audit by helping determine if modifier 54 is being used correctly and whether additional documentation might be required.

Modifier 54

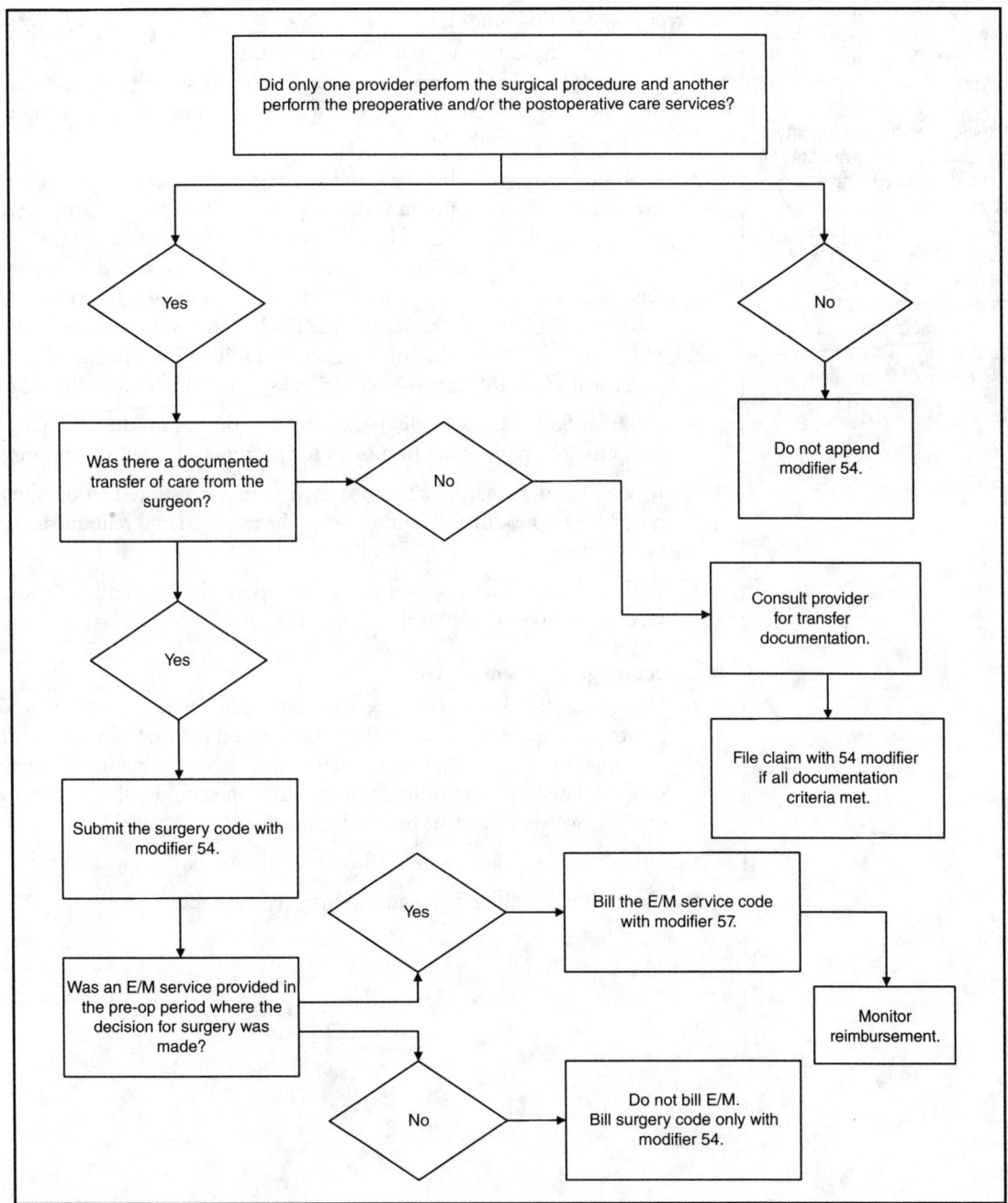

55   Postoperative Management Only

When one physician or other qualified health care professional performed the postoperative management and another performed the surgical procedure, the postoperative component may be identified by adding modifier 55 to the usual procedure number.

When to use this modifier:

Modifier 55 is used to identify the provider performing the postoperative management when one provider performs the postoperative management and another provider performs the surgical procedure.

Correct usage of this modifier:

- Use with surgical codes to indicate that only the postoperative care was performed (i.e., another provider performed the surgery). In this case, the postoperative component may be identified by adding modifier 55 to the CPT procedure code.

- Modifier 55 is appended if a physician or other qualified health care professional does not perform the surgery but does provide a portion of the postoperative care. List the assumed date in item 19 of the CMS-1500 claim form, the surgery code with modifier 55 in item 24d, the date of service in item 24a, and one unit of service in item 24g. Electronic billing software should have a narrative data field for this information in the HAO record. Be sure that information from item 19 is included so the payer will know the date the physician assumed the postoperative care.

- Modifier 55 is used after discharge of the patient from the hospital and only after the patient has been seen for postoperative follow-up care.

- If two providers share the postoperative care, each should report their portion with modifier 55 and indicate the assumed and relinquished dates on the claim.

- CPT codes for use with modifier 55 are appropriate codes in the surgery section (10004–69990) unless limited by the third-party payer.

Incorrect usage of this modifier:

- Using modifier 55 on the surgery code if a physician or other qualified health care professional other than the surgeon provides the inpatient postoperative care when the transfer of care occurs immediately after surgery. The physician other than the surgeon should bill these inpatient services using subsequent hospital care codes (99231–99233).

- Using modifier 55 on a surgical code with zero global days.

- Appending modifier 55 to an E/M procedure code.

The following flow chart can aid in an audit by helping determine if modifier 55 is being used correctly and whether additional documentation might be required.

Modifier 55

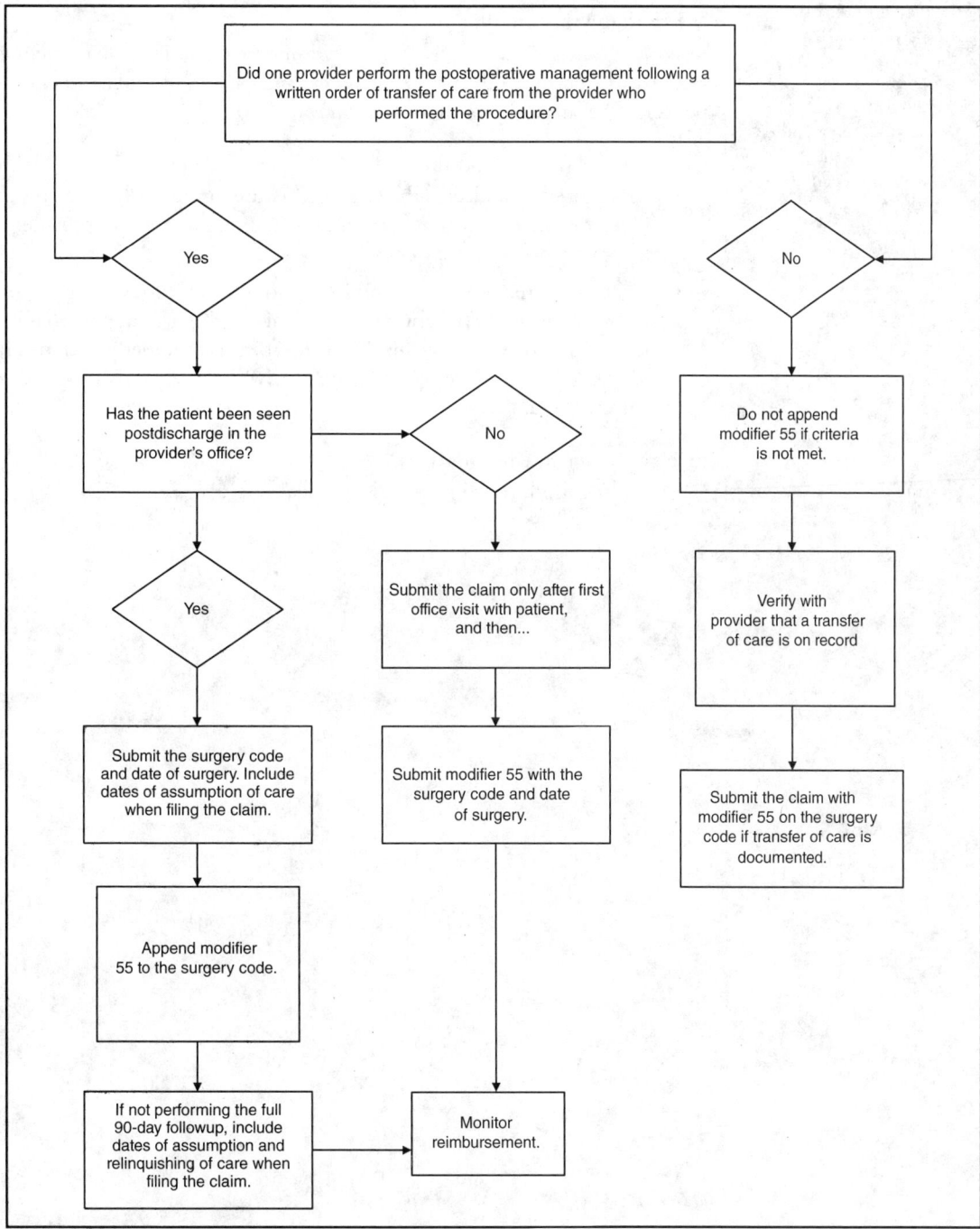

56   Preoperative Management Only

When one physician or other qualified health care professional performed the preoperative care and evaluation and another performed the surgical procedure, the preoperative component may be identified by adding modifier 56 to the usual procedure number.

When to use this modifier:

Modifier 56 identifies the provider performing preoperative management when one provider performs the preoperative care and evaluation and another provider performs the surgical procedure.

Correct usage of this modifier:

- Modifier 56 is added to the usual procedure number when one provider performs the preoperative care and evaluation but another provider performs the surgical procedure.

- Check with the Medicare contractor and other third-party payers for instructions on the appropriate use of this modifier. Modifier 56 is usually not used for Medicare claims. Payment for this modifier is included in the Medicare allowable for the surgery. Follow the payer's instructions for correct use of this modifier.

Incorrect usage of this modifier:

- Adding modifier 56 to an E/M service code.

The following flow chart can aid in an audit by helping determine if modifier 56 is being used correctly and whether additional documentation might be required.

Modifier 56

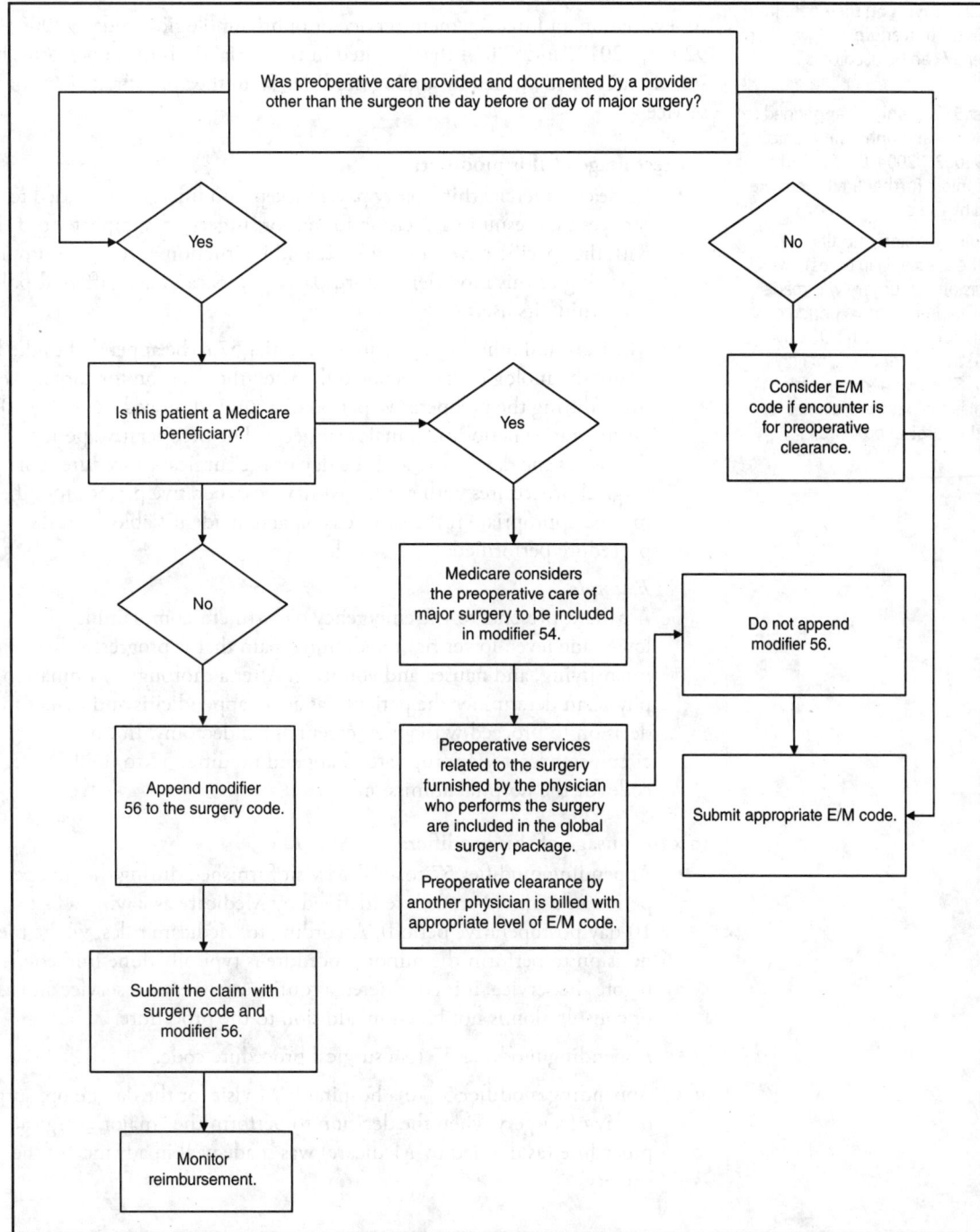

57   Decision for Surgery

An evaluation and management service that resulted in the initial decision to perform the surgery may be identified by adding modifier 57 to the appropriate level of E/M service.

When to use this modifier:

An evaluation and management service or ophthalmological codes 92002, 92004, 92012, and 92014 that resulted in the initial decision to perform the surgery may be identified by adding modifier 57 to the appropriate level of E/M service.

Correct usage of this modifier:

*   Some commercial third-party payers accept modifier 57 appended to E/M services that result in a decision for minor surgery. It is important to check with the specific payer for guidance and instruction as to the appropriate reporting of this modifier as third-party payers can have different policies concerning its use.

*   Medicare and other payers require modifier 57 to be appended to the E/M or ophthalmologic service code only when the decision for surgery was made during the preoperative period of a surgical procedure with a 90-day postoperative period (i.e., major surgery). The preoperative period is defined as the day before and the day of the surgical procedure. For surgical procedures with a 0- or 10-day postoperative period, modifier 25 may be appropriate if the service is separately identifiable from the procedure performed.

    Example
    A patient presents to the emergency department complaining of a low-grade fever, lower right abdominal pain that is progressively intensifying, and nausea and vomiting. After a thorough examination, the physician determines the patient has acute appendicitis and makes the decision to proceed with an emergent appendectomy. In this circumstance, it is appropriate to append modifier 57 to the E/M service code for the hospital admission.

Incorrect usage of this modifier:

*   Appending modifier 57 to an E/M visit furnished during the preoperative period of a minor procedure (defined by Medicare as having a 0- to 10-day postoperative period). According to Medicare rules, where the decision to perform the minor procedure is typically done immediately before the service, it is considered a routine preoperative service and a visit or consultation is not billed in addition to the procedure.

*   Appending modifier 57 to a surgical procedure code.

*   Appending modifier 57 to a hospital E/M visit for the day before surgery or day of surgery when the decision to perform the "major" surgical procedure (as defined by Medicare) was made well in advance of the surgery.

The following flow chart can aid in an audit by helping determine if modifier 57 is being used correctly and whether additional documentation might be required.

Modifier 57

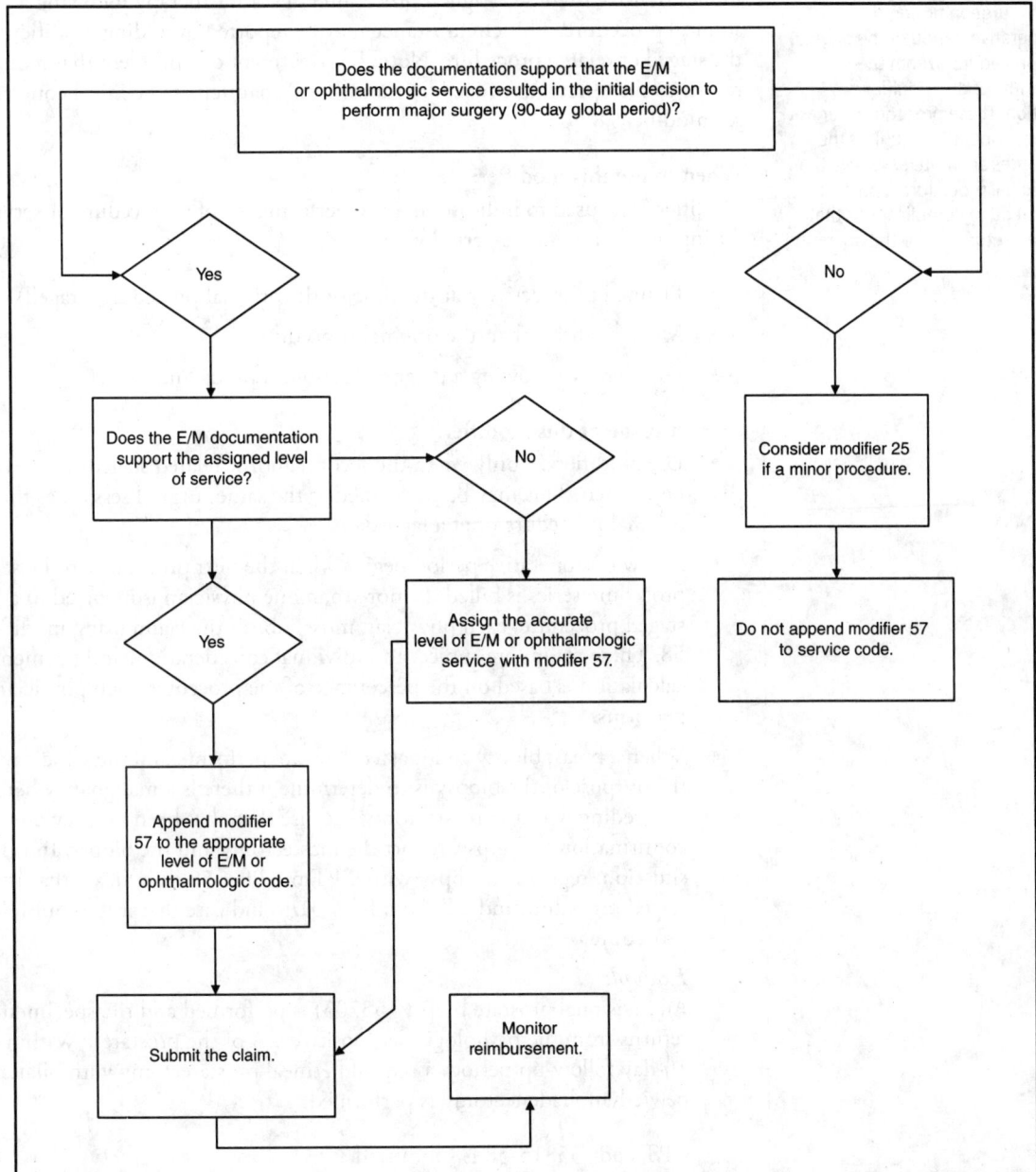

58 Staged or Related Procedure or Service by the Same Physician or Other Qualified Health Care Professional During the Postoperative Period

It may be necessary to indicate that the performance of a procedure or service during the postoperative period was: (a) planned or anticipated (staged); (b) more extensive than the original procedure; or (c) for therapy following a surgical procedure. This circumstance may be reported by adding modifier 58 to the staged or related procedure. **Note:** For treatment of a problem that requires a return to the operating/procedure room (e.g., unanticipated clinical condition), see modifier 78.

When to use this modifier:

Modifier 58 is used to indicate that the performance of a procedure or service during the postoperative period was:

- Planned prospectively at the time of the original procedure (staged)
- More extensive than the original procedure
- For therapy following a diagnostic surgical procedure

Correct usage of this modifier:

- Use modifier 58 only when the second and/or related staged services are performed. This may be performed at the same surgical session as the original procedure or at a later date.

- A new postoperative period begins when the next procedure in the staged procedure series is billed. If more than one physician is involved in a staged procedure, each physician must submit the claim using modifier 58. These claims are subject to individual consideration, and payment calculation is based on the percentage of the procedure each physician performs.

- When a breast biopsy and mastectomy are performed on the same day and the purpose of the biopsy is to determine if there is a malignancy before proceeding with the mastectomy because there has been no previous confirmation by biopsy, report the mastectomy and the biopsy. In this situation, report the biopsy with CPT modifier 58 to indicate that it is a staged procedure and CPT modifier 51 to indicate that it is a multiple procedure.

  Example

  An incisional prostate biopsy (55705) is performed and the specimen returns from the pathologist as "positive CA of the prostate." Within the 10-day follow-up period, a radical perineal prostatectomy with bilateral pelvic lymphadenectomy is performed.

  CPT code 55815-58 is submitted.

- Some injuries require multiple fracture debridement procedures and possibly staged fracture debridement. These procedures often are performed on open fractures that have not yet been treated to accommodate the reduction of the bones. When a staged procedure is performed, an initial fracture debridement may be performed to extend the wound for exploration or excisional debridement and irrigation of all tissue layers. Repeat debridement may be required for a heavily contaminated wound or for other reasons. In situations requiring repeat procedures following the initial debridement procedure, report the subsequent procedures with modifier 58.

Incorrect usage of this modifier:

- Using modifier 58 to report the treatment of an unexpected problem that requires a return to the operating room. See modifier 78.

- Do not use modifier 58 with procedures that describe a subsequent stage (i.e., 67208 Destruction of localized lesion of retina, one or more sessions)

- Using modifier 58 for unrelated procedures performed during the postoperative period of the original (first) procedure or service. See modifier 79 for unrelated procedures performed by the same physician or other qualified health care professional during the postoperative period or modifiers 51 and 59, as appropriate, for multiple procedures and distinct procedural service for procedures performed by another physician during the postoperative period of the original surgery. **Note:** For repeat procedures performed by another physician or other qualified health care professional, see modifier 77.

The following flow chart can aid in an audit by helping determine if modifier 58 is being used correctly and whether additional documentation might be required.

Modifier 58

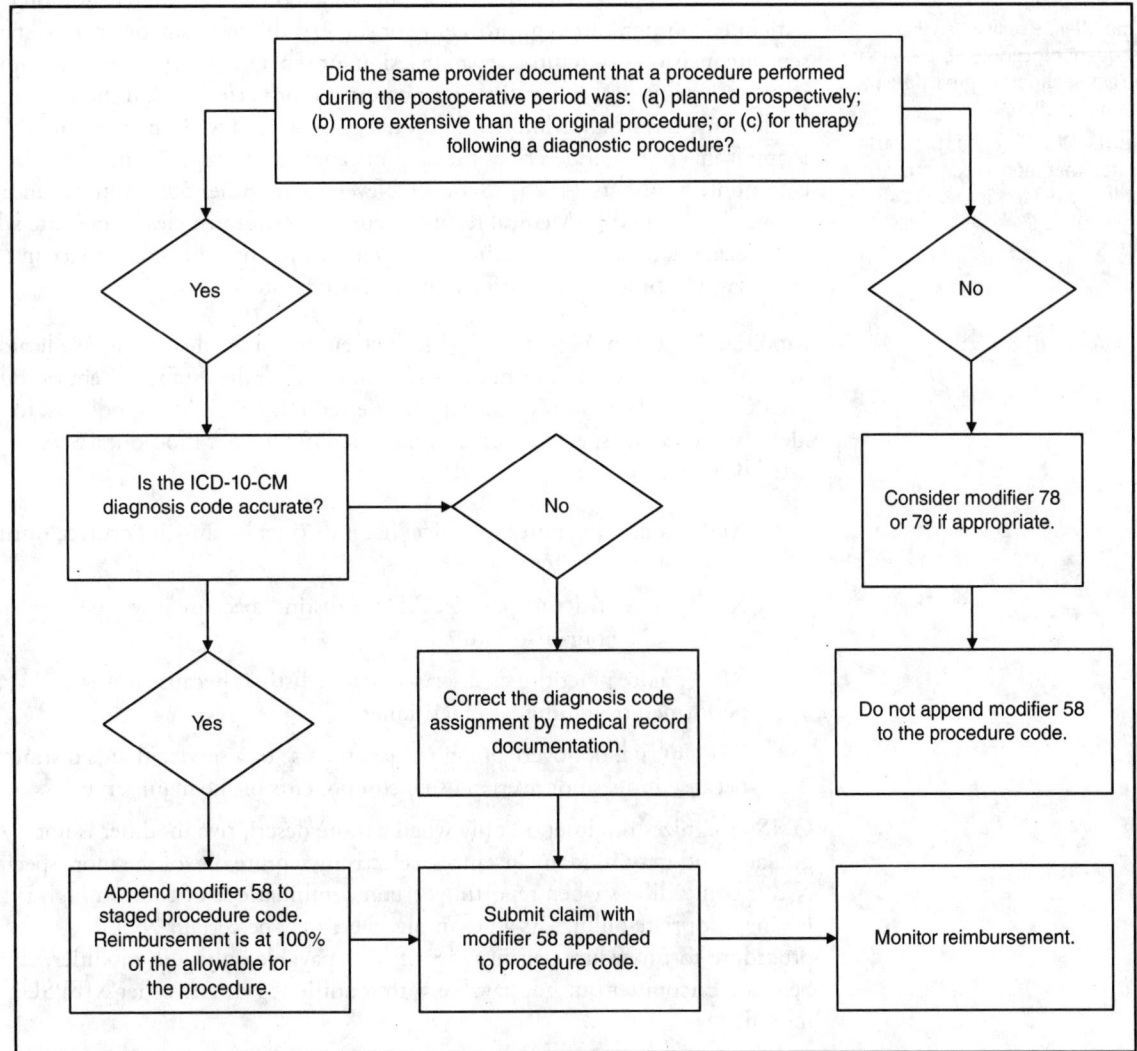

59   Distinct Procedural Service

Under certain circumstances, it may be necessary to indicate that a procedure or service was distinct or independent from other non-E/M services performed on the same day. Modifier 59 is used to identify procedures/services other than E/M services that are not normally reported together but are appropriate under the circumstances. Documentation must support a different session, different procedure or surgery, different site or organ system, separate incision/excision, separate lesion, or separate injury (or area of injury in extensive injuries) not ordinarily encountered or performed on the same day by the same individual. However, when another already established modifier is appropriate it should be used rather than modifier 59. Only if no more descriptive modifier is available, and the use of modifier 59 best explains the circumstances, should modifier 59 be used. **Note:** Modifier 59 should not be appended to an E/M service. To report a separate and distinct E/M service with a non-E/M service performed on the same date, see modifier 25.

When to use this modifier:

Use modifier 59 to indicate that a procedure or service was distinct or independent from other services performed on the same day. Modifier 59 is used to identify procedures or services that are not normally reported together, but are appropriate under the circumstances. This may represent a different session or patient encounter, different procedure or surgery, different site or organ system, separate incision or excision, separate lesion, or separate injury (or area of injury in extensive injuries) not ordinarily encountered or performed on the same day by the same physician. Modifier 59 should only be used when no other modifier is applicable or better describes the circumstances that occurred, most commonly modifiers 24, 25, 78, or 79. Never use modifier 59 simply as a means to override CCI edits. Medical record documentation must clearly indicate why the procedure or service is distinct. For example, if a patient is seen twice in the same day, the time of each visit should be documented.

Modifier Alert: On August 15, 2014, the Centers for Medicare and Medicaid Services (CMS) issued Transmittal 1422 announcing the establishment of four HCPCS Level II modifiers, collectively referred to as X{EPSU} modifiers, to identify and define specific subsets of modifier 59 Distinct Procedural Service, as listed below:

- XE Separate encounter, a service that is distinct because it occurred during a separate encounter

- XS Separate structure, a service that is distinct because it was performed on a separate organ/structure

- XP Separate practitioner, a service that is distinct because it was performed by a different practitioner

- XU Unusual nonoverlapping service, the use of a service that is distinct because it does not overlap usual components of the main service

CMS recognizes modifier 59 only when a more descriptive modifier is not available and may, in many instances, selectively require one of the more specific X{EPSU} modifiers when reporting certain combinations of codes at high risk for inappropriate billing. As an example, there may be certain NCCI procedure-to-procedure pairings identified as payable only with modifier XE Separate Encounter but not payable with modifier 59 or any other X{EPSU} modifiers.

Since these modifiers are more descriptive, specific versions of modifier 59, it is inappropriate to report both modifier 59 and one of the X{EPSU} modifiers on the same line item. CMS will accept either modifier 59 OR one of the more selective X{EPSU} modifiers since using both in combination would create an additional burden for both reporting and editing purposes.

CMS encourages providers to use these modifiers, as appropriate, whenever possible. Note that while national edits may not be in place, these modifiers are still considered active and valid; therefore, CMS contractors are permitted to begin requiring the use of these modifiers in place of the more general modifier 59 as necessitated by local integrity and program needs.

Correct usage of this modifier:
- Use modifier 59, XE, XP, XS, or XU when billing a combination of codes that would normally not be billed together. This modifier indicates that the ordinarily bundled code represents a service done at a different anatomic site or at a different session on the same date. This may represent:
  - different session or patient encounter (XE)
  - different practitioner/physician (XP)
  - different procedure or surgery on same day
  - different site or organ system (e.g., a skin graft and an allograft in different locations) (XS)
  - separate incision or excision (XS)
  - separate lesion (e.g., a biopsy of skin on the neck is performed at the same session as an excision of a benign 1.0 cm lesion of the face) (XS)
  - separate injury (XU)
- Use modifier 59, XE, XP, XS, or XU only on the procedure designated as a separate procedural service. The physician needs to document that the procedure or service was independent of other services rendered on the same day.
- Ensure that the medical record documentation is clear as to the separate and distinct procedure before appending modifier 59, XE, XP, XS, or XU to a code. This modifier allows the code to bypass edits; therefore, appropriate documentation must be present in the record. **Note:** Medicare uses the Correct Coding Initiative (CCI) screens when editing claims for possible unbundling. Under CCI screens, specific codes have been identified that should not be billed together. See the CCI and MUEs section earlier in this chapter for more information.
- Modifier 59 is used only if another modifier does not describe the situation more accurately.
- For Medicare billing purposes, it may be necessary to report one of the more specific X{EPSU} modifiers (XE, XS, XP, or XU) in lieu of appending general modifier 59.

Example:
When multiple approaches are taken to obtain a tissue sample (cytological or surgical), bill the most invasive procedure performed at the same session/site in order to obtain a specimen. For example, if a fine-needle aspiration (CPT codes 10004–10012, 10021) is attempted and is unsuccessful and the same physician proceeds to obtain a core biopsy using a cutting needle and ultimately finds it necessary to perform an open biopsy, all occurring at the same session, bill only the open biopsy. In the event that different lesions are biopsied using different methodologies,

even at the same session, use modifier 59, XE, XP, XS, or XU. If different biopsy procedures are necessary for different reasons (e.g., fine-needle aspiration for diagnosis and needle biopsy for receptors in breast carcinoma), bill both procedures.

- When a procedure or service designated as a separate procedure is carried out independently or considered to be unrelated from the other services provided at the same session, it may be reported by appending the modifier 59, XE, XP, XS, or XU to the specific separate procedure code. This indicates that the procedure is not considered a component of another procedure but instead is a distinct procedure.

  Example:
  A patient presents with a possible aspiration of a foreign body (food), and a diagnostic bronchoscopy is performed indicating a lobar foreign body. A decision is made to remove the foreign body by thoracotomy. The same-day open thoracotomy is reported in addition to the diagnostic bronchoscopy (separate procedure), which should be appended with modifier 59 or XE.

- CPT codes for use with modifier 59, XE, XP, XS, or XU unless limited by the payer are 00100–01999, 10004–69990, 70010–79999, 80047–89398, 90281–99199, and 99500–99607, when appropriate.

Incorrect usage of this modifier:

- Appending modifier 59 to E/M codes.

- Using modifier 59, XE, XP, XS, or XU as a replacement for modifiers 24, 25, 51, 78, and 79.

- Using modifier 59, XE, XP, XS, or XU when another modifier best describes the distinct service.

- Using modifier 59, XE, XP, XS, or XU simply as a method to bypass an appropriate CCI edit.

- Reporting modifier 59 in conjunction with one of the XE, XP, XS, or XU modifiers on the same line item.

© 2020 Optum360, LLC

The following flow chart can aid in an audit by helping determine if modifier 59 is being used correctly and whether additional documentation might be required.

Modifier 59

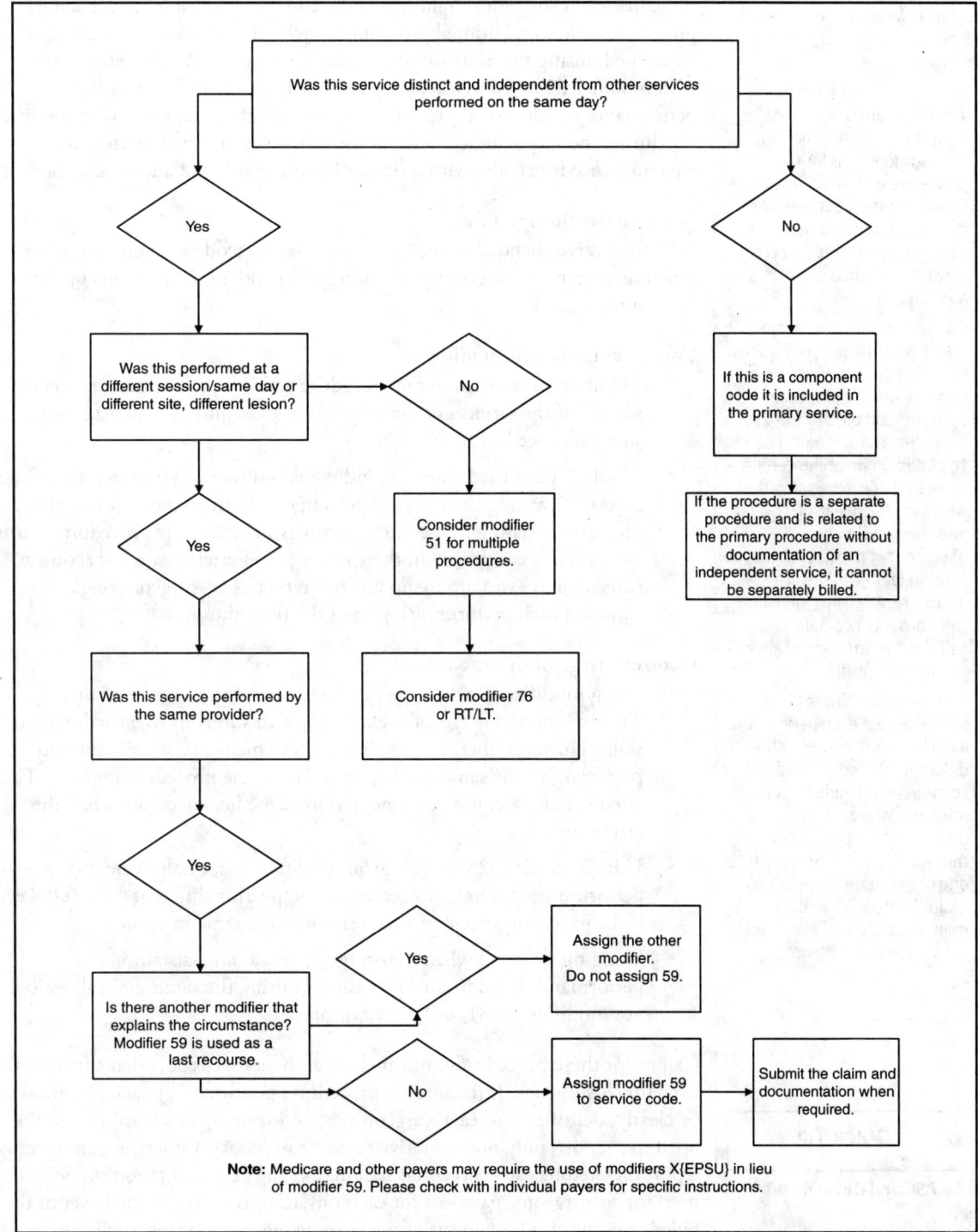

Was this service distinct and independent from other services performed on the same day?

Yes

No

Was this performed at a different session/same day or different site, different lesion?

No

If this is a component code it is included in the primary service.

Yes

Consider modifier 51 for multiple procedures.

If the procedure is a separate procedure and is related to the primary procedure without documentation of an independent service, it cannot be separately billed.

Was this service performed by the same provider?

Consider modifier 76 or RT/LT.

Yes

Is there another modifier that explains the circumstance? Modifier 59 is used as a last recourse.

Yes

Assign the other modifier.
Do not assign 59.

No

Assign modifier 59 to service code.

Submit the claim and documentation when required.

Note: Medicare and other payers may require the use of modifiers X{EPSU} in lieu of modifier 59. Please check with individual payers for specific instructions.

62   Two Surgeons

When two surgeons work together as primary surgeons performing distinct parts of a procedure, each surgeon should report his/her distinct operative work by adding modifier 62 to the procedure code and any associated add-on codes for that procedure as long as both surgeons continue to work together as primary surgeons. Each surgeon should report the co-surgery once using the same procedure code. If additional procedures, including add-on procedures, are performed during the same surgical session, separate codes may also be reported with modifier 62 added. **Note:** If a co-surgeon acts as an assistant in the performance of additional procedures other than those reported with modifier 62, during the same surgical session, those services may be reported using separate procedure codes with modifier 80 or modifier 82 added, as appropriate.

When to use this modifier:

Modifier 62 is appended to the appropriate service code when two surgeons function as primary surgeons performing independent components of the same procedure.

Correct usage of this modifier:

- Modifier 62 is added to the procedure code by each surgeon for reporting services if the services of two physicians are required to manage a specific surgical procedure.

- Modifier 62 is used when the individual skills of physicians with different specialties are required to perform surgery on the patient during the same operative session because of the complex nature of the procedure and/or the patient's condition. In these cases, the physicians are not acting as surgeon and assistant-at-surgery, but rather as co-surgeons (e.g., two surgeons each performing a part of the procedure).

Incorrect usage of this modifier:

- Using modifier 62 when the physicians are of the same specialty. Third-party payers typically expect the two surgeons to have different skills. However, there may be instances of medical necessity for two physicians of the same specialty to perform the procedure together. These circumstances require documentation of medical necessity when the claims are filed.

- Using modifier 62 when surgeons of different specialties are each performing a different procedure (i.e., reporting different CPT codes even if the procedures are performed through the same incision).

- Using modifier 62 when a co-surgeon acts as an assistant in the performance of additional procedures during the same surgical session. See modifier 80, 81, or 82, as appropriate.

Claims for these procedures must include an operative report that supports the need for co-surgeons. If the surgical procedures performed by each physician can be clearly identified and each surgeon's role is explicitly described within the operative report, only one operative report is necessary. Otherwise, an operative report dictated by each surgeon is required. If the documentation supports the need for co-surgeons, payment for each physician is based on the lower of the billed amount or 62.5 percent of the fee schedule amount for Medicare claims.

Although a procedure code may be on the list of procedures for which cosurgery may be covered, modifier 62 does not apply when two surgeons, regardless of their specialties, perform distinct procedures (different procedure codes). When modifier 62 for co-surgeons is deemed appropriate, payment for an assistant surgeon is usually not allowed (the same is true for team surgeons, modifier 66). However, if it is determined that it was medically necessary to have two surgeons and an assistant surgeon, payment for an assistant surgeon may be allowed.

Medicare has three classifications for cosurgery:

- Surgeries that may be paid as cosurgery but that require documentation to support the medical necessity for the two surgeons; these procedures are reported in the MPFSDB with a "1" in the cosurgery field.

- Surgeries that may be paid as cosurgery but do not require documentation, if the two-specialty requirement is met; these procedures are identified in the MPFSDB with a "2" in the cosurgery field.

- Procedures that may not be reported as cosurgery; these procedures are listed in the MPFSDB with cosurgery indicators of "0" or "9".

The following flow chart can aid in an audit by helping determine if modifier 62 is being used correctly and whether additional documentation might be required.

Modifier 62

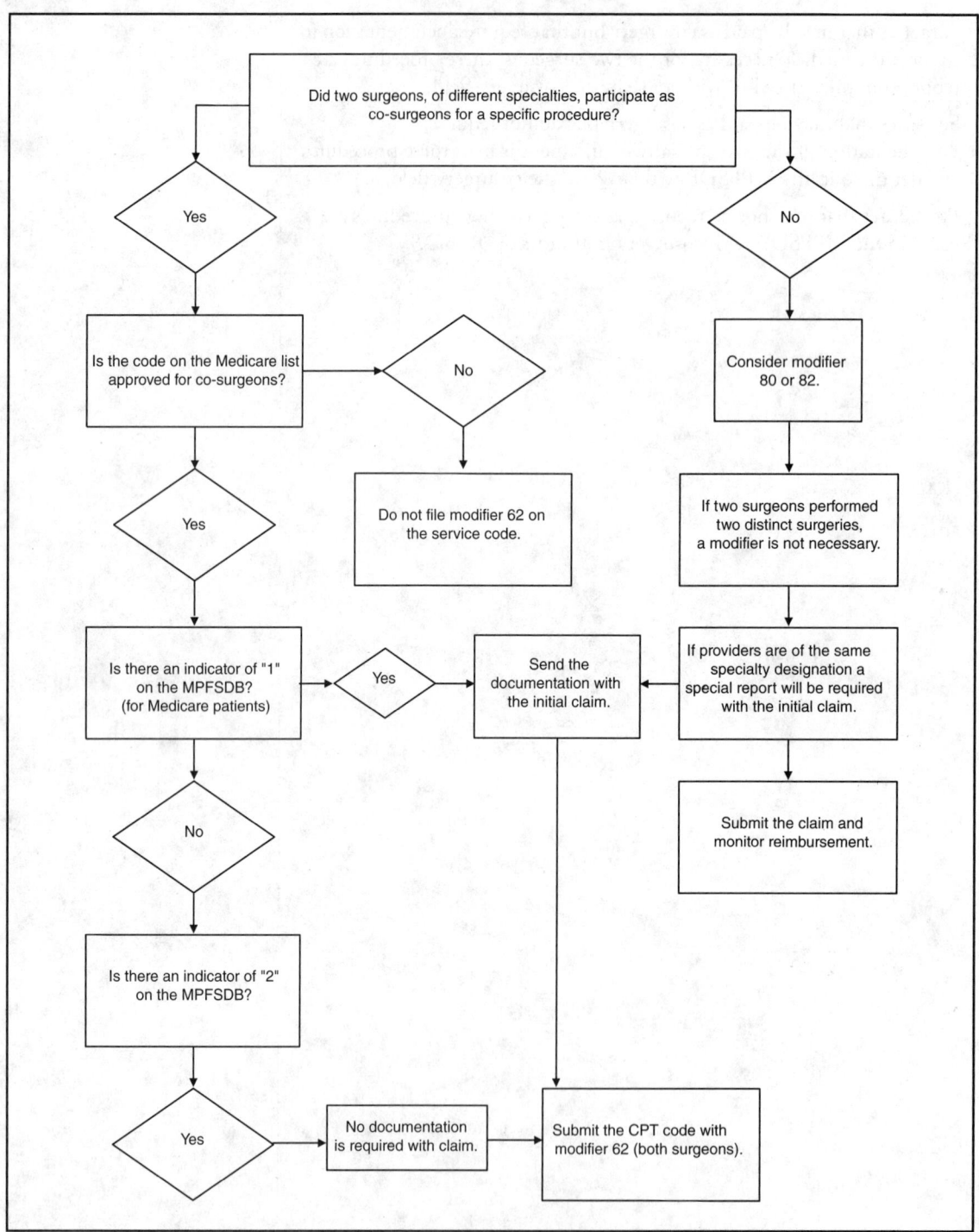

63   Procedures Performed on Infants Less Than 4 kg

Procedures performed on neonates and infants up to a present body weight of 4 kg may involve significantly increased complexity and physician or other qualified health care professional work commonly associated with these patients. This circumstance may be reported by adding modifier 63 to the procedure number. **Note:** Unless otherwise designated, this modifier may only be appended to procedures/services listed in the 20100–69990 code series and 92920, 92928, 92953, 92960, 92986, 92987, 92990, 92997, 92998, 93312, 93313, 93314, 93315, 93316, 93317, 93318, 93452, 93505, 93530, 93531, 93532, 93533, 93561, 93562, 93563, 93564, 93568, 93580, 93582, 93590, 93591, 93592, 93615, and 93616 from the Medicine/Cardiovascular section. Modifier 63 should not be appended to any CPT codes listed in the Evaluation and Management Services, Anesthesia, Radiology, Pathology/Laboratory, or Medicine sections (other than those identified above from the Medicine/Cardiovascular section).

When to use this modifier:

Modifier 63 is appended to the appropriate service code to indicate the additional work and difficulty associated with procedures performed on infants with a body weight of 4 kg or less.

Correct usage of this modifier:

- Append this modifier to services performed on infants weighing less than 4 kg.

Incorrect usage of this modifier:

- Do not append this modifier to services performed on infants weighing more than 4 kg.

- Do not append this modifier to any of the CPT codes listed in appendix F of the CPT book.

 FOR MORE INFO

Previously, modifier 22 Increased procedure service, was reported to describe services that were more complex due to the age and size of the patient; however, pediatricians and surgeons now report modifier 63. It is inappropriate to report modifier 22 in conjunction with modifier 63.

The following flow chart can aid in an audit by helping determine if modifier 63 is being used correctly and whether additional documentation might be required.

Modifier 63

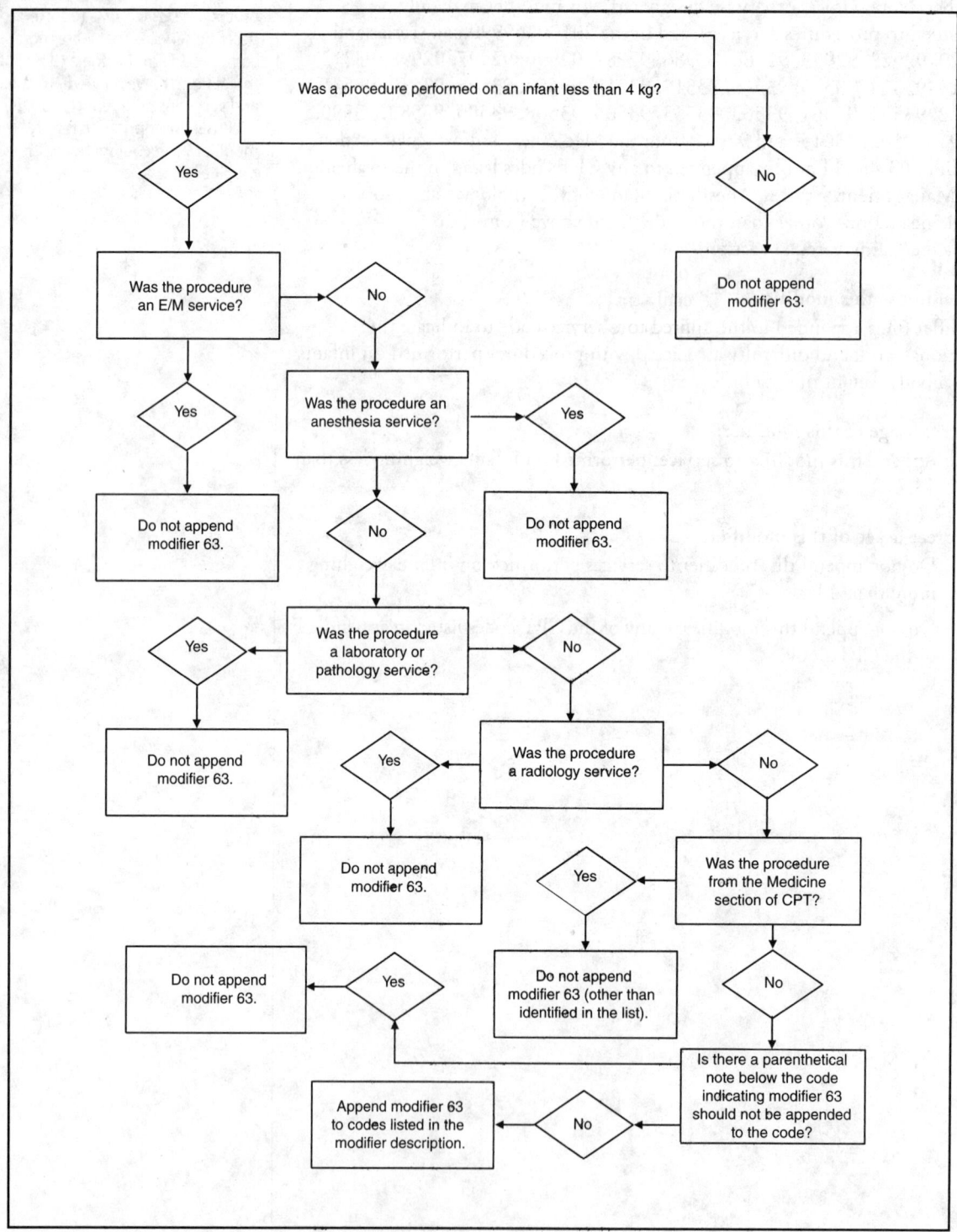

© 2020 Optum360, LLC

66   Surgical Team

Under some circumstances, highly complex procedures (requiring the concomitant services of several physicians or other qualified health care professionals, often of different specialties, plus other highly skilled, specially trained personnel, and various types of complex equipment) are carried out under the "surgical team" concept. Such circumstances may be identified by each participating individual with the addition of modifier 66 to the basic procedure number used for reporting services.

When to use this modifier:

Modifier 66 should be appended to the procedure code representing the services performed by each provider who participated in the operative session.

Correct usage of this modifier:

- Modifier 66 is added to the basic procedure when the concomitant services of several physicians or other qualified health care professionals, plus other highly skilled, specially trained personnel and various types of complex equipment, are required to perform a procedure.

- CPT codes for use with modifier 66 unless limited by the payer are 10004–69990, when appropriate.

Incorrect usage of this modifier:

- Using modifier 66 when other special equipment and trained personnel are not involved.

If the surgical procedures performed by each provider can be clearly identified and each surgeon's role is explicitly described within the operative report, only one operative report is necessary. Otherwise, an operative report dictated by each surgeon is required. Documentation should identify the role of other highly skilled, trained personnel and complex equipment and operators required for the procedure or procedures. All claims for team surgery must contain sufficient information to support the medical necessity for a surgical team. Copies of this documentation should be sent with claims.

> *Example*
>
> A patient is transported via life flight to the emergency department of a trauma hospital with severe injuries resulting from a multiple vehicle collision. The patient is immediately prepared for surgery to repair a ruptured spleen, a fractured femur requiring open reduction internal fixation (ORIF), and brain hemorrhaging and swelling. A general surgeon treats the ruptured spleen, an orthopaedic surgeon performs the ORIF, and a neurosurgeon operates to treat the brain injury. Each physician reports the appropriate service code that corresponds to the procedure performed and appends modifier 66 to identify the single operative session as requiring the special and distinct services of a surgical team.

The following flow chart can aid in an audit by helping determine if modifier 66 is being used correctly and whether additional documentation might be required.

Modifier 66

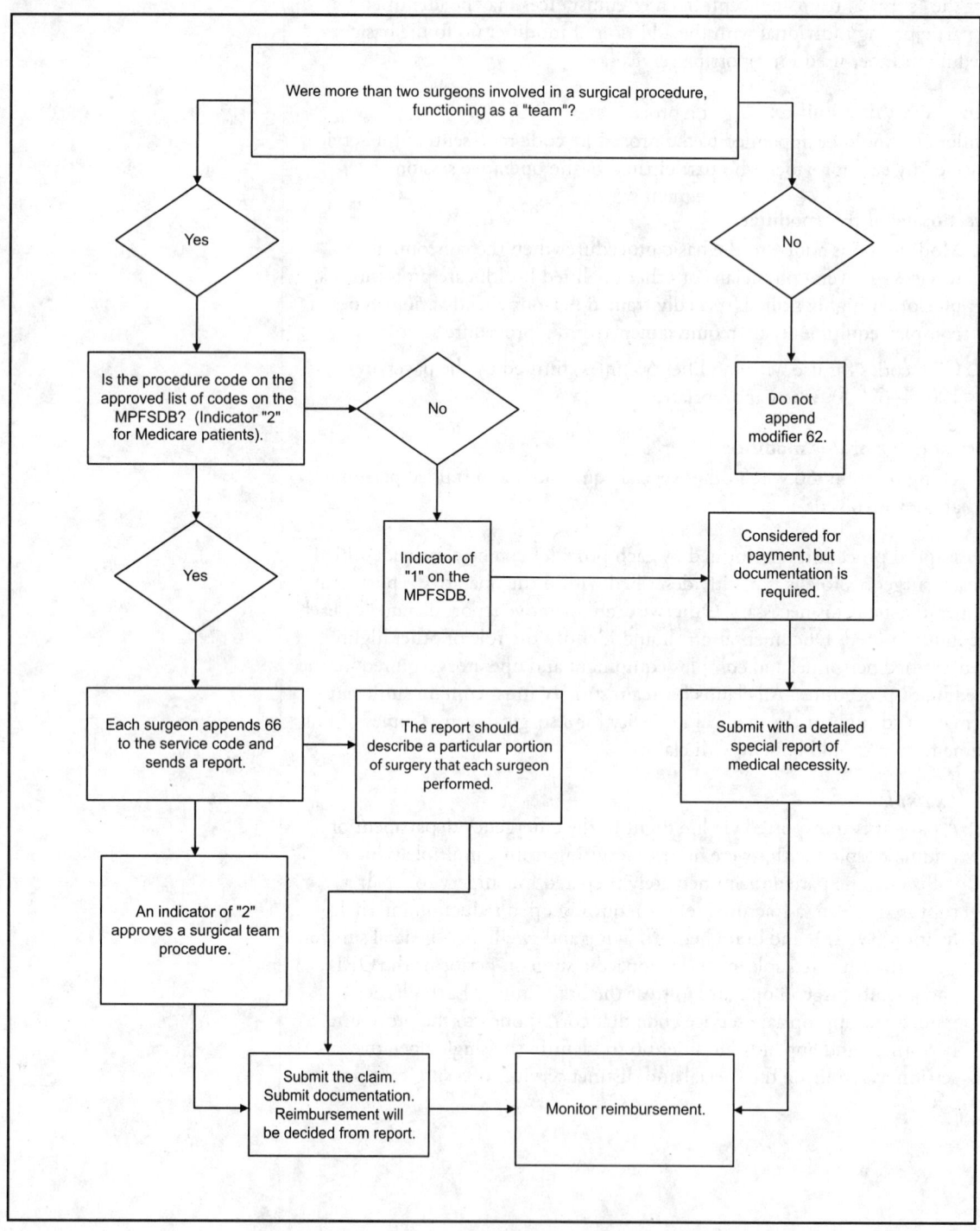

© 2020 Optum360, LLC

76 Repeat Procedure or Service by Same Physician or Other Qualified Health Care Professional

It may be necessary to indicate that a procedure or service was repeated by the same physician or other qualified health care professional subsequent to the original procedure or service. This circumstance may be reported by adding modifier 76 to the repeated procedure/service. **Note:** This modifier should not be appended to an E/M service.

When to use this modifier:

Modifier 76 is used to indicate that a procedure or service was repeated by the same physician or other qualified health care professional subsequent to the original procedure or service. The use of this modifier ensures that the payer does not erroneously deny the subsequent service as a duplicate when two of the same services are reported on the same date.

Correct usage of this modifier:

- Modifier 76 is appended to a code when the same provider repeats the same service, sometimes on the same day. This modifier can be used whenever the circumstances warrant the repeat procedure.

- Use this modifier to indicate that a repeat procedure was necessary and that it does not represent a duplicate bill for the original surgery or service.

- CPT codes for use with modifier 76, unless limited by the payer, are 10004–69990, 70010–79999, 90281–99199, and 99500–99607, when appropriate.

Incorrect usage of this modifier:

- Using modifier 76 to indicate repositioning or replacement 14 days after the initial insertion or replacement of an existing pacemaker or defibrillator. Modifier 76 is not reported with pacemaker or defibrillator codes after 14 days, as these are considered new, not repeat services.

- As an example, procedure codes such as 17000, 17003, and 17004 by description indicate multiple procedures on the same day and, therefore, use of modifier 76 would be inappropriate.

- Do not append modifier 76 on repeat services due to equipment or other technical failure or repeated procedures for quality control purposes.

Example

A 68-year-old female was in an assisted living center when fire erupted. She sustained severe inhalation burns. The patient was found to have extreme difficulty breathing and a suction bronchoscopy was performed. Due to the severity of her condition, the next day a suction bronchoscopy was performed at 7:30 a.m., and repeated at 5:30 p.m. by the same physician. Report 31645 for the initial bronchoscopy. On the second day, report 31646 for the first procedure and 31646-76 for the second bronchoscopy.

The following flow chart can aid in an audit by helping determine if modifier 76 is being used correctly and whether additional documentation might be required.

Modifier 76

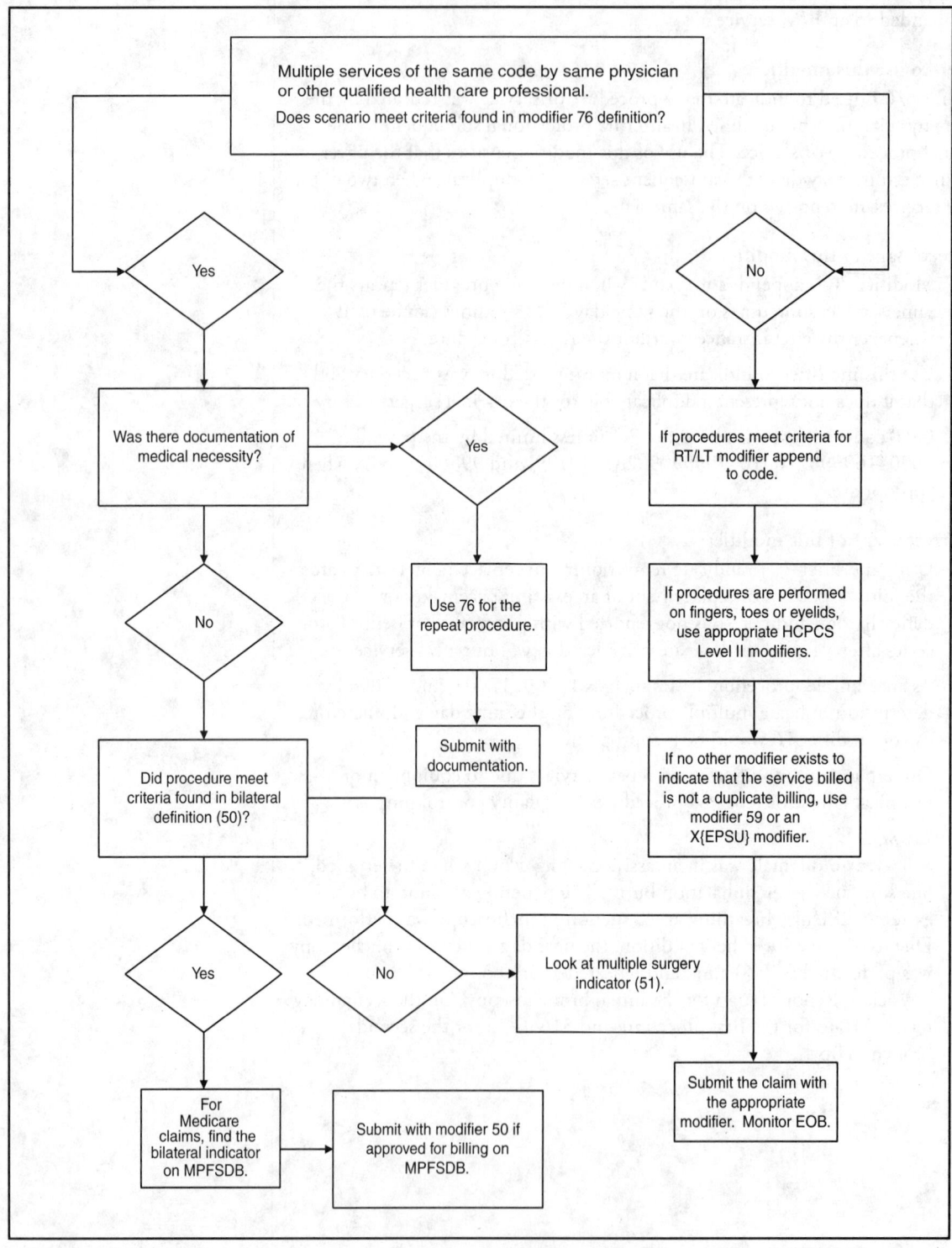

  © 2020 Optum360, LLC

77   Repeat Procedure by Another Physician or Other Qualified Health Care Professional

It may be necessary to indicate that a basic procedure or service was repeated by another physician or other qualified health care professional subsequent to the original procedure or service. This circumstance may be reported by adding modifier 77 to the repeated procedure or service. **Note:** This modifier should not be appended to an E/M service.

When to use this modifier:

Modifier 77 is used to indicate that a basic procedure or service was repeated by *another* physician or other qualified health care professional subsequent to the original procedure or service.

Correct usage of this modifier:

- Modifier 77 is appended to a CPT code when the same service (same CPT code) that was already performed by another provider is repeated by another provider. Sometimes this occurs on the same date of service. Modifier 77 can be used whenever the circumstances warrant this information. An explanation of the medical necessity for the repeat service is necessary.

- CPT codes for use with modifier 77, unless limited by the payer, are 10004–69990, 70010–79999, 90281–99199, and 99500–99607, when appropriate.

Incorrect usage of this modifier:

- Using modifier 77 to indicate repositioning or replacement 14 days after the initial insertion or replacement of an existing pacemaker or defibrillator. Modifier 77 is not reported with pacemaker or defibrillator codes after 14 days, as these are considered new, not repeat services.

The following flow chart can aid in an audit by helping determine if modifier 77 is being used correctly and whether additional documentation might be required.

Modifier 77

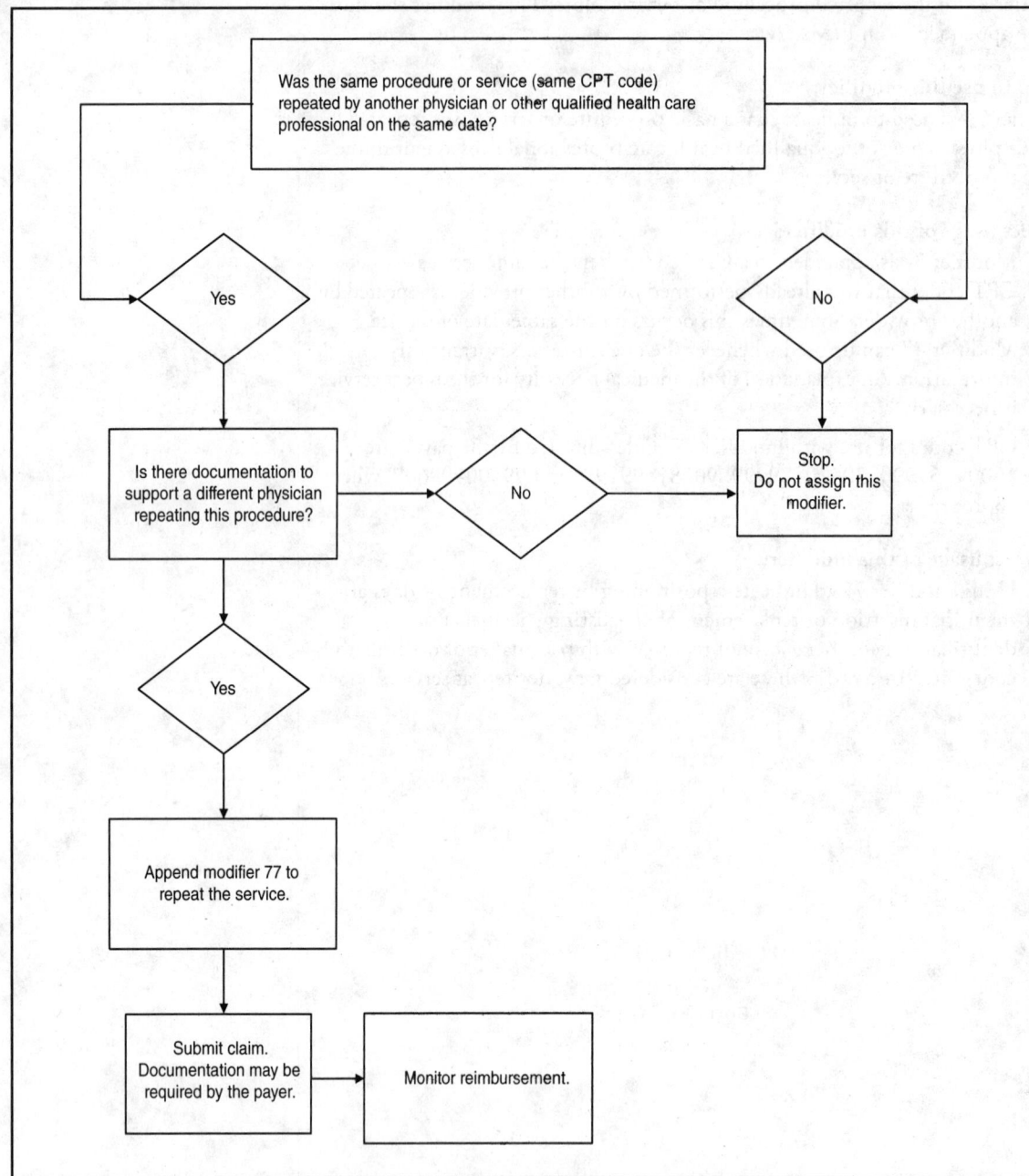

© 2020 Optum360, LLC

78 Unplanned Return to the Operating/Procedure Room by the Same Physician or Other Qualified Health Care Professional Following Initial Procedure for a Related Procedure During the Postoperative Period

It may be necessary to indicate that another procedure was performed during the postoperative period of the initial procedure (unplanned procedure following initial procedure). When this procedure is related to the first, and requires the use of an operating/procedure room, it may be reported by adding modifier 78 to the related procedure. (For repeat procedures, see modifier 76.)

When to use this modifier:

Modifier 78 should be used when a subsequent, unplanned but related procedure or service by the same provider during the postoperative period is performed. For example, a complication may arise during the postoperative period that requires a return to the operating room for treatment.

CMS defines an operating room as a place of service specifically equipped and staffed for the sole purpose of performing procedures. This includes cardiac catheterization, laser, and endoscopy suites. However, it does not include a patient's room, minor treatment room, recovery room, or the intensive care unit.

Correct usage of this modifier:

- Use modifier 78 when treatment for complications requires a return trip to the operating room. Use the CPT code that best describes the procedure performed during the return trip.

- If the patient is returned to the operating room after the initial operative session, even if on the same day as the original surgery, for one or more additional procedures as a result of complications from the original surgery, append modifier 78.

Incorrect usage of this modifier:

- Using modifier 78 on the procedure code when the original surgery is repeated. If the identical procedure was repeated by the same provider, use modifier 76.

- Only using modifier 78 for complications of surgery. The CPT book definition for this modifier does not limit its use to treatment for complications.

- Using this modifier to bill Medicare for a procedure not performed in the operating room (unless the patient's condition was so critical there would be insufficient time for transportation to an operating room).

SPECIAL ALERT

Modifier 78 is added to the procedure code when the subsequent procedure is related to the first and requires the use of an operating room. Failure to use modifier 78 when appropriate may result in denial of the subsequent surgery.

Do not use modifier 78 if treatment for postoperative complications did not require a return trip to the operating room. (For Medicare)

A new postoperative period does not begin with the use of modifier 78.

CODING AXIOM

Modifier 78, among others, was the target of an investigation by various Medicare contractors, under the direction of CMS, across the country. Errors in appropriately reporting modifier 78 occurred most often by ophthalmologists who were found to be misusing the modifier to bill for postoperative complications treated in the physician office setting. Only complications that require a return trip to the operating room are reportable with modifier 78; otherwise, treatment for those complications is included in the global surgery package as defined by Medicare.

KEY POINT

Categories T80–T88 in ICD-10-CM, Complications of surgical care, not elsewhere classified, identify many postoperative complications.

The following flow chart can aid in an audit by helping determine if modifier 78 is being used correctly and whether additional documentation might be required.

Modifier 78

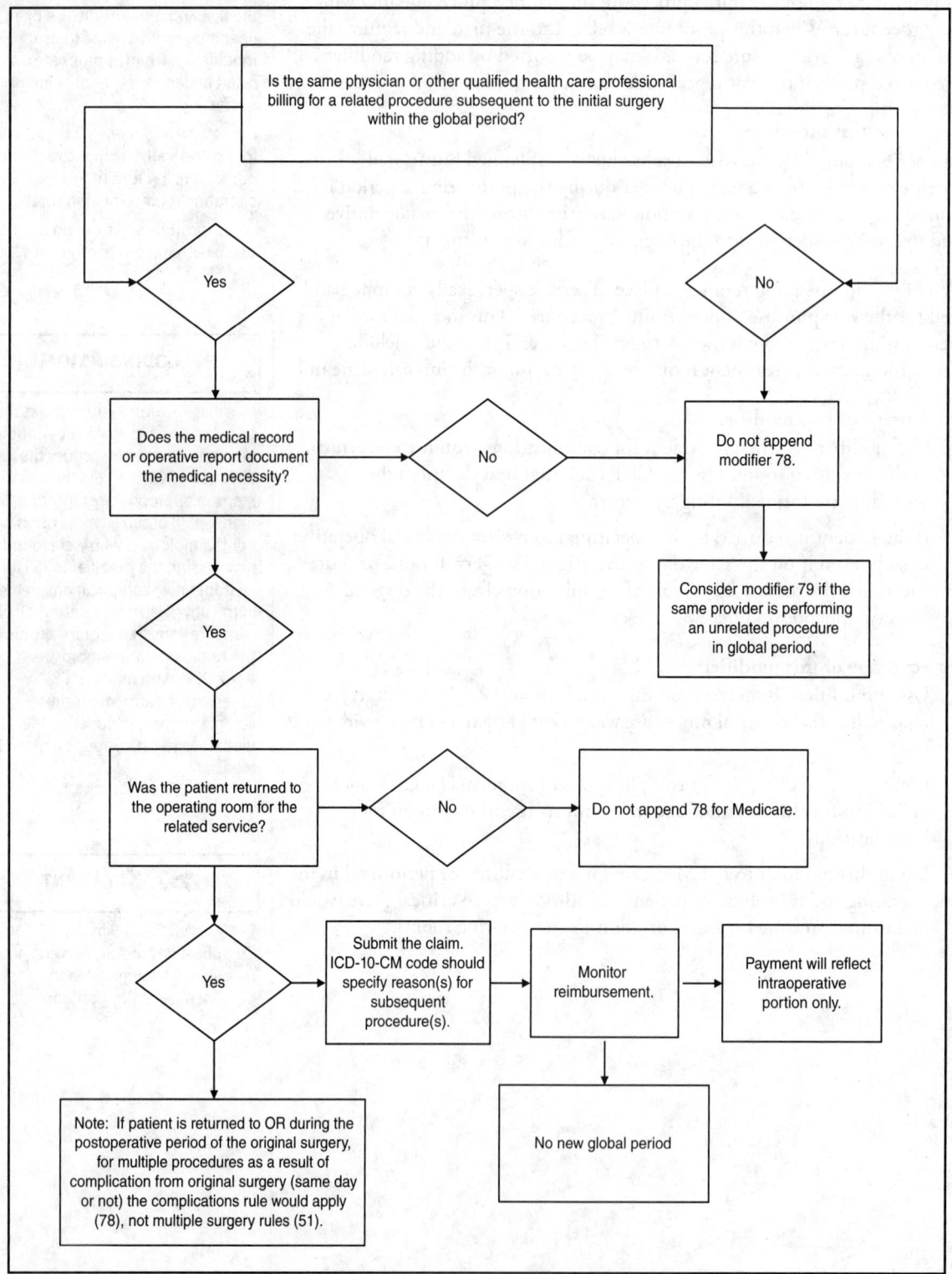

79 Unrelated Procedure or Service by the Same Physician or Other Qualified Health Care Professional During the Postoperative Period

The individual may need to indicate that the performance of a procedure or service during the postoperative period was unrelated to the original procedure. This circumstance may be reported by using modifier 79. (For repeat procedures on the same day, see modifier 76.)

When to use this modifier:

Modifier 79 is used when the patient is in the postoperative period for a specific procedure and has an unrelated condition or injury occur during that period that requires a return trip to the operating room for treatment by the same provider or other qualified health care professional who performed the initial procedure or service.

Correct usage of this modifier:

- Modifier 79 is used with surgical codes only to indicate that an unrelated procedure was performed by the same provider during the postoperative period of the original procedure.

Incorrect usage of this modifier:

- Using modifier 79 to describe a related or staged procedure performed in a postoperative period, by the same surgeon.

- Using this modifier to bill Medicare for a procedure not performed in the operating room (unless the patient's condition was so critical there would be insufficient time for transportation to an operating room).

🖥 SPECIAL ALERT

Modifier 79 is used to indicate that the procedure performed by the provider is unrelated to the original service or procedure and a different diagnosis code should be reported. Failure to use modifier 79 when appropriate may result in denial of the subsequent surgery.

It is important that each line item include the necessary modifier when appropriate.

☛ KEY POINT

When billing for an unrelated procedure by the same physician or other qualified health care professional during the postoperative period of an original procedure, a new postoperative period for the second procedure will automatically begin with the subsequent procedure.

The following flow chart can aid in an audit by helping determine if modifier 79 is being used correctly and whether additional documentation might be required.

Modifier 79

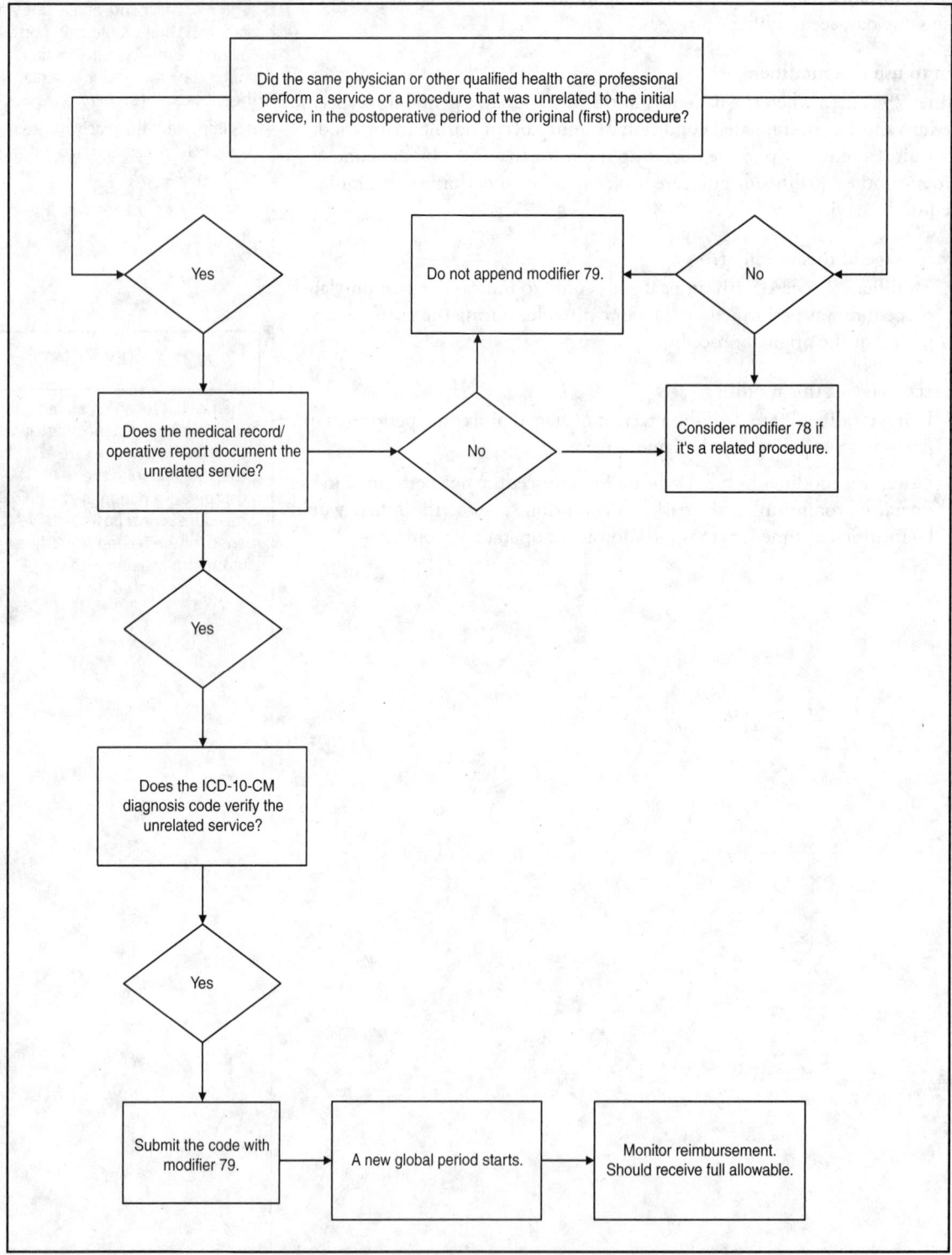

80 Assistant Surgeon

Surgical assistant services may be identified by adding modifier 80 to the usual procedure number(s).

When to use this modifier:

Modifier 80 is appended to the same service code as the primary surgeon and identifies the surgeon as a surgical assistant on the procedure performed.

Correct usage of this modifier:

- Use modifier 80 on the appropriate procedure codes. The codes must match those reported by the primary surgeon.

- If an assistant at surgery is used in a procedure also requiring the skills of two surgeons (modifier 62 or 66), report modifier 80 on the surgical assistant's claim, and submit documentation supporting the medical necessity for the surgical assistant.

- Modifier 80 can also be used on claims with other surgery modifiers, such as 50 and 51.

Incorrect usage of this modifier:

- Using modifier 80 with certain surgical procedures that are not covered for a surgical assistant. These procedures are not covered by Medicare Part B for surgical assistance, and providers cannot charge the patient for these services under any circumstances.

- Using modifier 80 when modifier 82 is more appropriate in a teaching setting. (See modifier 82.)

 SPECIAL ALERT

To determine if a surgical procedure is subject to the assistant-at-surgery restriction, refer to the MPFSDB.

- An indicator of "0" denotes procedures that would require medical necessity documentation in order for Medicare to pay for an assistant-at-surgery. A waiver should be signed (see modifier GA).

- An assistant surgery indicator of "1" identifies procedures that are restricted and not payable.

- An indicator of "2" denotes procedures that will allow payment for an assistant-at surgery.

- An indicator of "9" denotes that the concept does not apply to the procedure and an assistant-at-surgery is not payable.

✓ **QUICK TIP**

The Medicare physician fee schedule (MPFS) amount for an assistant at surgery is 16 percent of the amount allowed for an unassisted procedure. Medicare payment for assistant at surgery does not include preoperative or postoperative visits by the assistant surgeon. For nonparticipating assistant surgeons, the billed amount cannot exceed the limited charge (15 percent more than the MPFSDB amount) reduced to 16 percent.

The following flow chart can aid in an audit by helping determine if modifier 80 is being used correctly and whether additional documentation might be required.

Modifier 80

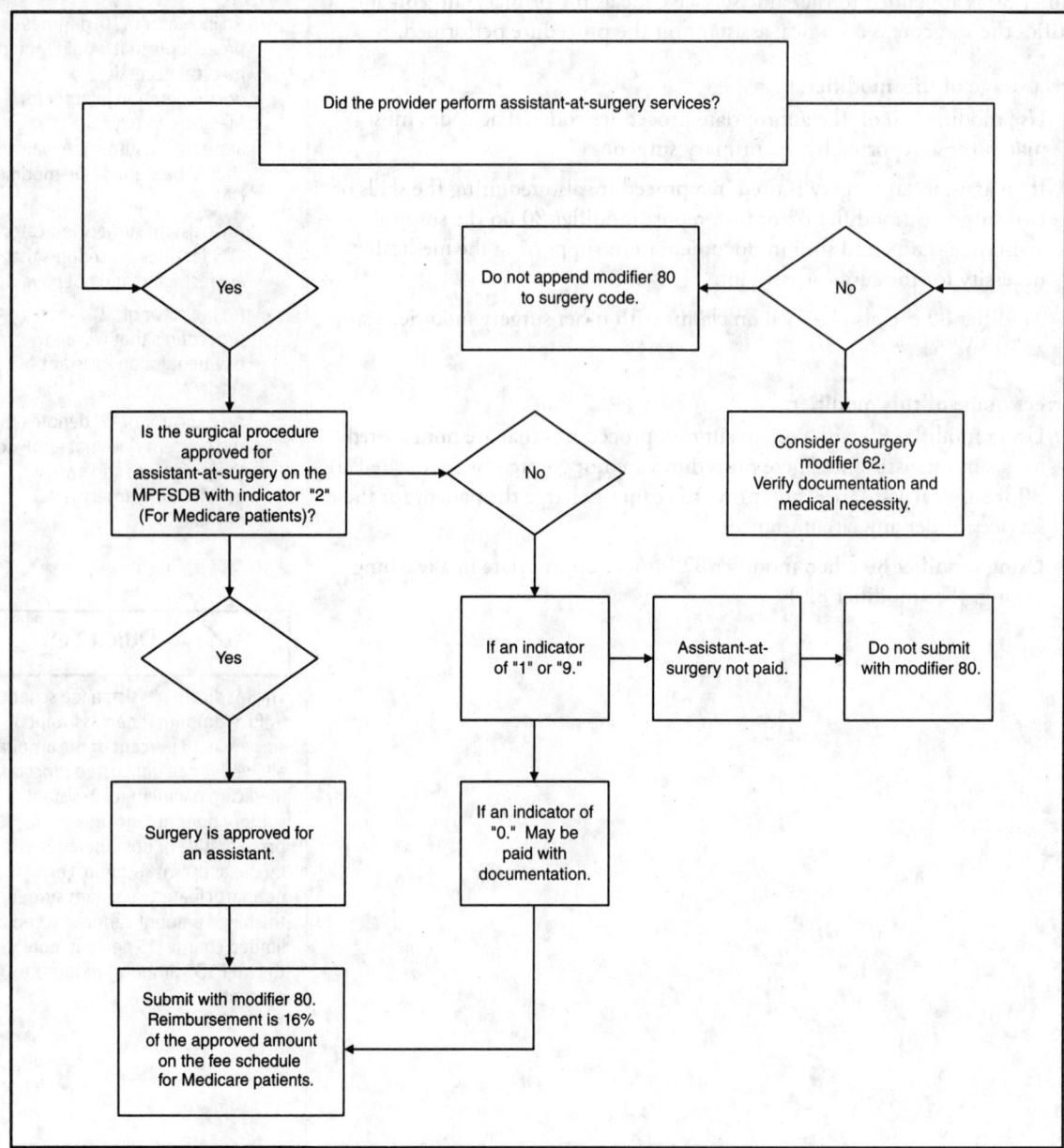

© 2020 Optum360, LLC

81   Minimum Assistant Surgeon

Minimum surgical assistant services are identified by adding modifier 81 to the usual procedure number.

When to use this modifier:

Modifier 81 should be appended to the procedure code representing the services performed by each provider who participated in the operative session. Typically, the assistant at surgery is not present for the entire procedure; rather, he or she assists with a specific part of the procedure only.

Correct usage of this modifier:

- Use modifier 81 when the assistant at surgery is not present for the entire procedure.

- Modifier 81 is used when the services of a second or third assistant surgeon are required during a procedure. Payers have varied interpretations of how, or even if, modifier 81 should be used and many do not recognize this modifier.

Incorrect usage of this modifier:

- Using modifier 81 to describe a full surgical assist. See modifiers 80 and 82.

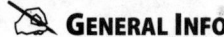 **GENERAL INFO**

Modifier 81 is not to be used to bill nonphysician assistants at surgery who do not meet criteria for payment as a provider under Medicare Part B. Medicare Part B does not recognize scrub technicians, certified surgical assistants, registered nurses, medical assistants, and similar care givers as assistants at surgery for payment. The payment for nonphysician assistants who do not qualify to bill Medicare Part B is considered included (bundled) in the payment to the hospital or ASC and should not be unbundled or billed to a contractor or a beneficiary.

The following flow chart can aid in an audit by helping determine if modifier 81 is being used correctly and whether additional documentation might be required.

Modifier 81

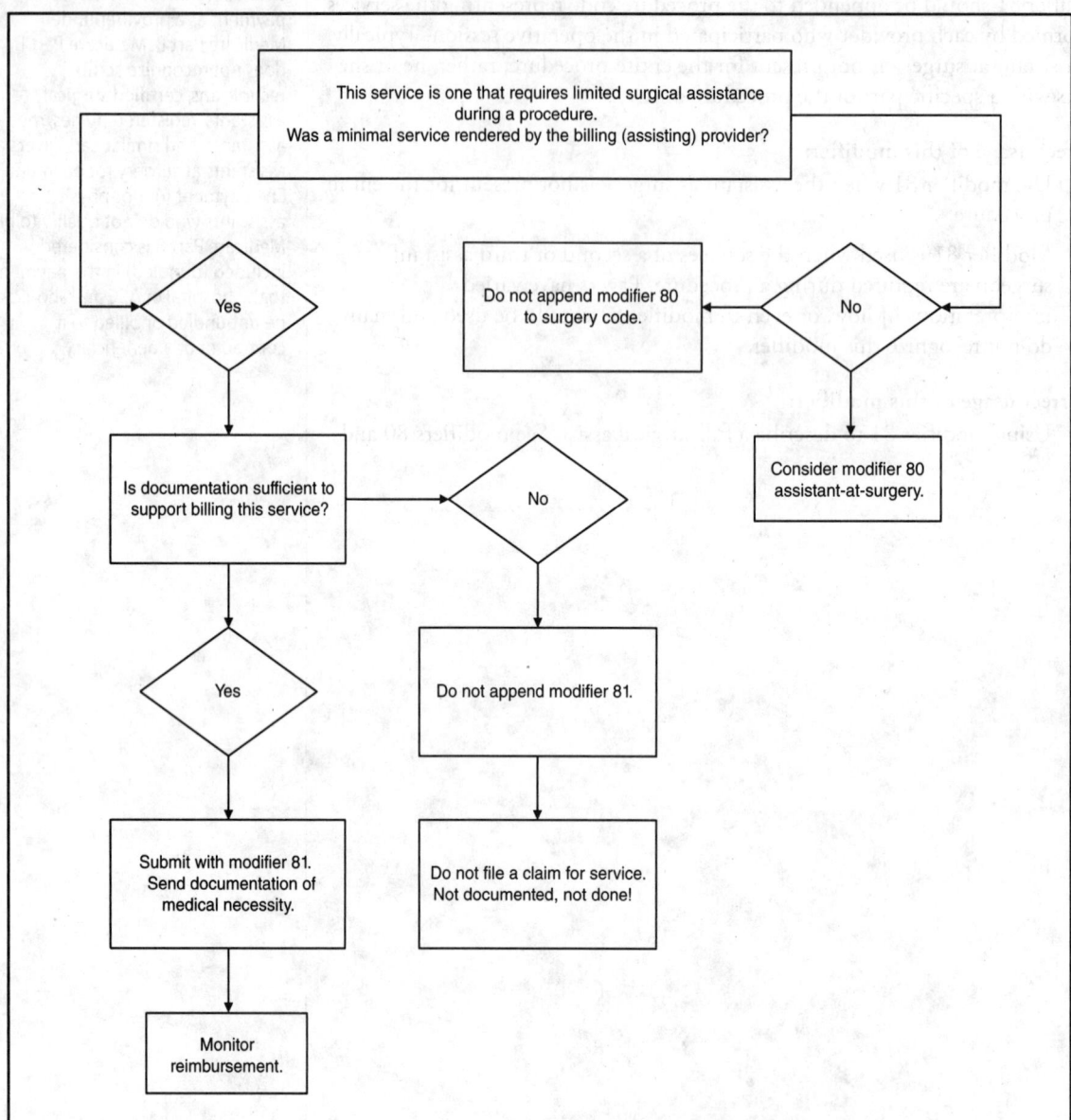

© 2020 Optum360, LLC

82   Assistant Surgeon (When Qualified Resident Surgeon not Available)

The unavailability of a qualified resident surgeon is a prerequisite for use of modifier 82 appended to the usual procedure number(s).

When to use this modifier:

Modifier 82 is limited to use in teaching hospitals to indicate that a qualified resident surgeon is unavailable. Typically in this environment, training programs allow qualified residents to function as the first assistant. However, when there is not a qualified resident available or in facilities without a teaching program for specific specialties, Medicare covers assistant-at-surgery services when modifier 82 is appended to the basic service code.

Note: In order to report modifier 82, the academic department is required to have a signed attestation form on file validating that no qualified residents are available.

Correct usage of this modifier:

- Modifier 82 is used to indicate a surgical assist when a qualified resident is not available. Medicare Part B does not pay when a resident is used as an assistant. Medicare Part B allows use of modifier 82 for services rendered only by a medical doctor not in a residency and/or fellowship program.

Incorrect usage of this modifier:

- Using an assistant-at-surgery modifier with surgical procedures that are not covered for a surgical assistant. These procedures are not covered by Medicare Part B for surgical assistance, and providers cannot charge the patient for these services under any circumstances.

- Repeated use of modifier 82 by physicians in teaching facilities. This practice raises a flag indicating potential abuse.

- Using modifier 82 when a qualified resident is available.

Note: Payment may be made for the services of an assistant at surgery, regardless of the availability of a qualified resident, when one of the following conditions exists:

- Exceptional medical circumstances (e.g., emergency life-threatening situations such as multiple traumatic injuries requiring immediate treatment).

- The primary surgeon has an across-the-board policy of never involving residents in the preoperative, operative, or postoperative care of his or her patients. (This often occurs when community physicians have no involvement in a hospital's graduate medical education program.)

- Complex medical procedures, including multistage transplant surgery, which may require a team of physicians.

The following flow chart can aid in an audit by helping determine if modifier 82 is being used correctly and whether additional documentation might be required.

Modifier 82

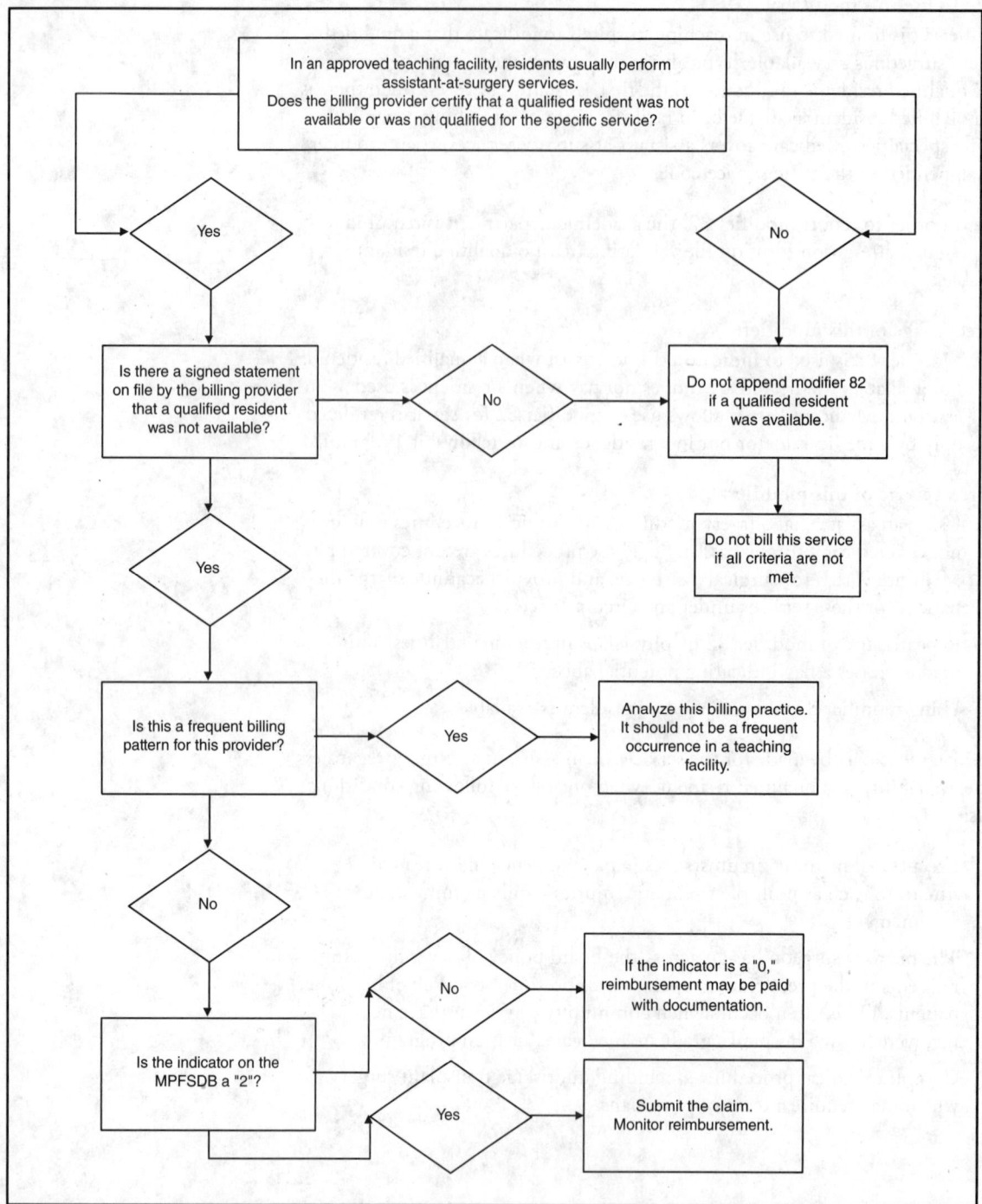

90   Reference (Outside) Laboratory

When laboratory procedures are performed by a party other than the treating or reporting physician or other qualified health care professional, the procedure may be identified by adding modifier 90 to the usual procedure number.

When to use this modifier:

Modifier 90 should be appended to the procedure code when the test is performed by an outside laboratory only.

Correct usage of this modifier:

- Modifier 90 is added to the procedure code when laboratory procedures are performed by a party other than the treating or reporting provider.

- Report modifier 90 only with clinical laboratory services paid according to the Medicare clinical laboratory fee schedule.

- Modifier 90 may be reported on claims that have been submitted only by independent laboratories (specialty code 69).

Incorrect usage of this modifier:

- Treating or reporting physician is completing the laboratory procedure.

- Reporting modifier 90 on anatomic pathology and lab services paid under the Medicare physician fee schedule.

The following flow chart can aid in an audit by helping determine if modifier 90 is being used correctly and whether additional documentation might be required.

Modifier 90

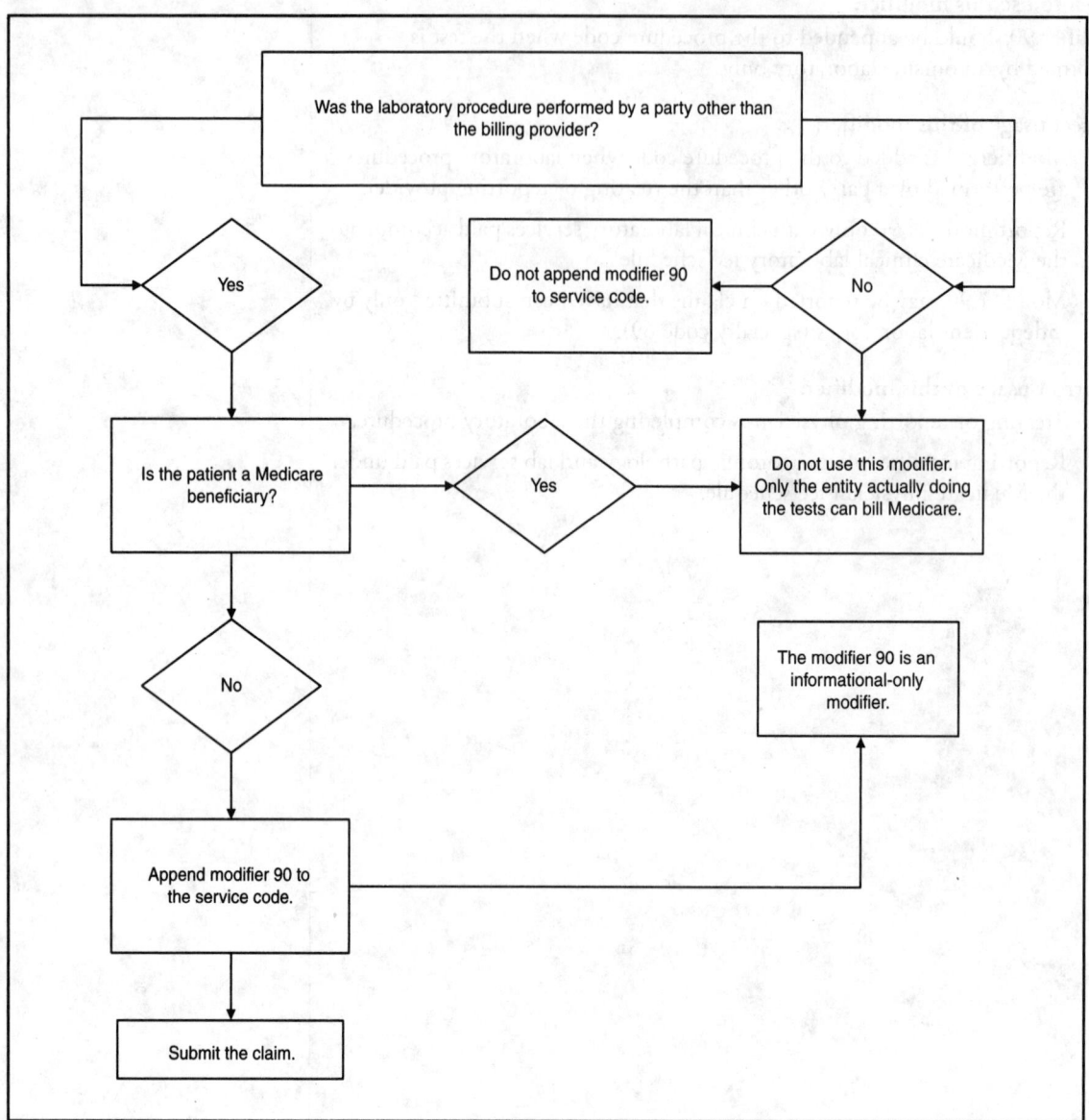

 © 2020 Optum360, LLC

91   Repeat Clinical Diagnostic Laboratory Test

In the course of treating the patient, it may be necessary to repeat the same laboratory test on the same day to obtain subsequent (multiple) test results. Under these circumstances, the laboratory test performed can be identified by its usual procedure number and the addition of modifier 91. **Note:** This modifier may not be used when tests are rerun to confirm initial results, due to testing problems with specimens or equipment, or for any other reason when a normal, one-time, reportable result is all that is required. This modifier may not be used when other codes describe a series of test results (e.g., glucose tolerance tests, evocative/suppression testing). This modifier may only be used for laboratory tests performed more than once on the same day on the same patient.

When to use this modifier:

Modifier 91 should be appended to the procedure code representing the service to properly identify a subsequent and medically necessary laboratory test being performed on the same day as the same previous laboratory test.

Correct usage of this modifier:

- Modifier 91 is added to the procedure codes that represent repeat laboratory tests or studies performed on the same day on the same patient.

- Add modifier 91 only when additional test results are to be obtained subsequent to the administration or performance of the same tests on the same day.

   Example

   An anxious appearing patient presents to the emergency department with complaints of confusion, shaking, and light-headedness. Additionally, the patient appears somewhat confused and appears to have difficulty speaking. Laboratory and other diagnostic studies are performed. The patient's glucose test reveals hypoglycemia. A nurse administers glucose to the patient, and another glucose test is performed approximately 20 to 30 minutes later. Modifier 91 is appended to the subsequent glucose test to indicate that the test is not a duplicate; rather it is a medically necessary repeat test performed on the same day as the initial test.

Incorrect usage of this modifier:

- Reporting modifier 91 on laboratory tests or studies that needed to be repeated due to an error or malfunction of equipment or damage to the specimen.

- Using modifier 91 for those services that already indicate that a series of test results are to be obtained, such as CPT code 82951 Glucose; tolerance test (GTT), three specimens (includes glucose).

The following flow chart can aid in an audit by helping determine if modifier 91 is being used correctly and whether additional documentation might be required.

Modifier 91

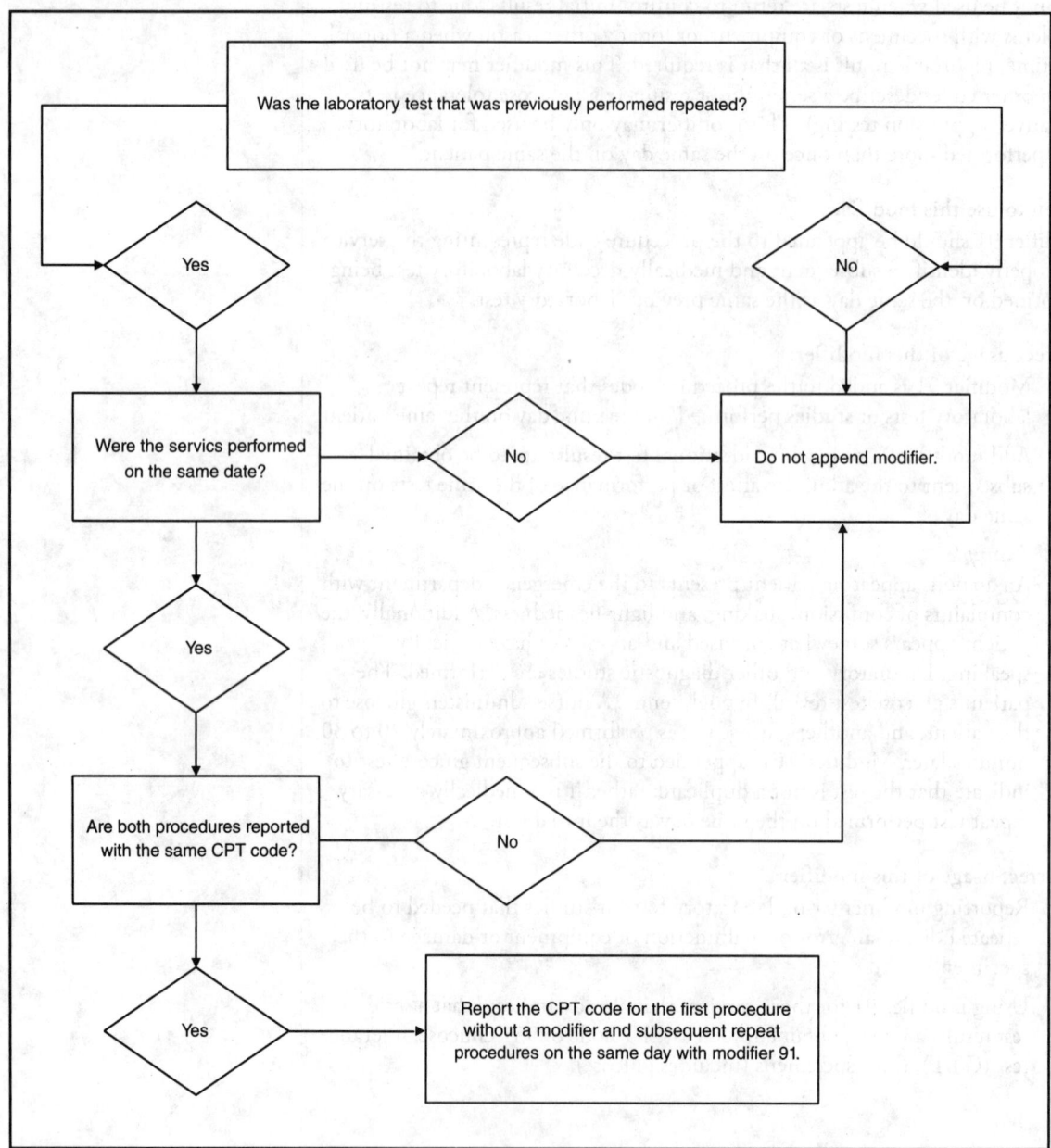

Was the laboratory test that was previously performed repeated?

Yes

No

Were the servics performed on the same date?

No

Do not append modifier.

Yes

Are both procedures reported with the same CPT code?

No

Yes

Report the CPT code for the first procedure without a modifier and subsequent repeat procedures on the same day with modifier 91.

95 Synchronous Telemedicine Service Rendered Via a Real-Time Interactive Audio and Video Telecommunications System

Synchronous telemedicine service is defined as a **real-time** interaction between a physician or other qualified health care professional and a patient who is located at a distant site from the physician or other qualified health care professional. The totality of the communication of information exchanged between the physician or other qualified health care professional and patient during the course of the synchronous telemedicine service must be of an amount and nature that would be sufficient to meet the key components and/or requirements of the same service when rendered via a face-to-face interaction. Modifier 95 may only be appended to the services listed in Appendix P of the CPT book. Appendix P lists the CPT codes for services that are typically performed face-to-face, but may be rendered via real-time (synchronous) interactive audio and video telecommunications system.

When to use this modifier:

This modifier should only be reported when real-time interaction is provided by a physician or other qualified health care professional. The documentation for the services provided with this modifier must be provided as if it was a face-to-face visit and include the required components or key components. A complete list of codes that modifier 95 can be appended to can be found in Appendix P of the CPT book.

Correct use of this modifier:

- Appending this modifier to services listed in Appendix P. These codes will be identified with in the CPT book with a ★ icon.

  Example

  A patient receives 30 minutes of psychotherapy while residing in a group home environment. The physician rendering the treatment is in an offsite inpatient psychiatric facility office. Report 90832 (a star icon identifies this code as a telemedicine service) and append modifier 95. The total amount of communication exchanged between the provider and the patient must be commensurate with the same requirements that would be in place had the service been provided in the more traditional face-to-face setting.

Incorrect use of this modifier:

- Appending this modifier to services other than those listed in Appendix P.

- Appending this modifier to codes for services not provided using a synchronous interactive audio and video telecommunications system.

The following flow chart can aid in an audit by helping determine if modifier 95 is being used correctly and whether additional documentation might be required.

Modifier 95

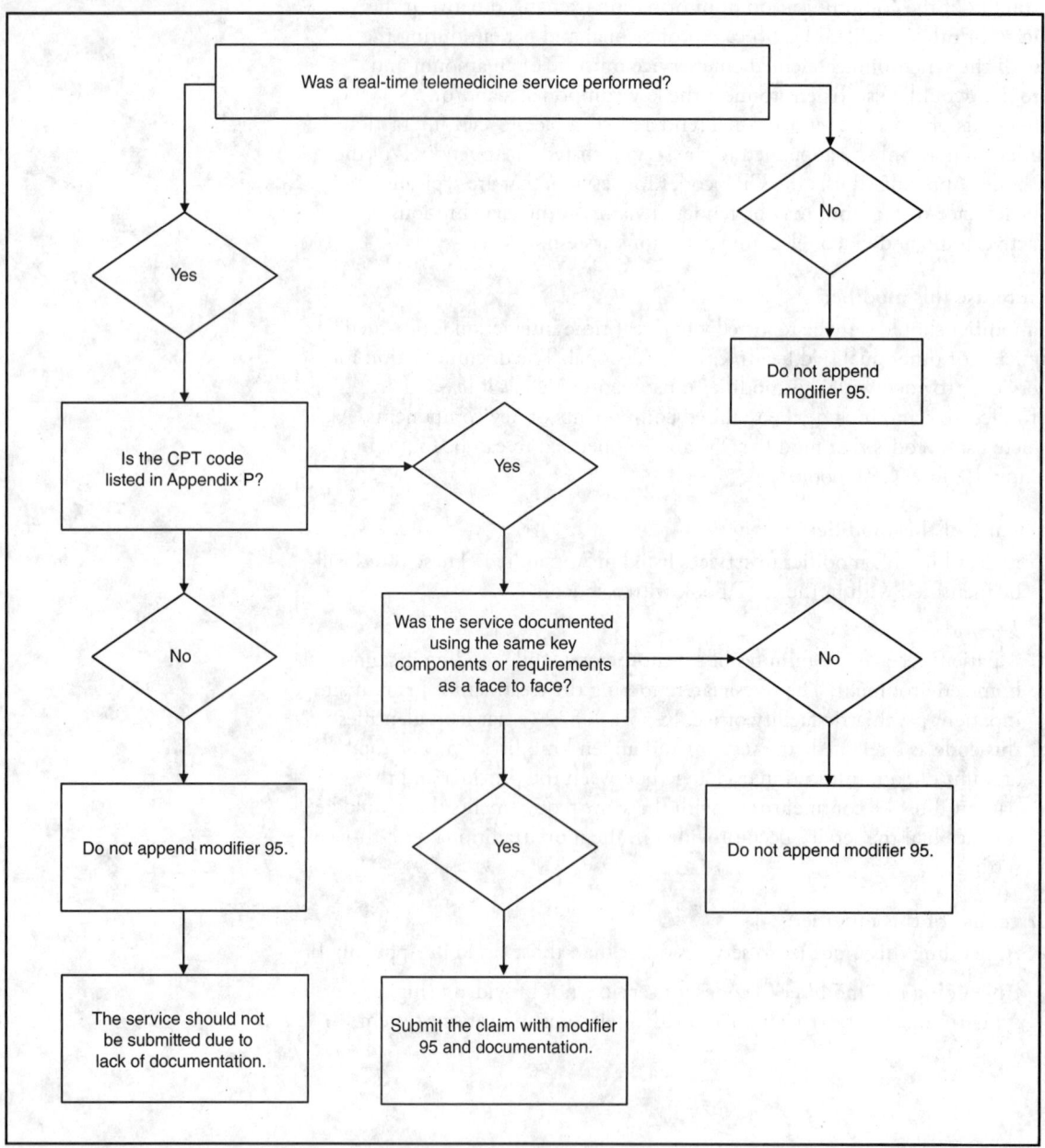

96   Habilitative Services

When a service or procedure that may be habilitative or rehabilitative in nature is provided for rehabilitative purposes, the physician or other qualified health care professional may add modifier 96 to the service or procedure code to indicate that the service or procedure provided was a habilitative service. Habilitative services help an individual learn skills and functioning for daily living that the individual has not yet developed, and then keep and/or improve those learned skills. Habilitative services also help an individual keep, learn, or improve skills and functioning for daily living.

When to use this modifier:

Modifier 96 should be appended to codes for services or procedures that are considered habilitative. Habilitative services describe medically needed services and/or devices that help a patient partly or fully learn, keep, and improve new skills or functioning required to perform daily living activities or manage a health condition. Habilitative services help patients acquire a skill for the first time.

Example:

A pediatric patient with a history of age-appropriate speech delay receives speech therapy on an outpatient basis. Report 92507 and append modifier 96 to indicate that the service was provided for habilitative purposes.

Correct use of this modifier:

- Modifier 96 should be reported with physical therapy, occupational therapy, speech therapy, and other therapy services, when applicable.

- Report modifier 96 with therapy services provided for the purpose of teaching the patient a new skill related to activities of daily living.

- Report modifier 96 with therapy services provided for the purpose of teaching the patient a new skill related to activities of daily living.

Incorrect use of this modifier:

- Appending this modifier to therapy services provided for reasons other than those related to introducing and/or improving skills and functioning related to daily living activities.

- Appending this modifier to services or procedures not defined as habilitative.

The following flow chart can aid in an audit by helping determine if modifier 96 is being used correctly and whether additional documentation might be required.

Modifier 96

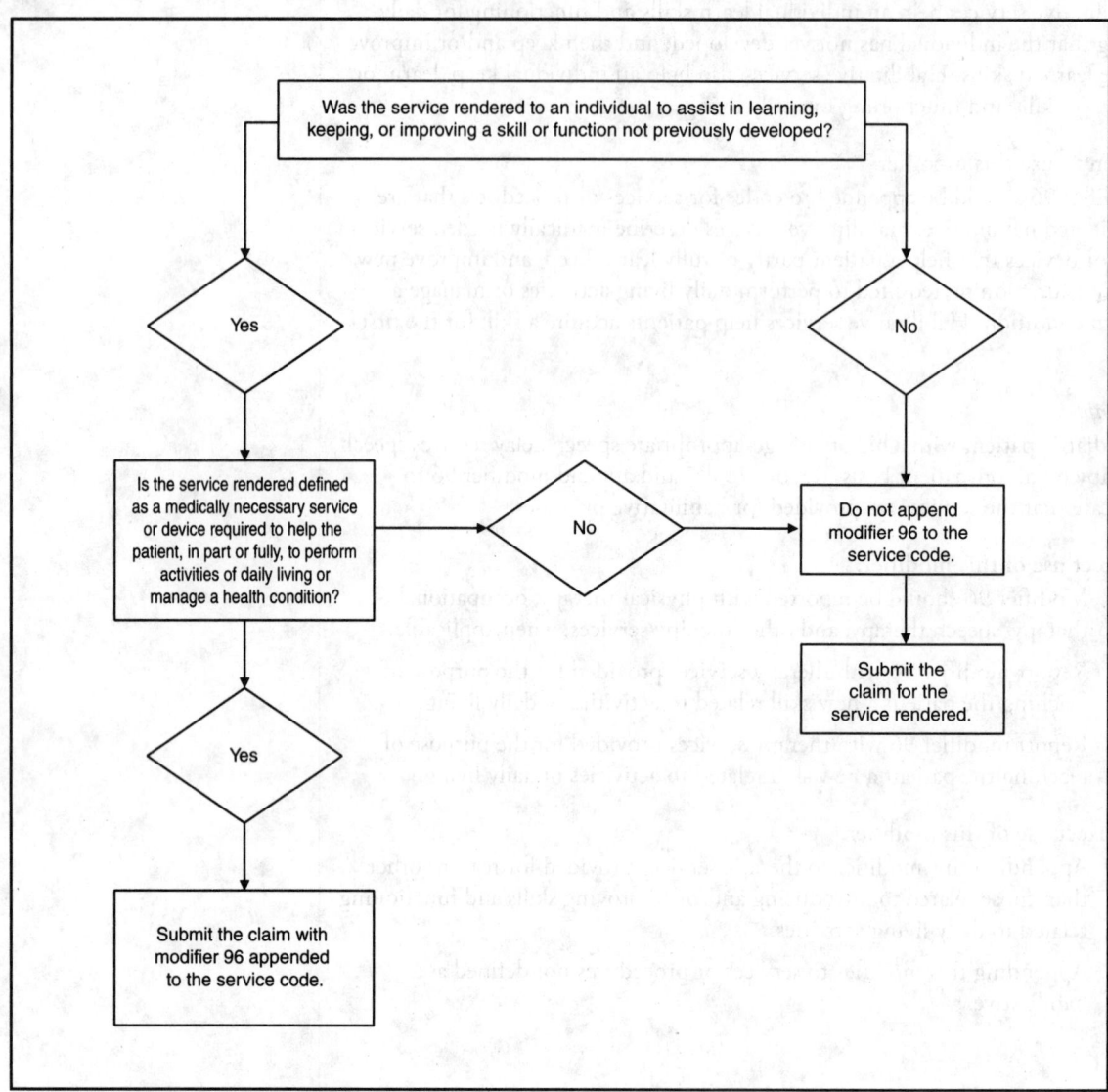

97   Rehabilitative Services

When a service or procedure that may be habilitative or rehabilitative in nature is provided for rehabilitative purposes, the physician or other qualified health care professional may add modifier 97 to the service or procedure code to indicate that the service or procedure provided was a rehabilitative service. Rehabilitative services help an individual keep, get back, or improve skills and functioning for daily living that have been lost or impaired because the individual was sick, hurt, or disabled.

When to use this modifier:

Modifier 97 should be appended to services or procedures that are considered rehabilitative. Rehabilitative services describe a diverse range of services—from complete specialized medically-based inpatient programs to outpatient therapy—provided in various settings, such as nursing homes or ambulatory centers, that encourage the best possible level of total well-being (physical, mental, emotional, psychological, social, and economic) of the patient to ensure he or she can function at the highest degree possible. Rehabilitative services are provided to help patients reacquire a skill that was lost or impaired due to an acquired condition.

Example

A patient with a history of previous automobile accident and multiple broken bones in both lower extremities requiring both legs to be immobilized and placed in casts receives rehabilitation services to help her learn to ambulate and climb stairs using a walker. Report 97116 and append modifier 97 to indicate that the services are rehabilitative in nature.

Correct use of this modifier:

- Modifier 97 should be reported with physical therapy, occupational therapy, speech therapy, and other therapy services, when applicable.

- Report modifier 97 with therapy services provided for the purpose of reteaching the patient a skill, related to activities of daily living, lost or impaired due to an acquired injury, illness, or disease.

Incorrect use of this modifier:

- Appending this modifier to therapy services provided for reasons other than those related to introducing and/or improving skills and functioning related to daily living activities.

- Appending this modifier to services or procedures not defined as rehabilitative.

The following flow chart can aid in an audit by helping determine if modifier 97 is being used correctly and whether additional documentation might be required.

Modifier 97

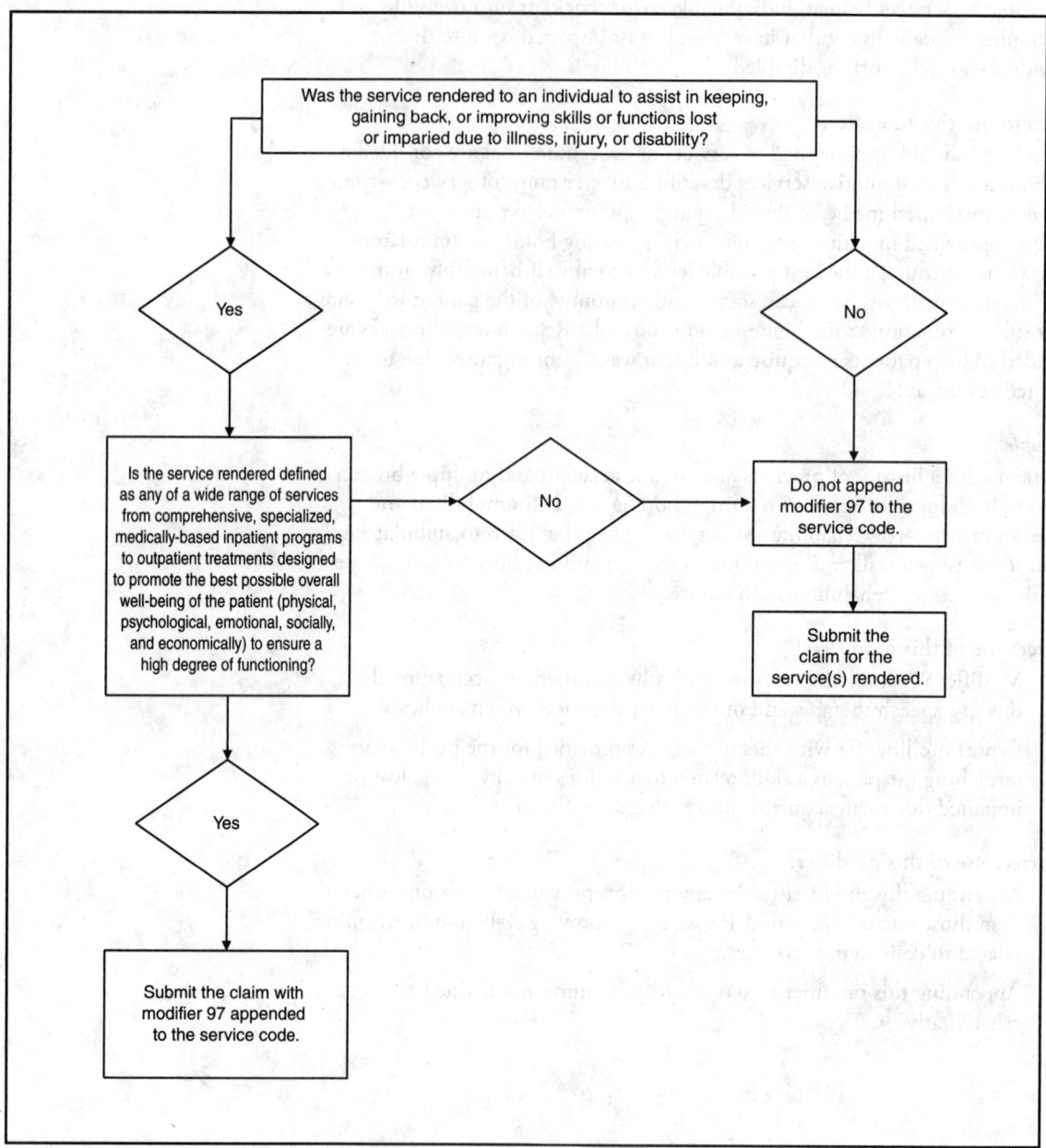

Was the service rendered to an individual to assist in keeping, gaining back, or improving skills or functions lost or imparied due to illness, injury, or disability?

Yes

No

Is the service rendered defined as any of a wide range of services from comprehensive, specialized, medically-based inpatient programs to outpatient treatments designed to promote the best possible overall well-being of the patient (physical, psychological, emotional, socially, and economically) to ensure a high degree of functioning?

No

Do not append modifier 97 to the service code.

Submit the claim for the service(s) rendered.

Yes

Submit the claim with modifier 97 appended to the service code.

HCPCS Level II Modifiers

The HCPCS Level II codes are alphanumeric codes developed by the Centers for Medicare and Medicaid Services as a complementary coding system to the AMA's CPT codes. HCPCS Level II codes describe procedures, services, and supplies not found in the CPT book.

Similar to the CPT coding system, HCPCS Level II codes also contain modifiers that further define services and items without changing the basic meaning of the CPT or HCPCS Level II code with which they are reported. However, the HCPCS Level II modifiers differ somewhat from their CPT counterparts in that they are composed of alpha characters or alphanumeric characters. HCPCS Level II modifiers range from A1 to XU and include such diverse modifiers as E1 Upper left, eyelid, AI Principal physician of record, and Q6 Service furnished by a locum tenens physician.

It is important to note that HCPCS Level II modifiers may be used in conjunction with CPT codes, such as 69436-LT Tympanostomy (requiring insertion of ventilating tube), general anesthesia, left ear. Likewise, CPT modifiers can be used when reporting HCPCS Level II codes, such as L5050-50 Ankle, Symes, molded socket, SACH foot, bilateral (this scenario can also be reported with modifiers RT and LT, depending on the third-party payer's protocol). In some cases, a report may be required to accompany the claim to support the need for a particular modifier's use, especially when the presence of a modifier causes suspension of the claim for manual review and pricing.

Below is a list of some of the most common HCPCS Level II modifiers.

A1   **Dressing for one wound**

A2   **Dressing for two wounds**

A3   **Dressing for three wounds**

A4   **Dressing for four wounds**

A5   **Dressing for five wounds**

A6   **Dressing for six wounds**

A7   **Dressing for seven wounds**

A8   **Dressing for eight wounds**

A9   **Dressing for nine or more wounds**

Modifiers A1, A2, A3, A4, A5, A6, A7, A8, and A9 wound dressings:

- Modifiers A1–A9 indicate that a primary or secondary dressing on a surgical or debrided wound is being applied. Primary dressings are defined as therapeutic or protective coverings, and secondary dressings are materials applied for a therapeutic or protective function.

- Documentation must indicate the number of wounds being dressed.

- The modifier number reported must correspond to the number of wound dressings applied, not necessarily the number of wounds treated. For example a patient with three previously debrided wounds may require a secondary dressing on only two wounds, which would be reported with modifier A2.

- Gradient compression stockings are not considered wound dressing and would not be reported with modifiers A1–A9 although A6531 and A6532 are covered for open venous stasis ulcers.

AA Anesthesia performed personally by anesthesiologist
- See chapter 5, Auditing Anesthesia Services, for detailed information.

AD Medical supervision by a physician; more than four concurrent anesthesia procedures
- See chapter 5, Auditing Anesthesia Services, for detailed information.

AE Registered dietician
- Used when reporting nutritional services to indicate that an appropriate provider performed the service

AF Specialty physician

AG Primary physician

Modifiers AF and AG physician designation:
- These modifiers are used as a physician designation for outpatient services provided in a critical access hospital (CAH) in a designated physician scarcity area (PSA) or health professional shortage area (HPSA).
- Primary care physicians are defined as general practice, family practice, internal medicine, and obstetrics/gynecology for modifier AG.
- Specialty care physicians are defined as specialties other than dental, optometry, chiropractic, or podiatry for modifier AF.

AH Clinical psychologist
- Medicare requires this modifier for services provided by a clinical psychologist who has met the required level of education (PhD) and hours of practice.
- These services are limited to CPT codes 90785–90899 and 96105–96146 or as limited by the specific state practice act.

AI Principal physician of record
- Modifier AI identifies the principal physician of record—the admitting or attending physician who is overseeing the patient's care while in an inpatient or nursing facility setting.

AJ Clinical social worker
- Medicare requires this modifier for services provided by a clinical psychologist who has met the required level of education and hours of practice per state regulations.
- These services are limited to CPT codes 90785–90899 or as limited by the state practice act. Some states may allow the clinical psychologist to administer the testing codes 96105–96146 but may not interpret.

AM Physician, team member service
- The physician member of a team is required to perform one out of every three visits made by a team member.
- Modifier AM should be used to indicate a team member visit was performed by the physician.
- Team member visits are denied if only one person rendering services is billing for team services, as this is inappropriate billing practice.

SPECIAL ALERT

If an anesthetist assists the physician in the care of a single patient, the service is considered personally performed by the physician. The anesthesiologist should report this service with modifier AA and the appropriate CPT code.

AS Physician Assistant, Nurse Practitioner or Clinical Nurse Specialist Services for Assistant-at-Surgery
- HCPCS Level II modifier AS is used to report nonphysician providers (NPP), advance practice providers (APP), or clinical nurse specialists (CNS) who assist in surgery.
- Append modifier AS to the CPT code for the procedure the NPP, APP, or CNS assisted with.
- When reporting modifier AS, the nonphysician practitioner should report the CPT code for the procedure using his or her own provider identification number with the appropriate site-of-service code.

CC Procedure code change
- Modifier CC is used by the contractor when the procedure code submitted had to be changed either for administrative reasons or because an incorrect code was filed.
- Payment rule: Payment determination will be based on the new code used by the contractor.

CS Cost-sharing waived for specified COVID-19 testing-related services that result in an order for, or administration of, a COVID-19 test and/or used for cost-sharing waived preventive services furnished via telehealth in Rural Health Clinics and Federally Qualified Health Centers during the COVID-19 public health emergency
- Modifier CS should be applied for certain evaluation and management services related to COVID-19 testing, regardless of whether they are performed in-person or via telehealth. These services are medical visits reported by outpatient providers, physicians, or other providers and suppliers who bill Medicare for Part B services, order, or administer a COVID-19 lab test. Cost-sharing does not apply for COVID-19 testing-related services, which are medical visits furnished between March 18, 2020, and the end of the PHE and one of the following:
  - Result in an order for or administration of a COVID-19 test;
  - Are related to furnishing or administering such a test or to the evaluation of an individual for purposes of determining the need for such a test;
  - Are in any of the following categories of HCPCS evaluation and management codes:
    - Office and other outpatient services
    - Hospital observation services
    - Emergency department services
    - Nursing facility services
    - Domiciliary, rest home, or custodial care services
    - Home services
    - Online digital evaluation and management services
  - Cost-sharing does not apply to the above medical visit services for which payment is made to:
    - Hospital Outpatient Departments paid under the Outpatient Prospective Payment System
    - Physicians and other professionals under the Physician Fee Schedule
    - Critical Access Hospitals (CAHs)

- Rural Health Clinics (RHCs)
- Federally Qualified Health Centers (FQHCs)

For services furnished on or after March 18, 2020, and through the end of the PHE, outpatient providers, physicians, and other providers and suppliers that bill Medicare for Part B services under these payment systems should use modifier CS on applicable claim lines to identify the service as subject to the cost-sharing waiver for COVID-19 testing-related services and should NOT bill Medicare patients for any co-insurance and/or deductible amounts for those services. Additionally, the CPT telehealth modifier, modifier 95, should be applied to claim lines that describe services furnished via telehealth. The billing practitioner should also report the POS code that reflects where the service would have been furnished if furnished in person.

E1   Upper left, eyelid

E2   Lower left, eyelid

E3   Upper right, eyelid

E4   Lower right, eyelid

Modifiers E1, E2, E3, and E4:
- These modifiers are used to identify services performed on separate eyelids.
- Modifiers LT and RT should be used for procedures on the eye globe or ocular adnexa.
- CMS and some private or third-party payers require these modifiers.

F1   Left hand, second digit

F2   Left hand, third digit

F3   Left hand, fourth digit

F4   Left hand, fifth digit

F5   Right hand, thumb

F6   Right hand, second digit

F7   Right hand, third digit

F8   Right hand, fourth digit

F9   Right hand, fifth digit

FA   Left hand, thumb

Modifiers F1, F2, F3, F4, F5, F6, F7, F8, F9, and FA:
- These modifiers are appended to procedures performed on the fingers.
- Report modifiers affecting reimbursement first (e.g., 51, 80).
- Procedures should be reported with these modifiers to identify the specific finger; it is not sufficient to simply increase the number of services in the unit box.

G8 **Monitored anesthesia care (MAC) for deep complex, complicated or markedly invasive surgical procedure**

G9 **Monitored anesthesia care for patient who has a history of severe cardiopulmonary condition**

Modifiers G8 and G9:

- See chapter 5, Auditing Anesthesia Services, for more information.

GA **Waiver of liability statement issued as required by payer policy, individual case**

- This modifier indicates that the physician's office has a signed advance beneficiary notice (ABN) retained in the patient's chart or has provided the notice to the patient and has documented the patient's refusal to sign the ABN.

- The purpose of the waiver of liability is to ensure that the provider will be paid for the services performed and to protect the beneficiary from receiving unnecessary services. Providers who acquire a waiver of liability for a service should use modifier GA directly following a procedure code to indicate that a beneficiary has signed a waiver of liability form. The provider should keep the form on file. No other statement regarding the waiver of liability is required when modifier GA is used. Modifier GA appended to a procedure code is sufficient evidence that the beneficiary has signed an advance notice and has agreed to pay for the service if it is denied as not medically necessary by Medicare. If the beneficiary subsequently requests a review of the denial, Medicare will request the physician to forward a copy of the notice for its files.

- An important preventive measure the physician can use to avoid most claim denials when the services are medically reasonable and necessary, is to fully complete claims. Medical necessity denials are often due to a lack of information on the claim to support the medical necessity of the service.

- An advance notice may be applied to an extended course of treatment, provided the notice identifies each service for which Medicare is likely to deny payment. A separate notice is required, however, if additional services for which Medicare is likely to deny payment are furnished later in the course of treatment.

- The Medicare beneficiary is never liable for payment of services that are unbundled from another service. Examples of unbundled services include two hospital visits on the same day by the same physician, removal of sutures by the same physician who performed the surgical procedure, and administration of an injection on the day of an evaluation and management service.

GC **This service has been performed in part by a resident under the direction of a teaching physician**

- When a teaching physician's services are billed using this modifier, the teaching physician is certifying that he or she was present during the key portions of the service and was immediately available during the other portions of the service.

- When an anesthesiologist uses modifier QK for two to four medically directed procedures, he or she would not also append modifier GC to the anesthesia code. Modifier QK only is used.

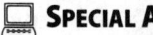
SPECIAL ALERT

A revised Advance Beneficiary Notice of Noncoverage (ABN), Form CMS-R-131, has been approved. Use will be mandatory starting 8/31/20. More information can be found at: https://www.cms.gov/Medicare/Medicare-General-Information/BNI/ABN

- When there is a one-on-one situation with a resident and a teaching anesthesiologist (teaching setting) the anesthesiologist appends modifier GC only.

GE **This service has been performed by a resident without the presence of a teaching physician under the primary care exemption**

- This modifier identifies services being billed under the primary care exception to the guideline for governing presence during the key portions of a service by the teaching physician.

  Note: On an interim basis for the duration of the COVID-19 public health emergency, residents furnishing services under the primary care exemption may provide an expanded set of services to beneficiaries. Generally, residents may only report 99202–99203, 99211–99213, G0402, and G0438–G0439. The interim rule allows resident services performed via telehealth and includes levels 4 and 5 of an office/outpatient E/M visit, telephone E/M, care management, and some communication technology-based services. The expanded set of services are CPT codes 99204–99205, 99214–99215, 99421–99423, 99452, 99441–99443, 99495–99496 and HCPCS codes G2010 and G2012. Additionally, when services are performed via telemedicine, code level selection is based on MDM or time. Append modifier GE to the service.

GN **Services delivered under an outpatient speech-language pathology plan of care**

GO **Services delivered under an outpatient occupational therapy plan of care**

GP **Services delivered under an outpatient physical therapy plan of care**

Modifiers GN, GO, and GP:

- Append the modifier to therapy services subject to a financial limitation as defined by CMS.

- Appending these modifiers does change the status of noncovered services.

- Assign the modifier based upon the type of service rendered; GN for speech-language pathology, GO for occupational therapy, and GP for physical therapy.

The following codes are subject to financial limitations and require the use of modifiers GN, GO, or GP, as applicable:

An "always therapy" service is a physical, speech-language, pathology, and occupational therapy service that must be performed by a qualified therapist under a certified therapy plan of care. A "sometimes therapy" service may be performed by an individual outside of a certified therapy plan of care.

When physicians or NPPs bill "always therapy" codes, they must follow the policies of the type of therapy they are providing (e.g., use a plan of care, bill with the appropriate therapy modifier [GP, GO, GN]). A physician or NPP shall not bill an "always therapy" code unless the service is provided under a therapy plan of care. When a "sometimes therapy" code is billed by a physician or NPP as a medical service and not under a therapy plan of care, the therapy modifier should not be used.

The following codes are subject to financial limitations and require the use of modifiers GN, GO, or GP, as applicable:

64550	90901	90912	90913	92507	92508
92520	92521	92522	92523	92524	92526
92597	92605	92606	92607	92608	92609
92610	92611	92612	92614	92616	92618
95851	95852	95992	96105	96111	96125
97010	97012	97016	97018	97022	97024
97026	97028	97032	97033	97034	97035
97036	97039	97110	97112	97113	97116
97124	97129	97130	97139	97140	97150
97161	97162	97163	97164	97165	97166
97167	97168	97530	97533	97535	97537
97542	97597	97598	97602	97605	97606
97607	97608	97610	97750	97755	97760
97761	97763	97799	98966	98967	98968
G0281	G0283	G0329	G0451	G2010	G2012
G2061	G2062	G2063			

The reimbursement limitations do not apply to audiologists, physicians, and NPPs.

GQ Via asynchronous telecommunications system

GT Via interactive audio and video telecommunication systems

Modifiers GQ and GT:
- These modifiers apply to telehealth services provided in an approved remote location as identified in CMS program memorandum AB-01-69.
- HCPCS code Q3014 Telehealth originating site facility fee, is reported at the patient site.
- The provider reports the service provided with the appropriate CPT code and modifier GQ or GT appended.
- Modifier GT is used to report an interactive session with audio and video portions.
- Modifier GQ indicates an asynchronous telecommunications system such as "store and forward" for transmission of medical files.

  Note: On an interim basis, for the duration of the COVID-19 public health emergency, when a provider delivers telehealth services using a cell phone and contacts the patient on their cell phone, modifiers GQ and GT would not be appended. Modifier 95 would still apply and should be appended to the service.

GY   Item or service statutorily excluded does not meet the definition of any Medicare benefit or, for non-Medicare insurers, is not a contract benefit

GZ   Item or service expected to be denied as not reasonable and necessary

Modifiers GY and GZ:

- Modifier GY should be used only when reporting a service that is statutorily excluded.
- Append modifier GZ to a service that may be denied for medical necessity.
- These modifiers are frequently misreported when a modifier is not required or in place of GA or other coverage modifiers.

LC   Left circumflex coronary artery

LD   Left anterior descending coronary artery

LM   Left main coronary artery

RC   Right coronary artery

RI   Ramus intermedius coronary artery

Modifiers LC, LD, LM, RC and RI:

- These codes are used when more than one intervention is required on a major vessel and its branches. CPT codes describe codes for coronary angioplasty, atherectomy, and stent procedures in terms of the "initial" vessel and a "subsequent" vessel.
- Note that modifiers LC, LD, and RC are included in the CPT book.
- Modifiers LM and RI are not in the CPT book but should be used to report these arteries.
- These modifiers may be used to bypass a CCI edit when correctly applied to an edit that allows a modifier.

LT   Left side
- This modifier indicates that side of the body on which a procedure is performed. It does not indicate a bilateral procedure. Lesion removal on the right and left arms should be coded with modifiers RT and LT.

P1   A normal healthy patient

P2   A patient with mild systemic disease

P3   A patient with severe systemic disease

P4   A patient with severe systemic disease that is a constant threat to life

P5   A moribund patient who is not expected to survive without the operation

P6   A declared brain-dead patient whose organs are being removed for donor purposes
- See chapter 5, Auditing Anesthesia Services, for more information

 © 2020 Optum360, LLC

QK **Medical direction of two, three or four concurrent anesthesia procedures involving qualified individuals**
- See chapter 5, Auditing Anesthesia Services, for more information.

QS **Monitored anesthesiology care service**
- See chapter 5, Auditing Anesthesia Services, for more information.

QW **CLIA-waived test**
- Modifier QW is to be used for all codes that were designated as waived tests after 1996. For codes approved prior to 1996, the existing codes should be used without the modifier.

QX **CRNA service with medical direction by a physician**
- See chapter 5, Auditing Anesthesia Services, for more information.

QY **Medical direction of one certified registered nurse anesthetist (CRNA) by an anesthesiologist**

QZ **CRNA service without medical direction by a physician**
- See chapter 5, Auditing Anesthesia Services, for more information.

RT **Right side**
- Many procedure codes require a physician to indicate the side of the body on which a procedure was performed by using modifiers RT and LT.
- When billing for a separately identifiable/unrelated surgical procedure performed during the postoperative period of another surgical procedure, procedure code modifiers RT (right) and LT (left) must be indicated on the claim as appropriate. In addition, modifier 79 Unrelated Procedure or Service by the Same Physician or Other Qualified Health Care Professional During the Postoperative Period, must be submitted on the subsequent claim.
- This modifier indicates the side of the body on which a procedure is performed. It does not indicate a bilateral procedure. Lesion removal on the right and left arms should be coded with modifiers RT and LT.

T1 **Left foot, second digit**

T2 **Left foot, third digit**

T3 **Left foot, fourth digit**

T4 **Left foot, fifth digit**

T5 **Right foot, great toe**

T6 **Right foot, second digit**

T7 **Right foot, third digit**

T8 **Right foot, fourth digit**

T9 **Right foot, fifth digit**

TA **Left foot, great toe**

Modifiers T1, T2, T3, T4, T5, T6, T7, T8, T9, and TA:
- These modifiers are appended to codes for procedures performed on the toes.
- Report modifiers affecting reimbursement first (e.g., 51, 80).

- Procedures should be reported with these modifiers to identify the toe; it is not sufficient to just increase the number of services in the unit box.

TC Technical component

- Under certain circumstances, a charge may be made for the technical component alone. In those cases, the technical component charge is identified by adding modifier TC to the usual procedure number. Technical component charges are institutional charges and are not billed separately by physicians. However, portable x-ray suppliers bill only for the technical component and should use modifier TC. The charge data from portable x-ray suppliers is then used to build customary and prevailing profiles.

- Modifier TC should be used to report only the technical component of a global procedure or service code. Remember, typically the technical component is provided by the facility or mobile x-ray unit. This modifier is never reported on evaluation and management service codes.

XE Separate encounter, a service that is distinct because it occurred during a separate encounter

XP Separate practitioner, a service that is distinct because it was performed by a different practitioner

XS Separate structure, a service that is distinct because it was performed on a separate organ/structure

XU Unusual non-overlapping service, the use of a service that is distinct because it does not overlap usual components of the main service

Modifiers XE, XP, XS and XU:

- See 59 Distinct Procedural Service in this chapter for more detailed information.

- Modifiers 59, XE, XP, XS, and XU indicate that a procedure or service was independent from other services performed on the same day.

- If a more descriptive modifier is not available and the use of modifier 59 best explains the circumstance, then report the service with this modifier.

- When a procedure or service designated as a separate procedure is carried out independently or considered to be unrelated from the other services provided at the same session, it may be reported by appending the modifier 59, XE, XP, XS, or XU to the specific separate procedure code. This indicates that the procedure is not considered a component of another procedure but instead is a distinct procedure.

- CPT codes for use with modifiers 59, XE, XP, XS, and XU unless limited by the payer are 00100–01999, 10004–69990, 70010–79999, 80047–89398, 90281–99199, and 99500–99607, when appropriate.

- Medicare and other payers may, in many instances, require that one of the four specific subsets of modifier 59 (X{EPSU} modifiers) be reported in lieu of simply reporting the more general modifier 59. In no circumstance should both modifier 59 and an X{EPSU} modifier be reported together.

🖥 SPECIAL ALERT

There are stand-alone procedure codes that describe technical component only (e.g., staff and equipment costs) diagnostic tests. They also identify procedures that are covered only as diagnostic tests and, therefore, do not have a related professional component. Do not use modifier TC on these codes. Technical component services only are institutional and should not be billed separately by physicians.

However, portable x-ray suppliers only bill for the technical component and should use modifier TC.

Chapter 4. **Auditing Evaluation and Management Services**

Evaluation and Management Codes

To make certain that evaluation and management (E/M) coding is reported correctly, it is essential to document the complete clinical picture in the medical record. Higher levels of service require more advanced documentation that supports not only the components of E/M codes but also the medical necessity of a higher level of service. In spite of years of examination and refining, E/M claims reviews remain a subjective endeavor. In simulated situations where documentation is borderline, justification to downcode the claim is as likely to be based on the time of day as it is the complexity of the medical decision. To be fair, recent studies show wide discrepancies when the same documentation was submitted to professional coders for code assignment as well. The physician specialty also has a bearing on code selection. A normal head and neck exam may involve something entirely different to an otolaryngologist than to an orthopedic surgeon.

From a coder's perspective, one of the most difficult instincts to curb is the desire to fill in missing information in the medical record to justify a code selection that seems intuitively or historically correct. As an auditor, determining that the documentation meets or exceeds the key components of the E/M code is imperative. Clearly, coders and auditors can never fill in, extrapolate, or assume that elements belong in the medical records that, in fact, do not appear there. If the documentation for a key E/M component does not meet or exceed the specified requirements for coding and reimbursement purposes, it should be viewed as if it was not performed.

Each E/M service is evaluated on the documentation for that service only; referring to information obtained from a prior history or exam is unacceptable grounds upon which to make a code assignment. The range of codes more accurately reflects the content and context of a visit than was ever remotely possible under the old levels of service codes.

As a result of these discrepancies and difficulties, E/M coding has ushered in an era of greater provider involvement in the coding process and increased clinical and technical demands on coding professionals.

Because evaluation and management (E/M) codes represent the most frequently reported services and comprise 70 to 80 percent of all billed services, they are the target of many payer audits and are also cited in the Office of the Inspector General (OIG) work plan every year. This chapter contains an overview of E/M services and includes guidance for auditing provider services.

DEFINITIONS

coordination of care. Care provided concurrently with counseling that includes treatment instructions to the patient or caregiver; special accommodations for home, work, school, vacation, or other locations; coordination with other providers and agencies; and living arrangements.

counseling. Discussion with a patient and/or family concerning one or more of the following areas: diagnostic results, impressions, and/or recommended diagnostic studies; prognosis; risks and benefits of management (treatment) options; instructions for management (treatment) and/or follow-up; importance of compliance with chosen management (treatment) options; risk factor reduction; and patient and family education.

E/M Levels of Service

The levels of E/M services define the wide variations in skill, effort, time, and medical knowledge required for preventing or diagnosing and treating illness or injury. They also include services promoting optimal health and prevention of health conditions. These codes are intended to denote provider work, including cognitive work. Because much of this work revolves around the thought process of the provider, and involves a large amount of provider training, experience, expertise, and knowledge, the true indications of the level of work may be difficult to recognize without some explanation.

The final E/M code is selected based upon a combination of the following factors:

- Location of the service
- Patient status
- Level of components provided

There are seven components used to define the level of evaluation and management service provided. The first three are considered key components. These key components are:

- History
- Examination
- Medical decision making

The other four are contributing components that may also affect the level of evaluation and management service provided, including:

- Time
- Counseling
- Coordination of care
- Nature of presenting problem

Location of Service

E/M codes are grouped according to the place where the service is rendered. Examples include:

- Office or other outpatient setting
- Inpatient hospital
- Emergency department
- Skilled nursing facilities

Status of Patient

E/M codes are further divided by new versus established patients and whether a visit is considered initial or subsequent. Examples include:

- New outpatient
- Established outpatient
- Initial inpatient hospital care
- Subsequent inpatient hospital care
- Observation care
- Consultations
- Emergency care
- Critical care
- Preventive medicine

The E/M section of the CPT® book includes a decision tree to help determine patient status as new or established. The following CPT definitions describe a new and established patient.

- A new patient is one who has not received any professional services from the provider/qualified health care professional or another physician/qualified health care professional of the exact same specialty and subspecialty who belongs to the same group practice within the past three years.

- An established patient is one who has received professional services from the physician/qualified health care professional or another physician/qualified health care professional of the exact same specialty and subspecialty who belongs to the same group practice within the past three years.
  Note: If a patient is seen by a physician/qualified health care professional who is covering for another physician/qualified health care professional, the patient will be considered the same as if seen by the physician/qualified health care professional who is unavailable.

 DEFINITIONS

Medicare contractor. Medicare Part A fiscal intermediary, Medicare Part B carrier, Medicare administrative contractor (MAC), or a durable medical equipment Medicare administrative contractor (DME MAC).

preventive medicine service. Evaluation and management service provided as a periodic health screening and/or prophylactic service that does not typically include management of new or existing diagnoses or problems.

Documentation

The E/M documentation guidelines published by CMS were first implemented in 1995 and extensively revised in May of 1997. Due to the indefinite delay of the implementation of the revised guidelines published in May 1997, providers have the option of using the original guidelines established in 1995 or the 1997 revised ones. Medicare contractors have been instructed by CMS to review claims in accordance with both sets of guidelines and not to penalize providers for inadvertent errors. Commercial payers may use one or the other, or both, so it is best to query the payer and determine which of the guidelines are used. Many components of both sets of guidelines are the same. However, the 1997 version particularly affects the history and examination components and may result in a different level of E/M code than when the 1995 guidelines are used. For this reason, whichever version of the guidelines (1995 or 1997) used by the payer should be used by the coder or auditor when assigning or reviewing E/M codes. The 1995 and 1997 guidelines for the history and examination components are included for clarification.

 QUICK TIP

CMS released two sets of guidelines for determining the level of physical exam. The 1995 guidelines are based upon the number of organ systems and body areas examined and documented. The 1997 guidelines are based upon identified listings of specific exam elements within the organ systems and body areas.

Commonly referred to as the 1995 and 1997 guidelines, the full documents can be found at https://www.cms.gov/Outreach-and-Education/Medicare-Learning-Network-MLN/MLNProducts/MLN-Publications-Items/CMS1243514.html. Some of the documentation guidelines (DG) stated in this section are examples of acceptable documentation.

2021 Changes to E/M Office/Other Outpatient and Prolonged Service Coding and Guidelines

Effective January 1, 2021, the AMA and CMS have adopted new guidelines and code descriptions for reporting E/M codes for new and established office or other outpatient services (99202–99215). In addition to these changes, code 99201 has been deleted and is no longer valid for dates of service after December 31, 2020.

Per the CMS CY2020 Physician Fee Schedule (PFS) Final Rule and CPT guidelines, the history and examination will no longer be used to select the code level for these services. These services will however still include a medically appropriate history and/or physical examination. The nature and extent of the history and/or physical examination will be determined by the treating provider based on clinical judgment and what is deemed as reasonable, necessary, and clinically appropriate. The history and physical examination should be documented in the medical record.

Selecting the level of office or other outpatient visit (99202–99205 and 99212–99215) should be based on the redefined levels of medical decision making (MDM) or total time spent by the provider on the day of the encounter, including face-to-face and non-face-to-face activities.

Medical Decision Making: Office or Other Outpatient E/M Services

MDM is used to establish diagnoses, assess the status of a condition, and select a management option(s). MDM for these services is defined by three elements detailed in the new MDM table published in the CPT E/M guidelines. Two significant changes in the MDM table are that new and established patient levels are scored the same and new and established codes both require two out of three elements for any given code.

The three elements of the table used in selecting an MDM are:

- Number and complexity of problems addressed
- Amount and/or complexity of data to be reviewed and analyzed
- Risk of complications and/or morbidity or mortality of patient management

Number and Complexity of Problems Addressed During the Encounter

CPT includes definitions to assist in the selection of the different levels of problems listed in the MDM table. It is important to review these definitions as some medical diagnoses or injuries may be classified in different categories using the new definitions. For example, a sinus infection with a fever and chest congestion would have been considered an acute illness with systemic symptoms on the previous Table of Risk, which would have been a moderate risk of complication and/or morbidity or mortality. Using the 2021 new MDM making table, an acute illness with systemic symptoms is defined as an illness that causes systemic symptoms and has a *high risk* of morbidity without treatment, which would be a moderate level illness. The correct classification for this illness now is an acute, uncomplicated illness or injury: A recent or new

 © 2020 Optum360, LLC

short-term problem with low risk of morbidity for which treatment is considered. There is little to no risk of mortality with treatment, and full recovery without functional impairment is expected, which would be a low-level illness using the new definitions.

The table below illustrates the Number and Complexity of Problems Addressed for a level 3 visit.

Level 3 – Number and Complexity of Problems Addressed

Code	Level of MDM	Number and Complexity of Problems Addressed at the Encounter
99203 99213	Low	**Low** • 2 or more self-limited or minor problems or • 1 stable, chronic illness or • 1 acute, uncomplicated illness or injury

Note: Each level has the same requirements for new or established patients.

Amount and/or Complexity of Data to be Reviewed and Analyzed

The second element listed for determining the level of service is no longer based on calculating points for each test category or specific task. Each level has the same requirements for new or established patients. There are four levels in this category, which are consistent with the current guidelines: minimal, limited, moderate, and extensive.

This MDM element includes medical records, tests, and other information that must be obtained, reviewed, ordered, and/or analyzed for the visit, including information obtained from multiple sources or interprofessional correspondence and interpretation of tests that are not reported separately. Ordering and subsequently reviewing test results are considered part of the current encounter, not a subsequent encounter.

CPT also includes new definitions of certain elements used within this category of the MDM table to assist with the interpretation of these elements.

The following table illustrates how the Amount and/or Complexity of Data Reviewed and Analyzed categories are organized for a level 3 visit.

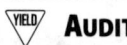 **AUDITOR'S ALERT**

See Appendix 1 for the audit worksheet for office or other outpatient visits.

Level 3 – Amount and/or Complexity of Data Reviewed and Analyzed

Code	Level of MDM	Amount and/or Complexity of Data to be Reviewed and Analyzed *Each unique test, order, or document contributes to the combination of 2 or combination of 3 in Category 1 below.*
99203 99213	Low	**Limited** *Must meet the requirements of at least 1 of the 2 categories* **Category 1: Tests and documents** • Any combination of 2 from the following: • review of prior external note(s) from each unique source* • review of the result(s) of each unique test* • ordering of each unique test* or **Category 2: Assessment requiring an independent historian(s)** *(For the categories of independent interpretation of tests and discussion of management or test interpretation, see moderate or high)*

Note: Each level has the same requirements for new or established patients.

Risk of Complications and/or Morbidity or Mortality of Patient Management

The third and final element listed for determining the level of service includes decisions made during the encounter associated with the patient's problems, diagnostic procedure(s), and treatment(s). This includes potential management options selected and those considered but not selected, after shared MDM with the patient and/or family.

There are four levels in this category that are consistent with the current guidelines: minimal, low, moderate, and high. The minimal and low categories no longer include clinical examples, and the examples for moderate and high risk have been revised.

CPT includes definitions for elements used within the data category of the MDM table to help with the interpretation of these elements.

The table below illustrates the Risk of Complications and/or Morbidity or Mortality of Patient Management column and the conditions listed for level 3 and 4 visits.

Level 3 and 4 – Risk of Complications and/or Morbidity or Mortality of
Patient Management

Code	Level of MDM	Risk of Complications and/or Morbidity or Mortality of Patient Management
99203 99213	Low	Low risk of morbidity from additional diagnostic testing or treatment
99204 99214	Moderate	Moderate risk of morbidity from additional diagnostic testing or treatment *Examples only:* • Prescription drug management • Decision regarding minor surgery with identified patient or procedure risk factors • Decision regarding elective major surgery without identified patient or procedure risk factors • Diagnosis or treatment significantly limited by social determinants of health

Note: Each level has the same requirements for new or established patients.

Time as the Basis for Code Selection

Effective January 1, 2021, time alone may be used to select the appropriate code
level for office or other outpatient visits (99202–99205 and 99212–99215).
Time alone may be used to report these services; the requirement that greater
than 50 percent of the encounter must be spent counseling and/or in
coordination of care has been removed. The new guidelines still require a
face-to-face encounter with the physician or other qualified health care
professional. The notable change is time includes both face-to-face and
non-face-to-face time personally spent by the provider on the day of the
encounter.

Prolonged Services

The AMA also revised guidelines in the 2021 CPT book for the current
prolonged services codes 99354–99355 (Prolonged E/M without Direct Patient
Contact) and 99358–99359 (Prolonged Service without Direct Patient Contact)
stating these codes will no longer be reported in conjunction with 99202–99205
or 99211–99215. Codes 99354-99355 may be used when a physician or
OQHCP provides prolonged services involving direct patient contact that is
provided beyond the usual service in the inpatient, observation, or outpatient
setting.

In addition, CMS will no longer reimburse separately for codes 99358–99359
in association with office E/M services (99202–99205 and 99212–99215).

For a detailed explanation of the changes for Office or Other Outpatient
Medical Services (99202–99215), refer to page 214.

Telehealth Services

As technology and health care advances, the way that providers render care has
also changed. Telemedicine continues to evolve as a way to deliver health care to
patients who might have difficulty accessing a physician or other qualified health
care provider in the traditional manner. It is also assisting patients in
underserved communities to gain access to health care as well as to patients who
desire traditional care delivered in a more modern, timely manner.

See "Temporary Expansion of Telehealth Services Due to Covid-19 Public Health Emergency" below for exemptions to these guidelines during the public health emergency (PHE).

Telehealth services are mostly evaluation and management services including, but not limited to, teleconsultations via telecommunication systems for patients. The teleconsultations most often involve a primary care practitioner with a patient at a remote site and a consulting medical specialist at an urban or referral facility. The primary care practitioner is usually requesting advice from the consulting physician about the patient's conditions or treatment.

Billing and Coding Rules

An originating site is the location of the eligible Medicare beneficiary at the time the service is being furnished via a telecommunications system. Originating sites authorized by law include the following:

- Physician or practitioner's office
- Hospital
- Community mental health center (CMHC)
- Critical access hospital (CAH)
- Federally qualified health center (FQHC)
- Homes of beneficiaries with End-Stage Renal Disease (ESRD) getting home dialysis
- Hospital-based or CAH-based renal dialysis center
- Mobile Stroke Units
- Renal Dialysis Facilities
- Rural health clinic (RHC)
- Skilled nursing facility (SNF)

Independent renal dialysis facilities are not eligible originating sites.

A physician, NP, PA, or CNS must provide at least one ESRD-related "hands on visit" (not using telehealth) per month to evaluate the patient's vascular access site.

Geographic eligibility for an originating site is established for each calendar year based upon the status of the area as of December 31 of the prior calendar year.

As a condition of Medicare payment for telehealth services, the physician or practitioner at the distant site must be licensed to provide the service. Medicare practitioners eligible to bill for covered telehealth services are:

- Physicians
- Nurse practitioners
- Physician assistants
- Certified registered nurse anesthetists
- Clinical nurse specialists
- Clinical psychologists
- Clinical social workers
- Nurse-midwives
- Registered dietitians or nutrition professional

Telehealth services are reimbursed when they are provided using technology that is designated as a real-time interactive audio and video telecommunications system. To demonstrate that the telehealth services furnished have been provided with this specific technology, CMS established two HCPCS Level II modifiers to be appended the CPT code of the service provided. The modifiers are GT Via interactive audio and video telecommunication systems, and GQ Via asynchronous telecommunications system.

When services are performed using asynchronous telecommunication, HCPCS Level II modifier GQ should be appended to the CPT code of the service provided. The use of asynchronous telecommunication is restricted to demonstration programs in Alaska and Hawaii. When using modifier GT, the provider is certifying the asynchronous medical file was collected and transmitted to the distant site from a federal telemedicine demonstration project conducted in Alaska or Hawaii.

For payers that do not recognize these HCPCS Level II modifiers, CPT modifier 95 Synchronous Telemedicine Service Rendered Via a Real-Time Interactive Audio and Video Telecommunications System, should be appended to the service provided. A list of applicable CPT codes for reporting real-time telehealth services with modifier 95 can be found in Appendix P of the CPT book.

The following is the CMS list of telehealth codes for 2020. (This is the most current list available at the time of printing.)

Note: This list does not include those codes that are temporarily approved for telehealth during the COVID-19 PHE.

Code	Short Descriptor
90785	Psytx complex interactive
90791	Psych diagnostic evaluation
90792	Psych diag eval w/med srvcs
90832	Psytx pt&/family 30 minutes
90833	Psytx pt&/fam w/e&m 30 min
90834	Psytx pt&/family 45 minutes
90836	Psytx pt&/fam w/e&m 45 min
90837	Psytx pt&/family 60 minutes
90838	Psytx pt&/fam w/e&m 60 min
90839	Psytx crisis initial 60 min
90840	Psytx crisis ea addl 30 min
90845	Psychoanalysis
90846	Family psytx w/o patient
90847	Family psytx w/patient
90951	ESRD serv 4 visits p mo <2yr
90954	ESRD serv 4 vsts p mo 2-11
90955	ESRD srv 2-3 vsts p mo 2-11
90957	ESRD srv 4 vsts p mo 12-19
90958	ESRD srv 2-3 vsts p mo 12-19
90960	ESRD srv 4 visits p mo 20+

 AUDITOR'S ALERT

Providers submitting codes for telehealth services to Medicare administrative contractors (MAC) should use telehealth POS code 02 to certify that the service performed was furnished as a professional telehealth service from a distant site.

 AUDITOR'S ALERT

The current list of Medicare's approved telehealth can be found at: https://www.cms.gov/Medicare/Medicare-General-Information/Telehealth/Telehealth-Codes.

Code	Short Descriptor
90961	ESRD srv 2-3 vsts p mo 20+
90963	ESRD home pt serv p mo <2yrs
90964	ESRD home pt serv p mo 2-11
90965	ESRD home pt serv p mo 12-19
90966	ESRD home pt serv p mo 20+
90967	ESRD home pt serv p day <2
90968	ESRD home pt serv p day 2-11
90969	ESRD home pt serv p day 12-19
90970	ESRD home pt serv p day 20+
96116	Neurobehavioral status exam
96156	Hlth bhv assmt/reassessment
96159	Hlth bhv ivntj indiv ea addl
96160	Pt-focused hlth risk assmt
96161	Caregiver health risk assmt
96164	Hlth bhv ivntj grp 1st 30
96165	Hlth bhv ivntj grp ea addl
96167	Hlth bhv ivntj fam 1st 30
96168	Hlth bhv ivntj fam ea addl
97802	Medical nutrition indiv in
97803	Med nutrition indiv subseq
97804	Medical nutrition group
99202	Office/outpatient visit new
99203	Office/outpatient visit new
99204	Office/outpatient visit new
99205	Office/outpatient visit new
99211	Office/outpatient visit est
99212	Office/outpatient visit est
99213	Office/outpatient visit est
99214	Office/outpatient visit est
99215	Office/outpatient visit est
99231	Subsequent hospital care
99232	Subsequent hospital care
99233	Subsequent hospital care
99307	Nursing fac care subseq
99308	Nursing fac care subseq
99309	Nursing fac care subseq
99310	Nursing fac care subseq
99354	Prolonged service office
99355	Prolonged service office
99356	Prolonged service inpatient
99357	Prolonged service inpatient
99406	Behav chng smoking 3-10 min
99407	Behav chng smoking > 10 min

Code	Short Descriptor
99495	Trans care mgmt 14 day disch
99496	Trans care mgmt 7 day disch
99497	Advncd care plan 30 min
99498	Advncd are plan addl 30 min
90785	Psytx complex interactive
G0108	Diab manage trn per indiv
G0109	Diab manage trn ind/group
G0270	Mnt subs tx for change dx
G0296	Visit to determ LDCT elig
G0396	Alcohol/subs interv 15-30mn
G0397	Alcohol/subs interv >30 min
G0406	Inpt/tele follow up 15
G0407	Inpt/tele follow up 25
G0408	Inpt/tele follow up 35
G0420	Ed svc ckd ind per session
G0421	Ed svc ckd grp per session
G0425	Inpt/ED teleconsult30
G0426	Inpt/ED teleconsult50
G0427	Inpt/ED teleconsult70
G0436	Tobacco-use counsel 3-10 min
G0437	Tobacco-use counsel>10min
G0438	PPPS, initial visit
G0439	PPPS, subseq visit
G0442	Annual alcohol screen 15 min
G0443	Brief alcohol misuse counsel
G0444	Depression screen annual
G0445	High inten beh couns std 30m
G0446	Intens behave ther cardio dx
G0447	Behavior counsel obesity 15m
G0459	Telehealth inpt pharm mgmt
G0506	Comp asses care plan CCM svc
G0508	Crit care telehea consult 60
G0509	Crit care telehea consult 50
G0513	Prolong prev svcs, first 30m
G0514	Prolong prev svcs, addl 30m
G2086	Off base opioid tx first m
G2087	Off base opioid tx, sub m
G2088	Off opioid tx month add 30

Temporary Expansion of Telehealth Services Due to Covid-19 Public Health Emergency

On March 17, 2020, the Centers for Medicare and Medicaid Services (CMS) announced the emergent and temporary expansion of telehealth services. CMS is expanding the telehealth benefit on a temporary and emergency basis under the 1135 waiver authority and Coronavirus Preparedness and Response Supplemental Appropriations Act. Beginning March 6, 2020 and through the duration of the Public Health Emergency (PHE), Medicare can reimburse telehealth services, including office, hospital, and other visits furnished by physicians and other practitioners to patients anywhere in the United States, including the patient's place of residence. Many services have been temporarily added to the Medicare list of eligible telehealth services, and some frequency limitations and other requirements have been removed. These changes have been made to encourage the substitution of in-person services, thus reducing exposure risks for patients, practitioners, and the community at large. These telehealth services are not limited to patients with COVID-19 but must be considered reasonable and necessary.

All health care practitioners who are authorized to bill Medicare for their services may also furnish and bill for telehealth services during the PHE including physical therapists, occupational therapists, speech language pathologists, licensed clinical social workers, and clinical psychologists. Telehealth services should include the same level of documentation that would ordinarily be provided if the services were furnished in person.

The following areas have been revised for the duration of the PHE Site of service:

- Originating site
  - Telehealth services can be provided to patients wherever they are located, including their home.
- Distant site
  - Physicians/practitioners should report the place-of-service (POS) code that would have applied if the service been provided in person. Provider are permitted to furnish the telehealth service from their home.

Telehealth technology requirements:

- For the duration of the COVID-19 pandemic, "interactive telecommunications system" is defined as multimedia communications equipment that includes, at a minimum, audio and video equipment permitting two-way, real-time interactive communication between the patient and distant-site physician or practitioner, including video-enabled phones.
- CMS is allowing some telehealth services to be provided using audio-only communications technology (telephones or other audio-only devices). They include telephone E/M services, certain counseling behavioral health care, and educational services, to name a few. For the duration of the PHE, Medicare is also reimbursing codes 99441–99443 for practitioners who can independently bill for E/M services. These CPT codes can be used for both new and established patients. Report the place of service code that would have applied if the service had occurred in

<table>
<tr><td>

☞ **KEY POINT**

For additional guidance regarding telehealth services during the public health emergency (PHE) due to COVID-19, refer to the Medicare FAQ, Section P, at: https://www.cms.gov/files/document/03092020-covid-19-faqs-508.pdf.

</td></tr>
</table>

© 2020 Optum360, LLC

person for these telephone-only telehealth service codes. Reimbursement for these codes was increased for dates of service on or after March 1 to align with the payment rates for levels 2–4 established office E/M services (99212–99214).

- Penalties will not be enforced for noncompliance with regulatory requirements under the Health Insurance Portability and Accountability Act (HIPAA) against physicians and other practitioners providing telehealth services to patients in good faith through everyday communication technologies, such as Facebook Messenger video chat, Google Hangouts video, FaceTime, or Skype.

During the PHE, CPT telehealth modifier 95 should be applied to claim lines that describe services furnished via telehealth. Modifiers CR (catastrophe/disaster related) and DR (disaster related) are not necessary for Medicare telehealth services.

Many Medicare services that are typically furnished in-person may be provided via telehealth during a waiver for the PHE, including emergency department codes (99281–99285), critical care codes (99291–99292), and observation codes (99217–99220, 99224–99226, and 99234–99236). CMS continues to evaluate and make appropriate additions of services to the Medicare telehealth list. This current and evolving list of services is available at: https://www.cms.gov/Medicare/Medicare-General-Information/Telehealth/Telehealth-Codes. The current list of audio-only services are included.

Teaching Physician Documentation

Medicare will cover professional services provided by attending physicians when they deliver personal direction to interns or residents participating in the care of their patients in teaching hospitals and in skilled nursing facilities with teaching programs. Payment is based on the physician fee schedule and is subject to strict guidelines.

Medicare guidelines for payment of physician services provided in a teaching setting require that the teaching physician be present during any services involving a resident for which payment will be sought under the Medicare program. Under Medicare's teaching physician reimbursement guidelines, the services provided by the teaching physician must be of the same character (in terms of responsibilities to the patient that are assumed and fulfilled) as the services rendered to other paying patients. These responsibilities by the teaching physician are demonstrated by:

- Reviewing the patient's history and conducting a physical examination
- Personally examining the patient within a reasonable period of time after admission
- Confirming or revising the diagnosis
- Determining the course of treatment to follow
- Assuring that any supervision needed by the interns and residents is furnished
- Making frequent review of the patient's progress

Teaching physicians and residents may both document in the patient's chart. However, a teaching physician who is billing Medicare must personally document "his or her participation in the management of the patient." This includes managing the patient or being present during the critical or key portions of the patient care. A statement by the resident that the attending physician was present is not sufficient (IOM Pub. 100-04, Chapter 12, Section 100.1.1, a).

Students may document in the medical record. However, the teaching physician must verify all portions of the medical record, including history, physical examination, and medical decision making. The teaching physician must personally perform or re-perform the physical examination and medical decision-making activities. However, these elements do not have to be re-documented by the teaching physician; verification of the student's documentation is sufficient (IOM Pub. 100-04, Chapter 12, Section 100.1.1, b).

Providers

The AMA advises coders that while a particular service or procedure may be assigned to a specific section, the service or procedure itself is not limited to use only by that specialty group (starting with paragraph 4 under "Instructions for Use of the CPT Codebook" on page xiv of the CPT book). Additionally, the procedures and services listed throughout the book are for use by any qualified physician or other qualified health care professional or entity (e.g., hospitals, laboratories, or home health agencies).

The use of the phrase "physician or other qualified health care professional" (OQHCP) was adopted to identify a health care provider other than a physician. This type of provider is further described in the CPT book as an individual "qualified by education, training, licensure/regulation (when applicable), and facility privileging (when applicable)." In addition, CPT guidelines indicate that the advanced practice nurses and physician assistant who work with physicians should practice in "the exact same specialty and exact same subspecialty as the physician." State licensure guidelines determine the scope of practice and a qualified health care professional must practice within these guidelines, even if more restrictive than the CPT guidelines. The qualified health care professional may report services independently or under incident-to guidelines. The professionals within this definition are separate from "clinical staff" and are able to practice independently. The CPT book defines clinical staff as "a person who works under the supervision of a physician or other qualified health care professional and who is allowed, by law, regulation, and facility policy to perform or assist in the performance of a specified professional service, but who does not individually report that professional service." Keep in mind that there may be other policies, guidance, or payer policies that can affect who may report a specific service.

Key Component Documentation

The 1995 guidelines placed great emphasis on the history and exam portions of the encounter. This focus led many providers and coders to become mired in the detail of history and exam elements and, in essence, miss the big picture when it came to true code selection.

This was further complicated by specialty society requests for revised guidelines that allowed the specialist to focus the physical exam within the systems related to his or her specialty. This led to the 1997 guidelines that focus on the exam portion. This version provides more quantification of the medical examination portion using finite elements or bullets.

The first three of the E/M components (i.e., history, examination, and medical decision making) are the key components in selecting the level of E/M services.

© 2020 Optum360, LLC

In the case of visits that consist predominantly (more than half of the visit time with the provider) of counseling or coordination of care, time is the controlling factor to qualify for a particular level of E/M service.

Because the level of E/M service is dependent on performance and documentation of more than one key component, one component (e.g., examination) documented and performed at the highest level does not necessarily mean that the encounter in its entirety qualifies for the highest level of E/M service.

Documentation of History

Effective January 1, 2021, the AMA and CMS have adopted new guidelines and code descriptions for reporting E/M codes for new and established office or other outpatient services (99202–99215). The history and physical exam elements are not required for code level selection for office and other outpatient services. However, a medically appropriate history and/or physical examination should still be documented. The nature and degree of the history and/or physical examination will be determined by the treating physician or other qualified health care professional reporting the service. Therefore, the following guidelines section does not apply to new and established office or other outpatient services (99202–99215).

There are four types of history, including problem-focused, expanded problem-focused, detailed, and comprehensive. Each type of history includes some or all of the following elements:

- Chief complaint (CC)
- History of present illness (HPI)
- Review of systems (ROS)
- Past, family, and social history (PFSH)

The extent of history of present illness (HPI), review of systems, and past, family, and social history that is obtained and documented is dependent upon clinical judgment and the nature of the presenting problem.

The table below shows the progression of the elements required for each type of history. To qualify for a given type of history, all three elements in the table must be met or exceeded. (A chief complaint is indicated at all levels.)

History of Element Progression

History of Present Illness	Review of Systems	Past, Family, and Social History	Type of History
Brief	N/A	N/A	Problem-focused
Brief	Problem-pertinent	N/A	Expanded problem-focused
Extended	Extended	Pertinent	Detailed
Extended	Complete	Complete	Comprehensive

DG: The CC, ROS, and PFSH may be listed as separate elements of history, or they may be included in the description of the HPI.

DG: A ROS and/or a PFSH obtained during an earlier encounter does not need to be re-recorded if there is evidence that the provider reviewed and updated the

DEFINITIONS

chief complaint. In medical documentation, the presenting problem bringing the patient to the health encounter.

family history. Record of the health of family members, including the health status or cause of death of parents, siblings, and children, and specific diseases related to the patient's chief complaint, history of present illness, and/or review of systems.

history of present illness. Chronological account of signs and symptoms of the present condition.

previous information. This may occur when a provider updates his or her own record or in an institutional setting or group practice where many providers use a common record. The review and update may be documented by:

- Describing any new ROS and/or PFSH information or noting there has been no change in the information

- Noting the date and location of the earlier ROS and PFSH

DG: The ROS and/or PFSH may be recorded by ancillary staff or on a form completed by the patient. To document that the provider reviewed the information, there must be a notation supplementing or confirming the information recorded by others by the provider.

DG: If the provider is unable to obtain a history from the patient or other source, the record should describe the patient's condition or other circumstance that precludes obtaining a history.

Definitions and specific documentation guidelines for each of the elements of history are listed below.

Chief Complaint

The chief complaint (CC) is a concise statement describing the symptom, problem, condition, diagnosis, provider recommended return, or other factor that is the reason for the encounter, usually stated in the patient's words.

DG: The medical record should clearly reflect the chief complaint.

History of Present Illness

The history of present illness (HPI) is a chronological description of the development of the patient's present illness from the first sign and symptom or from the previous encounter to the present. It includes the following elements:

- Location
- Quality
- Severity
- Duration
- Timing
- Context
- Modifying factors
- Associated signs and symptoms

Brief and extended HPIs are distinguished by the amount of detail needed to accurately characterize the clinical problem.

According to the 1995 guidelines, a brief HPI contains one to three elements. An extended HPI contains four or more elements of the present illness or associated comorbidities.

The 1997 documentation guidelines for HPI are defined as follows:

A *brief* HPI consists of one to three elements of the HPI.

DG: The medical record should describe one to three elements of the present illness (HPI).

AUDITOR'S ALERT

A review of systems and/or a personal, family, or social history obtained during a previous encounter does not need to be re-recorded and may be considered in code selection ONLY if there is evidence that the provider reviewed and updated the previous information.

An *extended* HPI consists of at least four elements of the HPI or the status of at least three chronic or inactive conditions.

DG: The medical record should describe at least four elements of the present illness (HPI), or the status of at least three chronic or inactive conditions.

Review of Systems

A review of systems (ROS) is an inventory of body systems obtained through a series of questions seeking to identify signs and symptoms that the patient may be experiencing or has experienced.

For purposes of ROS, the following systems are recognized:

- Constitutional symptoms (e.g., fever, weight loss)
- Eyes
- Ears, nose, mouth, throat
- Cardiovascular
- Respiratory
- Gastrointestinal
- Genitourinary
- Musculoskeletal
- Integumentary (skin and/or breast)
- Neurological
- Psychiatric
- Endocrine
- Hematologic/lymphatic
- Allergic/immunologic

A *problem-pertinent* ROS inquires about the system directly related to the problem identified in the HPI.

DG: The patient's positive responses and pertinent negatives for the system related to the problem should be documented.

An *extended* ROS inquires about the system directly related to the problem identified in the HPI and a limited number of additional systems.

DG: The patient's positive responses and pertinent negatives for two to nine systems should be documented.

A *complete* ROS inquires about the system directly related to the problem identified in the HPI plus all additional body systems.

DG: At least 10 organ systems must be reviewed. Those systems with positive or pertinent negative responses must be individually documented. For the remaining systems, a notation indicating all other systems are negative is permissible. In the absence of such a notation, at least 10 systems must be individually documented.

Past, Family, and Social History

The past, family, and social history (PFSH) consists of a review of three areas:

 AUDITOR'S ALERT

For established office or outpatient encounters, physicians may choose to document only the parts of the history that have changed since the last encounter, instead of rerecording a list of defined elements.

- Past history (the patient's past experiences with illnesses, operations, injuries, and treatments)

- Family history (a review of medical events in the patient's family, including diseases that may be hereditary or place the patient at risk)

- Social history (an age-appropriate review of past and current activities that includes military history)

For certain categories of E/M services that include only an interval history, it is not necessary to record information about the PFSH. Those categories are subsequent hospital care, subsequent observation care, and subsequent nursing facility care.

A *pertinent* PFSH is a review of the history area directly related to the problem identified in the HPI.

DG: At least one specific item from any of the three history areas must be documented for a pertinent PFSH.

A *complete* PFSH is a review of two or all three of the PFSH history areas, depending on the category of the E/M service. A review of all three history areas is required for services that by their nature include a comprehensive assessment or reassessment of the patient. A review of two of the three history areas is sufficient for other services.

DG: At least one specific item from two of the three history areas must be documented for a complete PFSH for the following categories of E/M services: office or other outpatient services, established patient; emergency department; domiciliary care, established patient; and home care, established patient.

DG: At least one specific item from each of the three history areas must be documented for a complete PFSH for the following categories of E/M services: office or other outpatient services, new patient; hospital observation services; hospital inpatient services, initial care; consultations; comprehensive nursing facility assessments; domiciliary care, new patient; and home care, new patient.

Documentation of Examination

1995 Guidelines

According to the 1995 guidelines, the following four types of examinations are recognized for purposes of E/M services:

- **Problem-focused.** A limited examination of the affected body area or organ system.

- **Expanded problem-focused.** A limited examination of the affected body area or organ system, as well as other symptomatic or related organ system.

- **Detailed.** Includes an extended examination of the affected body area and other symptomatic or related organ system.

- **Comprehensive.** A general multisystem examination or a complete examination of a single organ system.

Body areas and organ systems are defined by CMS and the AMA for purposes of documenting the examination. The recognized body areas include:

- Head, including the face

- Neck
- Chest, including breasts and axillae
- Abdomen
- Genitalia, groin, buttocks
- Back, including spine
- Each extremity

The recognized organ systems include:

- Psychiatric
- Eyes
- Ears, nose, mouth, and throat
- Cardiovascular
- Respiratory
- Gastrointestinal
- Genitourinary
- Musculoskeletal
- Skin
- Neurologic
- Constitutional (e.g., vital signs or general appearance)
- Hematologic/lymphatic/immunologic

The medical record for a general multisystem examination should include eight or more of the 12 organ systems. If a portion of an examination is deferred, such as a pelvic or rectal examination, document the reason for deferral.

1997 Guidelines

The 1997 documentation guidelines also recognize four types of examinations:

- **Problem-focused.** A limited examination of the affected body area or organ system
- **Expanded problem-focused.** A limited examination of the affected body area or organ system and any other symptomatic or related body area(s) or organ system(s)
- **Detailed.** An extended examination of the affected body area(s) or organ system(s) and any other symptomatic or related body area(s) or organ system(s)
- **Comprehensive.** A general multisystem examination or complete examination of a single organ system and other symptomatic or related body area(s) or organ system(s)

These types of examinations have been defined for general multisystem and the following single-organ systems:

- Cardiovascular
- Eyes
- Ears, nose, mouth, and throat
- Skin
- Hematologic/lymphatic/immunologic

 AUDITOR'S ALERT

Although constitutional signs are defined by CMS as an organ system for purposes of examination, the term "constitutional" was intentionally omitted in the list of organ systems in the CPT book since it is not considered to be a true organ system according to AMA guidelines.

 AUDITOR'S ALERT

When billing Medicare, a provider may choose either version (1995 or 1997) of the documentation guidelines, not a combination of the two, to document a patient encounter. However, beginning with services performed on or after September 10, 2013, physicians and other qualified health care professionals may use the documentation guidelines for an extended history of present illness along with other elements from the 1995 guidelines to document an evaluation and management service.

- Genitourinary (female)
- Genitourinary (male)
- Respiratory
- Musculoskeletal
- Neurological
- Psychiatric

A general multisystem examination or a single-organ system examination may be performed by any provider regardless of specialty. The type (general multisystem or single-organ system) and content of examination are selected by the examining provider and are based upon clinical judgment, the patient's history, and the nature of the presenting problem.

The content and documentation requirements for each type and level of examination are summarized in the following text and described in detail by CMS. In the documentation tables, organ systems and body areas recognized by the CPT coding system for purposes of describing examinations are shown in the left column. The content, or individual elements, of the examination pertaining to that body area or organ system are identified by bullets (•) in the right column.

Parenthetical examples "(e.g.,)" have been used for clarification and to provide guidance regarding documentation. Documentation for each element must satisfy any numeric requirements (such as "Measurement of any three of the following seven…") included in the description of the element.

Elements with multiple components but with no specific numeric requirement (such as "examination of liver and spleen") require documentation of at least one component. It is possible for a given examination to be expanded beyond what is defined here. When that occurs, findings related to the additional systems and areas should be documented.

DG: Specific abnormal and relevant negative findings of the examination of the affected or symptomatic body area or organ system should be documented. A notation of "abnormal" without elaboration is insufficient.

DG: Abnormal or unexpected findings of the examination of any asymptomatic body area or organ system should be described.

DG: A brief statement or notation indicating "negative" or "normal" is sufficient to document normal findings related to unaffected areas or asymptomatic organ systems.

General Multisystem and Single-organ System Examinations

Elements identified by a bullet with multiple components (e.g., "oral pharynx" in a multisystem examination) should be examined by the provider, but it is only necessary to document one of the multiple components per bullet (element). For example, for "hard and soft palate: normal," it is not required to document findings of oral mucosa, salivary glands, tongue, tonsil, and posterior pharynx, even though each site was examined.

General Multisystem Examinations

General multisystem examinations are described in detail on the following pages. To qualify for a given level of multisystem examination, the following content and documentation requirements should be met:

- **Problem-focused examination.** Should include performance and documentation of one to five elements identified by a bullet (•) in one or more organ system(s) or body area(s).

- **Expanded problem-focused examination.** Should include performance and documentation of at least six elements identified by a bullet (•) in one or more organ system(s) or body area(s).

- **Detailed examination.** Should include at least six organ systems or body areas. For each system/area selected, performance and documentation of at least two elements identified by a bullet (•) is expected. Alternatively, a detailed examination may include performance and documentation of at least 12 elements identified by a bullet (•) in two or more organ systems or body areas.

- **Comprehensive examination.** Should include at least nine organ systems or body areas. For each system or area selected, all elements of the examination identified by a bullet (•) should be performed, unless specific directions limit the content of the examination. For each area/system, documentation of at least two elements identified by a bullet is expected.

Single-Organ System Examinations

The single-organ system examinations recognized by CMS are described in detail in the guidelines. Variations among these examinations in the organ systems and body areas identified in the left columns and in the elements of the examinations described in the right columns reflect differing emphasis among specialties. Some of the specialty exams do not specifically identify elements in each of the other organ systems. To qualify for a given level of single-organ-system examination, the following content and documentation requirements should include:

- **Problem-focused examination.** Performance and documentation of one to five elements identified by a bullet (•), whether in a box with a shaded or plain border.

- **Expanded problem-focused examination.** Performance and documentation of at least six elements identified by a bullet (•), whether in a box with a shaded or plain border.

- **Detailed examination.** Performance and documentation of at least 12 elements identified by a bullet (•), whether in box with a shaded or plain border for all examinations other than eye and psychiatric. Eye and psychiatric examinations should include the performance and documentation of at least nine elements identified by a bullet (•), whether in a box with a shaded or plain border.

- **Comprehensive examination.** Should include performance of all elements identified by a bullet (•), whether in a shaded or plain box. Documentation of every element in a box with a shaded border and at least one element in each box with a plain border is expected.

The general multisystem examination guidelines are included in this text. Any of the specialty-specific guidelines may be referenced, but not all systems have identified elements on each exam. The coder cannot pick and choose across the exams but must select the most appropriate exam and define the documented elements.

General Multisystem Examination

System/Body Area	Elements of Examination
Constitutional	• Measurement of **any three of the following seven** vital signs: 1) sitting or standing blood pressure, 2) supine blood pressure, 3) pulse rate and regularity, 4) respiration, 5) temperature, 6) height, 7) weight (May be measured and recorded by ancillary staff) • General appearance of patient (e.g., development, nutrition, body habitus, deformities, attention to grooming)
Eyes	• Inspection of conjunctivae and lids • Examination of pupils and irises (e.g., reaction to light and accommodation, size and symmetry) • Ophthalmoscopic examination of optic discs (e.g., size, C/D ratio, appearance) and posterior segments (e.g., vessel changes, exudates, hemorrhages)
Ears, nose, mouth, and throat	• External inspection of ears and nose (e.g., overall appearance, scars, lesions, masses) • Otoscopic examination of external auditory canals and tympanic membranes • Assessment of hearing (e.g., whispered voice, finger rub, tuning fork) • Inspection of nasal mucosa, septum and turbinates • Inspection of lips, teeth and gums • Examination of oropharynx: oral mucosa, salivary glands, hard and soft palates, tongue, tonsils and posterior pharynx
Neck	• Examination of neck (e.g., masses, overall appearance, symmetry, tracheal position, crepitus) • Examination of thyroid (e.g., enlargement, tenderness, mass)
Respiratory	• Assessment of respiratory effort (e.g., intercostal retractions, use of accessory muscles, diaphragmatic movement) • Percussion of chest (e.g., dullness, flatness, hyperresonance) • Palpation of chest (e.g., tactile fremitus) • Auscultation of lungs (e.g., breath sounds, adventitious sounds, rubs)
Cardiovascular	• Palpation of heart (e.g., location, size, thrills) • Auscultation of heart with notation of abnormal sounds and murmurs Examination of: • Carotid arteries (e.g., pulse amplitude, bruits) • Abdominal aorta (e.g., size, bruits) • Femoral arteries (e.g., pulse amplitude, bruits) • Pedal pulses (e.g., pulse amplitude) • Extremities for edema and/or varicosities
Chest (Breasts)	• Inspection of breasts (e.g., symmetry, nipple discharge) • Palpation of breasts and axillae (e.g., masses or lumps, tenderness)

 © 2020 Optum360, LLC

System/Body Area	Elements of Examination
Gastrointestinal (Abdomen)	• Examination of abdomen with notation of presence of masses or tenderness • Examination of liver and spleen • Examination for presence or absence of hernia • Examination (when indicated) of anus, perineum and rectum, including sphincter tone, presence of hemorrhoids, rectal masses • Obtain stool sample for occult blood test when indicated
Genitourinary	**Male:** • Examination of the scrotal contents (e.g., hydrocele, spermatocele, tenderness of cord, testicular mass) • Examination of the penis • Digital rectal examination of prostate gland (e.g., size, symmetry, nodularity, tenderness) **Female:** Pelvic examination (with or without specimen collection for smears and cultures), including: • Examination of external genitalia (e.g., general appearance, hair distribution, lesions) and vagina (e.g., general appearance, estrogen effect, discharge, lesions, pelvic support, cystocele, rectocele) • Examination of urethra (e.g., masses, tenderness, scarring) • Examination of bladder (e.g., fullness, masses, tenderness) • Cervix (e.g., general appearance, lesions, discharge) • Uterus (e.g., size, contour, position, mobility, tenderness, consistency, descent or support) • Adnexa/parametria (e.g., masses, tenderness)
Lymphatic	Palpation of lymph nodes in **two or more** areas: • Neck • Groin • Axillae • Other

Musculoskeletal	• Examination of gait and station
	• Inspection and/or palpation of digits and nails (e.g., clubbing, cyanosis, inflammatory conditions, petechiae, ischemia, infections, nodes)
	• Examination of joints, bones and muscles of **one or more of the following six areas**: 1) head and neck; 2) spine, ribs and pelvis; 3) right upper extremity; 4) left upper extremity; 5) right lower extremity; and 6) left lower extremity. The examination of a given area includes:
	  • Inspection and/or palpation with notation of presence of any misalignment, asymmetry, crepitation, defects, tenderness, masses, effusions
	  • Assessment of range of motion with notation of any pain, crepitation or contracture
	  • Assessment of stability with notation of any dislocation (luxation), subluxation or laxity
	  • Assessment of muscle strength and tone (e.g., flaccid, cog wheel, spastic) with notation of any atrophy or abnormal movements

Skin	• Inspection of skin and subcutaneous tissue (e.g., rashes, lesions, ulcers) • Palpation of skin and subcutaneous tissue (e.g., induration, subcutaneous nodules, tightening)

System/Body Area	Elements of Examination
Neurologic	• Test cranial nerves with notation of any deficits • Examination of deep tendon reflexes with notation of pathological reflexes (e.g., Babinski) • Examination of sensation (e.g., by touch, pin, vibration, proprioception)

Psychiatric	• Description of patient's judgment and insight
	• Brief assessment of mental status, including:
	  • Orientation to time, place and person
	  • Recent and remote memory
	  • Mood and affect (e.g., depression, anxiety, agitation)

The CMS website includes many more specialty exams that can be used with the 1997 guidelines. The website is found at https://www.cms.gov/Outreach-and-Education/Medicare-Learning-Network-MLN/MLNEdWebGuide/Downloads/97Docguidelines.pdf.

Documentation of the Complexity of Medical Decision Making

Effective January 1, 2021, revised Medical Decision Making (MDM) criteria per the CPT Editorial Panel, including a new table for determining the appropriate level of MDM, will be adopted. The new table replaces the current CMS Table of Risk only for codes 99202–99205 and 99212–99215. The levels of E/M services recognize four types of medical decision making (straightforward, low complexity, moderate complexity, and high complexity). Medical decision making refers to the complexity of establishing a diagnosis and selecting a management option as measured by:

- The number of possible diagnoses and the number of management options that must be considered

- The amount and complexity of medical records, diagnostic tests, and other information that must be obtained, reviewed, and analyzed

- The risk of significant complications, morbidity, and mortality, as well as comorbidities, associated with the patient's presenting problem, the diagnostic procedure, and the possible management options

The following table shows the progression of the elements required for each level of medical decision making. To qualify for a given type of decision making, two of the three elements in the table must be met or exceeded.

Medical Decision Making Progression

Number of Diagnoses or Management Options	Amount and/or Complexity of Data to Be Reviewed	Risk of Complications and/or Morbidity or Mortality	Type of Decision Making
Minimal	Minimal or none	Minimal	Straightforward
Limited	Limited	Low	Low
Multiple	Moderate	Moderate	Moderate
Extensive	Extensive	High	High

Each element of medical decision making listed in the table is described below.

Number of Diagnoses or Management Options

The number of possible diagnoses and the number of management options that must be considered is based on the number and types of problems addressed during the encounter, the complexity of establishing a diagnosis, and the management decisions that are made by the provider.

Generally, decision making with respect to a diagnosed problem is easier than that for an identified but undiagnosed problem. The number and type of diagnostic tests employed may be an indicator of the number of possible diagnoses. Problems that are improving or resolving are less complex than those that are worsening or failing to change as expected. The need to seek advice from others is another indicator of complexity of diagnostic or management problems.

DG: For each encounter, an assessment, clinical impression, or diagnosis should be documented. It may be explicitly stated or implied in documented decisions regarding management plans and further evaluation.

- For a presenting problem with an established diagnosis, the record should reflect whether the problem is:
    - improved, well controlled, resolving, or resolved
    - inadequately controlled, worsening, or failing to change as expected
- For a presenting problem without an established diagnosis, the assessment or clinical impression may be stated in the form of differential diagnoses or as a "possible," "probable," or "rule out (R/O)" diagnosis.

DG: The initiation of, or changes in, treatment should be documented. Treatment includes a wide range of management options including patient instructions, nursing instructions, therapies, and medications.

DG: If referrals are made, consultations requested, or advice sought, the record should indicate to whom or where the referral or consultation is made or from whom the advice is requested.

The following table demonstrates how the number of diagnosis or management options is configured. This table (minimal, limited, multiple, or extensive) is then used with the Amount and Complexity of Data to Be Reviewed table to determine the level of service.

Number of Diagnosis or Management Options (Number x Points = Results)

Diagnosis or Management Options	Number	Points	Results
Self-limited or minor (stable, improved, or worsening) [max two]		1	
Established problem (to examiner); stable, improved		1	
Established problem (to examiner); worsening		2	
New problem (to examiner); no additional work-up planned		3	
New problem (to examiner); additional work-up planned		4	

Total points: Minimal = 1 Limited = 2 Multiple = 3 Extensive = 4 or more

Amount and Complexity of Data to Be Reviewed
The amount and complexity of data to be reviewed are based on the types of diagnostic testing ordered or reviewed. A decision to obtain and review old medical records and obtain history from sources other than the patient increases the amount and complexity of data to be reviewed.

Discussion of contradictory or unexpected test results with the provider who performed or interpreted the test is an indication of the complexity of data being reviewed. On occasion, the provider who ordered a test may personally review the image, tracing, or specimen to supplement information from the provider who prepared the test report or interpretation; this is another indication of the complexity of data being reviewed.

DG: If a diagnostic service (test or procedure) is ordered, planned, scheduled, or performed at the time of the E/M encounter, the type of service (e.g., lab or x-ray) should be documented.

DG: The review of lab, radiology, and other diagnostic tests should be documented. A simple notation such as "WBC elevated" or "chest x-ray unremarkable" is acceptable. Alternatively, the review may be documented by initialing and dating the report containing the test results.

DG: A decision to obtain old records or decision to obtain additional history from the family, caretaker, or other source to supplement that obtained from the patient should be documented.

DG: Relevant findings from the review of old records, and the receipt of additional history from the family, caretaker, or other source to supplement that obtained from the patient, should be documented. If there is no relevant information beyond that already obtained, that fact should be documented. A notation of "old records reviewed" or "additional history obtained from family" without elaboration is insufficient.

DG: The results of discussion of laboratory, radiology, or other diagnostic tests with the provider who performed or interpreted the study should be documented.

DG: The direct visualization and independent interpretation of an image, tracing, or specimen previously or subsequently interpreted by another provider should be documented.

The following table may be used to help determine the amount and complexity of data that was reviewed or planned during a patient encounter. This table (minimal, limited, multiple, or extensive) is then used with the Number of Diagnosis or Management Options table to determine the level of service.

Amount and Complexity of Data to Be Reviewed

Data to Be Reviewed	Points
Review and/or order of clinical lab tests	1
Review and/or order of tests in radiology section of the CPT book	1
Review and/or order of tests in the medicine section of the CPT book	1
Discussion of tests results with performing physician	1
Decision to obtain old records and/or obtaining history from someone other than patient	1
Review and summarization of old records and/or obtaining history from someone other than patient and/or discussion of case with another health provider	2
Independent visualization of image, tracing, or specimen itself (not simply care review of report)	2
Total points: Minimal = 1 Limited = 2 Multiple = 3 Extensive = 4 or more	

Risk of Significant Complications, Morbidity, and Mortality

The risk of significant complications, morbidity, and mortality is based on the risks associated with the presenting problem, the diagnostic procedure, and the possible management options.

DG: Comorbidities or underlying diseases or other factors that increase the complexity of medical decision making by increasing the risk of complications, morbidity, and mortality should be documented.

DG: A surgical or invasive diagnostic procedure ordered, planned, or scheduled at the time of the E/M encounter should document the nature of the specific type of procedure (e.g., laparoscopy).

DG: A surgical or invasive diagnostic procedure performed at the time of the E/M encounter should be documented as to the specific type of service provided.

DG: Referral for or decision to perform a surgical or invasive diagnostic procedure on an urgent basis should be documented or implied.

The Table of Risk may be used to help determine whether the risk of significant complications, morbidity, and mortality is minimal, low, moderate, or high. Because the determination of risk is complex and not readily quantifiable, the table includes common clinical examples rather than absolute measures of risk. The assessment of risk of the presenting problem is based on the risk related to the disease process anticipated between the present encounter and the next one. The assessment of risk of selecting diagnostic procedures and management options is based on the risk during and immediately following any procedures or treatment. The highest level of risk in any one category (presenting problem, diagnostic procedure, or management options) determines the overall risk.

Table of Risk Medical Decision Making

Level of Risk	Presenting Problem(s)	Diagnostic Procedure(s) Ordered	Management Options Selected
Minimal	One self-limited or minor problem (e.g., common cold, insect bite, tinea corporis)	• Laboratory test requiring venipuncture • Chest x-rays • EKG/EEG • Urinalysis • Ultrasound (e.g., echocardiography) • KOH prep	• Rest • Gargles • Elastic bandages • Superficial dressings
Low	• Two or more self-limited or minor problems • One stable chronic illness (e.g., well controlled hypertension, non-insulin-dependent diabetes, cataract, BPH) • Acute, uncomplicated illness or injury (e.g., cystitis, allergic rhinitis, simple sprain)	• Physiologic tests not under stress (e.g., pulmonary function tests) • Non-cardiovascular imaging studies with contrast (e.g., barium enema) • Superficial needle biopsies • Clinical laboratory tests requiring arterial puncture • Skin biopsies	• Over-the-counter drugs • Minor surgery with no identified risk factors • Physical therapy • Occupational therapy • IV fluids without additives
Moderate	• One or more chronic illnesses with mild exacerbation, progression or side effects of treatment • Two or more stable chronic illnesses • Undiagnosed new problem with uncertain prognosis (e.g., lump in breast) • Acute illness with systemic symptoms (e.g., pyelonephritis, pneumonitis, colitis) • Acute complicated injury (e.g., head injury with brief loss of consciousness)	• Physiologic tests under stress (e.g., cardiac stress test, fetal contraction stress test) • Diagnostic endoscopies with no identified risk factors • Deep needle or incisional biopsy • Cardiovascular imaging studies with contrast and no identified risk factors (e.g., arteriogram, cardiac catheterization) • Obtain fluid from body cavity (e.g., lumbar puncture, thoracentesis, culdocentesis)	• Minor surgery with identified risk factors • Elective major surgery (open, percutaneous or endoscopic) with no identified risk factors • Prescription drug management • Therapeutic nuclear medicine • IV fluids with additives • Closed treatment of fracture or dislocation without manipulation
High	• One or more chronic illnesses with severe exacerbation, progression or side effects of treatment • Acute or chronic illnesses or injuries that may pose a threat to life or bodily function (e.g., multiple trauma, acute MI, pulmonary embolus, severe respiratory distress, progressive severe rheumatoid arthritis, psychiatric illness with potential threat to self or others, peritonitis, acute renal failure) • An abrupt change in neurologic status (e.g., seizure, TIA, weakness, or sensory loss)	• Cardiovascular imaging studies with contrast with identified risk factors • Cardiac electrophysiological tests • Diagnostic endoscopies with identified risk factors • Discography	• Elective major surgery (open, percutaneous or endoscopic) with identified risk factors • Emergency major surgery (open, percutaneous, or endoscopic) • Parenteral controlled substances • Drug therapy requiring intensive monitoring for toxicity • Decision not to resuscitate or to de-escalate care because of poor prognosis

Documentation and the Pediatric Patient

Documentation guidelines developed by CMS for other outpatient and inpatient E/M procedures are based upon adolescent or adult patients. This has created problems for providers who treat newborn and pediatric patients.

A problem-oriented E/M service for an infant or neonate may not include an extensive history due to the patient's age and limited prior problems. It may be appropriate in these circumstances to include prenatal history, including any complications the mother had during the pregnancy and delivery. Any complications during birth or initial hospitalization and subsequent treatment should also be noted.

For most pediatric patients, the parent or caregiver is often the best source of an accurate history and can often answer questions based upon their own interaction with and observation of the patient. The provider may also use his or her own observations for history and exam elements where appropriate.

In those situations where a complete history is precluded or an exam is limited due to patient circumstances, the provider should document the level of history and exam obtained. In addition, the reason why a more complete medically necessary history and exam were not obtained should be documented. This is as important for continuity of patient care and liability issues as it is for supporting code selection.

Contributory Components

Effective January 1, 2021, the AMA and CMS have adopted new guidelines and code descriptions for reporting E/M codes for new and established office or other outpatient services (99202–99215). The following contributory components are not required for code level selection for office and other outpatient services. Therefore, the following guidelines section does not apply to new and established office or other outpatient services (99202–99215). When specific criteria are met, the contributory components may drive the selection of a level of E/M service. The contributory components are:

- Time
- Counseling
- Coordination of care
- Nature of presenting problem

Time

For services outside of the new and established office or other outpatient services (99202–99215), the previous time guidelines remain unchanged. Time is used in selecting an E/M code only when counseling or coordination of care represents more than 50 percent of the time the provider spent face-to-face with the patient and/or family (outpatient) or at the patient's beside and on the floor or unit with the patient or family (inpatient). Both time elements, total length of time for the visit and total length of time involved in counseling or coordination of care, as well as the nature of the counseling and coordination of care, must be documented explicitly in the medical record. Family, as used above, includes not just family members but also other parties that have assumed responsibility for the care of and/or decision making for the patient, whether or

 AUDITOR'S ALERT

Effective January 1, 2021, providers may base the level of office/other outpatient visit (99202 99205 and 99212 99215) solely on total time on the date of the encounter. For these specific services, time may be used regardless of whether counseling and/or coordination of care dominate the service.

not they are family (e.g., foster parents, person acting in locum parentis legal guardian).

Time is perceived by many payers to be used inappropriately. The documentation must clearly state the following:

- Total time spent with the patient and/or family, including:
  - face-to-face in the outpatient setting
  - bedside, floor, and/or unit time in the inpatient setting
- That at least 50 percent of that time was spent counseling or coordinating the patient's care
- The nature and extent of the counseling or coordination of care
- Start and stop time of the service.

When any of these elements are omitted or not contained in the documentation, time cannot be used as the controlling component in the selection of a code.

Counseling

Counseling is a discussion with the provider and the patient and/or family members.

It is performed when one or more of the following areas are discussed face-to-face with the patient and/or family:

- Diagnostic testing or procedure results, impressions, or recommended diagnostic studies
- Prognosis
- Risks and benefits of management (treatment) options
- Instructions for management (treatment) or follow-up
- Importance of compliance with chosen management (treatment) options
- Risk factor reduction
- Patient and family education

Counseling is usually considered an inherent component of E/M services and part of the decision-making process. In the case where counseling and coordination of care dominates (more than 50 percent) the provider/patient and family encounter (face-to-face time in the office or other outpatient setting, floor/unit time in the hospital or nursing facility), time is considered the key or controlling factor to qualify for a particular level of E/M services.

Counseling in this context is not synonymous with psychiatric counseling.

Coordination of Care

Coordination of care is frequently provided concurrently with counseling. This includes treatment instructions to the patient and or caregiver. It may also include special accommodations that must be made for home, work, school, vacation, or other locations, as well as coordination with other types of providers, agencies, and living arrangements.

Counseling and coordination of care are usually considered inherent components of medical decision making. In the case where counseling and coordination of care dominates (more than 50 percent) the provider/patient and family encounter (face-to-face time in the office or other outpatient setting, floor/unit time in the hospital or nursing facility), time is considered the key or controlling factor to qualify for a particular level of E/M services.

DG: If the provider elects to report the level of service based on counseling and coordination of care, the total length of time of the encounter (face-to-face or floor time, as appropriate) and the amount of counseling time should be documented and the record should describe the counseling and activities to coordinate care. The total time of the encounter is used to select the level of E/M service. Time spent coordinating care after the patient has left the office is not included in this time.

When coordination of care does not include a patient encounter on that day, the services should be reported using the case management codes. Note, however, that many payers do not cover case management services.

Nature of Presenting Problem

The nature of the presenting problem should be used by the provider to determine the amount and complexity of the three key elements that are required to appropriately treat the patient. The nature of presenting problem is described by one of the following five levels:

- **Minimal.** Problem that may not require the presence of the physician or other qualified health care professional, but service is provided under the physician's or other qualified health care professional's supervision.

- **Self-limited or minor.** Transient problem, low probability of permanently altered state; or good prognosis with management/compliance.

- **Low severity.** Problem that has a low risk of morbidity or little, if any, risk of mortality without treatment; full recovery is expected without functional impairment.

- **Moderate severity.** Problem that carries a moderate risk of morbidity or mortality without treatment, uncertain outcome, or increased probability of prolonged functional impairment.

- **High severity.** Problem that has a high to extreme risk of morbidity, moderate to high risk of mortality without treatment, or high probability of severe, prolonged functional impairment.

The first two categories, minimal and self-limited, are most often associated with the straightforward level of decision making. A provider is generally accorded the risk associated with the morbidity or mortality of differential diagnoses, not simply what is ruled in. The key principle when addressing provider cognitive work is that the condition or problem need not ultimately be found for it to be considered as the basis for the work-up, or the complexity of that work.

The level of the severity of the presenting problem may vary during the encounter, usually based on the presence or development of differential diagnoses. Medical record documentation should clearly define the findings and reflect the thought process of the physician or other qualified health care professional in ordering diagnostic or therapeutic services to support medical necessity for those services. This component is the foundation for establishing the level of service performed and documented based upon medical necessity and is inherent in the medical decision making process.

Modifiers

There are a number of situations that may require the assignment of a modifier to the E/M codes in order to identify the specific services performed. Modifiers 24, 25, 57, and AI may be appended to evaluation and management services only.

24	Unrelated Evaluation and Management Service by the Same Physician or Other Qualified Health Care Professional During a Postoperative Period
25	Significant, Separately Identifiable Evaluation and Management Service by the Same Physician or Other Qualified Health Care Professional on the Same Day of the Procedure or Other Service
32	Mandated Service
33	Preventive Service
57	Decision for Surgery
AI	Principal Physician of Record

Please see chapter 3 for a detailed explanation of these modifiers.

▽ DENIAL ALERT

Failure to append modifier AI Principal Physician of Record could result in delay or denial for E/M services.

Correct Coding Policies for Evaluation and Management Services

CPT codes for E/M services are principally included in the code range 99202–99499. The codes describe the site of service (e.g., office, hospital, home, nursing facility, emergency department, critical care), the type of service (e.g., new or initial encounter, follow-up, observation, or subsequent encounter), and various miscellaneous services (e.g., prolonged physician service, care plan oversight service). E/M services are further classified by the complexity of the relevant clinical history, physical examination, and medical decision making. Some E/M codes are based on the duration of the encounter (e.g., critical care services).

Effective January 1, 2010, Medicare does not recognize consultation codes 99241–99255 for billing and payment purposes. If a provider performs a consultation E/M, the provider may report the appropriate level of E/M service for the site of service where the consultation E/M occurs.

Rules governing the reporting of more than one E/M code for a patient on the same date of service are very complex and are not described herein. However, the NCCI contains numerous edits based on several principles including, but not limited to, those found below:

Allowed

- A provider may report only one "new patient" code on a single date of service.

- A provider may report only one code from a range of codes describing an initial E/M service on a single date of service.

- A provider may report only one "per diem" E/M service from a range of per diem codes on a single date of service.

- The prolonged service with direct face-to-face patient contact E/M codes (99354–99357) may be reported in conjunction with other evaluation and management codes and codes 90837 and 90847. These prolonged service E/M codes are add-on codes that may generally be reported with the E/M codes listed in the CPT instruction following each code in the code range 99354–99357.

Not Allowed:

- A provider should not report an "initial" per diem E/M service with the same type of "subsequent" per diem service on the same date of service.

- A physician should not double count time if reporting more than one E/M service for the same date of service or same monthly period.

- E/M codes describing observation/inpatient care services with admission and discharge on same date (99234–99236) should not be reported on the same date of service as initial hospital care per diem codes (99221–99223), subsequent hospital care per diem codes (99231–99233), or hospital discharge day management codes (99238–99239).

- Digital rectal examination for prostate screening (HCPCS Level II code G0102) is not reported separately with an evaluation and management code. CMS published this policy in the *Federal Register,* November 2, 1999, page 59414.

A number of other factors must be considered when evaluation and management services are reported:

- Since critical care (99291–99292) and prolonged E/M services (99354–99357) are reported based on time, providers should not include the time devoted to performing separately reportable services when determining the amount of critical care or prolonged provider E/M service time.

- Evaluation and management services, in general, are cognitive services, and significant procedural services are not included in evaluation and management services. Certain procedural services that arise directly from the evaluation and management service are included as part of the evaluation and management service. For example, cleansing of traumatic lesions, closure of lacerations with adhesive strips, application of dressings, counseling, and educational services are included in evaluation and management services.

- Because of the intensive nature of caring for critically ill patients, certain practitioner services in addition to patient history, examination, and medical decision making are included in the evaluation and management associated with critical and intensive care. Per CPT book instructions, services not reported separately by practitioners reporting critical care codes 99291 and 99292 include, but are not limited to, the interpretation of cardiac output measurements (93561 and 93562), chest x-rays (71045 and 71046), pulse oximetry (94760–94762), blood gases, data stored in computers (ECGs, blood pressures, hematologic data), gastric intubation (43752–43753), temporary transcutaneous monitoring (92953), ventilator management (94002–94004, 94660, 94662), and vascular access procedures (36000, 36410, 36415, 36591, 36600). However, facilities may individually report these services with critical care codes 99291 and 99292.

- Per CPT book instructions, practitioner inpatient neonatal and pediatric critical and intensive care services (99466–99467, #99485–#99486, 99468–99480) include the same services as critical care codes 99291 and 99292, as well as additional services listed in the CPT book specific to neonatal and pediatric critical and intensive care services. These services should not be reported separately by practitioners reporting codes 99466–99480 or 99485–99486. However, facilities may individually report these services with codes 99466–99480 or 99485–99486.

- Per Medicare rules, critical and intensive care codes include thoracic electrical bioimpedance (93701), which should not be reported separately.

- Certain sections of CPT include codes describing specialty-specific services that primarily involve evaluation and management services. When codes for these services are reported, a separate evaluation and management service from the range of codes 99202–99499 should not be reported on the same date of service. Examples of these codes include general and special ophthalmologic services and general and special diagnostic and therapeutic psychiatric services.

- The AMA published clarification regarding the appropriate reporting of an E/M service related to surgical procedures. When the decision for the surgical procedure is made during the encounter, the appropriate E/M service is billed with modifier 57 Decision for surgery. However, when an E/M service is provided after the decision for surgery has been made and is for the purpose of preoperative history and physical, it is included in the global surgery package regardless of the timeframe. For more information regarding E/M services and the global surgery package, see below.

Medicare global surgery rules define the rules for reporting E/M services with procedures. This section summarizes some of the rules.

- All procedures on the Medicare Physician Fee Schedule are assigned a global period of 000, 010, 090, MMM, XXX, YYY, or ZZZ. The global concept does not apply to XXX procedures. The global period for YYY procedures is defined by the carrier (A/B MACs processing practitioner service claims.) All procedures with a global period of ZZZ are related to another procedure, and the applicable global period for the ZZZ code is determined by the related procedure. Procedures with a global period of MMM are maternity procedures.

- Since NCCI edits are applied to same day services by the same provider to the same beneficiary, certain global surgery rules are applicable to NCCI. An E/M service is separately reportable on the same date of service as a procedure with a global period of 000, 010, or 090 days under limited circumstances.

- If a procedure has a global period of 090 days, it is defined as a major surgical procedure. If an E/M service is performed on the same date of service as a major surgical procedure for the purpose of deciding whether to perform this surgical procedure, the E/M service is separately reportable with modifier 57. Other preoperative E/M services on the same date of service as a major surgical procedure are included in the global payment for the procedure and are not separately reportable. NCCI does not contain edits based on this rule because MACs processing practitioner service claims have separate edits.

 © 2020 Optum360, LLC

- If a procedure has a global period of 000 or 010 days, it is defined as a minor surgical procedure (e.g., osteopathic manipulative therapy and chiropractic manipulative therapy have global periods of 000.) In general, E/M services on the same date of service as the minor surgical procedure are included in the payment for the procedure. The decision to perform a minor surgical procedure is included in the payment for the minor surgical procedure and should not be reported separately as an E/M service. However, a significant and separately identifiable E/M service unrelated to the decision to perform the minor surgical procedure is separately reportable with modifier 25. The E/M service and minor surgical procedure do not require different diagnoses. If a minor surgical procedure is performed on a new patient, the same rules for reporting E/M services apply. The fact that the patient is "new" to the provider is not sufficient alone to justify reporting an E/M service on the same date of service as a minor surgical procedure. NCCI contains many, but not all, possible edits based on these principles.

  Example
  If a provider determines that a new patient with head trauma requires sutures, confirms the allergy and immunization status, obtains informed consent, and performs the repair, an E/M service is not separately reportable. However, if the provider also performs a medically reasonable and necessary full neurological examination, an E/M service may be reported separately.

- For major and minor surgical procedures, postoperative E/M services related to recovery from the surgical procedure during the postoperative period are included in the global surgery package as are E/M services related to complications of the surgery that do not require additional trips to the operating room. Postoperative visits unrelated to the diagnosis for which the surgical procedure was performed unless related to a complication of surgery may be reported separately on the same day as a surgical procedure with modifier 24 Unrelated Evaluation and Management Service by the Same Physician or Other Qualified Health Care Professional During a Postoperative Period.

- Procedures with a global surgery indicator of "XXX" are not covered by these rules. Many of these "XXX" procedures are performed by providers and have inherent preprocedure, intra-procedure, and postprocedure work usually performed each time the procedure is completed. This work shall not be reported as a separate E/M code. Other "XXX" procedures are not usually performed by a provider and have no physician work relative value units associated with them. A provider shall not report a separate E/M code with these procedures for the supervision of others performing the procedure or for the interpretation of the procedure. With most "XXX" procedures, the provider may, however, perform a significant and separately identifiable E/M service on the same date of service, which may be reported by appending modifier 25 to the E/M code. This E/M service may be related to the same diagnosis necessitating performance of the "XXX" procedure, but cannot include any work inherent in the "XXX" procedure, supervision of others performing the "XXX" procedure, or time for interpreting the result of the "XXX" procedure. Appending modifier 25 to a significant, separately identifiable E/M service when performed on the same date of service as an "XXX" procedure is correct coding. Examples of "XXX" procedures include allergy testing and immunotherapy, physical therapy services, and neurologic and vascular diagnostic testing procedures.

- Pediatric and neonatal critical and intensive care codes (99466–99480) are per diem codes that can be reported by one provider on each day of service. These codes are reported by the provider directing the inpatient critical or intensive care of the patient. These codes should not be reported by other providers performing critical care services on the same date of service. Critical care services provided by a second provider of a different specialty may be reported with codes 99291 and 99292. However, if a neonate or infant becomes critically ill on a day when initial or subsequent intensive care service (99477–99480) has been performed by one provider and is transferred to a critical level of care provided by a different individual in a different group, the second provider may report a per diem critical care service (99468–99476).

- CPT codes 99238 and 99239 describe hospital discharge day management. These codes should not be reported with initial hospital care (99221–99223) or initial observation care (99218–99220) for the same date of service. If a physician or other qualified health care professional provides initial hospital care or observation care on the same day as discharge, the services should be reported with 99234–99236 (observation or inpatient hospital care with admission and discharge on the same date of service). Additionally, codes 99238 and 99239 include all provider services provided to the patient on the date of discharge. The provider should not report another E/M code (e.g., 99202–99215, 99281–99285) on the same date of service that the provider reports 99238 or 99239.

- HCPCS Level II codes G0396 and G0397 describe alcohol and/or substance (other than tobacco) abuse structured assessment and intervention services. These codes should not be reported separately with an evaluation and management (E/M), psychiatric diagnostic, or psychotherapy service code for the same work/time. If the E/M, psychiatric diagnostic, or psychotherapy service would normally include assessment and/or intervention of alcohol or substance abuse based on the patient's clinical presentation, HCPCS Level II code G0396 or G0397 should not be additionally reported. If a provider reports either of these G codes with an E/M, psychiatric diagnostic, or psychotherapy code utilizing an NCCI-associated modifier, the provider is certifying that the G code service is a distinct and separate service performed during a separate time period (not necessarily a separate patient encounter) than the E/M, psychiatric diagnostic, or psychotherapy service and is a service that is not included in the E/M, psychiatric diagnostic, or psychotherapy service based on the clinical reason for the E/M, psychiatric diagnostic, or psychotherapy service.

  CPT codes 99408 and 99409 describe services that are similar to those described by HCPCS codes G0396 and G0397 but are "screening" services not covered under the Medicare program. When codes 99408 and 99409 are covered by state Medicaid programs, the policies explained in the previous paragraph for G0396/G0397 also apply to 99408/99409.

- Transesophageal echocardiography (TEE) monitoring (93318) without probe placement is not reported separately by a physician performing critical care evaluation and management (E/M) services. However, if a physician places a transesophageal probe to be used for TEE monitoring on the same date of service as the date the physician performs critical care E/M services, code 93318 may be reported with modifier 59 or XU. The time necessary for probe placement should not be included in the critical care time reported with CPT codes 99291 and 99292 as is true for all separately reportable procedures performed on a patient receiving critical care E/M services. Diagnostic TEE services are separately reportable by a physician performing critical care E/M services.

- Practitioner ventilation management (94002–94005, 94660, 94662) and critical care (99291, 99292, 99466–99467, #99485–#99486, 99468–99480) include respiratory flow volume loop (94375), and breathing response to hypoxia (94450) testing if performed.

Office or Other Outpatient Medical Services (99202–99215)

New Patient (99202–99205)

These codes are used to report new patient encounters or visits with physicians or other qualified health care professionals (OQHCP) in the outpatient setting. This may include the office, clinic, urgent care center, or an outpatient seen in the emergency department or other ancillary department of the hospital. The level of service is determined by the extent of the medical decision making (MDM) performed or the time documented in the medical record. MDM levels or time amounts must be met to report a code in this section. The following table details the level of history, examination, medical decision making, and time that is required for each service.

 CODING AXIOM

It is important to document the start and stop times of an E/M service that is reported based on time.

Office or Other Outpatient Services—New Patient

Code	History & Exam	Medical Decision Making	Time in minutes
99202	Medically appropriate	Straightforward	15-29
99203	Medically appropriate	Low level	30-44
99204	Medically appropriate	Moderate level	45-59
99205	Medically appropriate	High level	60-74

Established Patient (99211–99215)

Established patient encounters or visits by the provider in the outpatient setting are identified by codes in this range. This may include the office, clinic, urgent care center, or an outpatient seen in the emergency department or other ancillary department of the hospital. The level of service is determined by the extent of the MDM or total amount of time documented in the medical record. The following table details the level of history, examination, medical decision making, and time that is required for each service.

Office or Other Outpatient Services—Established Patient[1]

Code	History & Exam	Medical Decision Making	Time in minutes
99211*	N/A	N/A	N/A
99212	Medically appropriate	Straightforward	10-19
99213	Medically appropriate	Low level	20-29
99214	Medically appropriate	Moderate level	30-39
99215	Medically appropriate	High level	40-54
99XXX			Each additional 15 minutes

* Physician presence is not required, presenting problems are minimal

Guideline Changes for Office or Other Outpatient E/M Services

As mentioned earlier in this chapter, new guidelines will be effective January 1, 2021 for this section of codes. In addition, code 99201 has been deleted and is no longer valid for dates of service after December 31, 2020.

Per the CMS CY2020 Physician Fee Schedule (PFS) Final Rule and CPT guidelines, the history and examination will no longer be used to select the code level for these services. These services will, however, still include a medically appropriate history and/or physical examination. The nature and extent of the history and/or physical examination will be determined by the treating provider based on clinical judgment and what is deemed as reasonable, necessary, and clinically appropriate. The history and physical examination should be documented in the medical record.

Selecting the level of office or other outpatient visit (99202–99205 and 99212–99215) should be based on the redefined levels of medical decision making (MDM) or total time spent by the provider on the day of the encounter, including face-to-face and non-face-to-face activities.

Medical Decision Making: Office or Other Outpatient E/M Services

The MDM is used to establish diagnoses, assess the status of a condition, and select a management option(s). MDM for these services is defined by three elements detailed in the new MDM table published in the CPT E/M guidelines. Two notable changes have been made in the MDM table: 1) new and established patient levels are scored the same, 2) new and established codes both require two out of three elements for any given code.

The three elements of the table used in selecting an MDM are:

- Number and complexity of problems addressed
- Amount and/or complexity of data to be reviewed and analyzed
- Risk of complications and/or morbidity or mortality of patient management

Number and Complexity of Problems Addressed During the Encounter

During a patient encounter, several new or established conditions may be addressed by the provider and may affect the medical decision making. The final diagnosis for a condition does not by itself determine the complexity or risk, as an extensive evaluation may be required to reach the conclusion that the signs or symptoms result in a lower level diagnosis. A notable change in the CPT guidelines is that a problem also includes consideration of further testing or treatment that may not be elected by virtue of risk/benefit analysis or patient/parent/guardian/surrogate choice.

Comorbidities or other underlying diseases should not be considered when selecting a level of service *unless* they are addressed during the patient encounter and their presence increases the amount and/or complexity of data to be reviewed and analyzed or the risk of complications and/or morbidity or mortality of patient management.

CPT includes definitions to assist in the selection of the different levels of problems listed in the MDM table. It is important to review the definitions of what is considered a problem, illness, or injury as some medical diagnoses or injuries may be classified in different categories. They are as follows:

- Minimal problem: A problem that may not require the presence of the physician or other qualified health care professional, but the service is provided under the physician's or other qualified health care professional's supervision (see 99211).

- Self-limited or minor problem: A problem that runs a definite and prescribed course, is transient in nature, and is not likely to permanently alter health status.

- Stable, chronic illness: A problem with an expected duration of at least one year or until the death of the patient.

- Acute, uncomplicated illness or injury: A recent or new short-term problem with low risk of morbidity for which treatment is considered. There is little to no risk of mortality with treatment, and full recovery without functional impairment is expected.

- Chronic illness with exacerbation, progression, or side effects of treatment: A chronic illness that is acutely worsening, poorly controlled, or progressing with an intent to control progression and requiring additional supportive care or requiring attention to treatment for side effects but that does not require consideration of hospital level of care.

- Acute illness with systemic symptoms: An illness that causes systemic symptoms and has a high risk of morbidity without treatment.

- Acute, complicated injury: An injury that requires treatment that includes evaluation of body systems that are not directly part of the injured organ, extensive injuries, or the treatment options are multiple and/or associated with risk of morbidity.

- Chronic illness with severe exacerbation, progression, or side effects of treatment: The severe exacerbation or progression of a chronic illness or severe side effects of treatment that have significant risk of morbidity and may require hospital level of care.

- Acute or chronic illness or injury that poses a threat to life or bodily function: An acute illness with systemic symptoms, or an acute complicated injury, or a chronic illness or injury with exacerbation and/or progression, or side effects of treatment that poses a threat to life or bodily function in the near term without treatment.

- Undiagnosed new problem with uncertain prognosis: A problem in the differential diagnosis that represents a condition likely to result in a high risk of morbidity without treatment.

 AUDITOR'S ALERT

Some diagnoses or injuries may be classified in different categories using the new 2021 definitions. For example, a sinus infection with a fever and chest congestion would have been considered an acute illness with systemic symptoms on the previous Table of Risk, which would have been a moderate risk of complication and/or morbidity or mortality. Using the 2021 new MDM making table, an acute illness with systemic symptoms is defined as an illness that causes systemic symptoms and has a *high risk* of morbidity without treatment, which would be a moderate level illness. The correct classification for this illness now is an acute, uncomplicated illness or injury: A recent or new short-term problem with low risk of morbidity for which treatment is considered. There is little to no risk of mortality with treatment, and full recovery without functional impairment is expected, which would be a low-level illness using the new definitions.

Level 4 – Number and Complexity of Problems Addressed

Code	Level of MDM	Number and Complexity of Problems Addressed at the Encounter
99204 99214	Moderate	**Moderate** • 1 or more chronic illnesses with exacerbation, progression, or side effects of treatment or • 2 or more stable chronic illnesses or • 1 undiagnosed new problem with uncertain prognosis or • 1 acute illness with systemic symptoms or • 1 acute complicated injury

Note: Each level has the same requirements for new or established patients.

Amount and/or Complexity of Data to be Reviewed and Analyzed

The second element is used for determining the level of service; it is no longer based on calculating points for each test category or specific task. The requirements for new or established patients are the same for each level. The four levels of this category are consistent with the current guidelines: minimal, limited, moderate, and extensive.

This MDM element includes medical records, tests, and other information that must be obtained, reviewed, ordered, and/or analyzed for the visit, including information obtained from multiple sources or interprofessional correspondence and interpretation of tests that are not reported separately. Ordering and subsequently reviewing test results are considered part of the current encounter, not a subsequent encounter.

CPT includes definitions of certain elements used within the data category of the MDM table to assist with the interpretation of these elements. They are as follows:

- Test: Imaging, laboratory, psychometric, or physiologic data. A clinical laboratory panel (e.g., basic metabolic panel [80047]) is a single test. The differentiation between single or multiple unique tests is defined in accordance with the CPT code set.

- External: Records, communications, and/or test results from an external physician, other qualified health care professional, facility, or health care organization.

- External physician or other qualified health care professional: Individual who is not in the same group practice or is a different specialty or subspecialty.

- Independent historian(s): Individual (e.g., parent, guardian, surrogate, spouse, witness) that provides a history in addition to a history provided by a patient who is unable to provide a complete or reliable history (e.g., due to developmental stage, dementia, or psychosis) or because a confirmatory history is judged to be necessary.

- Independent interpretation: Interpretation of a test for which there is a CPT code and an interpretation or report is customary. This does not apply when the physician or other qualified health care professional is reporting the service or has previously reported the service for the patient. A form of interpretation should be documented but need not conform to the usual standards of a complete report for the test.

- Appropriate source: For the purpose of the discussion of management data element, an appropriate source includes professionals who are not health care professionals but may be involved in the management of the patient (e.g., lawyer, parole officer, case manager, teacher). It does not include discussion with family or informal caregivers.

Level 4 – Amount and/or Complexity of Data Reviewed and Analyzed

Code	Level of MDM	Amount and/or Complexity of Data to be Reviewed and Analyzed *Each unique test, order, or document contributes to the combination of 2 or combination of 3 in Category 1 below.*

99204
99214
	Moderate	**Category 1: Tests, documents, or independent historian(s)**
		• **Any combination of 3 from the following:**
		  • review of prior external note(s) from each unique source*
		  • review of the result(s) of each unique test*
		  • ordering of each unique test*
		  • assessment requiring an independent historian(s)
		or
		Category 2: Independent interpretation of tests
		• Independent interpretation of a test performed by another physician/other qualified health care professional (not separately reported)
		or
		Category 3: Discussion of management or test interpretation
		• Discussion of management or test interpretation with external physician/other qualified health care professional/appropriate source (not separately reported)

*Note: Test panels such as 80047 are counted as a single laboratory test. The differentiation between single or multiple unique tests is defined in accordance with the CPT code set.

Note: Each level has the same requirements for new or established patients.

Risk of Complications and/or Morbidity or Mortality of Patient Management

The third element listed for determining the level of service includes decisions made during the encounter associated with the patient's problems, diagnostic procedure(s), and treatment(s). This includes potential management options selected and those considered, but not selected, after shared MDM with the patient and/or family. Shared MDM involves eliciting patient and/or family preferences, patient and/or family education, and explaining risks and benefits of management options.

There are four levels in this category that are consistent with the current guidelines: minimal, low, moderate, and high. The minimal and low categories no longer include examples, and the examples for moderate and high risk have been revised.

CPT includes definitions of certain elements used within the data category of the MDM table to help with the interpretation of these elements. They are as follows:

- Risk: The probability and/or consequences of an event. The assessment of the level of risk is affected by the nature of the event under consideration. Definitions of risk are based upon the usual behavior and thought processes of a physician or other qualified health care professional in the same specialty. For the purposes of MDM, level of risk is based upon consequences of the problem(s) addressed at the encounter when appropriately treated. Risk also includes MDM related to the need to initiate or forego further testing, treatment, and/or hospitalization.

- Morbidity: A state of illness or functional impairment that is expected to be of substantial duration during which function is limited, quality of life is impaired, or there is organ damage that may not be transient despite treatment.

- Social determinants of health: Economic and social conditions that influence the health of people and communities. Examples may include food or housing insecurity.

- Drug therapy requiring intensive monitoring for toxicity: A drug that requires intensive monitoring is a therapeutic agent that has the potential to cause serious morbidity or death. The monitoring is performed for assessment of these adverse effects and not primarily for assessment of therapeutic efficacy.

Level 3 and 4 – Risk of Complications and/or Morbidity or Mortality of Patient Management

Code	Level of MDM	Risk of Complications and/or Morbidity or Mortality of Patient Management
99203 99213	Low	Low risk of morbidity from additional diagnostic testing or treatment
99204 99214	Moderate	Moderate risk of morbidity from additional diagnostic testing or treatment *Examples only:* • Prescription drug management • Decision regarding minor surgery with identified patient or procedure risk factors • Decision regarding elective major surgery without identified patient or procedure risk factors • Diagnosis or treatment significantly limited by social determinants of health

Note: Each level has the same requirements for new or established patients.

		Medical Decision Making		
Code	Level of MDM (Based on 2 out of 3 Elements of MDM)	Number and Complexity of Problems Addressed	Amount and/or Complexity of Data to be Reviewed and Analyzed *Each unique test, order, or document contributes to the combination of 2 or combination of 3 in Category 1 below.*	Risk of Complications and/or Morbidity or Mortality of Patient Management
99211	N/A	N/A	N/A	N/A
99202 99212	Straight-forward	**Minimal** • 1 self-limited or minor problem	**Minimal or none**	**Minimal risk of morbidity from additional diagnostic testing or treatment**
99203 99213	Low	**Low** • 2 or more self-limited or minor problems; or • 1 stable chronic illness; or • 1 acute, uncomplicated illness or injury	**Limited** *(Must meet the requirements of at least 1 of the 2 categories)* **Category 1: Tests and documents** • **Any combination of 2 from the following:** • Review of prior external note(s) from each unique source* • Review of the result(s) of each unique test* • Ordering of each unique test* or **Category 2: Assessment requiring an independent historian(s)** *(For the categories of independent interpretation of tests and discussion of management or test interpretation, see moderate or high)*	**Low risk of morbidity from additional diagnostic testing or treatment**
99204 99214	Moderate	**Moderate** • 1 or more chronic illnesses with exacerbation, progression, or side effects of treatment; or • 2 or more stable chronic illnesses; or • 1 undiagnosed new problem with uncertain prognosis; or • 1 acute illness with systemic symptoms; or • 1 acute complicated injury	**Moderate** *(Must meet the requirements of at least 1 out of 3 categories)* **Category 1: Tests, documents, or independent historian(s)** • **Any combination of 3 from the following:** • Review of prior external note(s) from each unique source* • Review of the result(s) of each unique test* • Ordering of each unique test* • Assessment requiring an independent historian(s) or **Category 2: Independent interpretation of tests** • Independent interpretation of a test performed by another physician/other qualified health care professional (not separately reported) or **Category 3: Discussion of management or test interpretation** • Discussion of management or test interpretation with external physician/other qualified health care professional\appropriate source (not separately reported)	**Moderate risk of morbidity from additional diagnostic testing or treatment** *Examples only:* • Prescription drug management • Decision regarding minor surgery with identified patient or procedure risk factors • Decision regarding elective major surgery without identified patient or procedure risk factors • Diagnosis or treatment significantly limited by social determinants of health

* Note: Test panels such as 80047 are counted as a single laboratory test. The differentiation between single or multiple unique tests is defined in accordance with the CPT code set.

		Medical Decision Making		
Code	**Level of MDM (Based on 2 out of 3 Elements of MDM)**	**Number and Complexity of Problems Addressed**	**Amount and/or Complexity of Data to be Reviewed and Analyzed** *Each unique test, order, or document contributes to the combination of 2 or combination of 3 in Category 1 below.*	**Risk of Complications and/or Morbidity or Mortality of Patient Management**

99205 99215	**High**	**High**
		 • 1 or more chronic illnesses with severe exacerbation, progression, or side effects of treatment;
		 or
		 • 1 acute or chronic illness or injury that poses a threat to life or bodily function
			Extensive *(Must meet the requirements of at least 2 out of 3 categories)* **Category 1: Tests, documents, or independent historian(s)**
			 • **Any combination of 3 from the following:**
			   • Review of prior external note(s) from each unique source*;
			   • Review of the result(s) of each unique test*;
			   • Ordering of each unique test*;
			   • Assessment requiring an independent historian(s)
			 or
			 Category 2: Independent interpretation of tests
			 • Independent interpretation of a test performed by another physician/other qualified health care professional (not separately reported)
			 or
			 Category 3: Discussion of management or test interpretation
			 • Discussion of management or test interpretation with external physician/other qualified health care professional/appropriate source (not separately reported)
				High risk of morbidity from additional diagnostic testing or treatment *Examples only:*
				 • Drug therapy requiring intensive monitoring for toxicity
				 • Decision regarding elective major surgery with identified patient or procedure risk factors
				 • Decision regarding emergency major surgery
				 • Decision regarding hospitalization
				 • Decision not to resuscitate or to de-escalate care because of poor prognosis

* Note: Test panels such as 80047 are counted as a single laboratory test. The differentiation between single or multiple unique tests is defined in accordance with the CPT code set.

Time as the Basis for Code Selection

Effective January 1, 2021, time alone may be used to select the appropriate code level for office or other outpatient visits (99202–99205 and 99212–99215). Time alone may be used to report these services; the requirement that greater than 50 percent of the encounter must be spent counseling and/or in coordination of care has been removed. The new guidelines still require a face-to-face encounter with the physician or other qualified health care professional. The notable change is time includes both face-to-face and non-face-to-face time personally spent by the provider on the day of the encounter.

The following activities are included in the provider's time when performed:

- Preparing to see the patient (e.g., review of tests)
- Performing a medically appropriate examination and/or evaluation
- Care coordination (not reported separately)
- Counseling and educating the patient/family/caregiver
- Documenting clinical information in the electronic or other health record
- Independently interpreting results (not reported separately) and communicating results to the patient/family/caregiver

 AUDITOR'S ALERT

See Appendix 1 for the audit worksheet for time only reporting.

- Obtaining and/or reviewing separately obtained history
- Ordering medications, tests, or procedures
- Referring and communicating with other health care professionals

Along with the new guidelines, the times for each code have been revised. The table below illustrates the changes.

Code	History & Exam	Medical Decision Making	Time in Minutes
99202	Medically appropriate	Straightforward	15–29
99203	Medically appropriate	Low level	30–44
99204	Medically appropriate	Moderate level	45–59
99205	Medically appropriate	High level	60–74
99211*	N/A	N/A	N/A
99212	Medically appropriate	Straightforward	10–19
99213	Medically appropriate	Low level	20–29
99214	Medically appropriate	Moderate level	30–39
99215	Medically appropriate	High level	40–54

*Physician presence is not required; presenting problems are minimal

The time defined in the code descriptor is used for selecting the appropriate level of service. Applicable time spent on the date of the encounter should be documented in the medical record when it is used as the basis for code selection.

Under the new time guidelines, shared or split visits may still be performed. A shared or split visit is when a physician and other qualified health care professional(s) jointly provide the face-to-face and non-face-to-face work related to the encounter. When performing a shared or split visit and the time is used as the basis for code selection, the time personally spent by the physician and other qualified health care professional evaluating and managing the patient on the date of the encounter is summed to determine the total time. If two or more providers meet with or discuss the patient, only one provider should count this time toward the total time of the split/shared visit.

Prolonged Services (99417)

The AMA also revised guidelines in the 2021 CPT book for current prolonged services codes 99354–99355 (Prolonged E/M without Direct Patient Contact) and 99358–99359 (Prolonged Service without Direct Patient Contact) stating these codes will no longer be reported with 99202–99205 or 99211–99215. Codes 99354-99355 may be used when a physician or OQHCP provides a prolonged service involving direct patient contact that is provided beyond the usual service in the inpatient, observation, or outpatient setting.

In addition, CMS will no longer reimburse separately for codes 99358–99359 in association with office E/M services (99202–99205 and 99212–99215).

To report additional time spent by the provider, the AMA has created a new add-on code for prolonged office visits.

99417   Prolonged office or other outpatient evaluation and management service(s) beyond the minimum required time of the primary procedure which has been selected using total time, requiring total time with or without direct patient contact beyond the usual service, on the date of the primary service, each 15 minutes of total time (List separately in addition to codes 99205, 99215 for office or other outpatient Evaluation and Management services)

 AUDITOR'S ALERT

Effective January 1, 2021, prolonged service codes 99354–99355 and 99358–99359 should not be reported with Office or Other Outpatient codes 99202–99205 or 99211–99215.

 AUDITOR'S ALERT

CMS will no longer reimburse separately for codes 99358–99359 in association with office E/M services (99202–99205 and 99212–99215).

This code is reported only when the office or other outpatient service code level selection is based on time alone (including face-to-face and non-face-to-face time), and the total time of the highest-level service (99205 or 99215) has been exceeded by at least 15 additional minutes.

New Patient Office/Outpatient E/M Visit (Total Practitioner Time, When Time is Used to Select Code Level)	CPT Code
60–74 minutes	99205
75–89 minutes	99205 x1 and 99417 x1
90–104 minutes	99205 x1 and 99417 x2
105 or more minutes	99205 x1 and 99417 x3 or more for each additional 15 minutes

Established Patient Office/Outpatient E/M Visit (Total Practitioner Time, When Time is Used to Select Code Level)	CPT Code
40–54 minutes	99215
55–69 minutes	99215 x1 and 99417 x1
70–84 minutes	99215 x1 and 99417 x2
85 or more minutes	99215 x1 and 99417 x3 or more for each additional 15 minutes

AUDITOR'S ALERT

Per the 2021 PFS proposed rule, a single add-on code (GPC1X) will be added to the office/outpatient E/M visit code set to report visit complexity associated with certain office/outpatient evaluation and management codes.

Despite all the 2021 office/outpatient E/M code revisions, CMS does not feel that they adequately reflect resources used with certain primary care and specialty care services. So, they proposed an add-on code (GPC1X) CY2021 PFS proposed rule. This code would be used to report visit complexity associated with certain office/outpatient evaluation and management codes.

CY2021 PFS final rule was not released at the time of this publication, refer to https://www.cms.gov/Medicare/Medicare-Fee-for-Service-Payment/Physician FeeSched/PFS-Federal-Regulation-Notices to review final comments/changes to these proposals.

Incident To Services

It is important to note that "incident to" requirements need to be reviewed in an audit. This is especially true if a practice employs mid-level providers or has residents participating in physician services. CMS has specific guidelines that need to be followed. Other payers may vary, so it is best to check individual payer guidelines before reporting services.

DEFINITIONS

incident to. Provision of a service concurrently with another service. For example, additional covered supplies and materials that are furnished after surgery typically are billed as "incident to" a physician's services and not as hospital services. This term is used specifically for revenue codes for pharmacy, supplies, and anesthesia furnished along with radiology and other diagnostic services.

In general, for services to be covered under the "incident to" provision, specific conditions must be met, in addition to the standard coverage criteria, including:

- Services must be an integral, although incidental, part of a physician professional service.

- Services must be commonly rendered, without charge, or included in the physician bill.

- Services are those commonly furnished in physician offices or clinics.

- Services are furnished by the physician or by auxiliary personnel under the physician's direct supervision.

Biling Guidelines

Certain requirements must be met before a service can be billed under the "incident to" methodology, including:

- Services must be commonly furnished in a physician's office.
- The physician must have initially seen the patient.
- There has to be direct personal supervision by the physician of auxiliary personnel, regardless of whether the individual is an employee, leased staff, or independent contractor of the physician.
- The physician has an active part in the ongoing care of the patient.

Services performed by the nonphysician practitioner (NPP) "incident to" a physician's professional services include not only services typically rendered by a nurse or medical assistant (i.e., blood pressure and temperature measurements, injections, and dressing changes) but also services reserved for the physician such as minor surgery, casting, treating simple fractures, reviewing x-rays, and other activities that involve evaluation or treatment of a patient's condition. However, only those services that are within the individual's legal scope of practice, and for which the individual is qualified, may be furnished.

As stated above, direct supervision in the office setting does not mean that the physician must be present in the same room. However, the physician must be present in the office suite and available immediately to provide assistance and direction, when needed, while the service is being performed.

A patient must be established with the practice in order for a service to be reported as incident to. New patients should always have an initial visit with the physician.

"Incident to" services are reported on the claim when the billing physician or nonphysician provider has provided the service. The provider's NPI is also required on the claim.

Documentation Requirements

Documentation must indicate that the patient is established. That is, the patient has seen the physician previously and is not considered a new patient to the practice. The medical record should have the cosignature or legible identity and credentials of both the NPP and the supervising physician, when applicable. There should also be some indication in the documentation as to the level of involvement by the supervising physician, such as other dates of service linking the two providers.

In the case of allied health professionals, such as medical assistants etc., the allied health professional must be qualified under state law to perform the service.

Documentation must specify a physician was present to supervise the service. As always, the medical necessity should be clearly stated in the medical record.

Hospital "Incident To" Services

Services performed by auxiliary personnel in an inpatient or outpatient setting are **not** covered as "incident to" services. Likewise, services provided by auxiliary personnel not in the employ of the physician, even when provided by order of the physician, are not covered as "incident to." The law requires that, in addition to being those most commonly performed in a physician's office, the doctor must incur an expense resulting from providing the service or procedure.

CODING AXIOM

Payment for code 99211, with or without modifier 25, is not allowed if it is reported with a nonchemotherapy drug infusion code or a chemotherapy administration code.

CODING AXIOM

Direct supervision means the physician is in the office and able to provide assistance and direction as necessary. The physician does not have to be physically present in the room where the procedure or service is being performed.

Auxiliary personnel are defined as individuals who are acting under the supervision of the physician, regardless of whether that individual is an employee, leased staff, or independent contractor of the physician or legal entity that employs or contracts with the physician.

Shared Visits

E/M services provided in the office or clinic setting by the physician must be billed using the physician's NPI. When the E/M service is shared or split between the physician and an NPP, such as a nurse practitioner (NP), physician assistant (PA), clinical nurse specialist (CNS), or a certified nurse midwife (CNM), it may be reported in one of two ways:

- If the service is provided to an established patient, and the incident-to requirements are met, the service is billed using the physician's NPI.

- If the incident-to provisions are not met, the service must be billed using the NPI of the NPP.

Whenever an E/M service is shared by a physician and an NPP from the same group, and the physician provides any of the face-to-face portion of the service, the service may be reported using the physician's or the NPP's NPI. In a situation in which there is no face-to-face visit between the patient and the physician (e.g., the physician reviewed the patient's medical record only), the service must be billed using the NPP's NPI.

When the service is an inpatient, outpatient, or emergency department E/M service shared between the physician and NPP and the physician provides any face-to-face portion of the encounter, the service may be billed under the physician or NPP provider number when the NPP is a member of the same group practice. However, if no direct face-to-face encounter occurs between the provider and patient, the service must be billed under the NPP provider number.

For example, a patient is admitted for abdominal pain. During the admission, the patient is seen by the NPP. The physician employing the NPP reviews the medical record documentation and indicates that they are in agreement concerning the treatment plan. In this scenario, even though the physician has reviewed and amended the medical record, the encounter must be billed under the NPP provider number as there was no direct face-to-face contact between the physician and patient. However, if the physician discussed the current complaints and proposed treatment by the NPP directly with the patient, the encounter could be billed under either the physician's or the NPP's provider number.

Provider offices should perform random internal audits to verify "incident to" guidelines are being adhered to. Claims should be compared to the medical record documentation. The aforementioned requirements may be used to ensure that all "incident to" billing criteria have been followed.

Finally, medical records should be evaluated to validate the medically necessity of the codes assigned and reported.

In order to substantiate that the "incident to" guidelines were met, the medical record should contain at a minimum:

AUDITOR'S ALERT

For shared/split E/M services, each provider should document his or her portion of the E/M service. The documentation must support the face-to-face requirement and must clearly identify both providers involved in the service. Select the code for the level of E/M service based on the combined documentation.

- Cosignature or legible identity and credentials (i.e., MD, DO, NP, PA, etc.) of the practitioner who provided the service and the supervising physician.

- Some indication of the supervising physician's involvement with the patient's care. This indication could be satisfied by:

  - notation of supervising physician's involvement (the degree of which must be consistent with clinical circumstances of the care) within the text of the associated medical record entry   OR

  - documentation from other dates of service (e.g., initial visit, etc.) other than those requested, establishing the link between the two providers

Observation Hospital Services

Hospital Observation Services (99217–99220, 99224–99226, 99234–99236)

Hospital observation service codes are used to report services provided to patients designated as under observation status in an outpatient hospital. Observation services may be provided in an observation unit or other designated hospital area. There are 10 codes used to report observation services and they include counseling and/or coordination of care with other providers or agencies, and the patient or patient's family.

Hospitals have their own guidelines regarding how long a patient can remain in observation status. Many hospitals do not allow a patient to remain in observation for longer than 23 hours, although Medicare guidelines allow up to 48 hours for certain conditions.

According to CMS, in the *Medicare Claims Processing Manual,* Pub. 100-04, chapter 12, section 30.6.8, if the patient remains in observation after the first date following the admission to observation, it is expected that the patient would be discharged on that second calendar date. The provider bills CPT code 99217 for observation care discharge services provided on the second date.

In the rare circumstance when a patient is held in observation status for more than two calendar dates, the provider must bill subsequent services furnished before the date of discharge using the subsequent observation care codes (99224-99226). The provider may not use the subsequent hospital care codes since the patient is not an inpatient of the hospital.

These codes include review of the medical record, diagnostic studies, and patient status changes since the last assessment by the health care provider. Code level is based on the extent of interval history, exam, and medical decision making.

Patients admitted and discharged from observation status (or inpatient hospital status) on the same day should be reported with the single-day service codes, 99234-99236. The provider must satisfy the documentation requirements for both the admission to and discharge from inpatient or observation care to bill for these services. All services provided on this date by the same provider are combined into a single service regardless of where the service was rendered.

These services are based upon the three key components as a time element is not defined.

 DENIAL ALERT

Place of service code 22 for the outpatient setting must be reported on the claim to prevent denial of observation services.

Observation care discharge, code 99217, is not reported in conjunction with a hospital admission immediately following discharge from outpatient hospital observation status (i.e., subsequent to the patient being changed from observation status to hospital inpatient status). This change may or may not require the patient to be moved from a hospital observation unit to a hospital inpatient care unit.

Documentation must clearly indicate the change of status from outpatient hospital observation to hospital admission. The following tables detail the level of history, examination, and medical decision making that is required for each service.

Hospital Observation Services

E/M Code	History[1]	Exam[1]	Medical Decision Making[1]	Problem Severity	Coordination of Care; Counseling	Time Spent Bedside and on Unit/Floor (avg.)
99217	Observation care discharge day management					
99218	Detailed or comprehensive	Detailed or comprehensive	Straight-forward or low complexity	Low	Consistent with problem(s) and patient's needs	30 min.
99219	Comprehensive	Comprehensive	Moderate complexity	Moderate	Consistent with problem(s) and patient's needs	50 min.
99220	Comprehensive	Comprehensive	High complexity	High	Consistent with problem(s) and patient's needs	70 min.

1   Key component. All three components (history, exam, and medical decision making) are crucial for selecting the correct code.

Subsequent Hospital Observation Services[1]

E/M Code[2]	History[3]	Exam[3]	Medical Decision Making[3]	Problem Severity	Coordination of Care; Counseling	Time Spent Bedside and on Unit/Floor (avg.)
99224	Problem-focused interval	Problem-focused	Straight-forward or low complexity	Stable, recovering, or improving	Consistent with problem(s) and patient's needs	15 min.
99225	Expanded problem-focused interval	Expanded problem-focused	Moderate complexity	Inadequate response to treatment; minor complications	Consistent with problem(s) and patient's needs	25 min.
99226	Detailed interval	Detailed	High complexity	Unstable; significant new problem or significant complication	Consistent with problem(s) and patient's needs	35 min.

1   All subsequent levels of service include reviewing the medical record, diagnostic studies, and changes in the patient's status, such as history, physical condition, and response to treatment since the last assessment.

2   These codes are resequenced in CPT and printed following codes 99217–99220.

3   Key component. For subsequent care, at least two of the three components (history, exam, and medical decision making) are needed to select the correct code.

Observation or Inpatient Care Services (Including Admission and Discharge Services)

E/M Code	History[1]	Exam[1]	Medical Decision Making[1]	Problem Severity	Coordination of Care; Counseling	Time
99234	Detailed or comprehensive	Detailed or comprehensive	Straight-forward or low complexity	Low	Consistent with problem(s) and patient's needs	40 min.
99235	Comprehensive	Comprehensive	Moderate	Moderate	Consistent with problem(s) and patient's needs	50 min.
99236	Comprehensive	Comprehensive	High	High	Consistent with problem(s) and patient's needs	55 min.

1   Key component. All three components (history, exam, and medical decision making) are crucial for selecting the correct code.

Inpatient Services

In the inpatient setting, there are several types of services provided to patients, including:

- Initial inpatient hospital care
- Subsequent inpatient hospital care
- Hospital discharge
- Inpatient consultation

There are specific guidelines for reporting each type of inpatient service. These guidelines are covered in more detail below. Although these services are not outpatient, they rely on the same key and contributory components for code selection as those previously discussed. A few codes use time or other criteria that will be explained.

Initial Inpatient Hospital Care (99221–99223)

Initial inpatient care can be reported only for services provided by the admitting physician. Other physicians or other qualified health care providers providing initial inpatient E/M services should use consultation or subsequent hospital care codes, as appropriate. Combine all E/M services performed on the same date by the same provider that are related to the admission, regardless of where they were provided (e.g., emergency department, observation status, office, or nursing facility), and report the appropriate initial hospital care code.

The lowest level of initial hospital care should be reported when the admitting physician performed a detailed or comprehensive history and physical several days prior to admission and a lesser history and physical on the day of admission.

If a patient is admitted late in the evening on the first day and the physician does not see the patient until the next day, the admission history and physical (H&P), or initial inpatient service, is reported on the second day if that is when the service was performed. This E/M service is used to report the first face-to-face encounter between the patient and the provider in the inpatient setting.

 DENIAL ALERT

Inpatient services must report place of service code 21 for the inpatient setting to prevent claim denial.

The admitting physician should append modifier AI Principal physician of record, to the CPT code when reporting claims for Medicare beneficiaries.

The following table details the level of history, examination, and medical decision making that is required for each service.

Hospital Inpatient Services—Initial Care[1]

E/M Code	History[2]	Exam[2]	Medical Decision Making[2]	Problem Severity	Coordination of Care; Counseling	Time Spent Bedside and on Unit/Floor (avg.)
99221	Detailed or comprehensive	Detailed or comprehensive	Straight-forward or low complexity	Low	Consistent with problem(s) and patient's needs	30 min.
99222	Comprehensive	Comprehensive	Moderate complexity	Moderate	Consistent with problem(s) and patient's needs	50 min.
99223	Comprehensive	Comprehensive	High complexity	High	Consistent with problem(s) and patient's needs	70 min.

1 The admitting physician should append modifier AI, Principal physician of record, for Medicare patients
2 Key component. For initial care, all three components (history, exam, and medical decision making) are crucial for selecting the correct code.

Subsequent Inpatient Hospital Care (99231–99233)

Subsequent hospital care codes are reported for any inpatient E/M services provided after the first inpatient encounter, including reviewing diagnostic studies and noting changes in the patient's status. For the admitting provider this includes all E/M services provided to the patient on subsequent visits starting the calendar day after the initial encounter. For all other providers providing consultation or concurrent care, the subsequent hospital care codes are reported. These codes are also used to report preoperative medical evaluation and/or postoperative care before discharge when these services were provided by a physician other than the surgeon. This is one of the few code sets where an interval history is described. The specific elements of these histories are not defined in the CPT book or federal guidelines, but the labels of each level are suggestive. A problem-focused interval history would focus on history of present illness (HPI) since the last visit. The expanded-problem-focused version would include some review of systems (ROS). The detailed version would simply have more of the above in each area, but again is limited by what has occurred since the last visit.

Remember that these are daily visit codes and only one subsequent visit per day per provider should be reported. If other services or critical care are performed they may be reported separately.

Hospital Discharge Services (99238–99239)

The codes for hospital discharge services are appropriately assigned by the length of time devoted to performing the service, less than 30 minutes or more than 30 minutes. Use of these codes excludes services rendered on behalf of a patient who has been admitted and discharged from observation status or inpatient status on the same day.

The hospital discharge services include final examination of the patient, discharge instructions for continued care, and completion of the patient record.

> ⚠ **DENIAL ALERT**
>
> Payers may deny these services if the admitting provider inadvertently appends modifier AI to subsequent inpatient services.

To report 99239, the physician's time must be more than 30 minutes and should be clearly documented in the patient's medical record. The following table details the level of history, examination, and medical decision making that is required for each service.

Hospital Inpatient Services—Subsequent Care[1]

E/M Code	History[2]	Exam[2]	Medical Decision Making[2]	Problem Severity	Coordination of Care; Counseling	Time Spent Bedside and on Unit/Floor (avg.)
99231	Problem-focused interval	Problem-focused	Straight-forward or low complexity	Stable, recovering or Improving	Consistent with problem(s) and patient's needs	15 min.
99232	Expanded problem-focused interval	Expanded problem-focused	Moderate complexity	Inadequate response to treatment; minor complications	Consistent with problem(s) and patient's needs	25 min.
99233	Detailed interval	Detailed	High complexity	Unstable; significant new problem or significant complication	Consistent with problem(s) and patient's needs	35 min.
99238	Hospital discharge day management					30 min. or less
99239	Hospital discharge day management					> 30 min.

1 All subsequent levels of service include reviewing the medical record, diagnostic studies, and changes in the patient's status, such as history, physical condition, and response to treatment since the last assessment.

2 Key component. For subsequent care, at least two of the three components (history, exam, and medical decision making) are needed to select the correct code.

Consultations (99241–99255, 99446–99452)

A consultation is the provision of a physician's or OQHCP's opinion or advice about a patient for a specific problem at the request of another physician or other appropriate source. CPT also states that a consultation may be performed when a physician or OQHCP is determining whether to accept the transfer of patient care at the request of another physician or appropriate source.

If a consultant initiates diagnostic and therapeutic services at the request of the attending physician or OQHCP, the service still qualifies as a consultation. The consultant must document the recommended course of action to the attending provider or OQHCP and treatment being initiated as requested. When the consulting provider assumes responsibility for the continuing care of the patient, any subsequent service rendered ceases to be a consultation. Follow-up visits to the provider in an office setting are coded to 99211–99215, established patient office visit.

Note: Effective January 1, 2010, the consultation codes are no longer recognized for Medicare Part B payment. Physicians are instructed to code patient evaluation and management visits with E/M codes that represent where the visit occurred and that identify the complexity of the visit performed. In both the inpatient hospital and the nursing facility settings, all physicians (and qualified nonphysician practitioners where permitted) who perform an initial evaluation may bill the initial hospital care codes (99221–99223) or nursing facility care codes (99304–99306). The principal physician of record is identified as the physician who oversees the patient's total care as opposed to other physicians who may be furnishing specialty specific care. The principal physician of record should append modifier AI Principal Physician of Record, in addition to the reported E/M code. Follow-up visits in the facility setting should be billed as subsequent hospital care visits (99231–99233) and subsequent nursing facility care visits (99307–99310).

Physician Consultant Documentation Guidelines

The consulting physician or OQHCP should confirm that the attending physician or OQHCP requested an evaluation for the express purpose of rendering an opinion regarding a patient's specific problem. The statement must include both the name of the provider requesting the consultation and the reason why it was necessary.

Consultations should be documented according to guidelines developed for this specific purpose. Any recommendations made by the consultant should be made in writing.

In addition, a consulting physician or OQHCP should:

- Note in the patient record that the patient was advised to follow up with the requesting provider for ongoing and further care.

- Include a statement verifying that all information pertaining to the consultation was forwarded, in writing, to the requesting provider. Information regarding the consultation must always be furnished to the requesting provider in written form. It is always a good idea to communicate noteworthy or significant findings verbally, as well, and include a notation of the call or discussion in the medical record.

- Document the consultation directly in the patient chart whenever both providers have access to the chart. This usually occurs in a hospital or multi-specialty clinic setting.

- Avoid stating there will be continued involvement with the patient. A consultation is a single event unless the patient's provider makes a subsequent request. However, a single consult may require more than one evaluation of the patient.

- Provide therapy only at the request of the patient's attending provider. In other words, the consulting provider should not unilaterally decide to treat the patient. In the event this happens, the visit is no longer considered a consultation and the service should be reported as a treatment visit.

Consultations are valued higher than concurrent care and, as a result, every effort should be made to ensure that the provider is not simply providing concurrent care under the guise of a consultation. Claim reviewers are becoming more astute at detecting this. Therefore, consultations do not involve assuming responsibility for the management of any or all of the patient's care during the consultation encounter. A transfer of care occurs when the provider requests that another provider **take over the responsibility of managing the patient's complete care for a specific condition.** However, a consultant may initiate diagnostic services and treatment at the time of the initial consultation or subsequent visit.

After an initial consultation, any ensuing, ongoing management should be reported using the appropriate place of service and nonconsultative E/M code by level of care rendered.

In the hospital or nursing facility settings, the consultant should use the appropriate level of initial inpatient consultation codes (99251–99255). The

 CODING AXIOM

Consultations mandated by an insurance company or legal entity are identified by adding modifier 32 to appropriately convey the circumstances.

© 2020 Optum360, LLC

initial inpatient consultation codes may be reported once per consultant, per patient, per admission. Following the initial consultation service, the subsequent hospital care codes (99231–99233) should be reported as appropriate. In the nursing facility setting, following the initial consultation service, the subsequent nursing facility care codes (99307–99310) are reported for additional follow-up visits.

The consulting provider should use the appropriate office or other outpatient consultation (new or established patient) codes (99241–99245) to report an initial consultation provided in all other settings. Following the initial consultation service, the office or other outpatient established patient codes (99212–99215) should be reported for additional follow-up visits. CPT code 99211 should not be reported as a follow-up consultation visit. The descriptor for CPT code 99211 states that the presence of a provider is not required in order to report this service; therefore, it would not meet the follow-up service criteria according to Medicare policies.

If an additional request is received for an opinion or advice regarding a new or same problem with the same patient (same or different provider) and documented within the health record, the consultation codes may be reported again. However, if the consultant continues to provide care for the patient for the original condition following his or her initial evaluation, consultative services should no longer be reported during that period.

Concurrent Care
If a referral does not qualify as a consultation, it usually falls under concurrent care. Concurrent care involves sending a patient to another provider for management of a specific problem. It may also be referred to as a partial transfer of care. Once the treatment is complete, the patient returns to the care of the first provider. The two providers are participating simultaneously in the care of the patient.

Documentation and diagnosis codes must reflect the fact that each provider managed a separate medical problem. For example, an orthopedic surgeon manages care of a patient's knee following surgery while the internist oversees the care of diabetes. In order to avoid potential billing problems, each provider involved in concurrent care should only use diagnosis codes applicable to the problem that was treated. This may present some difficulties in cases where two providers are managing different aspects of the same problem. For example, a cardiothoracic surgeon and a cardiologist may simultaneously manage a patient with coronary artery disease. This disease may require the expertise of more than one specialty. The diagnostic coding would be the same in this scenario. The documentation, however, should clearly indicate the medical necessity of having more than one specialist involved in the management of a single medical problem. To avoid reimbursement delays or issues, submit a cover letter with the claim clearly outlining the medical necessity of two providers in similar specialties participating in the patient's care.

Transfer of Care
A transfer of care is defined as the assignment of care to a second provider who assumes complete responsibility for managing the specific condition of a patient permanently or for a specified period of time. When a provider opts to transfer the care of a patient to another provider, the patient should be given names of providers to choose from and that list should be noted in the medical record. If the provider transfers the care of a patient to a specific provider, the referring provider could potentially be held liable in the event the patient files a

malpractice claim against the other provider. Medical record documentation should also indicate the nature of the condition that the other provider will be managing. For example, if the primary care provider requests that a patient with brittle diabetes see Dr. Smith, an endocrinologist for the management of the diabetes, the medical record should indicate that the patient is referred to Dr. Smith for ongoing management of diabetes mellitus. Documentation for later dates of service may include discussions with the patient regarding the type of care Dr. Smith is providing, such as insulin dosages or nutritional counseling or any correspondences between the primary care provider and Dr. Smith.

Outpatient Consultation Services (99241–99245)

An office or other outpatient consultation is provided in the consultant's office, in the emergency department, or in an outpatient or other ambulatory facility, including hospital observation services, home services, domiciliary, rest home, or custodial care. Consultations rendered in the outpatient setting should include documentation indicating who requested the consultation and the intent of the consultation. A written report must be sent to the requesting provider or source to be placed in the patient's permanent medical record. The following table details the level of history, examination, and medical decision making that is required for each service.

Consultations—Office or Other Outpatient

E/M Code	History[1]	Exam[1]	Medical Decision Making[1]	Problem Severity	Coordination of Care; Counseling	Time Spent Face-to-Face (avg.)
99241	Problem-focused	Problem-focused	Straight-forward	Minor or self-limited	Consistent with problem(s) and patient's needs	15 min.
99242	Expanded problem-focused	Expanded problem-focused	Straight-forward	Low	Consistent with problem(s) and patient's needs	30 min.
99243	Detailed	Detailed	Low complexity	Moderate	Consistent with problem(s) and patient's needs	40 min.
99244	Comprehensive	Comprehensive	Moderate complexity	Moderate to high	Consistent with problem(s) and patient's needs	60 min.
99245	Comprehensive	Comprehensive	High complexity	Moderate to high	Consistent with problem(s) and patient's needs	80 min.

1   Key component. For office or other outpatient consultations, all three components (history, exam, and medical decision making) are crucial for selecting the correct code.

Inpatient Consultation Services (99251–99255)

An inpatient consultation is provided in the hospital, nursing facility, and partial hospital setting.

A written report must be sent to the requesting provider to be placed in the permanent shared medical record for that patient. When a common chart is used, a separate report to the requesting provider does not need to be sent. Required documentation includes the request for consultation, need for the consultation, consultant's opinion, and any services that were ordered or performed.

A transfer of care from one provider to another is reported using the new or established patient visit codes as appropriate. The initial visit of a transfer of care is not considered a consultation service.

Report only one inpatient consultation by a consultant for each admission to the hospital or nursing facility.

The following table details the level of history, examination, and medical decision making that is required for each service.

Consultations—Inpatient[1]

E/M Code	History[2]	Exam[2]	Medical Decision Making[2]	Problem Severity	Coordination of Care; Counseling	Time Spent Bedside and on Unit/Floor (avg.)
99251	Problem-focused	Problem-focused	Straight-forward	Minor or self-limited	Consistent with problem(s) and patient's needs	20 min.
99252	Expanded problem-focused	Expanded problem-focused	Straight-forward	Low	Consistent with problem(s) and patient's needs	40 min.
99253	Detailed	Detailed	Low complexity	Moderate	Consistent with problem(s) and patient's needs	55 min.
99254	Comprehensive	Comprehensive	Moderate complexity	Moderate to high	Consistent with problem(s) and patient's needs	80 min.
99255	Comprehensive	Comprehensive	High complexity	Moderate to high	Consistent with problem(s) and patient's needs	110 min.

1   These codes are used for hospital inpatients, residents of nursing facilities or patients in a partial hospital setting.

2   Key component. For initial inpatient consultations, all three components (history, exam, and medical decision making) are crucial for selecting the correct code.

Emergency Department Services (99281–99288)

The code range does not distinguish new or established patients. These codes are reserved to identify services provided in an emergency department, which is defined as "an organized 24-hour hospital-based facility that provides unscheduled services to patients needing immediate medical attention." Urgent care centers and ambulatory surgery centers are not considered to be emergency departments.

Effective January 1, 2010, a physician, other than the emergency physician, may see a patient in the emergency department and report emergency department visit codes. This includes consultations provided in the emergency department when the patient is not admitted. Physicians should report the service that best describes the visit performed. If a patient is admitted to the hospital as a result of the visit, the appropriate level of the initial hospital care (99221–99223) should be reported. All evaluation and management services provided by the provider in conjunction with that admission are considered part of the initial hospital care when performed on the same date as the admission.

Physician direction of emergency medical systems (EMS) emergency care (99288) is reported when a physician or OQHCP in a hospital emergency or critical care department is in two-way communication with ambulance or rescue personnel outside the hospital. The physician or OQHCP directs performance of necessary medical procedures taking place in the field, including telemetry,

 CODING AXIOM

Time is not mentioned in the description of these services and is not considered when making a final code selection in the emergency department.

cardiopulmonary resuscitation, intubation, administration of intravenous fluids and/or administration of intramuscular, intratracheal, or subcutaneous drugs, and/or defibrillation/electrical conversion of arrhythmia.

Medicare, as well as most other third-party payers, considers this service bundled into the E/M code reported by the emergency department physician at the time the patient arrives at the facility. Therefore, it would not typically be reported separately.

The following table details the level of history, examination, and medical decision making that is required for each service.

Emergency Department Services, New or Established Patient

E/M Code	History[1]	Exam[1]	Medical Decision Making[1]	Problem Severity[3]	Coordination of Care; Counseling	Time Spent[2] Face-to-Face (avg.)
99281	Problem-focused	Problem-focused	Straight-forward	Minor or self-limited	Consistent with problem(s) and patient's needs	N/A
99282	Expanded problem-focused	Expanded problem-focused	Low complexity	Low to moderate	Consistent with problem(s) and patient's needs	N/A
99283	Expanded problem-focused	Expanded problem-focused	Moderate complexity	Moderate	Consistent with problem(s) and patient's needs	N/A
99284	Detailed	Detailed	Moderate complexity	High; requires urgent evaluation	Consistent with problem(s) and patient's needs	N/A
99285	Comprehensive	Comprehensive	High complexity	High; poses immediate/ significant threat to life or physiologic function	Consistent with problem(s) and patient's needs	N/A
99288[4]			High complexity			N/A

1. Key component. For emergency department services, all three components (history, exam, and medical decision making) are crucial for selecting the correct code and must be adequately documented in the medical record to substantiate the level of service reported.

2. Typical times have not been established for this category of services.

3. NOTE: The severity of the patient's problem, while taken into consideration when evaluating and treating the patient, does not automatically determine the level of E/M service unless the medical record documentation reflects the severity of the patient's illness, injury, or condition in the details of the history, physical examination, and medical decision making process. Federal auditors will "downcode" the level of E/M service despite the nature of the patient's problem when the documentation does not support the E/M code reported.

4. Code 99288 is used to report two-way communication with emergency medical services personnel in the field.

Other Types of E/M Service

The E/M section also includes other types of evaluative services. Some of these are critical care, prolonged services, case management, care plan oversight, preventive medicine, and special services.

Critical Care Services (99291–99292)

Critical care codes are used to report the care of a critically ill or critically injured patient. A critical illness or injury acutely impairs one or more vital organ systems such that there is a high probability of imminent or life-threatening deterioration in the patient's condition.

Critical care is usually, but not always, given in a critical care area, such as the coronary care unit, intensive care unit, pediatric intensive care unit, respiratory care unit, or the emergency care facility. However, the patient's presence in one of these critical care areas does not alone constitute the requirements to provide critical care. Critical care codes should never be routinely applied just because the patient is in a designated critical care unit or bed.

The guidelines for time in *CPT 2021* state: "A unit of time is attained when the mid-point is passed. For example, an hour is attained when 31 minutes have elapsed (more than midway between zero and 60 minutes). A second hour is attained when a total of 91 minutes have elapsed. When codes are ranked in sequential typical times and the actual time is between two typical times, the code with the typical time closest to the actual time is used."

When additional procedures are performed on the same date as critical care services, the time involved in the procedures may not be included in total critical care time. For Medicare beneficiaries, the list of inclusive CPT codes for critical care may vary slightly from that published in the CPT book. Check with the Medicare contractor for a current listing of inclusive services when critical care is provided.

These services are reported based upon the time spent by the provider in activities directly related to the patient's care and does not need to be strictly spent at bedside, but on a patient's floor/unit. The time spent with the patient and the services provided should be documented in the patient's record. The documentation should clearly state the urgency of care and the critical nature of the patient's condition and required care. Time begins when the provider assumes responsibility for the patient care and ends when the provider no longer needs to provide constant care to the patient.

Since critical care is reported based on time, the total time spent providing critical care on a single date should be added together, even if care is rendered multiple times during the day. Only one provider may report critical care for the same episode of care.

Critical care of fewer than 30 minutes is not separately reported. Documentation must include all services and monitoring provided and the time spent by the provider. Some payers may require documentation of start and stop times.

Critical care includes services usually performed in conjunction with this level of care, including:

36000	Introduction of needle or intracatheter, vein
36410	Venipuncture, age 3 years or older, necessitating the skill of a physician or other qualified health care professional (separate procedure), for diagnostic or therapeutic purposes
36415	Collection of venous blood by venipuncture
36591	Collection of blood specimen from a completely implantable venous access device
36600	Arterial puncture, withdrawal of blood for diagnosis
43752	Naso- or oro-gastric tube placement, requiring physician's skill and fluoroscopic guidance

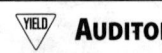 **AUDITOR'S ALERT**

See Appendix 1 for the critical care auditing worksheet.

43753	Gastric intubation and aspiration(s) therapeutic, necessitating physician's skill (e.g., for gastrointestinal hemorrhage), including lavage if performed
71045	Radiologic examination, chest; single view
71046	Radiologic examination, chest; 2 views
92953	Temporary transcutaneous pacing
93561	Indicator dilution studies such as dye or thermodilution, including arterial and/or venous catheterization; with cardiac output measurements
93562	Indicator dilution studies such as dye or thermodilution, including arterial and/or venous catheterization; subsequent measurement of cardiac output
94002	Ventilation assist and management, initiation of pressure or volume preset ventilators for assisted or controlled breathing; hospital inpatient/observation, initial day
94003	Ventilation assist and management, initiation of pressure or volume preset ventilators for assisted or controlled breathing; hospital inpatient/observation, each subsequent day
94004	Ventilation assist and management, initiation of pressure or volume preset ventilators for assisted or controlled breathing; nursing facility, per day
94660	Continuous positive airway pressure ventilation (CPAP), initiation and management
94662	Continuous negative pressure ventilation (CNP), initiation and management
94760	Noninvasive ear or pulse oximetry for oxygen saturation; single determination
94761	Noninvasive ear or pulse oximetry for oxygen saturation; multiple determinations (e.g., during exercise)
94762	Noninvasive ear or pulse oximetry for oxygen saturation; by continuous overnight monitoring

Note: Outpatient critical care performed (e.g., provider's office or emergency department) on a neonatal patient through age 71 months is reported with 99291 and 99292.

The following table details what is required for each service.

Critical Care

E/M Code	Patient Status	Physician Attendance	Time[1]
99291	Critically ill or critically injured	Constant	First 30–74 minutes
99292	Critically ill or critically injured	Constant	Each additional 30 minutes beyond the first 74 minutes

1 Per the guidelines for time in CPT 2021, "A unit of time is attained when the mid-point is passed. For example, an hour is attained when 31 minutes have elapsed (more than midway between zero and 60 minutes)."

Coding Tips

- As an "add-on" code, 99292 and is not subject to multiple procedure rules. No reimbursement reduction or modifier 51 is applied. Add-on codes describe additional intraservice work associated with the primary procedure and performed by the same provider on the same date of service as the primary service/procedure. An add-on code must never be reported as a stand-alone code.

Prolonged Services (99354–99359, 99415–99416, and 99417)

The code range contains two groups of codes that describe services performed by a physician or OQHCP: direct patient contact (face-to-face) services (99354–99357) and prolonged services without patient contact (99358–99359). Prolonged services with patient contact are broken down further by services performed in an outpatient setting and services performed in the inpatient or observation setting. Prolonged care without direct patient contact is used for services before and after direct patient care (e.g., review of extensive records and tests, communication with other professionals, and the patient/family) and must be related to a previous or future face-to-face service. Services are reported by the first hour with an additional code for each 30-minute block of time. Fewer than 30 minutes of prolonged care is not reported separately. Codes 99354–99357 may be reported in addition to outpatient, inpatient, or observation service or psychotherapy codes 90837 and 90847. These services cannot be reported in addition to new or established office or other outpatient services (99202–99215).

Add-on codes 99415–99416 report prolonged services provided by clinical staff. To report these services they must be performed under the direct supervision of a physician or OQHCP. Clinical staff services may not be provided for more than two patients concurrently. Fewer than 30 minutes of prolonged care is not reported separately as this time would be included in the primary E/M service. Services are reported by the first hour with an additional code for each 30-minute block of time. The highest total time in the time range for the code reported is used to determine when prolonged service time begins. For example, when reporting 99214 the highest total time is 39 minutes, so in order to report 99415, at least 69 minutes must pass. These codes may be reported only with E/M service codes 99202–99205 and 99212–99215.

Regardless of who performs the service, the documentation for all prolonged services must establish that the reason for the service was for continuing patient care. Prolonged services should be documented separately from other services reported at the same encounter. Time spent performing separately reportable services should not be used to meet the time thresholds for these codes.

A new code was created for 2021 that is used to report prolonged services used in conjunction with codes 99205 and 99215. This code is reported only when the provider is using time as the determining factor for code selection. The time spent on the date of the encounter may include face-to-face and non-face-to-face activities and must extend 15 minutes past the minimum time described in the code descriptions for 99205 and 99215. Prolonged services of fewer than 15 minutes should not be reported.

Other services provided during prolonged service periods may be reported separately. Time involved performing these activities should not be counted toward prolonged service times.

 AUDITOR'S ALERT

Effective January 1, 2021, prolonged service codes 99354–99355 and 99358–99359 should not be reported with Office or Other Outpatient codes 99202–99205 or 99211–99215.

 AUDITOR'S ALERT

When additional time is spent by the provider performing an office or other outpatient service, add-on code 99417 should be reported. Code 99417 is reported only when the office or other outpatient service code level selection is based on time (including face-to-face and non-face-to-face time), and the total time of the highest-level service (99205 or 99215) has been exceeded by at least 15 additional minutes.

When prolonged services are not performed on the same date as an office or outpatient service (99202–99215), codes 99358 and 99359 may be reported.

Coding Tips

- As add-on codes, 99415, 99416, and 99417 are not subject to multiple procedure rules. No reimbursement reduction or modifier 51 is applied. Add-on codes describe additional intraservice work associated with the primary procedure performed by the same provider on the same date of service as the primary service/procedure. An add-on code must never be reported as a stand-alone code.

- It should be noted that many codes in this section now have a ★ icon. This indicates that they are telemedicine codes and should be reported with modifier 95 Synchronous Telemedicine Service Rendered Via a Real-Time Interactive Audio and Video Telecommunications System. Please see chapter 3 for more information on this modifier. A complete list of these codes can be found in Appendix P in the CPT book.

Provider Standby Services (99360)

This code should be used to report services such as stand-by for cesarean or high-risk delivery, monitoring electroencephalograms (EEG), and standby for frozen section that are at the request of another provider. The physician or OQHCP may not be taking care of other patients when reporting standby time. This code is used for standby services that require prolonged physician or OQHCP attendance and when a surgeon on standby performs a procedure; only the procedure code is reportable. Standby services should not be reported with other procedure codes. According to CPT guidelines, the global surgical package rule applies; the standby code is not reported and is considered bundled with the procedure. Report only standby time exceeding 30 minutes.

Medical Team Conferences (99366–99368)

This section describes the physician or OQHCP process of coordinating and controlling access to other third-party services needed by the patient using medical team conferences.

Medical team conferences (99366–99368) are defined as the face-to-face collaboration of at least three qualified health care professionals from different specialties or disciplines who actively participate in the development, revision, coordination, and implementation of health care services for the patient. These codes should not be reported when the conference is part of a service that is contractually provided by an organizational or facility provider.

Appropriate code selection is dependent upon a number of criteria. First and foremost, the provider must have provided face-to-face evaluation and/or treatment, independent of the team, to the patient within the previous 60 days. The provider must also have an active role in the development, revision, and coordination of the patient's treatment plan.

A physician or OQHCP should report a medical team conference, in which the patient and/or patient's family is present, with the appropriate E/M code using time as the determining factor in selecting the level. When an E/M code is used, the provider must have provided face-to-face contact with the patient outside of the medical team conference. Be certain that the medical record documentation supports an E/M service, if selected.

There are two categories of medical team conferences: direct face-to-face contact with patient and/or family (reported by a nonphysician provider) (99366) and medical team conference without direct face-to-face contact with patient and/or family. The latter is further divided into two individual codes: physician (99367) and nonphysician health care professional (99368). Codes in this range require the service be a minimum of 30 minutes in duration. Anything less than 30 minutes is not reported separately.

Record keeping and report generation time are not used to determine the amount of time spent in a team conference; however, time is not limited to the time that a participant is presenting. Furthermore, time reported as part of the medical team conference may not be used as a determination for other timed services.

Care Plan Oversight Services (99374–99380)

This section includes care plan codes for physician or OQHCP supervision of patients under the care of home health agencies, hospice, or nursing facilities requiring complex or multidisciplinary care modalities involving regular provider development and revision of care plans; review of subsequent reports of patient status; review of related laboratory and other studies; communication with other health care professionals involved in the patient's care; integration of new information into the medical treatment plan; and adjustment of medical therapy, within a 30-day period. Only one provider may report services for a given period of time to reflect that individual's sole or predominant supervisory role with a particular patient. Care plan oversight codes are broken down by time (15–29 minutes or 30 minutes or more) and the place of service. Services performed must be documented in the patient's medical record.

Preventive Medicine Services (99381–99429)

This section reports preventive medicine, counseling and risk factor reduction intervention, and behavior change interventions.

Preventive medicine services (99381–99397) provide for evaluation of the patient and counseling or risk factor reduction. Appropriate use of these codes report E/M services provided to a patient who presents without complaints. If an abnormality is encountered, or if a pre-existing condition is treated by the provider and the service is significant enough to warrant a separate service, an appropriate E/M visit from the office or other outpatient section may be reported in addition to the preventive medicine code with modifier 25 appended to designate a separately identifiable service. The documentation must clearly identify both services. CPT guidelines further state: "An insignificant or trivial problem/abnormality that is encountered in the process of performing the preventive medicine evaluation and management service and which does not require additional work and the performance of the key components of a problem-oriented E/M service should not be reported."

The CPT book specifically states that an "age and gender appropriate" history and examination should be performed and documented during this comprehensive encounter. Preventive care includes counseling and/or risk factor reduction intervention.

The preventive medicine service code selection is based upon the patient's age and status of new or established at the time of the encounter. The same E/M definition applies for identifying new and established patients.

 DEFINITIONS

BMI. Body mass index. Tool for calculating weight appropriateness in adults. The Centers for Disease Control and Prevention places adult BMIs in the following categories: below 18.5, underweight; 18.5–24.9, normal; 25.0–29.9 overweight; 30.0 and above, obese. BMI may be a factor in determining medical necessity for bariatric procedures.

IPPE. Initial preventive physical examination. Evaluation and management service that enables new Medicare beneficiaries to receive important screenings and vaccinations, as well as allows the provider to evaluate and review the patient's health. Initially slated to be performed within the fist six months of the beneficiary's effective date of Medicare coverage, legislation extended the eligibility period from six months to 12 months for beneficiaries with effective dates on or after January 1, 2009.

One difference that should be noted for the preventive medicine section is that the extent of the history and examination is variable dependent upon the age of the patient. A comprehensive history and exam is not calculated based upon the documentation guidelines for other outpatient or inpatient services. Rather, the comprehensive exam is reflective of the age and gender of the pediatric patient. In addition, administration of immunizations, toxoid and vaccine products, screening services, lab tests, and radiology services are reported separately.

These services also include counseling, anticipatory guidance, and risk factor reduction interventions provided at the time of the preventive medicine examination.

If a significant problem is encountered or a pre-existing problem is addressed that requires additional work during the course of the preventive medicine service, the appropriate problem-oriented E/M code (e.g., 99202–99215) may be reported in addition to the preventive medicine code. A problem-oriented E/M code should not be reported if the problem encountered does not require additional work and the performance of key components required for code selection.

To report that a separately identifiable E/M service was performed by the same physician/qualified health care professional on the same day as a procedure or service, modifier 25 should be appended to the E/M service code. Only the work associated with the separate E/M service should be considered when selecting the E/M code.

Counseling risk factor reduction intervention and behavior change intervention services (99401–99412) services are divided into sections. Codes 99401–99404 and 99411–99412 are used to report services provided face-to-face by a physician or other qualified health care professional to healthy individuals to promote health status and prevent illness. These services should be reported at an encounter separate from the preventive medicine service. Risk-factor reduction services are reported for persons without a specific illness and where counseling might otherwise be used as part of the treatment process. Counseling patients with symptoms or complaints requires the use of codes from the office, hospital, consultation, or other appropriate coding section.

Codes 99401–99404 are reported for individual preventive medicine counseling for things such as diet and exercise, dental health, injury prevention, to name a few. These codes are defined by time, so it is important for the provider to document a start and stop time for the encounter.

Codes 99411–99412 are reported for group counseling and risk factor reduction.

Behavior change intervention services are reported with codes 99406–99409. The services are for patients who have a behavior that is often considered an illness unto itself, including tobacco or substance abuse or misuse and obesity. These services may be reported when performed as part of the treatment of a condition related to, or potentially exacerbated by, the behavior or when performed to modify harmful behavior that has not yet resulted in illness. These services involve assessing readiness for change and barriers to change; advising a change in behavior; assisting by providing specific suggested actions and motivational counseling; and arranging for services and follow-up. Per *CPT Assistant*, these codes may be reported in addition to other E/M services; however, the additional E/M service that it is reported with must be distinct, and the time spent performing the other services may not be used as a basis to select the E/M code selection.

Preventive medicine services (99381–99429) are specifically excluded from Medicare coverage. However, Medicare does provide beneficiaries with a one-time initial preventive physical exam (IPPE) benefit.

Medicare provides coverage of the IPPE for all newly enrolled beneficiaries who receive the IPPE within the first 12 months after the effective date of their Medicare Part B coverage. The IPPE is covered only as a one-time benefit per Medicare Part B enrollee. Medicare beneficiaries who cancel their Medicare Part B coverage but later re-enroll in Medicare Part B are not eligible for the IPPE benefit.

The IPPE is a preventive evaluation and management (E/M) service that includes seven components:

- Review of medical and social history
- Review of potential risk factors for depression or other mood disorders
- Review of functional ability and level of safety
- An examination to include:
  - measurement of the beneficiary's height, weight, blood pressure
  - measurement of body mass index
  - a visual acuity screen
  - other factors as deemed appropriate by the physician or qualified nonphysician practitioner, based on the beneficiary's medical and social history and current clinical standards
- End-of-life planning, upon the patient's consent
- Education, counseling, and referral based on the previous five components
- Education, counseling, and referral for other preventive services including a brief written plan, such as a checklist, provided to the patient for obtaining a screening EKG, if appropriate, and the appropriate screenings and other preventive services that are covered as separate Medicare Part B benefits

HCPCS Level II codes that should be used when reporting these services:

- G0402 Initial preventive physical examination; face-to-face visit, services limited to new beneficiary during the first 12 months of Medicare enrollment
- G0403 Electrocardiogram, routine ECG with 12 leads; performed as a screening for the initial preventive physical examination with interpretation and report
- G0404 Electrocardiogram, routine ECG with 12 leads; tracing only, without interpretation and report, performed as a screening for the initial preventive physical examination
- G0405 Electrocardiogram, routine ECG with 12 leads; interpretation and report only, performed as a screening for the initial preventive physical examination
- G0468 Federally qualified health center (FQHC) visit, IPPE or AWV; a FQHC visit that includes an initial preventive physical examination (IPPE) or annual wellness visit (AWV) and includes a typical bundle of medicare-covered services that would be furnished per diem to a patient receiving an IPPE or AWV

HCPCS Level II codes that should be used when reporting annual wellness visits (AWV) for Medicare patients.

- G0438 Annual wellness visit, includes a personalized prevention plan of service (PPS), initial visit
- G0439 Annual wellness visit, includes a personalized prevention plan of service (PPS), subsequent visit
- G0468 Federally qualified health center (FQHC) visit, IPPE or AWV; a FQHC visit that includes an initial preventive physical examination (IPPE) or annual wellness visit (AWV) and includes a typical bundle of medicare-covered services that would be furnished per diem to a patient receiving an IPPE or AWV
- 99497 Advance care planning including the explanation and discussion of advance directives such as standard forms (with completion of such forms, when performed), by the physician or other qualified health care professional; first 30 minutes, face-to-face with the patient, family member(s), and/or surrogate
- 99498 Advance care planning including the explanation and discussion of advance directives such as standard forms (with completion of such forms, when performed), by the physician or other qualified health care professional; each additional 30 minutes (List separately in addition to code for primary procedure)

These services are covered for a patient who has been enrolled in Medicare for more than 12 months and has not received an initial preventive physical examination (IPPE) or an annual wellness visit (AWV) within the preceding 12-month period. Visits are to include a health risk assessment, as well as a personalized prevention plan, including:

- Health risk assessment, including:
  - demographic data
  - self-assessment of health status
  - psychosocial risks
  - behavioral risks
  - activities of daily living (ADL), such as dressing, bathing, and walking
  - instrumental ADLs, such as shopping, housekeeping, managing own medications, and handling finances
- Individual medical and family history
- Current providers, suppliers, and medications
- Height, weight, BMI or waist circumference, blood pressure reading
- Review of beneficiary's potential risk factors for depression, including current or past experiences with depression or other mood disorders
- Review of beneficiary's functional ability and level of safety
- Cognitive impairment evaluation
- Advanced care planning
- List of risk factors and conditions
- Personalized health education and appropriate referrals, if necessary
- Establishment of a written screening schedule for the beneficiary, such as a checklist for the next five to 10 years, as appropriate

© 2020 Optum360, LLC

The subsequent visit, G0439, builds upon this initial visit, following up on the services performed initially to continue to promote wellness. Advance Care Planning is treated as an optional preventive service when furnished with an AWV.

Online and Telephone Evaluation and Management Services (99421–99423 and 99441–99443)

These services are initiated by the patient and must be provided by a physician or OQHCP. These are services provided to an established patient who may have a new problem and include the evaluation, assessment, and management of patient's condition. These services should not be reported if a related E/M service has been provided within the prior seven days or if the service falls within the postoperative period of a previously performed procedure. When a separately reportable E/M service occurs within seven days of initiation of the online service, the work devoted to the online service is counted into the separately reportable E/M service.

The telephone services are non face-to-face services. The online digital E/M services must be initiated through a HIPAA-compliant platform and require permanent storage of documentation (electronic or hard copy) of the encounter. Online services are for cumulative time over a seven-day period and include initial inquiry, records review, physician interaction with clinical staff regarding the patient's problem, development of management plans, generation of prescriptions, ordering tests, and subsequent communication with the patient either online, via telephone, email, or other supported digital communication. These codes should not be used to review test results or schedule appointments. For both types of services, if the encounters are fewer than five minutes they should not be reported.

Online digital E/M services performed by nonphysician providers are reported with codes 98970–98972.

The following table details the intent of service and the time required to report each service.

E/M Code	Intent of Service	Type of Communication	Time
99421	Online E/M service at the request of established patient	Online digital	5–10 min.
99422	Online E/M service at the request of established patient	Online digital	11–20 min.
99423	Online E/M service at the request of established patient	Online digital	At least 21 min.

Interprofessional Consultations Via Telephone, Internet, or Electronic Health Record (99446–99452)

In urgent or complex situations, an interprofessional telephone, internet, or electronic health record consultation (99446–99449) may be performed. Six levels are available depending on the time spent, but time must be documented. Consultations of fewer than five minutes are not reported. In these consultations a physician or other qualified health care provider requests an opinion and/or treatment from another provider who may have a specific specialty expertise. These codes do not require a face-to-face visit with the patient because many times the consultant may be in a different geographical area. There is no designation between new or established patient as in the face-to-face

FOR MORE INFO

Detailed information regarding AWVs and IPPEs can be found at IOM Pub. 100-04, Chapter 12, Section 30.6.1.1.

consultation codes discussed above. These services may be provided by the consultant for a new patient, an established patient with a new problem, or an exacerbation of an existing problem. As with other consultation codes, the verbal or written request and reason for the request must be documented in the patient chart. Correct code selection depends on the amount of time involved, including the provision of a verbal AND written report to the requesting provider, detailing the reason for the request and the consulting provider's opinion and/or advice regarding patient management. It is important to note that at least 50 percent of the time must be spent performing the verbal/internet consult. It is inappropriate for the consultant to report these codes if the patient has been seen within 14 days prior to the consult or the consult leads to a transfer of the patient's care within 14 days.

Code 99452 is reported for the time a provider spends, on a service day, preparing for or communicating with the consultant.

Codes 99446–99451 should not be reported more than once in a seven-day period. Code 99452 can be reported only once during a 14-day period. Communications between the consultant and the patient and/or family may be reported using telephone or online E/M service codes 98966–98968, 99421–99423, and 99441–99443, but the time associated with these calls should not be factored in when reporting these interprofessional telephone/internet consultation services.

In addition, if consultation exceeds 30 minutes and the patient is physically present and available to the *requesting provider*, the provider may report prolonged services (99354–99357) for his/her time spent while on the telephone or internet with the consulting provider. If the patient is not present, the requesting provider may report non-face-to-face prolonged services (99358–99359).

The following table details the intent of service and the time that is required to report each service.

Telephone, Internet or Electronic Health Record Consultations (99446–99542)

E/M Code	Intent of Service	Time Spent
99446	Consultation, including verbal and written report, at the request of another provider via the telephone, internet, or EHR	5–10 min
99447	Consultation, including verbal and written report, at the request of another provider via the telephone, internet, or EHR	11–20 min.
99448	Consultation, including verbal and written report, at the request of another provider via the telephone, internet, or EHR	21–30 min.
99449	Consultation, including verbal and written report, at the request of another provider via the telephone, internet, or EHR	31 min. or more
99451	Consultation, including written report, at the request of another provider via the telephone, internet, or EHR	5 min. or more
99452	Interprofessional telephone, internet, or electronic health record referral services provided by a requesting or treating provider	30 min.

 AUDITOR'S ALERT

Qualified nonphysician health care professional online digital evaluation and management services can be reported with 98970–98972. These codes are reported by time and used only for established patients.

Digitally Stored Data Services/Remote Physiologic Monitoring and Physiologic Monitoring Treatment Management Services (99453–99454, 99091, 99473–99474, 99457–99458)

Codes 99453–99454 report physiologic monitoring services that are performed remotely. To report these services, the device used must be a medical device as defined by the FDA. The services must be ordered by a physician or other qualified health care professional. Code 99453 reports the setup and education provided to the patient on the device that the patient will use to transmit health-related data to the provider. Code 99454 reports daily recordings or program alert transmissions. Time spent monitoring a more specific physiological condition, such as continuous glucose monitoring (95250), should not be included in the time needed to report 99453 or 99454. These codes should not be used for monitoring services of fewer than 16 days.

Code 99091 reports the collection and interpretation of health-related data (e.g., blood pressure, glucose) collected using a remote patient monitoring system and includes education and training. When a patient is seen for another E/M service on the same date of service, services provided in 99091 are considered an integral component of the E/M service and should not be reported separately. Code 99091 should not be reported in addition to 99339–99340, 99374–99380, 99457, or 99491 when provided in the same calendar month.

Codes 99453–99454 and 99091 are provided and reported once for each 30-day period.

Resequenced codes 99473–99474 report self-measured blood pressure using a device that has been validated for accuracy. Code 99473 also includes device calibration, patient education, and training. Code 99473 should not be reported more than once per device. Code 99474 is used to report separate self-measurements done twice, one minute apart, twice daily, in a 30-day period. A minimum of 12 readings per 30-day period is required to report this code. When a patient is seen for another E/M service on the same date of service, the services provided in 99474 are considered an integral component of the E/M service and should not be reported separately. These codes should not be reported in addition to 93784–93790, 99091, 99439, 99453, 99454, 99457, 99487–99491 when provided in the same calendar month.

Codes 99457–99458 require live, interactive communication with the patient or caregiver and the first-completed 20 minutes of provider or staff time within a calendar month. These codes also require an order from a physician or OQHCP. Code 99457 should only be reported when requirements for a more specific treatment management service have not been met. It may be reported in addition to 99439, 99487–99491, 99495, 99496, 99484, and 99492–99494 when performed during the same reporting period. However, time spent performing those services should not be included in the time needed to report code 99457. Code 99457 should not be reported on days when other separate and distinct services are provided, including 99202–99215, 99221–99223, 99231–99233, 99251–99255, 99324–99328, 99334–99337, and 99341–99350. Code 99457 should not be reported in addition to 99091.

Newborn Care (99460–99465)

Codes 99460 through 99465 are used to report services to normal and high-risk newborns. Many high-risk newborns are healthy at birth and do not meet the requirements for more intensive treatment.

Code 99460 is used for the initial evaluation of a normal and healthy infant, including birthing room deliveries. This includes documentation and preparation of hospital records.

Code 99461 is used to report an initial evaluation of a normal newborn outside of a hospital or birthing room setting. This code may be used for planned home deliveries or nonfacility deliveries and includes conferring with the parents.

Subsequent hospital care of a normal newborn is reported with 99462 and includes completion of chart notes and discussion of the newborn evaluation with the parents.

Some newborns are delivered and discharged on the same date. These newborn evaluations are reported with 99463 and include all services provided on that date.

Code 99464 is used for attendance at delivery when requested by the delivering provider. It should not be reported with the provider or OQHCP standby code 99360 or 99465, but may be reported with code 99460 for evaluation of the newborn. If the provider on standby subsequently performs resuscitation only, report the resuscitation. If the newborn's condition is stable upon delivery, report 99464 with 99460. Physician standby is not reported if the newborn requires surgical intervention.

Additional guidelines for the correct reporting of 99465 Newborn resuscitation, were contained in the *CPT Assistant,* March 2009, pages 3-4 and 7. In that edition, guidance was provided that stated this code is inclusive of ventilation and chest compressions with suctioning if necessary. All other resuscitation procedures medically necessary to stabilize the newborn are reported separately. It also notes that the procedures should be performed in the delivery room and prior to admitting the newborn. All procedures performed must be medically necessary and documented in the patient record. Intubation or other procedures performed as a convenience prior to admission to the NICU are considered part of the NICU daily service.

The following table details what is required for each service.

Newborn Care Services

E/M Code	Patient Status	Type of Visit
99460	Normal newborn	Inpatient initial inpatient hospital or birthing center per day
99461	Normal newborn	Inpatient initial treatment not in hospital or birthing center per day
99462	Normal newborn	Inpatient subsequent per day
99463	Normal newborn	Inpatient initial inpatient and discharge (on the same date) in hospital or birthing center
99464	Unstable newborn	Attendance at delivery
99465	High-risk newborn at delivery	Resuscitation, ventilation, and cardiac treatment

Pediatric Critical Care Transport (99466–99467, and 99485–99486)

Codes 99466–99467 describe critical care provided during transport of a pediatric patient and are used to report physician face-to-face services. Supervising physicians may not report this code for other members of the transport team. This must be an interfacility transport of the patient and not just from one specialized area of a facility to another. The pediatric patient is 24 months or younger. For physician services during transport of a critical patient over 24 months, see 99291 and 99292.

Time is calculated beginning when the physician assumes responsibility at the referring center and ends when the receiving facility accepts responsibility for the patient.

A critical illness or injury acutely impairs one or more vital organ systems such that there is a high probability of imminent or life-threatening deterioration in the patient's condition. Critical care involves high-complexity decision making to assess, manipulate, and support vital system functions to treat single or multiple vital organ system failure and/or to prevent further life-threatening deterioration of the patient's condition.

Codes 99466–99467 are reported based upon the face-to-face time spent by the physician. Only one provider may report critical care transport for the same episode of care. In addition, a transport of less than 30 minutes is not reported separately. Documentation must include all services and monitoring provided and the time spent by the physician.

Codes 99485–99486 represent the physician's role in interfacility transport of a critically ill or injured patient less than 24 months of age. These codes are for non-face-to-face contact; the physician is directing the transport services during an interfacility transport. The control physician uses a two-way radio to communicate treatment advice to the transport team providing the patient care. Additionally, a non-face-to-face transport of less than 15 minutes is not reported separately. Documentation must include all services provided and the time spent by the physician.

Do not report codes 99485–99486 with 99466–99467 for services provided on the same day when performed by the same provider or for patients older than 24 months of age that are not critically ill or injured.

Pediatric critical care transport (99466–99467) includes services usually performed in conjunction with this level of care, including:

36000 Introduction of needle or intracatheter, vein

36400 Venipuncture, younger than age 3 years, necessitating the skill of a physician or other qualified health care professional, not to be used for routine venipuncture; femoral or jugular vein

36405 Venipuncture, younger than age 3 years, necessitating the skill of a physician or other qualified health care professional, not to be used for routine venipuncture; scalp vein

36406 Venipuncture, younger than age 3 years, necessitating the skill of a physician or other qualified health care professional, not to be used for routine venipuncture; other vein

36415 Collection of venous blood by venipuncture

36591	Collection of blood specimen from a completely implantable venous access device
36600	Arterial puncture, withdrawal of blood for diagnosis
43752	Naso- or oro-gastric tube placement, requiring physician's skill and fluoroscopic guidance
43753	Gastric intubation and aspiration(s) therapeutic, necessitating physician's skill (eg, for gastrointestinal hemorrhage), including lavage if performed
71045	Radiologic examination, chest; single view
71046	Radiologic examination, chest; 2 views
92953	Temporary transcutaneous pacing
93562	Indicator dilution studies such as dye or thermodilution, including arterial and/or venous catheterization; subsequent measurement of cardiac output
94002	Ventilation assist and management, initiation of pressure or volume preset ventilators for assisted or controlled breathing; hospital inpatient/observation, initial day
94003	Ventilation assist and management, initiation of pressure or volume preset ventilators for assisted or controlled breathing; hospital inpatient/observation, each subsequent day
94660	Continuous positive airway pressure ventilation (CPAP), initiation and management
94662	Continuous negative pressure ventilation (CNP), initiation and management
94760	Noninvasive ear or pulse oximetry for oxygen saturation; single determination
94761	Noninvasive ear or pulse oximetry for oxygen saturation; multiple determinations (e.g., during exercise)
94762	Noninvasive ear or pulse oximetry for oxygen saturation; by continuous overnight monitoring (separate procedure)

There are no absolute limits on the amount of critical care transport time that can be billed per day as long as the medical records can support the need for all critical care services provided. Payment is dependent upon carrier policies for critical care.

Pediatric Critical Care Transport

E/M Code	Patient Status	Physician Attendance	Time
99466	Critically ill or critically injured	Face to face	First 30–74 minutes[1]
99467	Critically ill or critically injured	Face to face	Each additional 30 minutes beyond the first 74 minutes
99485	Critically ill or critically injured	Non face to face	First 30 minutes
99486	Critically ill or critically injured	Non face to face	Each additional 30 minutes beyond the first 45 minutes

1 The first hour of critical care transport can be reported only once per day.

Coding Tips

- As add-on codes, 99467 and 99486 and are not subject to multiple procedure rules. No reimbursement reduction or modifier 51 is applied. Add-on codes describe additional intraservice work associated with the primary procedure and performed by the same provider on the same date of service as the primary service/procedure. An add-on code must never be reported as a stand-alone code.

Neonatal and Pediatric Critical Care Services (99468–99472 and 99475–99476)

Critical care may be provided to a patient in critical care or other area of the facility. Critical care of the neonate or pediatric patient is reported by day of care. Separate codes are used to report an initial day of critical care and subsequent days of care. Only one initial day of critical care may be reported per admission to the facility. All other days of care are subsequent to the admission to the facility. Documentation must include all services and monitoring provided by the physician or OQHCP.

Code selection is based upon specific criteria. Critical care for a neonate (birth to 28 days) is reported with 99468 and 99469. Codes 99471 and 99472 should be used to report critical care provided to patients 29 days to 24 months of age and 99475 through 99476 for patients ages 2 to 5 years.

Neonatal and pediatric critical care includes services usually performed in conjunction with this level of care, including:

31500	Intubation, endotracheal, emergency procedure
36000	Introduction of needle or intracatheter, vein
36140	Introduction of needle or intracatheter; upper or lower extremity artery
36400	Venipuncture, younger than age 3 years, necessitating the skill of a physician or other qualified health care professional, not to be used for routine venipuncture; femoral or jugular vein
36405	Venipuncture, younger than age 3 years, necessitating the skill of a physician or other qualified health care professional, not to be used for routine venipuncture; scalp vein
36406	Venipuncture, younger than age 3 years, necessitating the skill of a physician or other qualified health care professional, not to be used for routine venipuncture; other vein
36410	Venipuncture, younger than age 3 years, necessitating the skill of a physician or other qualified health care professional, not to be used for routine venipuncture; femoral or jugular vein
36415	Collection of venous blood by venipuncture
36420	Venipuncture, cutdown; younger than age 1 year
36430	Transfusion, blood or blood components
36440	Push transfusion, blood, 2 years or younger
36510	Catheterization of umbilical vein for diagnosis or therapy, newborn
36555	Insertion of non-tunneled centrally inserted central venous catheter; younger than 5 years of age
36591	Collection of blood specimen from a completely implantable venous access device

36600	Arterial puncture, withdrawal of blood for diagnosis
36620	Arterial catheterization or cannulation for sampling, monitoring, or transfusion; (separate procedure) percutaneous
36660	Catheterization, umbilical artery, newborn, for diagnosis or therapy
43752	Naso or orogastric tube placement, requiring physician's skill and fluoroscopic guidance
43753	Gastric intubation and aspiration(s) therapeutic, necessitating physician's skill (eg, for gastrointestinal hemorrhage), including lavage if performed
51100	Aspiration of bladder; by needle
51701	Insertion of nonindwelling bladder catheter (eg, straight catheterization for residual urine)
51702	Insertion of temporary indwelling bladder catheter; simple (eg, Foley)
62270	Spinal puncture, lumbar, diagnostic
71045	Radiologic examination, chest; single view
71046	Radiologic examination, chest; 2 views
92953	Temporary transcutaneous pacing
93561	Indicator dilution studies such as dye or thermal dilution, including arterial and/or venous catheterization; with cardiac output measurement (separate procedure)
93562	Indicator dilution studies such as dye or thermal dilution, including arterial and/or venous catheterization; subsequent measurement of cardiac output
94002	Ventilation assist and management, initiation of pressure or volume preset ventilators for assisted or controlled breathing; hospital inpatient/observation, initial day
94003	Ventilation assist and management, initiation of pressure or volume preset ventilators for assisted or controlled breathing; hospital inpatient/observation, each subsequent day
94004	Ventilation assist and management, initiation of pressure or volume preset ventilators for assisted or controlled breathing; nursing facility, per day
94375	Respiratory flow volume loop
94610	Intrapulmonary surfactant administration by a physician or other qualified health care professional through endotracheal tube
94660	Continuous positive airway pressure ventilation (CPAP), initiation and management
94662	Continuous negative pressure ventilation (CNP), initiation and management
94760	Noninvasive ear or pulse oximetry for oxygen saturation; single determination
94761	Noninvasive ear or pulse oximetry for oxygen saturation; multiple determinations (eg, during exercise)
94762	Noninvasive ear or pulse oximetry for oxygen saturation; by continuous overnight monitoring

94780   Car seat/bed testing for airway integrity, for infants through 12 months of age, with continual clinical staff observation and continuous recording of pulse oximetry, heart rate and respiratory rate, with interpretation and report; 60 minutes

94781   Car seat/bed testing for airway integrity, for infants through 12 months of age, with continual clinical staff observation and continuous recording of pulse oximetry, heart rate and respiratory rate, with interpretation and report; each additional full 30 minutes (List separately in addition to code for primary procedure)

Neonatal and pediatric critical care services also include the following management, monitoring, and treatment services, which cannot be reported separately:

- Cardiac
- Respiratory
- Pharmacologic control of the circulatory system
- Enteral and parenteral nutrition
- Metabolic and hematologic maintenance
- Parent/family counseling
- Case management
- Personal direct supervision of the health care team in the performance of cognitive and procedural activities

When additional procedures not identified above are medically necessary and documented, they may be reported in addition to the neonatal and pediatric critical care.

In the event that a subsequent physician or other qualified health care provider of another specialty from the same or different group provides care to a critically ill neonate, report services with the hourly critical care codes 99291 and 99292. If the patient improves and is transferred to a lower level of care, the transferring provider will not report a per day critical care service. In that instance, the provider may report a subsequent hospital care visit (99231–99233) or a time-based critical care service (99291–99292) as appropriate.

The following table details what is required for each service.

Inpatient Neonatal and Pediatric Critical Care

E/M Code	Patient Status	Type of Visit
99468	Critically ill neonate, aged 28 days or less	Inpatient initial per day
99469	Critically ill neonate, aged 28 days or less	Inpatient subsequent per day
99471	Critically ill infant or young child, aged 29 days to 24 months	Inpatient initial per day
99472	Critically ill infant or young child, aged 29 days to 24 months	Inpatient subsequent per day
99475	Critically ill infant or young child, 2 to 5 years	Inpatient initial per day
99476	Critically ill infant or young child, 2 to 5 years	Inpatient subsequent per day

Initial and Continuing Intensive Care Services (99477–99480)

Initial care of a newborn that is not critical but does not meet the guidelines of a normal newborn is reported with 99477. This patient is a neonate (birth to 28 days) and requires intensive observation, frequent interventions, or other intensive care services, but does not meet the requirements for critical care. As with other daily pediatric and neonatal services, this is reported per day and is inclusive of other commonly performed intensive care procedures.

These patients may be normal neonates at birth who develop complications not requiring intensive care, but requiring observation, intervention, or other services. According to *CPT Assistant,* the normal newborn code may be reported for the initial care and 99477 may be reported for the care of the patient after development of a complication that is not considered to be critical care.

Codes 99478 through 99480 are for subsequent intensive care services for low birth weight neonates. The neonates must still require intensive observation along with frequent interventions, monitoring, and other intensive care services. The codes are reported by weight, per day:

- 99478   Very low birth weight (VLBW) (<1500 grams)
- 99479   Low birth weight (LBW) (1500–2500 grams)
- 99480   Normal birth weight (2501–5000 grams)

Codes 99477 through 99480 also include the following management, monitoring, and treatment services that cannot be billed separately:

- Cardiac
- Respiratory
- Pharmacologic control of the circulatory system
- Enteral and parenteral nutrition
- Metabolic and hematologic maintenance
- Parent/family counseling
- Case management
- Personal direct supervision of the health care team in the performance of cognitive and procedural activities

Codes 99477 through 99480 include the same list of procedures as identified with 99468 through 99476.

Note: When a neonatal or pediatric patient no longer needs the level of care provided within this section of daily critical care codes, the physician or OQHCP may transfer the patient to a lower level of care. In this case, the transferring physician or OQHCP should not report critical care services for that day, but instead report subsequent hospital care (99231–99233) or normal newborn codes (99460 or 99462), based on the condition of the neonate/infant. If the transfer to a lower level of care occurs on the same date of service that an initial intensive care code was reported by the transferring provider, 99477 may be reported by the transferring provider. If the patient's health declines and requires critical care services, the transferring provider may report critical care services (99291–99292) or subsequent intensive care services (99478–99480). Both codes should not be reported. The provider taking over the care of the patient should then report initial subsequent neonatal or pediatric intensive care services (99468–99476) as appropriate for the age of the patient and whether this is the first or subsequent admission to critical care for the patient's current hospital stay.

The following table details what is required for each service.

Initial and Continuing Intensive Care Services

E/M Code	Patient Status	Type of Visit
99477	Neonate, aged 28 days or less	Inpatient initial per day
99478	Infant with present body weight of less than 1500 grams, no longer critically ill	Inpatient subsequent per day
99479	Infant with present body weight of 1500-2500 grams, no longer critically ill	Inpatient subsequent per day
99480	Infant with present body weight of 2501-5000 grams, no longer critically ill	Inpatient subsequent per day

Cognitive Assessment and Care Plan Services (99483)

This service is a detailed and thorough face-to-face examination of a patient who is demonstrating signs and/or symptoms of a cognitive impairment in order to determine the diagnosis, cause, and severity of the impairment. As part of the examination, the clinician assesses a number of factors that could impact cognitive function, including, but not limited to:

- Cognition-relevant history
- Factors contributing to cognitive impairment, including:
  - chronic pain syndrome
  - depression
  - infection
  - other brain disease such as stroke, tumor, or normal hydrocephalus
  - psychoactive medications

In order to report this service, all of the following elements must be documented:

- Assessment of activities of daily living (ADL), including decision-making abilities
- Caregiver identification and assessment of caregiver's knowledge and willingness to take on needed tasks, in addition to the caregiver's needs and social supports
- Dementia staging via a standardized instrument (FAST, CDR)
- Developing, updating, or revising an advance care plan, and creating a written care plan to deal with cognitive symptoms, any limitations in function, and referrals to
- Review and reconciliation of medication, including high-risk medications
- Safety evaluation
- Screening for neuropsychiatric and behavioral conditions, including depression using standardized instrument

Medical-decision making for this service must include the patient's prognosis, rehabilitation needs, personal assistance services such as financial, social, and legal, or community-based assistance (meals, transportation), as well as other types of personal assistance services. The clinician usually spends approximately 50 minutes with the patient and/or caregiver in providing this service. This service should not be reported if all of the required elements are not performed or felt to be necessary for the patient; instead, assign the correct E/M service code. This service should not be reported more than once per 180-day period.

Care Management Services (99439, 99487–99491)

Care management services are generally provided for chronically ill patients who have continuous or episodic health conditions. These patients live in an assisted living facility, or at home, domiciliary, or rest home. The services are not reported by location as are other coordination services and are in part performed by clinical staff.

These services are reported when the provider establishes a comprehensive plan of care for a patient who has medical and/or psychosocial requirements. This plan is then implemented, revised, or monitored by the clinical staff under the direction of the physician or OQHCP or the provider may perform the services themselves. The care plan should be very specific and include goals that are achievable for each condition. In addition, the goals should be measurable and updated intermittently based on the progress of the patient.

Some items that may be included in a care plan are below; keep in mind that each care plan is patient-specific and may not include all elements. A plan of care must be documented and must indicate that it was communicated to the patient and/or caregiver. The medical record documentation should include, but is not limited to, the following components:

- Problem list
- Expected outcomes
- Prognosis
- Measurable treatment goals
- Cognitive/functional assessment
- Management of symptoms
- Planned interventions
- Medical management
- Assessment of caregivers
- Interaction/coordination plan of agencies and specialties not connected with the provider performing the complex care management service
- Revisions to care plan as necessary
- Environmental evaluation
- Summary of advance directives

Unlike the care plan oversight services (99374–99380), these codes are supported only if the patient has two or more chronic continuous or episodic conditions that are expected to last at least 12 months, or until the death of the patient. Patients receiving this service are also at a significant risk of death due their health conditions, or at risk of acute exacerbation/decompensation or functional decline.

The services that may be provided by the physician, OQHCP, or the clinical staff include:

- Assessment and support for treatment regimen adherence and medication management

- Collection of health outcomes data and registry documentation
- Communication with home health agencies and other community services the patient may use
- Communication and engagement with patient, family members, caretaker or guardian, surrogate decision makers, and/or other professionals regarding aspects of care
- Development, communication, and maintenance of a comprehensive care plan
- Education of patient and/or family/caretaker to support self-management, independent living, and activities of daily living
- Facilitating access to care and services needed by the patient and/or family
- Identification of available community and health resources
- Management of care transitions not reported as a component of codes 99495–99496
- Ongoing review of patient status, including review of laboratory and other studies not reported as an E/M service

To report these services, the office/practice providing them must:

- Provide 24-hour, seven-days-a-week access to the providers or clinical staff
- There must be a physician or OQHCP that oversees care team activities
- All care team members must be clinically integrated
- Use a standardized method to identify patients who require care management services
- Have an internal process so that when a patient meets the requirements for these services they can receive them in a timely manner
- Use a standardized form and format to document these services in the medical record within the practice
- Be able to engage and educate patients and caregivers in addition to coordinating care among all service professionals, for each patient, when necessary
- Provide continuity of care with a designated member of the care team with whom the patient is able to schedule successive routine appointments
- Provide timely access and management for follow-up after an emergency department visit or a facility discharge
- Use an electronic health record system to enable providers to have timely access to clinical information

The following services may not be reported in the same 30-day period by a physician or OQHCP as 99439, 99487–99490:

- Care plan oversight (99339–99340, 99374–99380)
- End-stage renal disease services (90951–90970)
- Medication therapy management (99605–99607)

There are two categories in this section: chronic care management services and complex chronic care coordination services. Codes in both sections are reported according to the amount of time spent in a month and certain elements required.

Chronic care management services (99439, 99490–99491) are reported per calendar month. Code 99490 requires at least 20 minutes of clinical staff time that is provided under the direction of the physician or other qualified health care provider. In addition, the following services may not be reported with 99439 and 99487–99490 during the same service time:

- Analysis of data (99091)
- Education and training (98960–98962, 99071, 99078)
- Home and outpatient INR monitoring (93792–93793)
- Medical team conferences (99366–99368)
- Preparation of special reports (99080)
- Prolonged services without direct patient contact (99358–99359)
- Online and telephone services (99421–99423, 99441–99443, 98966–98968)
- Medication therapy management services (99605–99607)

Codes 99439 and 99487–99490 should also not be reported during the same service time as 98970–98972. Code 99491 should not be reported during the same service time as 99495–99495.

If fewer than 20 minutes are documented in a calendar month, the service should not be reported. Code 99491 is performed by the physician or OQHCP and represents at least 30 minutes involved with care management activities per month.

Add-on code 99439 should be reported in conjunction with code 99490 for each additional 20 minutes of clinical staff time provided. This code should not be reported more than twice per 30-day period; code 99490 may be reported only one time in a 30-day period.

To report these codes, the following elements are required and should be documented in the medical record:

- The patient must have two or more chronic continuous or episodic health conditions. The duration of the conditions is expected to be at least 12 months or until the death of the patient.
- Chronic conditions place the patient at a significant risk of death, acute exacerbation/decompensation, or functional decline.
- Comprehensive care plan has been established, implemented, or revised, or is being monitored.

Complex chronic care management services (99487–99489) encompass the same services required in chronic care management services in addition to the establishment of or substantial revision to the patient's plan of care, including medical, functional, and when appropriate psychosocial difficulties. Medical decision making is moderate or high in complexity. Clinical staff care management services must be provided for at least 60 minutes and under the direction of the physician or other qualified health care provider.

Codes 99487–99489 are reported based on the amount of time spent providing the service per calendar month. When 60 to 89 minutes of care are documented in the medical record, code 99487 is reported. Code 99489 indicates each additional 30 minutes of care provided during the calendar month. Complex chronic care management of less than 60 minutes in a calendar month is not reported separately. The time involved in other evaluation and management service should not be considered when selecting a complex care management code.

Practices may establish practice-specific guidelines that can be used to determine the patients who meet the requirements for these services. There also are algorithms that have been developed using criteria such as:

- Multiple illnesses
- Multiple medication usage
- Difficulties performing activities of daily living
- Necessity of a caregiver
- Repeat inpatient or emergency department admissions

Typically, the patients who require these services have complex disease processes and morbidities with one or more of the following:

- The patient's conditions require the coordination of multiple providers across different specialties and multiple services.
- The patient is likely not to adhere to a treatment plan without the assistance of a caregiver because of an inability to perform activities of daily living or as the result of a cognitive impairment.
- The patient has psychiatric (e.g., dementia, substance abuse) or other medical comorbidities (chronic obstructive pulmonary disease, diabetes) that complicate care.
- The patient has difficulty with access to care because of a lack of social support.

To report these codes, the following elements are required (in addition to the time element) and should be documented in the medical record:

- The patient has two or more chronic continuous or episodic health conditions. The duration of the conditions is expected to be at least 12 months or until the death of the patient.
- Chronic conditions place the patient at a significant risk of death, acute exacerbation/decompensation, or functional decline.
- A comprehensive care plan has been established, implemented, or revised or is being monitored.
- Moderate or high complexity.

Coding Tips
- If the physician or OQHCP provides one or more face-to-face visits during the reporting month, the visits can be reported with the appropriate E/M code.
- These services are reported only one time per month. It is important to note that time spent coordinating care for patients in the emergency room may be counted toward the time required to report these codes. However, as soon as the patient is admitted to hospital observation or inpatient, time may not be reported using these codes.
- Only the time of one clinical staff person may be counted if multiple members of the provider's staff are meeting about a patient.
- Codes 99490 and 99491 should be reported only once per month.

 AUDITOR'S ALERT

If a patient resumes care following a discharge within the same month, the provider may choose to resume care coordination services or report transitional care management (99495-99496). If the discharge occurs in a new month, a new care coordination period may be started. However the provider may not report both services.

- Code 99439 may be reported twice per month.
- If a physician or qualified health care professional performs any of the clinical staff activities these codes describe, his or her time may be counted towards the clinical staff time to meet the requirements of the elements of the code.

Coding Trap

- Chronic care management (99439, 99490–99491) should not be reported with complex chronic care management (99487, 99489).
- Codes 99439 and 99490 should not be reported in the same month as code 99491.
- Care management services should not be reported in the same month as end-stage renal disease services (90951–90970).
- Clinical staff time should not be counted on the same date of service that a physician or OQHCP reports an E/M service code.
- Online digital E/M services (99421–99423) should not be reported concurrently with care management services.

Psychiatric Collaborative Care Management Services (99492–99494)

These services describe care reported by the treating physician or OQHCP overseeing a behavioral health care manager and psychiatric consultant providing a behavioral health assessment, including establishing, starting, revising, or monitoring a plan of care as well as providing brief interventions to a patient diagnosed with a mental health disorder. The psychiatric consultant contracts directly with the physician or OQHCP to render the consultation portion of the service. Patients are generally directed to a behavioral health care manager for assistance in receiving treatment for newly diagnosed conditions that have been unresponsive to traditional or standard care provided in a nonpsychiatric environment or who need additional examination and evaluation before a referral to a psychiatric care setting.

The following elements are required in order to report 99492:

- Outreach and engagement in the patient's treatment
- Initial patient assessment that involves the administration of a validated rating scale and development of an individual patient care plan
- Psychiatric consultant review and modifications, as needed
- Input of patient data into a registry, tracking of patient progress, follow-up, and weekly caseload participation with psychiatric consultant
- Provision of brief interventions using evidence-based techniques

In 99493, the elements required are as follows:

- Tracking patient follow-up and progress via registry
- Weekly caseload participation with psychiatric consultant
- Collaboration and coordinating with the physician or OQHCP and any other treating mental health providers
- Additional review of patient's progress and recommendations for treatment changes, as needed, including medications recommended by the psychiatric consultant
- Provision of brief interventions with the use of evidence-based techniques

- Monitoring patient outcomes using validated rating scales
- Relapse prevention planning

Each patient is treated for an episode of care that is defined as the time when the patient first was directed to the behavioral health care manager by the treating physician or OQHCP and ends when the treatment goals have been reached, the goals were not reached and the patient was referred to another provider for ongoing treatment, or no psychiatric collaborative care management was provided for a period of six consecutive months.

These codes do not differentiate between new or established patient status. Code 99492 should be reported for the initial 70 minutes of psychiatric collaborative care management in the first month. Code 99493 should be reported for the first 60 minutes of care in a subsequent month. When the time thresholds of 99492 or 99493 are surpassed, report add-on code 99494 for each additional 30 minutes of initial or subsequent care in a calendar month.

Transitional Care Management Services (99495–99496)

These services are provided to new or established patients who are transitioning from an inpatient facility, partial hospital, observation status, or skilled nursing facility to an assisted living facility, home, domiciliary, or rest home. The medical and psychological issues these patients may have necessitate a moderate or high level of medical decision making.

The 30-day transitional care management (TCM) period begins on the date the beneficiary is discharged from the inpatient hospital setting and continues for the next 29 days. During the 30-day period, the following three TCM components must be furnished, according to CMS:

- Interactive contact—The provider is required to attempt to have interactive contact with the beneficiary and/or caregiver, as appropriate, within two business days following the patient's discharge. The contact may be via telephone, email, or face-to-face. For Medicare purposes, attempts to communicate should continue after the first two attempts in the required two business days until they are successful. If two or more separate attempts are made in a timely manner and documented in the medical record but are unsuccessful, and if all other TCM criteria are met, TCM services may be reported. However, CMS stresses that they expect attempts to communicate to continue until they are successful. Do not report TCM services if the face-to-face visit is not furnished within the required timeframe.

- Non-face-to-face services—The provider must furnish non-face-to-face services to the patient, unless they are determined to be not medically indicated or necessary. Certain non-face-to-face services (listed below) may be furnished by licensed clinical staff under the provider's direction.

- Face-to-face visit—One face-to-face visit must be furnished within certain timeframes as described by codes 99495 (14 days) and 99496 (7 days)

Determining a level of medical necessity is also required to report these codes. Medical decision making (MDM) is determined by considering the following factors:

- The number of possible diagnoses and/or the number of management options that must be considered

- The amount and/or complexity of medical records, diagnostic tests, and/or other information that must be obtained, reviewed, and analyzed

- The risk of significant complications, morbidity, and/or mortality as well as comorbidities associated with the patient's presenting problem(s), selecting the diagnostic procedure(s), and/or selecting the possible management options

Code 99495 requires at least moderate complexity MDM; code 99496 requires high complexity MDM. For more detail on the selection of the medical decision making level, see the discussion earlier in this chapter titled "Documentation of the Complexity of Medical Decision Making."

Services that may be provided by the physician or OQHCP include:

- Assistance in scheduling any required follow-up with community providers and services

- Education of the patient, family, caregiver, and/or guardian

- Establishment or re-establishment of referrals and arranging for needed community resources

- Interaction with other providers who will assume or reassume care of the patient's system-specific problems

- Obtaining and reviewing the discharge information (discharge summary or continuity of care documents)

- Reviewing the need for or follow-up on pending diagnostic tests and treatments

Services that may be provided by the clinical staff include:

- Assessing and supporting treatment regimen adherence and medication management

- Helping the beneficiary and/or family access needed care and services.

- Communicating with home health agencies and other community services the patient may use

- Communicating with patient, family members, caretaker or guardian, surrogate decision makers, and/or other professionals regarding aspects of care

- Identifying available community and health resources

- Providing patient and/or family/caretaker education to support self-management, independent living, and activities of daily living

Coding Tips

- These codes should not be reported by a surgeon if the services rendered are within a global surgery period of the surgical procedure performed.

- If another provider reports these services during a postoperative period of a surgical procedure, modifier 54 is not required.

- If the physician or OQHCP provides more than one face-to-face visit in a month, additional visits should be reported with the appropriate E/M code.

- These services may be reported only one time within 30 days of discharge and by only one provider.

Due to the complexity of these codes and the many components that are required, it is crucial that practices audit these on a regular basis.

General Behavioral Health Integration Care Management Service (99484)

These services are provided face-to-face by clinical staff under the direction of a supervising physician or OQHCP to a patient with a diagnosed health care condition, including substance abuse issues requiring care management services for a minimum of 20 minutes per month. Specific elements must be provided and documented, including:

- Initial assessment or follow-up monitoring involving the use of validated rating scales

- Behavioral health care planning related to the patient's behavioral or mental health problems with revisions in cases where a patient is not responding to treatment or has a status change

- Organizing and coordinating all aspects of the patient's mental health care, such as counseling and/or psychiatric consultations, medications, and therapy

- Continuing ongoing care in conjunction with a designated care team member

The clinician does not need to provide a comprehensive assessment and treatment plan nor is it required to have all chronic care management (99439, 99487–99490) components documented. The patient may receive these services in any outpatient setting once certain criteria are established, namely that the clinician maintains a relationship with the patient and clinical staff and clinical staff be available to provide the patient with face-to-face services.

The provider may also report other E/M services, including care management services (99487, 99489, 99490, 99495–99496, and 90785–90899), in the same time period as long as the documentation supports the need of the service. These additional services do not count toward the required elements of code 99484.

Advanced Care Planning (99497–99498)

These services are used to report that the provider met with the patient, family members, or surrogate and discussed advance directives. Counseling is an integral part of the service. The provider may or may not complete the necessary legal forms. Examples of written directives include but are not limited to health care proxy, durable power of attorney for health care, living will, and medical orders for life-sustaining treatment (MOLST). Advanced care planning services may be reported in addition to other E/M services when the documentation supports the E/M service.

Chapter 5. **Auditing Anesthesia Services**

Anesthesia services are distinctive in the manner in which they are billed; therefore, when the need arises to audit anesthesia services, it must be conducted in a unique way.

While most payers, including Medicare, reimburse anesthesia services under a fee schedule, the calculation used is different because anesthesia services are paid on a base unit and the amount of time spent providing the service. Additionally, the geographically specific conversion factor or dollar value used to convert the total relative value (base and time unit together) is different from that used to compute payment for other types of services. Since anesthesia codes are based on time units, documentation must include the start and stop time of the service and who provided the anesthesia. Other factors such as the type of anesthesia provided (general, monitored anesthesia care, conscious sedation), if the anesthesia service was personally performed or medically directed, type of provider, modifiers assigned, and code selection also affect anesthesia coding, billing, and payments.

The Reimbursement Process

Appropriate reimbursement for anesthesia services can sometimes be difficult because of the myriad of rules and paperwork involved. The following guidelines outline the various requirements utilized in these types of claims.

Coverage Issues

First, it is important to know which services are covered. Covered services are those payable by the insurer in accordance with the terms of the benefit-plan contract. Such services must be documented and medically necessary for payment to be made.

When in doubt, providers should consult with the specific payer or refer to national policies, national coverage determinations (NCD), and local coverage determinations (LCD) that address the reasonable and necessary provisions of a service.

Typically, payers define medically necessary services or supplies as:

- Services established as safe and effective
- Services consistent with the symptoms or diagnosis
- Services necessary and consistent with generally accepted medical standards
- Services furnished at the most appropriate, safe, and effective level

Documentation must be provided to support the medical necessity of a service, procedure, and/or other item. This documentation should show:

- What service or procedure was rendered
- To what extent the service or procedure was rendered
- Why the service, procedure, or other item was medically warranted

Services, procedures, and/or other items that may not be considered medically necessary include:

- Services not furnished by a qualified provider
- Services that do not require the skills of a qualified provider
- Services not typically accepted as safe and effective in the setting where they are provided
- Services not generally accepted as safe and effective for the condition being treated
- Services not proven to be safe and effective based on peer review or scientific literature
- Experimental or investigational services
- Services furnished at a duration, intensity, or frequency that is not medically appropriate
- Services not furnished in accordance with accepted standards of medical practice
- Services not furnished in a setting appropriate to the patient's medical needs and condition

Most providers have to deal with a number of different payers and plans, each with its own specific policies and methods of payment. For that reason, it is important to become familiar with the guidelines for each payer the practice has contact with.

Anesthesia Reimbursement

While most payers, including Medicare, reimburse anesthesia services under a fee schedule, the computation used is different. This is because anesthesia services are paid based on a base unit, as well as the amount of time spent providing anesthesia services. Additionally, the conversion factor, or dollar value, used to convert relative value units into dollar amounts differs for anesthesia codes. Other factors that can influence billing and payment of anesthesia services include:

- Code selection
- Monitored anesthesia care
- Personally performed anesthesia service
- Medically directed anesthesia services
- Medical supervision of four or more concurrent procedures
- Directing a certified registered nurse anesthetist (CRNA) in solo cases
- Teaching situations
- Modifier usage
- Qualifying circumstances

Code Selection

The type of code assigned on the claim is dependent upon the payer. Some payers require the use of a CPT® surgical code that describes the procedure; however, most payers require a code from the anesthesia section of the CPT book be reported. Medicare requires that the appropriate anesthesia code be identified on the claim.

The American Society of Anesthesiologists (ASA) publishes a crosswalk that directs the provider from the surgical code to the appropriate anesthesia code. For example, if the patient is placed under anesthesia for the laparoscopic removal of a gallbladder (CPT code 47562), the provider can find code 47562 in the anesthesia crosswalk and see that code 00790 is the anesthesia code that corresponds with this service.

When auditing code selection, it must be determined if the appropriate type (surgical or anesthesia) of code was indicated. Once this is confirmed, verify that the code correctly describes the service provided.

Modifier Selection

Anesthesia claims must have a modifier assigned indicating provider type (anesthesiologist or certified registered nurse anesthetist [CRNA]), and whether the anesthesia was personally performed, medically directed, or under direct supervision. The correct use of these modifiers is important as they affect payment amounts.

Personally Performed, Medical Direction, and Medical Supervision

The following definitions assist in the appropriate assignment of modifiers.

Anesthesia services differ from other physician services in that the anesthesiologist may personally perform the service, may share a single service with a CRNA, may direct one or more CRNAs while two or three services are being performed, or may supervise four or more concurrent procedures. A clear understanding of what is required for each one of these situations is critical for correct modifier assignment.

Personally Performed Anesthesia Service

According to the *Medicare Claims Processing Manual*, Pub. 100-4, chapter 12, sec. 50, an anesthesia service is considered to be personally performed by an anesthesiologist when the physician personally performs the entire anesthesia service alone or when one of the following occurs:

- The physician is involved with one anesthesia case with a resident, meeting the teaching physician requirements.

- The physician is involved in the training of physician residents in a single anesthesia case, two concurrent anesthesia cases involving residents, or a single anesthesia case involving a resident that is concurrent to another case that meets the requirements for payment at the medically directed rate. This also meets the teaching physician requirements.

- The physician is continuously involved in a single case involving a student nurse anesthetist.

DEFINITIONS

CRNA. Certified registered nurse anesthetist. Nurse trained and specializing in the administration of anesthesia.

- The physician is involved with a single case with a qualified nonphysician anesthetist (a certified registered nurse anesthetist [CRNA] or an anesthesiologist's assistant [AA]). Contractors may pay the physician service and the qualified nonphysician anesthetist service in accordance with the requirements for payment at the medically directed rate.

OR

- The physician and the CRNA (or AA) are involved in one anesthesia case and the services of each are found to be medically necessary. Documentation must be submitted by the CRNA and the physician to support payment of the full fee for each of the two providers. The physician reports modifier AA and the CRNA reports modifier QZ.

Payments for services that are "personally performed" are made at 100 percent of the fee schedule amount.

Medically-Directed Anesthesia Services

Anesthesia services may also be performed under medical direction. A service is considered medically directed when the physician medically directs qualified individuals (all of whom could be CRNAs, anesthesiologist assistants, interns, residents, or a combinations of these individuals) in two, three, or four concurrent cases. However, it should be noted that the physician must perform the components below in order for the procedure to be considered directed by the physician:

- The physician performs a preanesthetic examination and evaluation.

- The physician prescribes the anesthesia plan.

- The anesthesiologist personally participates in the most demanding procedures in the anesthesia plan, including induction and emergence when indicated.

- The anesthesiologist must ensure that any procedures in the anesthesia plan not performed by that physician are performed by a qualified anesthetist.

- The anesthesiologist must monitor the course of anesthesia administration at frequent intervals.

- The physician must be physically present and available for immediate diagnosis and treatment of emergencies.

- The anesthesiologist provides indicated postanesthesia care.

- Physicians must document in the medical record that they performed the preanesthetic examination and evaluation, provided the indicated postanesthesia care, were present during some portion of the anesthesia monitoring, and were present during the most demanding procedures in the anesthesia plan, including induction and emergence, where indicated.

Medicare billing rules do allow a physician who is concurrently providing medical direction to attend to an emergency of short duration (when in the immediate area) or perform other services that do not require a great amount of time, such as the administration of an epidural or periodic monitoring of an obstetrical patient.

In addition, an anesthesiologist providing medical direction may also receive patients entering the operating suite for the next surgery, check or discharge patients in the recovery room, or handle scheduling matters without affecting payment.

However, an anesthesiologist providing medical direction may not leave the immediate area of the operating suite for other than short durations. Furthermore, if the anesthesiologist has to devote an extensive amount of time to another patient, such as in the case of an emergency, or is otherwise not available to attend to the immediate needs of the patients under anesthesia, the requirements for medical direction have not been met. In these cases, the anesthesiologist services are considered supervision.

If anesthesiologists are in a group practice, one physician member may provide the preanesthesia examination and evaluation while another fulfills the other criteria. Similarly, one physician member of the group may provide postanesthesia care while another member of the group furnishes the other component parts of the anesthesia service. However, the medical record must indicate that the services were furnished by physicians and identify the physicians who furnished them.

When filing claims for medically directed services, the physician must report modifier QK Medical direction of two, three or four concurrent anesthesia procedures involving qualified individuals. A CRNA claim must have modifier QX CRNA service: with medical direction by a physician. The physician fee schedule is split at 50 percent for each provider when requirements for physician payment are met. However, since interns and residents are not eligible to receive Medicare payment, the split fee is not applicable to these physicians.

Medical Supervision

Medical supervision of anesthesia services is defined as when the anesthesiologist is involved in more than four concurrent procedures or is performing other services while directing the concurrent procedures, such as when the anesthesiologist has to devote a significant amount of time to an emergency procedure elsewhere and is unable to attend to the immediate needs of the surgical patients. When billing for the medically supervising physician, indicate HCPCS Level II modifier AD Medical supervision by a physician: more than four concurrent anesthesia procedures.

Medicare contractors base payment on a three base unit amount multiplied by the anesthesia conversion factor. An additional time unit can be recognized if the physician can document he or she was present at induction. In these instances, medical record documentation must accompany the claim.

Directing a CRNA in Solo Cases

There are times when the physician and the CRNA (or AA) are involved in one anesthesia case and the services of each are found to be medically necessary. In these instances, the physician should submit the claim with the appropriate CPT code for the services and modifier AA Anesthesia services performed personally by the anesthesiologist. The CRNA should report the same CPT code with modifier QZ CRNA service without medical direction by a physician. In these cases, both the anesthesiologist and the CRNA are fully involved in the case and for this reason, full payment is made to each. These cases require supporting documentation indicating required presence of both providers. In addition, the physical status modifiers should be used to indicate any other physical conditions complicating the anesthesia care.

When the CRNA (qualified nonphysician anesthetist) and the anesthesiologist are involved in a single case and the physician is only performing medical direction, claims are submitted by the physician appending modifier QY Medical direction of one certified registered nurse anesthetist (CRNA) by an

 SPECIAL ALERT

If an anesthetist assists the physician in the care of a single patient, the service is considered personally performed by the physician. The anesthesiologist should report this service with modifier AA and the appropriate CPT code.

When the physician and a CRNA or an AA are involved in one anesthesia case and the services of each are found to be medically necessary, this modifier may be billed. The CRNA or AA would report the same procedure code with modifier QZ. Payers will usually require documentation substantiating the need for both anesthesia providers.

anesthesiologist, to the appropriate CPT code. The CRNA appends modifier QX CRNA service: with medical direction by a physician. In these instances, each provider receives 50 percent of the full fee schedule amount.

For general information regarding the reporting of modifiers or for information regarding modifiers that are not specific to anesthesia services, see chapter 3. Modifiers applicable to anesthesia services and associated guidelines are included in the following discussion. Modifiers 23 and 47, modifiers describing physical status (P1, P2, P3, P4, P5, and P6), and HCPCS Level II modifiers AA, AD, G8, G9, GC, QK, QS, QX, QY, and QZ may be appended only to identify anesthesia services.

23   **Unusual anesthesia**

47   **Anesthesia by surgeon**

These modifiers are discussed in detail in chapter 3.

HCPCS Level II Modifiers

The HCPCS Level II modifiers indicate the type of provider and, when appropriate, the level of direction or supervision provided.

AA   **Anesthesia services performed personally by anesthesiologist**

AD   **Medical supervision by a physician; more than four concurrent anesthesia procedures**

G8   **Monitored anesthesia care (MAC) for deep complex, complicated, or markedly invasive surgical procedures**

G9   **Monitored anesthesia care for patient who has a history of severe cardiopulmonary condition**

GC   **This service has been performed in part by a resident under the direction of a teaching physician**

Payment may be made under the regular fee schedule amount if the teaching anesthesiologist is involved in the training of a resident in a single anesthesia case, two concurrent anesthesia cases involving residents, or a single anesthesia case involving a resident that is concurrent to another case paid under the medical direction rules. To qualify for payment, the teaching anesthesiologist, or different anesthesiologists in the same anesthesia group, must be present during all critical or key portions of the anesthesia service or procedure involved. The teaching anesthesiologist (or another anesthesiologist with whom the teaching physician has entered into an arrangement) must be immediately available to furnish anesthesia services during the entire procedure. The documentation in the patient's medical records must indicate the teaching physician's presence during all critical or key portions of the anesthesia procedure and the immediate availability of another teaching anesthesiologist as necessary.

If different teaching anesthesiologists are present with the resident during the key or critical periods of the resident case, the National Provider Identifier (NPI) of the teaching anesthesiologist who started the case must be indicated in the appropriate field on the claim. The teaching anesthesiologist should report modifier AA and certification modifier GC in these cases.

Note: Modifier GC has no effect on payment. Modifier GC should not be used as a second modifier to the anesthesia code when an anesthesiologist uses modifier QK to reflect two to four medically directed procedures.

 AUDITOR'S ALERT

Most claims for MAC are denied for medical necessity reasons. Medicare and other third-party payers will not provide coverage for these services if, for example, it appears the gastroenterologist could have provided moderate sedation for the patient undergoing endoscopy.

 DEFINITIONS

monitored anesthesia care. Sedation, with or without analgesia, used to achieve a medically controlled state of depressed consciousness while maintaining the patient's airway, protective reflexes, and ability to respond to stimulation or verbal commands. In dental conscious sedation, the patient is rendered free of fear, apprehension, and anxiety through the use of pharmacological agents.

QK   Medical direction of two, three or four concurrent anesthesia procedures involving qualified individuals

QS   Monitored anesthesiology care services

If the service is usually performed under moderate sedation by the surgeon, determine what extenuating services occurred that necessitated the presence of an anesthesiology provider. The appropriate physical status modifier should be appended to inform the payer of the circumstance. If the physical status modifiers do not provide the necessary information, a special report should be attached. It is also necessary to confirm the medical necessity of MAC in these situations by the diagnosis listed on the claim, which may indicate a contraindication to other forms of anesthesia or the need for monitoring by the anesthesiologist. Check with third-party payers, as most have a list of diagnoses that substantiate the use of MAC. MAC is discussed in further detail later in this chapter.

Note: Modifier QS can be used by a physician or a qualified nonphysician anesthetist and is for informational purposes. Providers must report actual anesthesia time and one of the payment modifiers on the claim.

QX   CRNA Service: With Medical Direction By a Physician

QY   Medical Direction of One Certified Registered Nurse Anesthetist (CRNA) By an Anesthesiologist

QZ   CRNA Service: Without Medical Direction by a Physician

Payment may be made under Part B Medicare to a teaching CRNA who supervises a single case involving a student nurse anesthetist where the CRNA is continuously present. The CRNA reports the service using modifier QZ. This modifier designates that the teaching CRNA is not medically directed by an anesthesiologist. No payment is made under Part B Medicare for the service provided by a student nurse anesthetist.

The teaching CRNA, not under the medical direction of a physician, can also be paid for his or her involvement in each of two concurrent cases with student nurse anesthetists. Payment will be made at the regular fee schedule rate in these cases. The CRNA must document his or her involvement in the cases and report the anesthesia services using modifier QZ.

To bill the anesthesia base units, the CRNA must be present with the student nurse anesthetist during the pre- and postanesthesia care for each of the two cases. The teaching CRNA must continue to devote his or her time to the two concurrent cases and not be involved in other activities. The teaching CRNA can decide how to allocate his or her time to optimize patient care in the two cases based on the complexity of the anesthesia case, the experience and skills of the student nurse anesthetist, the patient's health status, and other factors.

The teaching CRNA must document his or her involvement in the cases with the student nurse anesthetists.

 AUDITOR'S ALERT

Whenever the documentation indicates that MAC services have been provided, verify that modifier QS Monitored anesthesiology care services, has been appended to the procedure code.

 AUDITOR'S ALERT

A common error in anesthesia documentation is the failure to note the presence of the physician during intubation and extubation. If medical record documentation does not support the physician's presence, then medical direction may not be billed.

The following table may be used as a tool when auditing anesthesia modifier assignment.

HCPCS Level II Modifiers for Anesthesia Services

Modifier	Description	When to Use	Payment
AA	Anesthesia performed personally by anesthesiologist	This modifier indicates that the anesthesiologist personally performed the service.	When this modifier is used, no reduction in physician payment is made.
AD	Medically supervised by a physician; more than four concurrent procedures	Modifier AD is appended to physician claims when a physician supervises four or more concurrent procedures.	In these instances, payment is made on a 3 base unit amount.
G8	Monitored anesthesia care (MAC) for deep complex, complicated, or markedly invasive surgical procedures	For use with the following anesthesia codes only: 00100, 00160, 00300, 00400, 00532, and 00920.	No payment reductions are made for MAC; this modifier is for informational purposes only.
G9	Monitored anesthesia care for patient who has a history of severe cardiopulmonary condition	This modifier should be reported whenever MAC is used due to a history of advanced cardiopulmonary disease.	No payment reductions are made for MAC; this modifier is for informational purposes only.
GC	Services performed in part by a resident under the direction of a teaching physician	Modifier GC is reported by the teaching physician to indicate he or she rendered the service as a teaching physician. A payment modifier must be used with GC.	No payment reductions are made for teaching physicians. This modifier is for informational purposes only.
QK	Medical direction of two, three, or four concurrent anesthesia procedures involving qualified individuals	This modifier is used on physician claims to indicate that the physician provided medical direction of two to four concurrent anesthesia services.	Physician payment is reduced to 50% of the fee schedule amount.
QS	Monitored anesthesiology care service	This modifier can be used by the anesthesiologist or the CRNA and indicates that the type of anesthesia performed was monitored anesthesiology care (MAC).	No payment reductions are made for MAC; this modifier is for informational purposes only.
QX	CRNA service: with medical direction by a physician	This modifier is appended to CRNA or anesthetist assistant (AA) claims. This informs an insurance payer that a CRNA or AA provided the service with direction by an anesthesiologist.	The CRNA receives 50 percent of the fee schedule amount or the amount billed, whichever is less.
QY	Medical direction of one Certified Registered Nurse Anesthetist (CRNA) by an anesthesiologist	This modifier is used by the anesthesiologist when directing a CRNA in a single case.	Payment is made at 50 percent to the physician and 50 percent to the CRNA.
QZ	CRNA service: without medical direction by a physician	When a CRNA performs the anesthesia without any direction by a physician, modifier QZ should be indicated on the claim.	In these instances, CRNA or AA payment is based on 100 percent of the fee.

 © 2020 Optum360, LLC

Physical Status Modifiers P1, P2, P3, P4, P5, and P6

Physical status modifiers reflect the patient's state of health. Individuals undergoing surgery may be healthy or may have varying degrees of systemic disease. A patient's health status affects the work related to providing the anesthesia service. Use modifiers P1–P6 to report the patient's health status.

These physical status modifiers are consistent with the American Society of Anesthesiologists' (ASA) ranking of patient physical status, except for the exclusion of modifier P6. Physical status is included in the CPT book to distinguish among various levels of complexity of the anesthesia service provided.

P1	A normal healthy patient
P2	A patient with mild systemic disease
P3	A patient with severe systemic disease
P4	A patient with severe systemic disease that is a constant threat to life
P5	A moribund patient who is not expected to survive without the operation
P6	A declared brain-dead patient whose organs are being removed for donor purposes

Note: Medicare does not recognize physical status modifiers for reporting anesthesia services.

Appropriate Use of Physical Status Modifiers
Below are further examples of correct physical status modifier usage:

- Physical status modifiers are to be reported with an anesthesia procedure code (00100–01999).
- Physical status modifiers should only be used on claims being submitted to commercial insurance carriers.

Inappropriate Use of Physical Status Modifiers
- Reporting physical status modifiers for anesthesia services provided to Medicare patients.

Regulatory and Coding Guidance for Physical Status Modifiers
- Anesthesia services should be reported with the physical status modifier consistent with the American Society of Anesthesiologists' ranking of the patient's physical status.
- Anesthesiologist/CRNAs should document the patient's physical status within the anesthesia record as P1 through P6 accordingly.
- Verify specific coverage requirements for the use of this modifier with the specific private payer.
- Medicare, many state Medicaid programs, as well as some commercial carriers do not recognize physical status modifiers.

Physical Status Modifiers: Clinical Examples of Appropriate Use

Example #1:

A 31-year-old AIDS patient presents to the hospital for surgical treatment of an intestinal blockage. AIDS is considered a severe systemic disease—one that affects many organs or affects the entire body. The anesthesiologist will append physical status modifier P3 to the anesthesia service code.

Example #2:

A sheriff's deputy responds to a domestic dispute call and upon arriving at the residence, begins to walk toward the front door. The door opens and the officer is confronted by an angry male presumed to be the perpetrator. The man opens fire on the officer, shooting him in the head. Emergency medical services are contacted and respond to the scene. The officer is immediately taken to surgery with life-threatening injuries. The anesthesiologist would append modifier P5 to the anesthesia service code to indicate a moribund or dying patient who requires immediate surgical intervention if he is to have any hope of survival.

Anesthesia Physical Status Modifiers

Modifier	Description	When to Use	Payment
P1	A normal healthy patient	This modifier indicates a healthy individual.	No additional payment is made.
P2	A patient with mild systemic disease	Use this modifier when the patient has a mild systemic disease, such as diabetes.	No additional payment is made
P3	A patient with severe systemic disease	This modifier is appended when the patient has a severe systemic disease that affects the care of the patient. Examples include diabetes with complications of body systems, severe heart disease, etc.	Most payers reimburse an additional one to three base units when this modifier is appended.
P4	A patient with severe systemic disease that is a constant threat to life	A patient with severe systemic disease that is a constant threat to life. Use this modifier when the patient's condition is life threatening and thus, makes administration of anesthesia more difficult.	Most payers reimburse an additional one to three base units when this modifier is appended.
P5	A moribund patient who is not expected to survive without the operation	This modifier is often used to identify critically injured patients who must undergo emergency surgery in order to survive.	Most payers will reimburse an additional one to three base units when this modifier is appended.
P6	A declared brain-dead patient whose organs are being removed for donor purposes	This modifier is used when anesthesia is provided during organ harvesting.	No additional payment is made.

Qualifying Circumstance Codes

The qualifying circumstance codes, although not modifiers, are included here because many health care and insurance professionals think of them as five-digit modifiers for anesthesia claims. Four circumstances have been specifically identified as significantly impacting the anesthesia service provided. These procedures are not reported alone. More than one qualifying circumstance may apply and each is reported separately. These codes, which are listed below, indicate that anesthesia services were provided under difficult circumstances.

Qualifying Circumstance Codes for Anesthesia Claims

Code	Description	Payment
99100	Anesthesia for patient of extreme age, younger than 1 year and older than 70	No additional payment is made.
99116	Anesthesia complicated by utilization of total body hypothermia	Many payers allow separate payment for this code.
99135	Anesthesia complicated by utilization of controlled hypotension	Many payers allow separate payment for this code.
99140	Anesthesia complicated by emergency conditions (specify)	No additional payment is made.

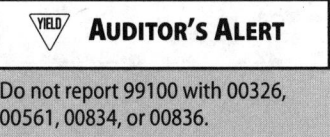

AUDITOR'S ALERT

Do not report 99100 with 00326, 00561, 00834, or 00836.

Correct Coding Policies for Anesthesia Services

One principle of CPT coding is that if a service is routinely provided as part of a more comprehensive service, then it should be included in and be considered part of (or bundled into) the service.

The advances in technology allow for intraoperative monitoring of a variety of physiological parameters. The following preparation or monitoring services are integral to anesthesia services in general and are not to be separately reported.

- Transporting, positioning, prepping, and draping the patient for satisfactory anesthesia induction/surgical procedures

- Placement of devices necessary for cardiac monitoring, oximetry, capnography, temperature, Doppler flow, electroencephalogram (EEG), and central nervous system (CNS) evoked responses (e.g., BSER)

- Placement of peripheral intravenous lines necessary for fluid and medication administration

- Placement of airway (e.g., endotracheal tube, orotracheal tube) or laryngoscopy (direct or endoscopic) for placement of airway (e.g., endotracheal tube)

- Placement of nasogastric or orogastric tube

- Intraoperative determination of monitored functions (blood pressure, heart rate, respirations, oximetry, capnography, temperature, EEG, BSER, Doppler flow, CNS pressure)

- Interpretation of laboratory determinations (arterial blood gases such as pH, pO_2, pCO_2, bicarbonate, blood chemistries, lactate) by the anesthesiologist/CRNA

- Nerve stimulation for determination of level of paralysis or localization of nerve

- Blood sample procurement through existing lines or requiring only venipuncture or arterial puncture

- Insertion of urinary bladder catheter

When certain CPT codes are billed with an anesthesia code, it is assumed that these services are being billed as part of the anesthesia service, and they will be bundled into the primary anesthesia code. Many of these procedures may occur on the same date of surgery and are not performed in the course of the anesthesia provision for the day. Therefore, the codes in the list below are separately paid only if accompanied by modifier 59 or XE, indicating that the service rendered was independent of the anesthesia service. The following is a partial list of CPT codes describing services that, when performed as part of the anesthesia service, would be considered bundled into the anesthesia code:

- Laryngoscopy (31505, 31515, 31527)

- Bronchoscopy (31622, 31645, 31646)

- Introduction of needle into vein (36000, 36010–36015)

- Venipuncture/transfusion (36400–36440)

- Injection of diagnostic or therapeutic substance—bolus, intermittent bolus, or continuous infusion (62320–62327)

- Peripheral nerve blocks—bolus injection or continuous infusion (64400–64530)

  Codes 62320–62327 and 64400–64530 may be reported on the date of surgery if performed for postoperative pain relief only if the operative anesthesia is general anesthesia, subarachnoid injection, or epidural injection and the adequacy of the intraoperative anesthesia does not depend on the peripheral nerve block. Peripheral nerve block codes should not be reported separately on the same date of service as a surgical procedure if used as the primary anesthetic technique or as a supplement to the primary anesthetic technique. Modifier 59 or XU may be used to indicate that a peripheral nerve block injection was performed for postoperative pain management, rather than intraoperative anesthesia. A procedure note should be included in the medical record.

- Retrobulbar injection medication (67500)

- Performance and interpretation of laboratory tests (80345, 81000–81015, 82013, 82270–82271)

- Gastric intubation (43753–43755)

- Special otorhinolaryngologic services (92511–92520, 92537–92538)

- Cardiopulmonary resuscitation (92950)

- Temporary transcutaneous pacemaker (92953)

- Cardioversion (92960–92961)

- Electrocardiography (93000–93010, 93040–93042)

- Transthoracic echocardiography when used for monitoring purposes (93303–93308)

- Transesophageal echocardiography when used for monitoring purposes (93312–93317)

When performed for diagnostic purposes with documentation including a formal report, echocardiography codes 93303–93308 and 93312–93317 may be considered significant, separately identifiable, and separately reportable services.

- Transesophageal echocardiography for monitoring purposes (93318)
- Transesophageal echocardiography for guidance for transcatheter intracardiac or great vessels structural interventions (93355)
- Indicator dilution studies (93561–93562)
- Thoracic electrical bioimpedance (93701)
- Extremity arterial and venous studies (93922–93981)

  When performed diagnostically with a formal report, codes 93922–93981 may be considered a significant, separately identifiable, and, if medically necessary, reimbursable service.

- Inhalation/IPPB treatment (94640)
- Ventilation management/CPAP (94002–94004, 94660–94662)

  If codes 94002–94004 and 94660–94662 are performed as management for maintenance ventilation during a surgical procedure, this is part of the anesthesia service. It is separately reimbursable if performed after transfer out of postanesthesia recovery to a hospital unit or the intensive care unit. Modifier 59 or XU would be necessary to signify that this was a separate service.

- Inhalation (94664)
- Expired gas analysis (94680–94690)
- Oximetry (94760–94762)
- Drug administration (96360–96377)
- Evaluation and management (99202–99499)

Anesthesia for Endoscopic Procedures

There are five anesthesia codes specifically for endoscopy: 00731-00732 and 00811-00813. Each code has specific uses.

Code 00731 should be reported with procedures 43180-43206 and 43213-43232. Esophagogastroduodenoscopies (EGD) (43210, 43233, 43235-43259, 43266, and 43270) may also be reported with this anesthesia code if the duodenum is not examined. If the duodenum is included in the endoscopy, see 00811.

Code 00732 should be reported when endoscopic retrograde cholangiopancreatography (ERCP) procedures are performed (43260-43265 and 43273-43278).

Code 00811 should be reported when lower endoscopies are performed, including:

- Colonoscopy (45378-45393 and 45398)
- Colonoscopy through a stoma (44388-44408)

 AUDITOR'S ALERT

If an esophagogastroduodenoscopy is performed (43210, 43233, 43235-43259, 43266, and 43270) and the duodenum is not examined, append modifier 52 or 53 to the CPT code. These modifiers are used when the duodenum is intentionally not examined (modifier 52) or when a medical issue exists that puts the safety of the patient at risk (modifier 53).

- Esophagogastroduodenoscopy (including duodenum) (43210, 43233, 43235-43259, 43266, and 43270)
- Ileoscopy through a stoma (44380-44386)
- Proctosigmoidoscopy (45300-45327)
- Sigmoidoscopy (45330-45342 and 45346-45350)

Report 00812 when a colonoscopy is scheduled as a screening colonoscopy. Modifier 33 is not necessary when the service is identified as screening. In the case of a Medicare patient, modifier PT Colorectal cancer screening test; converted to diagnostic test or other procedure, should be appended to the diagnostic or surgical procedure code instead of the colorectal cancer screening if an additional procedure is performed. Report 00812 regardless of whether an additional procedure is performed. If the procedure was scheduled as a screening colonoscopy, it remains a screening when reporting anesthesia.

Code 00813 is reported when an upper and lower endoscopy is performed in the same operative setting on the same date of service. This code is a combination code used instead of reporting 00731 and 00811, which is inappropriate billing.

Coding Tips
- Code 00812 should be reported for any screening colonoscopy regardless of the final outcome.
- When a procedure is a combined upper and lower gastrointestinal endoscopy, report 00813.

Anesthesia for Radiological Procedures

In keeping with Medicare's standard anesthesia billing guidelines, only one anesthesia code may be billed for anesthesia services provided in conjunction with radiological procedures. Radiological supervision and interpretation (S&I) codes usually are applicable to radiological procedures being performed.

The appropriate S&I code may be billed by the appropriate provider (e.g., radiologist, cardiologist, neurosurgeon, radiation oncologist, etc.). Accordingly, S&I codes are not bundled into anesthesia codes that relate to these procedures; however, only the appropriate provider may bill for S&I services.

CPT code 01920 Anesthesia for cardiac catheterization including coronary arteriography and ventriculography, not to include Swan-Ganz catheter, may be billed for MAC in patients who are critically ill or critically unstable. If the physician performing the radiologic service places a catheter as part of that service and, through the same site, a catheter is left and used for monitoring purposes, it is inappropriate for the anesthesiologist or anesthetist, or the physician performing the radiologic procedure, to bill for placement of the monitoring catheter (e.g., codes 36500, 36555–36556, 36568–36569, 36580, 36584, 36597).

Monitored Anesthesia Care

CMS recognizes MAC services as payable when medically reasonable and necessary. MAC may be performed by an anesthesiologist or anesthetist who administers sedatives, analgesics, hypnotics, and other anesthetic agents but only to the level that the patient remains responsive and is able to breathe on his or her own. MAC provides relief of anxiety, pain, amnesia, and comfort. Appropriate patient monitoring is required that allows for the anticipation of a possible need to administer general anesthesia during a surgical or other procedure. Conscientious and continuous evaluation of various vital physiologic functions and the recognition and treatment of any adverse changes is necessary.

MAC involves the intraoperative monitoring by a physician (or a qualified individual under the medical direction of a physician) of the patient's vital physiological signs in anticipation of the need for administration of general anesthesia, as well as the occurrence of any adverse physiological reaction to the surgical procedure. It also includes:

- Performance of a preanesthetic examination and evaluation
- Prescription of anesthesia care
- Administration of any required oral or parenteral medications
- Providing necessary postoperative anesthesia care.

Medical necessity issues are addressed by national and local contractor medical review policies.

General Policy Statements

The term "physician" (unless indicated differently) is applicable to all practitioners, hospitals, providers, or suppliers eligible to bill the relevant HCPCS/CPT codes pursuant to applicable portions of the Social Security Act (SSA) of 1965, the *Code of Federal Regulations* (CFR), and Medicare rules. In some instances, the term "physician" would not include some of these entities because specific rules do not apply to them. For example, anesthesia rules and global surgery rules in the CMS Internet-Only Manual, Publication 100-04, chapter 12, sections 40 and 50 do not apply to hospitals.

Physicians should not report codes 96360–96377 for anesthetic agents or other drugs administered between the patient's arrival at the operative center and discharge from the postanesthesia care unit.

With few exceptions, Medicare anesthesia rules prohibit separate payment for anesthesia for a medical or surgical service when provided by the physician who also performs the service. In addition, physicians should not unbundle anesthesia procedures and report component codes individually. For instance, the following services should not be reported when related to the delivery of an anesthetic agent:

- Introduction of a needle or intracatheter into a vein (36000)
- Venipuncture (36410)
- Drug administration (96360–96377)
- Cardiac assessment (93000–93010, 93040–93042)

 AUDITOR'S ALERT

Anesthesiologists use modifier QS to report monitored anesthesia care cases, in addition to reporting the actual anesthesia time and one of the payment modifiers on the claim.

In some instances, Medicare may allow separate payment for moderate sedation services (99151–99153) when provided by the same physician performing the medical or surgical procedure.

Intraoperative neurophysiology testing (95940, 95941, G0453) should not be reported by the physician/anesthesia practitioner performing an anesthesia procedure since it is integral to the primary service code. The physician/ anesthesia practitioner performing an anesthesia procedure should not report other neurophysiology testing codes for intraoperative neurophysiology testing (e.g., 95822, 95860, 95861, 95867, 95868, 95870, 95907–95913, 95925–95937) since they are integral to the primary service code. However, when performed by a different physician during the procedure, intra-anesthesia neurophysiology testing may be reported separately by the second physician.

Units of Service Indicated

Computing Fees
The system that third-party payers most commonly use to calculate professional anesthesia payment is one that combines time units with the base unit values (BUV). The American Society of Anesthesiologists (ASA), as well as CMS, each developed a system of BUV. The combined units are multiplied by a payer-specific conversion factor (dollar amount). This formula for fee calculation is as follows:

> Base unit value (BUV) + Time units (TU)
> x Conversion factor (CF)
> = Payment

Base Units
Each anesthesia code is assigned a base unit by the American Society of Anesthesiologists (ASA) that reflects the difficulty of the procedure and inherent risks. Base units range from three to 30 units. It should be noted, however, that some payers may revise the base units of certain procedures. CMS also developed base units for anesthesia codes. Base units are used to help calculate payment and should not be included when determining the number of units to be indicated on the claim. Both the CMS and ASA base unit value represent the entire usual anesthesia services, with the exception of the time actually spent in anesthesia care, as well as any modifying factors that may occur.

The following are included in the BUV:

- Pre- and postoperative visits
- Administration of fluids and/or blood as incident to the anesthesia care
- Interpretation of noninvasive monitoring such as electrocardiogram, temperature, blood pressure, oximetry, capnography, and mass spectrometry

AUDITOR'S ALERT

The BUV is created for most of the anesthesia codes included in the CPT book. Services that are rarely performed may not have an assigned base unit value. When a service that does not have a BUV is provided, attach a special report describing the services and medical necessity. The payer then assigns a BUV after giving the encounter individual consideration.

KEY POINT

When indicating the number of units or the total time on the claim form, do not include the number of base units. Payers will compute payment using the appropriate number of base units.

The CMS base units are very similar to the ASA base units, with the exceptions shown in the following table.

Code	ASA Base Units	CMS Base Units
00147	6	4
00326	8	7
00537	10	7
01924	6	5
01925	8	7
01926	10	8
01932	7	6
01933	8	7
01963	10	8
01968	3	2

Medicare, as well as many other third-party payers, do not recognize the physical status and qualifying circumstance indicators.

Time Units

Most payers require the anesthesia provider to indicate the number of time units in item 24G of the CMS-1500 claim form. Most payers use 15-minute increments; however, be advised that the amount of time that constitutes a single unit may vary from payer to payer. The following is an example of how to compute the number of time units for a payer who uses a 15-minute increment:

Start time:	9:15
End time:	10:30
Total time:	1 hour 15 min or 75 min
75 Minutes	5- 15 units
Total time	5 Time units

Anesthesia time begins when the provider begins to prepare the patient in the operating room or an equivalent area and ends when the patient is placed under postoperative care, such as transfer to the recovery room. Blocks of time should be rounded using the appropriate mathematical formula. For example, seven minutes or less are not included when determining the total number of time units. Eight to 14 minutes are considered a unit when computing time units. Individual payer guidelines should be followed.

Anesthesia time is a continuous time from the start of anesthesia to the end of an anesthesia service. When billing for anesthesia services, it is appropriate to add blocks of time around an interruption as long as continuous anesthesia care is provided around the interruption. For example, an anesthesiologist is providing general anesthesia to a patient. The anesthesiologist must leave the room to start an intravenous (IV) line and then returns to the operating suite. The time spent providing anesthesia care before and after the interruption may be added together to determine the total anesthesia time. For instance, the provider is out of the operating suite for 15 minutes starting the IV. The start time for the procedure is 10:00 and the end time is 11:00. This means that 60 minutes of

 AUDITOR'S ALERT

Most often anesthesia services are denied as not medically necessary when provided during a procedure or service that does not usually warrant anesthesia. In these instances, the medical record documentation must support the use of anesthesia and modifier 23 Unusual anesthesia, should be appended second to the HCPCS modifier identifying the type of provider and anesthesia service provided (AA, QX, etc.).

A special report indicating the special need should be written.

total time less the 15 minutes spent with another patient for a total of 45 minutes or three time units is indicated on the claim.

For Medicare purposes, the actual anesthesia time (total number of minutes) must be reported on the anesthesia claim in item 24G of the CMS-1500 claim (the units column). Medicare then computes the time units as one unit per 15-minute time period. For fractions of the 15-minute units, Medicare rounds the time unit to one decimal place as shown in the following table.

Anesthesia Time Conversion Table, 15-Minute Increments

Minute	Unit
1–2	.1
3	.2
4–5	.3
6	.4
7–8	.5
9	.6
10–11	.7
12	.8
13–14	.9
15	1.0

If the ending time on one anesthesia service and the starting time for a second anesthesia service are identical, Medicare considers these procedures to be two concurrent procedures, which should be reported using modifier QK.

Because the amount of time spent with the patient is so important, the provider should document the start and stop time of anesthesia, the stop and start time that they are present when providing medical direction or supervision, and the amount of time spent providing other services, such as monitoring the patient in the recovery room.

Depending upon the payer the claim is being filed to, CPT code requirements may be either the surgical CPT code that appropriately describes the procedure being performed or the anesthesia CPT code that describes the type and anatomical location of procedure being performed.

For Medicare claims, a CPT anesthesia code must be identified on the claim. For example, if a patient is placed under anesthesia for the laparoscopic removal of a gallbladder, the correct CPT code that should be indicated on the Medicare claim would be 00790.

However, many commercial payers require the use of the surgical procedure code. In that case, the code used on a claim in the example provided above would be 47562. No matter which type of CPT code is used, a HCPCS Level II modifier indicating that the anesthesia was provided by an anesthesiologist or CRNA, and whether or not the anesthesia was medically directed or provided under supervision, is necessary. HCPCS Level II modifiers are discussed in chapter 3.

No matter which CPT code is required, it is important to select that code from the final anesthesia record and/or operative report and not from preoperative information.

General Anesthesia

The American Medical Association (AMA) includes a section of anesthesia codes in the CPT book immediately following the evaluation and management section. In addition, the CPT book includes four add-on codes to report qualifying circumstances for anesthesia (99100–99140) located in the medicine section.

The anesthesia section of the CPT book is arranged according to:

- Body region (e.g., head, neck, thorax, intrathoracic, spine, abdomen, perineum, pelvis, leg, shoulder, arm)
- Radiological procedures (e.g., hysterosalpingography, ventriculography, pneumoencephalography, cardiac catheterization, angioplasty, noninvasive imaging)
- Other procedures (e.g., physiological support for harvesting organs, regional IV administration of local anesthetic, daily management of epidural drug administration)

Most anesthesia codes are associated with surgery. These are first arranged by the anatomic surgical site and, second, by the surgical procedure involved. It is important to remember that even when multiple surgeries are performed, all that is often necessary is a single CPT anesthesia code with the appropriate modifier. In most circumstances, a CPT anesthesia code must be accompanied by a modifier.

A patient is considered under general anesthesia when rendered unconscious and has lost his or her reflexes secondary to the administration of drugs. In adults, an injection of anesthetic medicines through an intravenous catheter begins the anesthetic state. After the patient is rendered unconscious, the anesthetic state is maintained by a combination of inhalation agents and intravenous medications. The appropriate modifier indicating the type of provider (i.e., physician, CRNA), as well as the type of service being rendered (i.e., personally performed, medical direction), should be appended to the procedure code. Modifiers indicating the physical status of the patient should also be appended when required by the third-party payer. Note that Medicare does not recognize physical status modifiers.

Monitored Anesthesia Care General Guidelines

Monitored Anesthesia Care (MAC) is many times mistaken for moderate/conscious sedation (99151–99157) yet is distinct from moderate sedation in a few ways. MAC may include the administration of similar sedatives and/or analgesics as moderate sedation but provides a much deeper sedation. Deep sedation/analgesia is included in MAC.

Deep sedation/analgesia is a drug-induced depression of consciousness during which patients cannot be easily aroused but respond purposefully following repeated or painful stimulation. The ability to independently maintain ventilatory function may be impaired. Patients may require assistance in maintaining a patent airway and spontaneous ventilation may be inadequate. Cardiovascular function is usually maintained. The provider must assess and manage the patient's actual or anticipated physiological derangements or medical problems that could interfere with sedation. Additionally, the provider's training is crucial. In the event that the patient cannot maintain his or her airway due to sedation compromise, the provider must be qualified to convert the sedation to general anesthesia. Moderate sedation does not usually induce a sedation deep enough to impair the patient's ability to maintain the integrity of his or her airway. If the patient loses control of the airway, it is considered unconscious sedation and not MAC.

According to CMS guidelines, which most third-party payers follow, in order for care to be considered MAC the following criteria must be met:

- Intraoperative monitoring of the patient's vital signs in anticipation of the need for administration of general anesthesia or treatment of the development of adverse physiological patient reaction to the surgical procedure
- Provision of a preanesthesia examination and evaluation
- Prescribing required anesthesia care
- Administration of any needed oral or parental medications such as Atropine, Demerol, or Valium
- Postoperative anesthesia care as indicated

Most claims for MAC are denied for medical necessity reasons. Medicare and other third-party payers will not provide coverage for these services if, for example, it appears the gastroenterologist could have provided intravenous (IV) sedation for the patient undergoing endoscopy.

One method some payers use to allow the anesthesia provider to indicate medical necessity is use of physical status modifier P3 A patient with severe systemic disease. Be aware that not all payers accept the physical status modifiers so check with each before using.

When MAC is provided, report the appropriate anesthesia code and append HCPCS Level II modifier QS Monitored anesthesiology care services.

This modifier should not be reported by providers of other specialties.

Most often, however, MAC is determined medically necessary not so much by the service being performed but by the patient's diagnosis, which may indicate a

DEFINITIONS

moderate sedation. Medically controlled state of depressed consciousness, with or without analgesia, while maintaining the patient's airway, protective reflexes, and ability to respond to stimulation or verbal commands.

© 2020 Optum360, LLC

contraindication to other forms of anesthesia. Check with third-party payers, as most have a list of diagnoses that substantiate the use of MAC.

Regional Anesthesia

Regional anesthesia is the provision of pain relief for one segment or portion of the body. That portion is usually considered to be an extremity or some portion of the trunk or combination of the above. The patient may receive sedation in addition to the regional anesthesia medications for anxiety. If the patient is sedated to the extent that they lose their protective airway reflexes, it is considered general anesthesia. The following are examples of regional anesthesia:

- Brachial plexus block
- Femoral, sciatic blocks
- Wrist block
- Ankle block
- Spinal block
- Epidural

Regional intravenous administration of local anesthetic or other medication in an upper or lower extremity when performed by an anesthesiologist and used as the anesthetic for the surgical procedure should be reported with the appropriate anesthesia code for the surgical procedure performed.

If the anesthesiologist performs regional anesthesia with the usual pre- and postoperative care and monitors the patient throughout the procedure, the anesthesia code that describes the surgical procedure should be reported along with time and modifying units.

When the anesthesiologist administers a regional or local anesthetic and does not provide the monitoring associated with anesthesia care, only the injection should be reported using a code from the surgical section of the CPT book. These services are reimbursed at the same rate as for a surgeon and are based upon surgical values and conversion factors. Time units and other anesthesia modifiers may not be reported.

Epidural Analgesia

The formula for reporting epidural analgesia for labor and delivery may differ from the standard formula in some geographical areas. When epidural analgesia is administered, an anesthesiologist may attend to more than one patient. The anesthesiologist may insert the epidural catheter, start the continuous anesthetic, and leave the patient's bedside. The anesthesiologist periodically returns to check on the patient or to adjust the amount of anesthetic while attending to other patients who are also receiving epidurals for vaginal deliveries. For this reason, epidural analgesia for labor and delivery may be reimbursed at a reduced rate.

The CPT book includes a section of anesthesia codes (01958–01969) for vaginal delivery, cesarean delivery, urgent hysterectomy following delivery, cesarean hysterectomy without labor, analgesia care, abortion procedures, and neuraxial codes.

Note: Most third-party payers allow the following:

- One time unit per hour of labor for patients receiving continuous infusion.
- One time unit for each 15 minutes of actual delivery time

The following general guidelines apply to epidural anesthesia:

- When provided as anesthesia for a surgical procedure, the appropriate anesthesia or surgical procedure code (whichever is required by the payer) should be identified. Payment is determined by the number of base and time units. No additional payment is made for the epidural insertion. Since these codes are time based, documentation includes the start and stop time of the service.
- When provided for relief of pain, the appropriate code from range 62320–62327 should be identified. Diagnoses should identify the type of pain as well as the condition causing the pain.
- Payment is based upon the fee schedule amount or actual charge, whichever is lower.
- When providing epidural anesthesia for obstetrical care, the appropriate anesthesia (or surgical) code should be identified.
- For Medicare payers, if the anesthesiologist inserts an epidural catheter during the surgical procedure and initiates postoperative pain management, code 01996 may be reported.
- For non-Medicare payers, reporting epidural catheter placement for postoperative pain management may be appropriate, when provided separately from other anesthesia purposes. See codes 62324–62327.
- When both sides of the same spinal level are injected, modifier 50 should be appended to indicate that the procedure was performed bilaterally.
- Codes 62320–62327 are reported once per level, per side, regardless of the number or type of injections provided.

Nerve Block Anesthetics

Nerve blocks involve the injection of an anesthetic agent into or around a nerve. These procedures may be performed for diagnostic or therapeutic purposes. Code selection is determined by the specific nerve injected and the level of a spinal injection. The following general coding guidelines apply.

- If the block is performed primarily for anesthesia during a surgical procedure, then the appropriate anesthesia code should be used.
- If the block is performed for postoperative pain management by the same physician at the time of the procedure, then the appropriate code from this range may be reported with modifier 59 appended. Payer guidelines regarding postoperative pain management varies. Check with the payer in question for specific guidelines.
- See codes 64505–64530 for injection of anesthetic agents into sympathetic nerves.

Distinguish between a single-level block (codes 64420, 64483, 64490, and 64493) or a multiple-level/regional block (assigned add-on codes of somatic nerves):

- **Single-level block.** Interruption of a nerve function at a single dermatomal level (e.g., the skin area that a single nerve supplies).

- **Multiple-level block.** Interruption of nerve function of more than one dermatomal level.

- **Regional block.** Interruption of nerve function from a limb or area of the body, achieved by placement of local anesthetics along the course of the nerve or into the spinal space.

Note: Image guidance and localization are required for performance of 64490–64495, and are inclusive components of these codes.

Coding Tips

- As add-on codes, 64421, 64462, 64480, 64484, 64491, 64492, 64494, and 64495 are not subject to multiple procedure rules. No reimbursement reduction or modifier 51 is applied. Add-on codes describe additional intraservice work associated with the primary procedure. They are performed by the same provider on the same date of service as the primary service/procedure, and must never be reported as a stand-alone code. The following table provides additional information for these codes as found in the Medicare Physician Fee Schedule Database.

Parent Code	Add-On	GLOB DAYS	MULT PROC	BILAT SURG	ASST SURG	CO-SURG	TEAM SURG
64420		000	2	0	1	0	0
	64421		2	1	1	0	0
64461		000	2	1	1	0	0
	64462	ZZZ	0	1	1	0	0
64479		000	2	1	1	0	0
	64480	ZZZ	0	1	1	0	0
64483		000	2	1	1	0	0
	64484	ZZZ	0	1	1	0	0
64490		000	2	1	2	0	0
	64491	ZZZ	0	1	2	0	0
	64492	ZZZ	0	1	2	0	0
64493		000	2	1	2	0	0
	64494	ZZZ	0	1	2	0	0
	64495	ZZZ	0	1	2	0	0

- Codes 64400–64455, 64461, 64462, 64463, 64479, 64480, 64483, 64484, and 64490–64495 are unilateral procedures, if performed bilaterally, some payers require that the service be reported twice with modifier 50 appended to the second code, while others require identification of the service only once with modifier 50 appended. Check with individual payers.

- When add-on codes 64421, 64462, 64480, 64484, 64491, 64492, 64494, and 64495 are reported bilaterally, they should be reported twice. Modifier 50 does not apply to these codes.

- Localization and imaging guidance may be reported separately with 64455.
- Contrast injections and imaging guidance are included with 64451, 64455, 64461–64463, 64479, 64480, 64483, 64484, and 64486–64489 should not be reported separately.
- Injections performed in the epidural or subarachnoid areas should be reported with 62320–62327.

Coding Traps
- Do not report these codes in addition to anesthesia codes from range 01991–01992.
- Do not report 01996 with codes that include continuous infusion by catheter, in their code description, such as 64416 or 64446, or 64448–64449.

Patient-Controlled Anesthesia

Patient-controlled anesthesia (PCA) involves placing a catheter so that the patient may self-administer intravenous drugs through an infusion device. Guidelines for PCA include:

- Non-Medicare payers often allow payment for the insertion of the catheter when not performed as part of the surgical procedure.
- No base or time units apply to the catheter insertion. Payment is made from the fee schedule amount or actual charge, whichever is lower.
- Management of the PCA should be reported using the appropriate evaluation and management code.
- Medicare bundles the insertion of the PCA catheter, when inserted in the recovery room by the anesthesiologist, as part of the anesthesia time.
- The initial set up of the PCA is incorporated in the total time of anesthesia units.
- Any follow-up services provided for monitoring the PCA are included in the postoperative portion of the surgical procedure and will not be paid separately, regardless of who performs the service.
- Since these codes are time based, the documentation includes the start and stop time of the service.

Postoperative Pain Management

Normally postoperative pain management is provided or supervised by the surgeon and oral, intramuscular, or intravenous medications are provided. Postoperative pain management provided by the surgeon is included in the global fee for the surgical procedure. Some procedures and patients require more than the usual type of postoperative pain management, and this is frequently provided or supervised by an anesthesiologist.

These services are additional procedures and are reported as follows:

- Epidural or subarachnoid pain management is reported with procedure codes 62320–62327 for placement of the epidural or subarachnoid catheter, which includes the initial day of pain management. Many payers will deny the placement of the epidural or subarachnoid catheter if used in providing general anesthesia.

- Subsequent management is reported with 01996 and is reported per day.

- Postoperative pain management services are not calculated based on time. These services are reported as a single, daily charge.

Anesthesia-Specific Documentation Recommendations

Anesthesia documentation varies from all other specialties in the basic requirements. There are also variations between the attending anesthesiologist, medical directing anesthesiologist, and teaching physician (anesthesiologist). The basic documentation requirements include the preoperative evaluation, presurgery review, discussion, questions answered, attendance during surgery, and postanesthesia care unit evaluation and attendance as necessary.

The basic information that should be readily available from the anesthesia record includes:

- Preanesthesia
  - the reason for the procedure or service requiring anesthesia (diagnosis)
  - any additional conditions warranting the use of anesthesia (such as age, mental status of the patient, etc.)
  - a preanesthesia examination and evaluation
  - a written anesthesia plan
- Perianesthesia (time-based record of events)
  - indication that the anesthesiologist was present (or in the case of medical direction, personally participated in the most demanding procedures of the anesthesia plan including, if applicable, induction and emergence)
  - intraoperative re-evaluation of the patient
  - check of equipment, drugs, etc.
  - intraoperative monitoring of patient
  - patient vital signs including temperature, oxygenation, ventilation, and circulation
  - amounts of all drugs and agents used including the times given
  - unusual events occurring during the anesthesia monitoring period
  - total time
  - provision of indicated postanesthesia care
- Postanesthesia
  - evaluation on admission and discharge from postanesthesia
  - time based record of vitals signs and level of consciousness
  - drugs provided to the patient including the dosage and time
  - any unusual postanesthesia events or complications
  - postanesthesia visits and follow-up
  - initiation of any pain management services such as patient controlled anesthesia

The preanesthesia examination and evaluation should include a review of the patient's past medical history, medications, family history, social history, and adverse reactions to previous anesthesia.

The current lab work should be reviewed and the patient's desire regarding blood and blood product transfusions should be noted on the anesthesia preoperative evaluation and anesthesia record.

Anesthesia time starts when the provider begins to prepare the patient for anesthesia service in the operating room or an equivalent area and ends when the patient is placed under postoperative care, such as when transferred to the recovery room. Anesthesia time is a continuous time from the start of anesthesia to the end of an anesthesia service. The anesthesia provider can add blocks of time around an interruption as long as continuous anesthesia care is provided around the interruption. For example, an anesthesiologist provides general anesthesia to a patient. The anesthesiologist must leave the room to start an IV line, and then returns to the operating suite. The time spent providing anesthesia care before and after the interruption may be added together to determine the total anesthesia time.

Line placement must be noted, including location of placement, who performs the placement, and any complications regarding the placement. The lines placed include Swan-Ganz, central venous line (CVL), and arterial line (A-line). The placement of a Swan-Ganz and CVL should not both be reported unless noted on the anesthesia record that a second CVL was placed, where it was placed, and the reason for placement.

Medically Directed

The medically directing physician must document that he or she performed the preanesthesia evaluation, prescribed the plan of care, and was present and available for the "key portions," which include induction and emergence, if applicable.

The recommendation is that the anesthesiologist notes his or her presence at induction and emergence, initials the anesthesia record when monitoring the case, and makes sure the anesthesia record is complete. In addition, many payers require that the physician have on file each procedure performed and the name of each anesthetist directing for the service.

Teaching Physician

Medicare requires that medical record documentation for a teaching physician indicate that the physician was present "during all critical (or key) portions of the procedure." It is very important to note that the teaching physician's physical presence during only the preoperative or postoperative visits with the beneficiary is not sufficient to receive Medicare payment. If an anesthesiologist is involved in concurrent procedures with more than one resident or with a resident and a nonphysician anesthetist, the medical direction guidelines should be followed.

© 2020 Optum360, LLC

Monitored Anesthesia Care

It is recommended that the following items be documented when providing monitored anesthesia care:

- Preanesthesia evaluation
  - patient interview to include medical history, anesthesia history, medication history
  - appropriate physical exam
  - review of objective diagnostic data (e.g., laboratory, electrocardiogram (EKG), x-ray)
  - assignment of physical status (e.g., American Society of Anesthesiologists (ASA) physical status protocols)
  - formulation and discussion of an anesthesia plan with the patient and/or responsible adult and the patient's attending surgeon
- Perianesthesia (time-based record of events)
  - immediate review prior to initiation of anesthetic procedure
    - patient re-evaluation
    - check of equipment, drugs, gas supply
  - monitoring of the patient
    - qualified anesthesia personnel shall be present in the room throughout (MAC)
    - the patient's oxygenation, ventilation, circulation, and temperature shall be continually evaluated.
  - amounts of all drugs and agents used, and times given
  - the type and amounts of any/all intravenous fluids used, including blood and blood products, and times given
  - the technique used
  - all unusual events during the anesthesia-monitoring period
  - status of patient at conclusion of anesthesia and procedure
- Postanesthesia
- Patient evaluation on admission and discharge from postanesthesia
- A time-based record of vital signs and level of consciousness
  - all drugs administered and their dosages
  - types and amounts of intravenous fluids administered
  - any unusual events including postanesthesia or postprocedural complications
  - postanesthesia visits and any follow-up prescribed

Treatment Plan Documentation

Documentation should reflect any treatment failure or a change in diagnosis and/or a change in treatment plan, including the treatment of acute, chronic, or postoperative pain management. There should also be evidence of any initiation or reinstitution of a drug regime, which requires close and continuous skilled medical observation. Treatment plan goals and objectives must be well defined and signed by the attending physician, and progress notes must clearly demonstrate that the patient displays evidence of improvement or regression.

In addition, the physician must review the results of diagnostic tests, evaluate rehabilitation potential, advise staff members of the goals to be achieved, review the patient's progress at least every 30 days, and update the plan of treatment as needed. These records must be documented and available for review, upon request.

Providers should be certain that sufficient documentation is provided in the medical records to accurately verify any description of services rendered. Additionally, records should be legible and signed with the appropriate name and title of the provider of service. Adequate medical record documentation of services is essential to substantiate the service provided.

Chapter 6. **Auditing Surgical Procedures**

Auditing surgical services requires a unique approach. There are a number of coding, reporting, and payment guidelines that must be considered before determining if the claim is correct and supported by the medical record documentation.

When auditing surgical services, not only must the reviewer determine if the date of service, place of service, number of units, modifier application, and code selection is correct, the reviewer must also determine if the coder:

- Was in compliance with the global surgical package definition (items that are included in the surgical package, and should not be reported separately).
- Reported follow-up care unrelated to the surgical procedure, when applicable.
- Submitted additional, separately identifiable services with the appropriate modifier appended.
- Followed separate procedure guidelines.
- Billed supplies over and above the usual, when appropriate.
- Identified whether the provider was the surgeon, cosurgeon, or member of a surgical team.

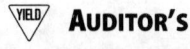 **AUDITOR'S ALERT**

See Appendix 1 for auditing worksheets for procedures in this chapter.

Date of Service

The date of service on the claim must correspond with the date of service in the medical record. For services that extend beyond a single calendar day, such as an emergency appendectomy started at 11:45 p.m. and completed at 1:15 a.m. the next day, the date the procedure was started is usually indicated on the claim.

Medical Necessity

Medical necessity dictates that one would never do more than is necessary. The medical record documentation should describe the patient's condition and complaints; thereby, indicating the need for the service. These conditions are then translated into ICD-10-CM codes and reported on the claim form. It is the responsibility of the auditor to determine that what the clinician has documented as the patient's condition has been appropriately reported on the claim. ICD-10-CM codes should never be selected simply to ensure payment. See chapter 1 for more information on medical necessity and ICD-10-CM codes.

Complications and Unusual Services

Any intraoperative misadventure should be summarized in the complications section of the operative report. Specific information about the complication and the steps taken to remedy it are to be thoroughly documented in the procedure section of the medical report. Examine the medical record documentation to determine the amount of time the provider spent addressing the complication and its relation to the overall length of the surgery to determine if the complication affects code assignment. For instance, if one hour of a nine-hour surgery was spent performing lysis of adhesions, this should be stated in the medical documentation. Not only will this ensure comprehensive and precise documentation, it provides the details necessary to support a higher level of coding. The use of main terms like difficult, complicated, increased, or unusual can help to substantiate the higher level of service reported.

Number of Units

The number of times a service is performed and reported is critical when determining that a procedure has been reported correctly, particularly when reporting such procedures as removal of lesions. Some CPT® codes indicate that a procedure may be performed for two or more, each additional, up to four, etc. When auditing these types of services the auditor should:

- Read the operative report carefully to determine the number of times the service was performed.
- Compare to the CPT code narrative to determine the number of times the service is to be performed per the description.
- Confirm against the claim to ensure the appropriate code has been reported.

Documentation

Operative Reports

The operative report is a written account of the surgical procedure. As with any clinical documentation, the focus is on patient care and the outcome. The information, first and foremost, is a tool that enables the physician and nursing staff to care for the patient during the postoperative period.

In-office procedures, as well as many minor surgeries performed in the outpatient setting, permit the surgeon to dictate the operative report immediately following the session. In more complex cases, the lead surgeon documents the session with the individual surgical specialists dictating their portions of the surgery separately. Timeliness may vary slightly, but in general the operative report must be completed and entered into the medical record before the patient is transferred to another facility or discharged.

A number of physician offices and clinics now have the capability to electronically interface with hospital systems that permit access to the operative report, discharge summary, and other documents to assist with coding and billing. When information is not readily available via these means and must be reviewed at a later time, perhaps in the form of a special summary, the document should contain:

- Pre- and postoperative diagnoses
- Name of surgeon, cosurgeon(s), assistant surgeon(s)
- Type and amount of anesthetic and duration
- Name of anesthesiologist

- Complications and unusual services
- Immediate postoperative condition
- Estimate of blood loss and replacement
- Fluids given and invasive tubes, drains, and catheters used
- Hardware or foreign objects left intentionally in the operative site

Operative report summaries may not necessarily contain all of these elements or completely describe the service. For this reason, coders may find it necessary to rely on other types of documentation to assign diagnoses and procedure codes. Therefore, it is essential that when this occurs, the other forms or types of documentation referenced be included in the medical record.

When coding for surgical procedures, key terms within the operative report are instrumental in identifying the appropriate code. Terms such as incision, excision, removal, debridement, etc. aid the coder in understanding exactly what has occurred.

Equally important, for coding purposes, is to determine the specifics and detail precisely what occurred and by whom during procedures involving more than one physician in order to facilitate the appropriate use of modifiers, if applicable.

Global Surgical Package Definition

CMS and most other third-party payers consider specific services to be included in the global surgical package and are, therefore, not reported separately. The services that are bundled into the surgical package include:

- Preoperative visits after the decision is made to operate beginning with the day before surgery for major procedures and the day of surgery for minor procedures
- Intra-operative services that are normally a usual and necessary part of the surgical procedure
- Complications following surgery treated during the postoperative period that do not require additional trips to the operating room. **Note:** Some payers may allow treatment of complications following surgery that do not require a return trip to the operating room separately
- Follow-up visits during the postoperative period of the surgery that are related to recovery from the surgery
- Postsurgical pain management provided by the surgeon
- Supplies except for those identified as exclusions
- Miscellaneous services including dressing changes; local incisional care; removal of operative pack; removal of cutaneous sutures and staples, lines, wires, tubes, drains, casts, and splints; insertion, irrigation, and removal of urinary catheters, routine peripheral intravenous lines, nasogastric and rectal tubes; and changes and removal of tracheostomy tubes

According to CMS, services that are NOT included in the global surgical package include:

- The initial consultation or evaluation by the surgeon that determines the need for surgery. This policy only applies to major surgical procedures. An

DEFINITIONS

debride. To remove all foreign objects and devitalized or infected tissue from a burn or wound to prevent infection and promote healing.

excision. Surgical removal of an organ or tissue.

incision. Act of cutting into tissue or an organ.

initial evaluation is always included in the allowance for a minor surgical procedure.

- Services of other providers except where the surgeon and the other provider(s) agree on the transfer of care. This agreement may be in the form of a letter or an annotation in the discharge summary, hospital record, or ASC record.

- Visits unrelated to the diagnosis for which the surgical procedure is performed, unless the visits occur due to complications of the surgery.

- Treatment for the underlying condition or an added course of treatment that is not part of normal recovery from surgery.

- Diagnostic tests and procedures, including diagnostic radiological procedures.

- Clearly distinct surgical procedures during the postoperative period (not re-operations or treatment for complications). A new postoperative period would begin with the subsequent procedure. This includes procedures done in two or more parts for which the decision to stage the procedure is made prospectively or at the time of the first procedure. Examples of this are procedures to diagnose and treat epilepsy (codes 61533–61536, 61539, 61541, and 61543), which may be performed in succession within 90 days of each other.

- Postoperative complications that require a return trip to the operating room (OR). An OR, for this purpose, is defined as a place of service specifically equipped and staffed for the sole purpose of performing procedures. The term includes a cardiac catheterization suite, a laser suite, and an endoscopy suite. It does not include a patient's room, a minor treatment room, a recovery room, or an intensive care unit (unless the patient's condition was so critical there would be insufficient time for transportation to an OR).

- If a less extensive procedure fails, and a more extensive procedure is required, the second procedure is payable separately.

- For certain services performed in a physician's office, separate payment can no longer be made for a surgical tray (code A4550). This code is assigned a Status B on the Medicare physician fee schedule and is not separately reimbursed. However, splints and casting supplies are covered and paid under the reasonable charge payment methodology.

- Immunosuppressive therapy for organ transplants.

- Critical care services (codes 99291 and 99292) unrelated to the surgery where a seriously injured or burned patient is critically ill and requires constant attendance of the physician.

While preoperative care is not specifically identified in the CPT book as included in the surgical package, most payers have strict guidelines for payment of preoperative services. Non-Medicare payers may identify a specific preoperative period (24 hours to three days) during which no additional reimbursement is made for E/M services. Medicare's global surgical package includes a one-day preoperative period.

Preoperative E/M services to establish the need for surgery are usually reimbursed separately as are services provided during the period before the decision for surgery. The visit at which the need for surgery is determined should be reported with the documented, appropriate level of E/M service and modifier 57. Medicare requires this modifier only if the visit is the day of or day prior to the surgery; other payer guidelines may vary. Reimbursement of E/M

AUDITOR'S ALERT

Staged procedures should be reported with modifier 58 Staged or related procedure or service by the same physician or other qualified healthcare professional during the postoperative period, appended to the surgical CPT code.

AUDITOR'S ALERT

Postoperative complications that require a trip to the operating room should be reported with modifier 78 Unplanned return to the operating/procedure room by the same physician or other qualified healthcare professional following initial procedure for a related procedure during the postoperative period, appended to the surgical CPT code.

© 2020 Optum360, LLC

services may be denied for care provided after the decision for surgical intervention has been made when related to the condition for which the surgery is required.

Postoperative complications (e.g., wound dehiscence, more than localized infection, or extensive bleeding resulting in a return trip to the operating room) are not included in the surgical package and are reported separately. However, it should be noted that Medicare coverage policies are to reimburse only for postoperative complications that require a return trip to the operating room. Any postoperative complications that are treated in the physician's office or treatment room at the hospital are not separately payable. An ICD-10-CM diagnosis code should be assigned to reflect the nature of the complication when billing for services rendered to treat the complication. Unrelated care is always reported. Report services unrelated to the operative problem, such as care for other diseases or injuries, with an appropriate inpatient or outpatient E/M code and modifier 24 if performed by the surgeon during the global period. Also report the corresponding diagnosis ICD-10-CM code that identifies concurrent problems other than the surgical diagnosis.

Diagnostic Procedures

Diagnostic procedures are performed to evaluate the patient's complaints or symptoms. These procedures help the provider establish the nature of the patient's disease or condition so that definitive care can be provided. Diagnostic procedures include endoscopy, arthroscopy, injection procedures, and biopsies. A diagnostic procedure is one in which the patient is still being diagnosed with consideration for possible treatment. Care related to recover from diagnostic procedures is included in the appropriate diagnostic procedure code. Ongoing care for the condition or symptoms that prompted the diagnostic procedure or other conditions is not included and may be listed separately. In other words, with completion of the diagnostic procedure, so ends the reportable postprocedure care and any further "treatment" may be reported separately. However, caution should be taken to confirm this because certain guidelines do include care and treatment for the condition following the diagnostic examination.

Therapeutic Surgical Procedures

A therapeutic procedure is one that provides a therapy or treatment for the patient's condition. Such therapy may be surgical. If complications, exacerbations, or the recurrence or presence of other conditions or injuries require additional services during the postoperative period of the original therapeutic surgical service, those services may be reported individually.

Major vs. Minor Surgical Procedures

Medicare distinguishes between major and minor surgical procedures. This is important not only because it affects billing for the decision for surgery, it also determines when a provider can start billing for care provided after surgery.

Minor and Endoscopic Surgical Procedures

According to CMS guidelines, visits by the same physician or OQHCP on the same day as a minor surgery or endoscopy are included in the payment for the procedure, unless a significant, separately identifiable service is also performed. For example, a visit on the same day could be properly billed in addition to suturing a scalp wound if a full neurological examination is made for a patient with head trauma. Billing for a visit would not be appropriate if the provider only identified the need for sutures and confirmed allergy and immunization status.

Minor surgical procedures have a postoperative period of 0 or 10 days assigned. The postoperative period for a given procedure can be located in the Physician Fee Schedule Database. When a 10-day postoperative or global period is assigned, Medicare contractors do not allow separate payment for postoperative visits or services within 10 days of the surgery when those visits are related to recovery from the procedure. However, when a diagnostic biopsy with a 10-day global period precedes a major surgery on the same day or in the 10-day period, the major surgery is payable separately.

When the minor or endoscopic surgical procedure is assigned a postoperative period of 0, any visit performed after the date of the surgery is separately billable and will be paid if all other requirements are met (i.e., medical necessity).

Major Surgical Procedures

Major surgical procedures contain a postoperative period of 90 days. The global package begins the day before the major surgical procedure. Billing guidelines for major surgical procedures permit a surgeon to bill for the decision to perform surgery as stated above. Modifier 57 Decision for surgery, must be appended to the E/M code in these instances or payment will be denied.

Generally, all services related to the surgical procedure within the 90-day global period are not billable. However, complications requiring a return trip to the operating room and, in some instances, critical care may be reported. Other exceptions are defined above.

Supplies and Materials Supplied by Physician

Many payers reimburse only for supplies that are excessive or extraordinarily expensive. Do not report supplies that are customarily included in surgical packages, such as gauze, sponges, applicators, staples, sutures, or Steri-strips. Surgical services do not include the supply of medications and sterile trays, which may be coded and billed separately. Separately list and identify drugs, trays, supplies, and materials provided with code 99070 or the appropriate HCPCS Level II supply code. These additional charges are only permitted in a nonfacility setting.

Many payers prefer or require the use of HCPCS Level II codes to report supplies. When reporting supplies to a payer, a statement for the supply should be attached to the claim form. Include a description of the supply and state the provider's cost.

Explanations of benefits should be audited on a regular basis to ensure charges for supplies are allowed and reimbursed by various payers. Note those payers that recognize HCPCS Level II codes.

Fragmentation and Unbundling

To understand unbundling and fragmentation, look at the term "bundle." A bundle is a defined set of items or services wrapped together in a group, bunch, or package. The items in the bundle can be related or unrelated, but all defined elements must be present to make a specific bundle. In medical coding,

© 2020 Optum360, LLC

unbundling pertains to surgical CPT codes and the global or package concept. Unbundling or fragmentation commonly occurs in two ways.

First, minor integral services are reported separately or in addition to a major procedure. All minor components of a procedure are not typically explicitly listed. It is sometimes difficult to determine which services are integral to a given procedure. One approach is to ask what services are normally performed with a procedure. A simple example is excision of an appendix. An incision must be made to excise an appendix and is always integral to such procedures. However, an incision is not described in the appendectomy CPT code descriptions. It is implicit—performed with every excision—and is not reported separately.

Second, unbundling occurs when a single procedure with two or more explicitly described components is broken into its component parts and reported by several CPT codes instead of the single CPT code for the combined service. A simple example of this type of unbundle is illustrated by the procedure for a combined abdominal hysterectomy with colpourethrocystopexy. Because the two components of this procedure are frequently performed together, the combined code 58152 was developed to report this service. However, each of the components may be performed separately with 58150 Abdominal hysterectomy, and 51840–51841 Vesicourethropexy. When the combined procedure is performed during a single surgical session, it must be reported with the bundled code 58152. When code 58150 is reported in conjunction with 51840 or 51841, it is considered unbundled or fragmented billing.

Unbundling, whether intentional or not, is considered by payers to be a form of fraudulent or careless billing. The rationale is simple: unbundled services frequently net higher reimbursement than the single bundled CPT code.

CMS implemented the Correct Coding Initiative (CCI) January 1, 1996. It was developed to control improper coding that leads to inappropriate and increased payment for Part B claims. The CCI was also designed to promote correct coding nationwide and assist providers in correctly coding their services for payment. The policies are based on established coding conventions, including those found in the AMA's CPT book, national and local policies and edits, coding guidelines developed by national societies, analyses of standard medical and surgical practice, and reviews of current coding practice.

An additional category of edits was added to the CCI edit file, the medically unlikely edits (MUE). They establish maximum daily allowable units of service. The edits will be applied to the services provided to the same patient, for the same CPT or HCPCS Level II code, on the same date of service when billed by the same provider. Edits are based on medically reasonable expectations and anatomical considerations.

MUE edits are released quarterly and are available on the CMS website at: http://www.cms.gov/Medicare/Coding/NationalCorrectCodInitEd/MUE.html. Edits can be determined when providers review the Medicare remittance advice.

Assistants at Surgery

The names of all surgeons involved with any procedure should always be listed, including the primary surgeon and any co- or assistant surgeons. For surgical procedures involving more than one surgeon, the primary surgeon is responsible for dictating the procedural note. In the teaching environment, a resident, intern, or assistant may dictate the note but the primary surgeon must indicate agreement by reading and signing off on it with a teaching addendum. That verifies that the teaching physician performed the critical or key portion(s) of the service and that he/she was directly involved in the management of the patient.

Co-surgeons, usually called in to manage a particular area of expertise, have shared responsibility in the procedure and must record their involvement. On the other hand, assistant surgeons only provide assistance when asked and needed. They do not have specific responsibilities during the surgery and do not dictate any part of the operative note.

Documentation must clearly support the need and medical necessity of involving a co-surgeon or assistant surgeon. Medicare regulations state that payment will only be made for assistant-at-surgery procedures when a physician is used as an assistant at surgery in more than 5 percent of cases nationally. Medicare determines this through manual reviews.

CPT modifiers 80 Assistant surgeon, 81 Minimum assistant surgeon, and 82 Assistant surgeon (when qualified resident surgeon not available), as well as any procedures submitted with modifier AS Physician assistant, nurse practitioner, or clinical nurse specialist services for assistant at surgery, are subject to Medicare's assistant surgeon policy as indicated in the Medicare Physician Fee Schedule Database (MPFSDB).

Medicare reimbursement for assistant-at-surgery services performed by a physician is 16 percent of the global surgery payment. Physicians may not bill a Medicare patient for assistant-at-surgery services when that procedure is subject to the assistant-at-surgery limit.

More information on modifiers can be found in chapter 3.

Separate Procedures

There are some procedures within the CPT coding system that have the designation of "separate procedure." Medicare and many other payers interpret this designation to prohibit the reporting of a separate procedure when it is performed at the same surgical session as a related procedure, i.e., with another procedure that is anatomically related (approached through the same incision, orifice, or surgical approach).

However, according to the Correct Coding Initiative, any procedure containing the separate procedure designation may be reported separately when performed at a different encounter (including two encounters on the same date of service) or are unrelated, often requiring a separate skin incision, orifice, or other surgical approach. In these instances, modifier 59, the appropriate X{EPSU} modifier, or another more specific modifier such as an anatomic modifier should be appended to the code reporting the separate procedure.

Multiple Procedures

Multiple surgical procedures may be performed at the same operative session. When multiple codes are needed to report all of the services rendered, the primary procedure (i.e., the procedure with the higher relative value) is sequenced first on the claim and reported without a modifier. The additional procedures are listed next in ascending order based upon relative value units and may require modifier 51 to indicate that additional services were performed at the same session. An exception would be add-on codes which should be reported immediately following the parent code with no modifier appended. It is inappropriate to assign modifier 51 to an E/M service. Clear documentation in the operative report should accompany the claim to ensure appropriate payment consideration.

Most payers have multiple payment reduction policies and apply the reductions to the second and subsequent procedures. However, the CPT book does exempt certain codes from the modifier 51 (multiple procedure) policy. These codes are identified in the CPT book with the ⊘. Modifier 51 is not to be appended to add-on codes (discussed below) or those identified as modifier 51 exempt. The exempt codes are identified in appendix E of the CPT code book.

Add-on Codes

Add-on codes permit the reporting of significant supplemental services commonly performed in addition to the primary procedure. Add-on codes can never be billed alone and must always be reported with another CPT code. The add-on code always has notes following the code description to indicate the specific range of codes to which it applies. In all cases, the code will state, "List separately in addition to code for primary procedure." The multiple procedure modifier 51 should not be appended to add-on codes, and the multiple procedure payment reduction does not apply to add-on codes. Report bilateral add-on procedures as two separate line items. Do not report modifier 50 with bilateral add-on procedure codes. Designated add-on codes are identified in Appendix D of the CPT book. Please reference CPT 2021 for the most current list of add-on codes.

Moderate (Conscious) Sedation

When it is medically necessary, moderate (conscious) sedation may be reported when provided by the performing physician with 99151–99153; when provided by another physician, report 99155–99157. However, other anesthesia services (CPT codes 00100–01999) may be billed separately when performed by a physician (or other qualified provider) other than the physician performing the procedure.

Unlisted Procedures

Another important area to audit in surgical coding is unlisted procedures. Not all medical services or procedures are assigned CPT codes. Each code section contains one or more codes that have been set aside specifically for reporting unlisted procedures. The guidelines at the beginning of each section, as well as in sequence among the codes, contain unlisted procedure codes.

The CPT book should be reviewed carefully before choosing an unlisted procedure code to ensure that a more specific code is not available. HCPCS Level II or Category III codes should be reported for Medicare and other providers when available. Carriers generally require additional documentation or report (e.g., progress notes, operative report, consultation report, or history and physical) before considering claims with unlisted procedure codes. The documentation should be precise and contain pertinent information including a description of the procedure, the extent and need for the procedure, as well as the effort, time, and equipment used. The claim should have a letter attached explaining the reasoning behind the fee (e.g., was it compared to a similar procedure and how was it different?).

Modifiers for Surgical Procedures

In order to correctly report all of the necessary details regarding a surgical procedure, it is often necessary to append a modifier to the surgical procedure code. A modifier is necessary to indicate that the procedure was altered in some way (e.g., that only a portion of the global surgical package was provided, that a procedure was discontinued, etc.). When auditing surgical claims, strict attention to any modifier requirements should be maintained.

The following modifiers apply to surgical procedures:

22	Increased procedural services
26	Professional component
32	Mandated services
33	Preventive service
47	Anesthesia by surgeon
50	Bilateral procedure
51	Multiple procedures
52	Reduced services
53	Discontinued procedure
54	Surgical care only
55	Postoperative management only
56	Preoperative management only
57	Decision for surgery
58	Staged or related procedure or service by the same physician or other qualified health care professional during the postoperative period
59	Distinct procedural service
62	Two surgeons
63	Procedure performed on infants less than 4kg
66	Surgical team
76	Repeat procedure or service by same physician or other qualified health care professional

 © 2020 Optum360, LLC

77	Repeat procedure by another physician or other qualified health care professional
78	Unplanned return to the operating/procedure room by the same physician or other qualified health care professional following initial procedure for a related procedure during the postoperative period
79	Unrelated procedure or service by the same physician or other qualified health cae professional during the postoperative period
80	Assistant surgeon
81	Minimum assistant surgeon
82	Assistant surgeon (when qualified resident surgeon not available)
99	Multiple modifiers
LT	Left side
RT	Right side

For more information regarding the use of modifiers, see chapter 3.

Procedures Performed on the Integumentary System

The integumentary section includes codes for procedures performed on the skin, nails, and breasts, including repair of lacerations, excision and destruction of lesions, removal of subcutaneous contraceptive devices, grafts, treatment of decubitus ulcers, breast surgeries, and reconstruction.

The type of treatment rendered (e.g., destruction, excision, incision) should be determined along with the anatomical location and, when appropriate, size of the lesion or repair.

The following is a discussion of some of the more difficult areas in this section that an auditor may want to consider in a review.

DEFINITIONS

dermis. Skin layer found under the epidermis that contains a papillary upper layer and the deep reticular layer of collagen, vascular bed, and nerves.

epidermis. Outermost, nonvascular layer of skin that contains four to five differentiated layers depending on its body location: stratum corneum, lucidum, granulosum, spinosum, and basale.

General Procedures Performed

This section contains the CPT code for fine needle aspiration (FNA) biopsies. Correct code assignment is dependent upon whether guidance imaging was used and, if so, the type of guidance utilized.

Fine Needle Aspiration (FNA) Biopsies (10004–10021)

A fine needle aspiration (FNA) biopsy is the aspiration of a suspected lesion using a fine needle. The cytological examination of the cells is reported using the appropriate code from the Laboratory and Pathology section of the CPT book.

Fine needle aspiration biopsy procedures 10004–10012 and 10021 are reported once *per lesion* sampled in a single session. A FNA biopsy may be performed with or without imaging guidance. Imaging codes 76942, 77002, 77012, and 77021 may not be reported with 10004–10012 and 10021 when performed with imaging guidance. However, in the instance when more than one FNA biopsy is performed on separate lesions during the same session and using the same imaging modality, the appropriate imaging modality add-on code for the second and subsequent lesion(s) may be reported. Furthermore, when more than one FNA biopsy is performed on separate lesions during the same session but using different imaging modalities, report the appropriate primary code with modifier 59 for each additional imaging modality and corresponding add-on codes for subsequent lesions biopsied. According to the AMA, this instruction applies irrespective of whether the lesions are ipsilateral (unilateral) or contralateral (bilateral) to each other, and/or if they are in the same or different organs/structures.

Procedure Differentiation

FNA is a diagnostic percutaneous procedure that uses a fine gauge needle (often 22 or 25 gauge), and a syringe to sample fluid from a cyst or remove clusters of cells from a solid mass. If a lump can be felt, the radiologist or surgeon guides a needle into the area by palpating the lump. If the lump is nonpalpable, the FNA procedure is performed using ultrasound, fluoroscopy, computed tomography (CT), or MR imaging with the patient positioned according to the area of concern.

Report 10021 for fine needle aspiration of the initial lesion performed without imaging guidance; for each subsequent lesion, report 10004. Each modality is differentiated by a code for the first lesion and another for each additional lesion biopsied.

Ultrasound-guided aspiration biopsy (10005–10006) involves inserting an aspiration catheter needle device through the accessory channel port of the echoendoscope; the needle is placed into the area to be sampled under endoscopic ultrasonographic guidance. After the needle is placed into the region of the lesion, a vacuum is created and multiple in and out needle motions are performed. Several needle insertions are usually required to ensure that an adequate tissue sample is taken.

In fluoroscopic guidance (10007–10008), intermittent fluoroscopy guides the advancement of the needle. CT image guidance (10009–10010) allows computer-assisted targeting of the area to be sampled. At the completion of the procedure, the needle is withdrawn and a small bandage is placed over the area.

MR image guidance (10011–10012) involves the use of a magnetic field, radio waves and computer-assisted targeting to identify the area for biopsy without the use of ionizing radiation.

Key Documentation Terms

Documentation should indicate the type of modality used, the location of the biopsy and whether subsequent biopsies are performed. Terms include ultrasound guidance, fluoroscopic guidance, MR image guidance, or without guidance, provide the needed information to ensure correct code assignment.

Coding Tips
- Local infiltration, digital blocks, or topical anesthesia are usually considered an integral part of the FNA and are not reported separately.
- When both an FNA and core needle biopsy are both performed on the same lesion during the same session and using the same type of imaging guidance, do not separately report the imaging guidance for the core needle biopsy.

- When documentation indicates that during the same surgical session a FNA biopsy is performed on one lesion and a core needle biopsy is performed on a separate lesion using the same type of imaging guidance, both the core needle biopsy and the appropriate imaging guidance code for the core needle biopsy may be reported separately with modifier 59.

- When a FNA biopsy is performed on one lesion using imaging and a core needle biopsy is performed during the same surgical encounter on a separate lesion using a different type of guidance imaging, the core needle biopsy and the imaging guidance for the core needle biopsy may be reported with modifier 59.

- Codes 10004, 10006, 10008, 10010, and 10012 are used to report each additional lesion a FNA was performed on during the same session. The same type of guidance imaging is required.

- As "add-on" codes, 10004, 10006, 10008, 10010, and 10012 are not subject to multiple procedure rules. No reimbursement reduction or modifier 51 is applied. The following table provides additional information for these codes as found in the Medicare Physician Fee Schedule Database.

Parent Code	Add-On	GLOB DAYS	MULT PROC	BILAT SURG	ASST SURG	CO-SURG	TEAM SURG
	10004	ZZZ	0	0	0	0	0
10005		XXX	2	0	0	0	0
	10006	ZZZ	0	0	0	0	0
10007		XXX	2	0	0	0	0
	10008	ZZZ	0	0	0	0	0
10009		XXX	2	0	0	0	0
	10010	ZZZ	0	0	0	0	0
10011		XXX	2	0	0	0	0
	10012	ZZZ	0	0	0	0	0
10021		XXX	2	0	0	0	0

Debridement Procedures (11000–11047)

When auditing encounters in which debridement (11000–11047) was performed, pay close attention to the code descriptions as they are differentiated by the type of debridement, as well as the amount of tissue debrided.

Note: The debridement codes report services that describe the deepest level of tissue removed. If debridement of the skin, epidermis, and/or dermis only is performed, the service would be reported with active wound care management codes 97597 and 97598.

Procedure Differentiation

When reporting debridement of a single wound, the deepest level of tissue removed determines the correct code. The debridement of multiple wounds at the same tissue level may be added together to determine the appropriate code. Different tissue depths should not be added together for code selection.

Codes 11000 and 11001 describe the debridement of *extensive* eczematous or infected skin and are reported based on the percentage of body surface. The key word in this section is extensive. Documentation must specifically indicate the percentage of body surface that was debrided.

DEFINITIONS

devitalized. Deprivation of vital necessities or of life itself.

dislocation. Displacement of a bone in relation to its neighboring tissue, especially a joint.

eczema. Inflammatory form of dermatitis with red, itchy breakouts of exudative vesicles that leads to crusting and scaling that occurs as a reaction to internal or external agents.

fascia. Fibrous sheet or band of tissue that envelops organs, muscles, and groupings of muscles.

gangrene. Death of tissue, usually resulting from a loss of vascular supply, followed by a bacterial attack or onset of disease.

necrotic. Pathological condition of death occurring in a group of cells or tissues within a living part or organism.

open fractures. Exposed break in a bone, always considered compound due to its high risk of infection from the open wound leading to the fracture. Broken bone ends may protrude through the skin and contaminants or foreign bodies are often embedded in the tissues.

osteomyelitis. Inflammation of bone that may remain localized or spread to the marrow, cortex, or periosteum, in response to an infecting organism, usually bacterial and pyogenic.

pemphigus vulgaris. Most common, severe form of a group of chronic, relapsing skin diseases that may become fatal. Beginning around age 40, easily ruptured bullae appear on otherwise normal skin and mucous membranes, spreading more generally and becoming large, open, weeping areas with some crusting, but no tendency to heal. The affected areas may cause sepsis, electrolyte imbalances, or cachexia and become fatal.

subcutaneous tissue. Sheet or wide band of adipose (fat) and areolar connective tissue in two layers attached to the dermis.

ulcer. Open sore or excavating lesion of skin or the tissue on the surface of an organ from the sloughing of chronically inflamed and necrosing tissue.

Codes 11004–11006 for debridement of necrotizing skin, subcutaneous tissue, muscle, and fascia are also differentiated by area treated. Code 11004 is reported for the external genital and perineum; 11005 reports the abdominal wall; and 11006 is a combination code and reports external genital, perineum, and the abdominal wall. It would be inappropriate to report 11004 in conjunction with 11005 during the same operative setting. Code 11008 is an add-on code that describes the removal of mesh or prosthetic material due to an abdominal wall infection.

Medical Necessity

The following conditions may warrant extensive debridement (this list is not all inclusive):

- Actinomycotic infections
- Autoimmune skin diseases (such as pemphigus)
- Extensive skin trauma
- Pyoderma gangrenosum
- Rapidly spreading necrotizing process (e.g., aggressive streptococcal infections)
- Severe eczema

Key Documentation Terms

The key terms for these procedures include eczematous or infected. Documentation for these procedures should include the indications for the procedure and narrative that describes the wound and details the debridement procedure. The record should also include the presence and extent of necrotic, devitalized, or nonviable tissue and the percentage of the body surface debrided. It is crucial to document the specific type of disease; for instance, there are many types of eczema (e.g., allergic, irritant, cutaneous). With I-10 documentation, it is very important to provide enough information to code the diagnosis to the highest specificity.

Procedure Differentiation

Codes from range 11010–11012 apply to debridement associated with open fractures or dislocations. The code choice depends on the depth of debridement.

Key Documentation Terms

Documentation should indicate the surgical procedure that was performed. Terms such as open fracture, open dislocation, bone, fascia, muscle, skin, and subcutaneous provide the guidance needed to ensure correct code assignment. Above all else the documentation should support the medical necessity of the procedure.

Procedure Differentiation

Codes 11042–11047 describe debridement of the subcutaneous tissues, muscle, and/or fascia and bone. The codes are further classified by add-on codes for each additional 20 square centimeters treated.

Medical Necessity

The following conditions may warrant debridement (this list is not all-inclusive):

- Gangrene
- Injuries resulting in deep-seated debris

- Necrotizing fasciitis
- Nonhealing surgical wound
- Osteomyelitis
- Skin ulcers

Key Documentation Terms

When debridement is reported, the debridement documentation should include which tissue was removed. Key terms should include skin, full or partial thickness, subcutaneous tissue, and muscle and/or bone; the method used (i.e., hydrostatic, sharp, abrasion, etc.); and the condition of the wound before and after debridement (including dimensions, description of necrotic material present, description of tissue removed, degree of epithelialization, etc.). In addition, the patient's response to wound treatment at each visit should also be included. The documentation should reflect the depth of the wound and the size of the area debrided. When documenting the diagnosis, be specific in the type of osteomyelitis (e.g., chronic, due to another disease). Also note that there are many types of skin ulcers and they can occur in many locations, making documentation specificity crucial when coding accurately.

Coding Tips

- Local infiltration, digital blocks, or topical anesthesia are an integral part of debridement and are not reported separately.
- As "add-on" codes, 11001, 11008, and 11045-11047 are not subject to multiple procedure rules. No reimbursement reduction or modifier 51 is applied. The table below identifies the appropriate add-on code. The following table provides additional information for these codes as found in the Medicare Physician Fee Schedule Database.

Parent Code	Add-On	GLOB DAYS	MULT PROC	BILAT SURG	ASST SURG	CO-SURG	TEAM SURG
10180		010	2	0	1	0	0
11000		000	2	0	1	0	0
	11001	ZZZ	0	0	1	0	0
11004		000	2	0	1	0	0
11005		000	0	0	0	0	0
11006		000	2	0	1	0	0
	11008	ZZZ	0	0	0	0	0
11042		000	2	0	1	0	0
11043		000	2	0	1	0	0
11044		000	2	0	1	0	0
	11045	ZZZ	0	0	0	0	0
	11046	ZZZ	0	0	0	0	0
	11047	ZZZ	0	0	0	0	0

Coding Traps

- Do not report 11042-11047 in conjunction with active wound care management codes when performed on the same wound during the same operative session.
- Do not report these codes for debridement of burns; see 16020–16030.

Excision of Benign Hypertrophic Skin Lesions (11055–11057)

In order for these codes to be supported, medical record documentation must indicate that the provider removed tissue by the cutting away of the edge or surface of a lesion, such as corns and callosities. A hyperkeratotic lesion refers to overgrowth of skin. Report only one code from this series based on the number of lesions removed.

Medical Necessity

The lesion that is removed must be symptomatic; otherwise, they are considered to have been removed for cosmetic purposes and, therefore, not medically necessary.

The following conditions may warrant these procedures (this list is not all inclusive):

- Inflammation (e.g., purulence, oozing, edema, erythema, etc.)
- Lesion is located in an area that is subject to recurrent physical trauma and there is documentation that such trauma has in fact occurred.
- Lesion obstructs an orifice or restricts vision
- Questionable diagnosis; in particular when the lesion may be malignant based on lesion appearance, strong family history of melanoma, dysplastic nevus syndrome, or prior melanoma
- Symptoms and/or signs include, but are not limited to, bleeding, burning, irritation, itching, or significant change in color or size

It should be noted that Medicare generally excludes these services and includes them under routine foot care services. However, there are specific indications or exceptions under which Medicare provides benefits. These include:

- Routine foot care when the patient has a systemic disease, such as metabolic, neurologic, or peripheral vascular disease, of sufficient severity that performance of such services by a nonprofessional person would put the patient at risk (e.g., a systemic condition that has resulted in severe circulatory embarrassment or areas of desensitization in the patient's legs or feet).
- Treatment of warts on foot is covered to the same extent as services provided for the treatment of warts located elsewhere on the body.
- Services normally considered routine may be covered if they are performed as a necessary and integral part of otherwise covered services, such as diagnosis and treatment of ulcers, wounds, or infections.
- Treatment of mycotic nails may be covered under the exceptions to the routine foot care exclusion. An ambulatory patient is covered only when the provider documents that:
  - there is clinical evidence of mycosis of the toenail
  - the patient has marked limitation of ambulation, pain, or secondary infection resulting from the thickening and dystrophy of the infected toenail plate

A nonambulatory patient is covered only when the provider documents that:

  - There is clinical evidence of mycosis of the toenail
  - The patient suffers from pain or secondary infection resulting from the thickening and dystrophy of the infected toenail plate

Key Documentation Terms

Medical records must clearly document the medical necessity for lesion removal(s). Documentation must contain a written description of each surgically treated lesion in terms of location and physical characteristics. The description should support a suspicion of malignancy, if present. Although not required for coding, the size of the lesion should also be noted. Key terms may include benign, corn, callus, or malignant.

Coding Trap

- When this procedure is performed for cosmetic reasons it will be deemed not medically necessary and denied coverage.

Surgical Biopsy of Skin, Subcutaneous Tissue, and Mucous Membranes (11102–11107)

Codes within the 11102–11107 range are used to report the removal of tissue for pathological examination. When performed at the time of a more extensive procedure, the biopsy is only reported when carried out for the immediate pathological diagnosis that resulted in the decision to proceed with the more extensive procedure, e.g., when a frozen section of a lesion is performed and, because of the pathological interpretation, a lesion is excised. However, if a suspected skin cancer is biopsied for pathologic diagnosis prior to proceeding with Mohs micrographic surgery (17311-17315), the biopsy (11102-11107) and frozen section pathology (88331) may be reported separately. When reporting biopsies separately, CMS requires that modifier 58 be reported to indicate that the biopsy and the more extensive procedure were planned or staged procedures. Documentation must clearly indicate that the biopsy was used for determining that the more extensive procedure was necessary. There are times when a single lesion may have to be biopsied multiple times due to the size, location, or preoperative diagnosis. In this situation, the appropriate code for the biopsy is only reported once with "1" for the unit. When biopsies of multiple lesions of the same kind are obtained, the appropriate add-on code may be reported for EACH lesion.

Partial-thickness biopsies are those that sample a portion of the thickness of skin or mucous membrane and do not penetrate below the dermis or lamina propria. Full- thickness biopsies enter the deep tissue to include the dermis or lamina propria, and the subcutaneous or submucosal space. A biopsy of stratum corneum only, by any modality, does not qualify as a skin biopsy and is not reported separately.

Procedure Differentiation

Correct code assignment is dependent upon the type of biopsy performed.

Codes 11102–11103 describe the tangential technique which is a biopsy performed via a sharp blade to obtain a superficial, epidermal tissue specimen that may or may not include sections of underlying dermis and does not involve a full-thickness biopsy. Report 11102 for the initial lesion; each additional lesion should be reported with 11103.

A punch biopsy (11104–11105) involves the use of a specific punch tool to obtain a full-thickness, barrel-shaped or columnar shaped specimen and is usually performed to collect a sample of a cutaneous lesion for diagnostic pathologic examination. Simple closure including manipulation of the biopsy defect is included in the service and should not be reported separately. Report 11104 for the initial lesion; each additional lesion should be reported with 11105.

Documentation for an incisional biopsy (11106–11107) should describe a biopsy utilizing a scalpel to remove a full-thickness sample of tissue via a vertical incision or wedge. This technique type may involve specimens of subcutaneous fat. Closure of an incisional biopsy, other than simple closure, is reported separately. This type of biopsy is usually performed to obtain a full- thickness tissue sample of a skin lesion for the purpose of diagnostic pathologic examination. Incisional biopsies usually require closure and include simple closure. Report 11106 for the initial lesion; each additional lesion should be reported with 11107.

Multiple Biopsies

When multiple biopsy techniques are performed during the same encounter, only one primary lesion biopsy code is reported.

When two or more biopsies of the same technique (e.g., tangential, punch, or incisional) are performed on separate lesions, use the appropriate add-on code identifying the type of biopsy (11103, 11105, 11107) to specify each additional biopsy. When two or three different biopsy techniques (i.e., tangential, punch, or incisional) are performed to biopsy separate lesions, select the appropriate biopsy code (11102, 11104, 11106) for the first lesion and an additional add-on code (11103, 11105, 11107) for each additional biopsy performed. Additional biopsy codes should be selected based on the following guidelines:

- When multiple biopsies of the same type are performed, the primary code for that biopsy should be used along with the corresponding add-on code(s).

- When an incisional biopsy is performed, report 11106 and the appropriate add-on code for the additional biopsy procedure(s) (i.e., tangential [11103], punch [11105], or incisional biopsy [11107]).

- When a punch biopsy is performed with a tangential or punch biopsy, report 11104 as the primary procedure and the add-on codes for tangential (11103), or punch (11105), for the additional biopsy procedures.

The following table provides an illustration of the appropriate use of these codes for multiple biopsies:

Procedures Performed	CPT Code(s) Reported
tangential biopsies x 2	11102 X 1, 11103 X 1
punch biopsies x 3	11104 X 1, 11105 X 2
incisional biopsies x 2	11106 X 1, 11107 X 1
1 incisional biopsy, 1 tangential biopsy and 1 punch biopsy	11106 X 1, 11103 X 1, 11105 X 1
1 punch biopsy and 2 tangential biopsies	11104 X 1, 11103 X 2

Medical Necessity

Multiple indications for these services exist for them to be performed; verify coverage with the payer.

Key Documentation Terms

Medical record documentation must indicate that a section of the lesion was removed for the sole purpose of examination and not as a means of removing the entire lesion. Key terms include single or multiple lesions as well as the type of biopsy performed.

A common documentation error is one in which the provider fails to document the exact number of lesions biopsied when performed on more than one lesion. When this occurs, the claim should indicate only the number of lesions clearly documented or, in some cases, only one lesion. Provider education should be performed to prevent this from occurring.

Coding Tips

- As "add-on" codes, 11103, 11105, and 11107 are not subject to multiple procedure rules. No reimbursement reduction or modifier 51 is applied. The following table provides additional information for these codes as found in the Medicare Physician Fee Schedule Database.

Parent Code	Add-On	GLOB DAYS	MULT PROC	BILAT SURG	ASST SURG	CO-SURG	TEAM SURG
11102		000	2	0	1	0	0
	11103	ZZZ	0	0	1	0	0
11104		000	2	0	1	0	0
	11105	ZZZ	0	0	1	0	0
11106		000	2	0	1	0	0
	11107	ZZZ	0	0	1	0	0

- To report the removal of a lesion by shave technique, see 11300–11313.
- To report the complete removal of a lesion in toto (including margins), see 11400–11646.
- To report the biopsy of the lip see, 40490.
- To report the biopsy of the vestibule of mouth, see 40808.
- To report the biopsy of a nail unit, see 11755.

Skin Lesion Removal: Shaving (11300–11313)

These codes are used to report the sharp removal of epidermal or dermal lesions by a transverse or horizontal slicing method (shaving).

Procedure Differentiation

Appropriate code selection is determined by the location and size of the lesion. Shaving is a method of removal that would not require a suture closure. The codes include chemical or electrocauterization. When measuring the size of the lesion, the borders around the area are not considered part of the lesion diameter.

Medical Necessity

The following conditions may warrant these procedures (this list is not all inclusive):

- Actinic keratosis
- Inflamed seborrheic keratosis
- Molluscum contagiosum
- Viral and plantar warts

Key Documentation Terms

Terms such as dermal, epidermal, and shaving provide the guidance needed to ensure correct code assignment. Documentation for these procedures must indicate that the provider removed a single, elevated epidermal or dermal lesion

 DEFINITIONS

actinic keratosis. Flat, scaly precancerous lesions appearing on dry, sun-aged, and overexposed skin, including the eyelids.

seborrheic keratosis. Common, benign, noninvasive, lightly pigmented, warty growth composed of basaloid cells that usually appear at middle age as soft, easily crumbling plaques on the face, trunk, and extremities.

by placing a scalpel blade against the skin, adjacent to the lesion, and, using a horizontal slicing motion, excised the lesion from its base. When a lesion is removed by this method, the wound does not require suturing and bleeding is controlled by chemical or electrical cauterization. Correct reporting of the procedure involves knowing the size and anatomical location of the lesion.

Coding Tips

- The removal of skin tags by shaving should not be reported with a code from this range, see 11200–11201.

- Chemical or electrical cauterization of the wound is included in these services.

- If a specimen is transported to an outside laboratory, report 99000 for handling or conveyance.

Skin Lesion Removal (11400–11646)

Codes for the excision of skin lesions include:

- Biopsy of same lesion

- Full thickness removal including margins

- Lesion measurement before excision at largest diameter plus margin

- Local anesthesia

- Simple, nonlayered closure

Measurements must be precise because being off by just one millimeter can result in the selection of an incorrect code. When more than one dimension of a lesion is provided, indicate the largest side. For example, if the dimensions are described as 2 x 1.2 x 0.5 cm, the lesion should be listed as 2 cm.

In order to determine if the excision of a lesion was reported appropriately, the following information must be extrapolated from the medical record documentation:

- Morphology (benign or malignant)

- Size of the lesion

- Size of margins

- Anatomical site.

Procedure Differentiation

Codes 11400–11446 report excision of benign lesions. Codes 11600–11646 report excision of malignant lesions. The appropriate code is reported according to anatomical site and size of the lesion, including margins.

Codes 11450–11471 report excisions of skin and subcutaneous tissue for hidradenitis. The appropriate code is reported according to anatomical site and whether a complex repair is necessary.

Medical Necessity

The following conditions may warrant excision of a **benign** lesion (this list is not all inclusive):

- Hemangioma

- Keloid scar

- Lipoma

- Lymphangioma
- Molluscum contagiosum
- Plantar or viral wart

The following conditions may warrant excision of a **malignant** lesion (this list is not all inclusive):

- Basal cell carcinoma
- Malignant melanoma
- Other malignant lesions of the skin
- Squamous cell carcinoma

Key Documentation Terms

Documentation should indicate the surgical procedure that was performed. Terms that describe an anatomical location and morphology (benign or malignant) provide the guidance needed to ensure correct code assignment. Above all else, the documentation should support the medical necessity of the procedure.

Documentation for these procedures should include the indications for the procedure and the narrative of the procedure that describes the excision, including anatomical site, morphology, size of the lesion, and size of margins.

Coding Tips

- When a biopsy is performed as part of a lesion removal, the biopsy is a component of the overall procedure and is not reported separately.

- After lesion excision, the defect may require simple, intermediate, or complex closure and, in unusual circumstances, tissue transfer procedures. Bandaging, strip closure, or simple closure is considered to be a component of the excision and should not be reported separately. Intermediate, complex, or other types of complicated repair services must be thoroughly documented in the medical record to be reported separately.

- When a malignant lesion has been excised and a re-excision is performed to ensure that the entire lesion has been removed, the malignant lesion excision code is assigned to the second procedure, even though the pathology report may indicate no further evidence of malignancy at the margins. According to the AMA, because the patient had a previous malignancy at this site, the procedure should be coded as excision of a malignancy.

- Removal of a lesion from a previous mastectomy site would be assigned to the anatomic site "trunk," not "breast," since the breast is no longer present.

- For destruction of premalignant lesions, by any method, including laser, see 17000–17004; benign, see 17106–17111.

- For excision of a cicatricial lesion that is full thickness, see 11400-11406.

- For removal of skin tags, see 11200–11201.

- For destruction of extensive cutaneous neurofibroma lesions, see 0419T for more than 50 lesions of the face, head, and neck and 0420T for more than 100 lesions of the trunk and extremities.

DEFINITIONS

curettage. Removal of tissue by scraping.

distal. Located farther away from a specified reference point or the trunk.

frostbite. Damage to skin, subcutaneous, and possibly deeper tissue caused by exposure to low temperatures, resulting in ischemia, thrombosis, even gangrene, and the loss of affected body parts.

onychauxis. Congenital condition in which the nails are hypertrophied.

Nail Trimming (11719)

Code 11719 describes fingernail or toenail trimming, usually with scissors, nail cutters, or other instruments. This code is reported when the nails are not defective from nutritional or metabolic abnormalities and can be used for one or more nails.

Coding Tips

- This code is reported only once regardless of the number of nails that are trimmed.

- Some non-Medicare payers may require that HCPCS Level II code S0390 be reported for this service when provided as routine foot care or as preventive maintenance in specific medical conditions.

- For diabetic patients with diabetic sensory neuropathy resulting in a loss of protective sensation (LOPS), see G0247.

- For trimming of nondystrophic nails, see 11719. For trimming of dystrophic nails, see G0127.

Debridement (11720–11721)

Procedure Differentiation

Codes from range 11720–11721 are reported for debridement of finger or toenails, including tops and exposed undersides, by any method. The cleaning is performed manually with cleaning solutions, abrasive materials, and tools. The nails are shortened and shaped. For one to five nails, see 11720; six or more nails, see 11721.

Medical Necessity

The following conditions may warrant nail debridement (this list is not all inclusive):

- Crushing injury
- Frostbite
- Infection
- Ingrown toenail
- Mycosis of the toenail
- Onychauxis
- Onychogryphosis

Coding Tip

- Correct Coding Initiative (CCI) edits prohibit separate reporting of code 11720 Nail debridement by any method, one to five nails, with code 11719 Trimming of nondystrophic nails. This edit is often bypassed by using modifier 59. According to CMS, the use of modifier 59 to bypass this edit is only appropriate when the trimming and debridement of the nails are performed on different nails or if the two procedures are performed at separate patient encounters.

- Correct Coding Initiative (CCI) edits prohibit reporting codes 11055-11057 for removal of hyperkeratotic skin on the same digit a nail is also debrided (11720-11721).

Nail Avulsion/Excision/Evacuation/Biopsy (11730–11765)

Procedure Differentiation

Codes 11730–11732 for nail avulsion involve the forcible separation and removal of a portion of, or the entire nail from, the nail bed matrix using other than topical anesthesia. Simple cutting of a portion of the toenail distal to the eponychium, without injected local anesthesia, should be considered routine foot care and not reported as nail avulsion.

Code 11740 is reported when blood from a hematoma located beneath a fingernail or toenail is drained. The nail plate is pierced using an electrocautery tool or large gauged needle creating a large enough opening to allow the hematoma to drain.

Code 11750 (nail excision) involves the performance of standard techniques for the removal of a portion of the nail or the entire nail. The nail plate is bluntly dissected and lifted away from the nail bed. The nail plate is detached from the matrix using a scalpel. The matrix is destroyed using chemical ablation, CO_2 laser, or electrocautery. The procedure code applies to one or both sides of the nail or entire nail (sides of the same nail should not be reported separately).

Code 11755 is reported when a portion of the nail unit is removed for biopsy. Sections may be taken from the hard nail itself, the nail bed, lateral skin, or underlying soft tissue. The specimen may be excised by clippers or with a scalpel.

Code 11760 is used to report the repair of the nail bed. The removal of the nail is considered part of the service and is not reported separately. The physician may place the nail back onto the bed to act as a stent. Code 11762 is used when the physician uses a graft to reconstruct part of the nail bed.

Code 11765 Wedge excision of skin of nail fold, should be assigned when a Winograd or Frost nail surgery is performed and documented in the medical record.

Medical Necessity

The following conditions may warrant the above procedures (11730–11765) (this list is not all inclusive):

- Cellulitis
- Dermatophytosis of nail (onychomycosis)
- Felon
- Hemangioma
- Infection
- Onychia and paronychia
- Other specified disease of nail (dystrophia unguium, dystrophic nail)

It should be noted that Medicare generally excludes these services and includes them under routine foot care services. However, there are specific indications or exceptions under which Medicare provides benefits. These include:

- Routine foot care when the patient has a systemic disease, such as metabolic, neurologic, or peripheral vascular disease, of sufficient severity that performance of such services by a nonprofessional person would put the patient at risk (e.g., a systemic condition that has resulted in severe circulatory embarrassment or areas of desensitization in the patient's legs or feet).

 DEFINITIONS

dermatophytosis. Superficial parasitic fungal infections occurring in the skin, hair, or nails that involve the corneal stratum, or outermost layer of cells, commonly referring to as ringworm and athlete's foot.

eponychium. Thin layer of epidermis or skin found at the proximal portion and sides of the nail or the cuticle.

felon. Painful abscess on the palmar side of a distal fingertip, usually occurring after inoculation of a disease-causing microorganism, such as *Staphylococcus aureus* in the closed space of the terminal phalanx.

onychia. Inflammation or infection of the nail matrix leading to a loss of the nail.

paronychia. Infection or cellulitis of nail structures.

- Treatment of warts on foot is covered to the same extent as services provided for the treatment of warts located elsewhere on the body.
- Services normally considered routine may be covered if they are performed as a necessary and integral part of otherwise covered services, such as diagnosis and treatment of ulcers, wounds, or infections.
- Treatment of mycotic nails may be covered under the exceptions to the routine foot care exclusion. An ambulatory patient is covered only when the provider documents that:
  - there is clinical evidence of mycosis of the toenail
  - the patient has marked limitation of ambulation, pain, or secondary infection resulting from the thickening and dystrophy of the infected toenail plate

A nonambulatory patient is covered only when the provider documents that:

  - there is clinical evidence of mycosis of the toenail
  - the patient suffers from pain or secondary infection resulting from the thickening and dystrophy of the infected toenail plate

Key Documentation Terms

Documentation should indicate the surgical procedure that was performed. Terms such as avulsion, biopsy, excision, evacuation, and removal provide the guidance needed to ensure correct code assignment. Above all else, documentation should support the medical necessity of the procedure.

Coding Tip

- As an add-on code, 11732 is not subject to multiple procedure rules. No reimbursement reduction or modifier 51 is applied. The following table provides additional information for these codes as found in the Medicare Physician Fee Schedule Database.

Parent Code	Add-On	GLOB DAYS	MULT PROC	BILAT SURG	ASST SURG	CO-SURG	TEAM SURG
11730		000	2	0	1	0	0
	11732	ZZZ	0	0	1	0	0

Suturing of Wounds (12001–13160)

Code selection depends on the anatomic site, length of the wound (in centimeters), and type of repair.

Procedure Differentiation

There are three categories of wound repairs: simple, intermediate, and complex. They are defined in the following discussion.

Suturing of Superficial Wounds (12001–12021)

Codes for the repair of superficial wounds (simple closure) include:

- Administration of local anesthesia
- Routine debridement and decontamination
- Simple one-layer closure
  - superficial tissues
  - sutures, staples, tissue adhesives
  - exploration of nerves, blood vessels, tendons not resulting in substantial dissection or repair

- – vessel ligation, in wound
- Cauterization without closure

Wound repair should be measured and reported in centimeters. If the provider performs a simple, one-layer repair of the same complexity and in the same anatomical area, the length of all wounds sutured is summed and reported as one total length.

Wounds involving cleansing, irrigation, and control of bleeding by electrocautery or chemical cauterization qualify as a simple repair even if sutures are not used. It should be noted that some payers may not follow this guideline and simply include wound closure by other means as part of the evaluation and management service. Check with specific third-party payers for coverage determinations.

Wounds repaired with adhesive strips (e.g., Steri-strips or butterfly strips) are included in the appropriate E/M code (99202–99499). Do not report wounds repaired without the use of sutures separately. Skin adhesives, such as Dermabond, are a newer alternative to sutures or Steri-strips in the treatment of minor skin lacerations. The AMA recommends assigning the appropriate code for a simple repair when Dermabond or skin adhesive is used to close a wound.

Suturing of Intermediate Wounds (12031–12057)
Codes for the intermediate repair of a wound include:

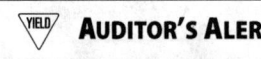

AUDITOR'S ALERT

See Appendix 1 for the audit worksheet for wound repair.

- Administration of local anesthesia
- Closure of contaminated single-layer wound
  - – layered closure (e.g., subcutaneous tissue, superficial fascia)
  - – removal of foreign material (e.g. gravel, glass)
  - – routine debridement and decontamination
  - – exploration of nerves, blood vessels, tendons in wound not resulting in substantial dissection or repair
  - – limited undermining, a distance that is at least one entire edge of the defect but less than the maximum width of the defect, measured perpendicular to the closure line
  - – vessel ligation, in wound

More complex lacerations require deeper subcutaneous or layered suturing techniques. Multiple wounds in the same repair category and anatomic site are reported as one total length by adding together the lengths of all wounds sutured.

Suturing of Complicated Wounds (13100–13160)
Codes for the complicated repair of a wound include:

- Administration of local anesthesia
- Creation of a limited defect for repair
- At least one of the following is required:
  - – exposure of bone, cartilage, tendon, or a named neurovascular structure
  - – extensive undermining that is at least one entire edge of the defect but a distance greater than or equal to the maximum width of the defect, measured perpendicular to the closure line

– involvement of free margins of helical rim, nostril rim, or vermilion border in which retention sutures are placed

Complex repairs do not include excision of benign or malignant lesions.

Coding guidelines instruct that when multiple wounds are repaired, wounds of the same anatomical site requiring the same type of closure (i.e., simple, intermediate, complex) be added together and the sum is used to determine correct code assignment. For example, a patient presents with three lacerations on the leg. Laceration A is 1.0 cm and laceration B is 1.5 cm, both lacerations are on the arm, and require simple closure. Laceration C is 3.6 cm and requires layered closure. To determine correct code assignment, lacerations A and B are added together, and the correct code for simple repair of a 2.5 cm lesion is assigned. If the lacerations are in different anatomical areas described by separate code ranges, the appropriate code from each range would be assigned. This is true regardless of the shape of the wound.

In addition to the three categories listed above, the provider may also perform a secondary closure of a wound. This is most commonly performed due to a wound dehiscence. When the wound dehiscence is requires a simple repair, see codes 12020–12021. When a complex repair is required, see 13160.

When two types of sutures are used to close a wound, verify with the provider whether an intermediate repair code is appropriate. At times, two kinds of sutures are used to repair an irregularly shaped wound (e.g., elliptical) and closure is really a simple repair. If two sutures are used and one is absorbable (e.g., Vicryl, chromic, gut or Dexon), an intermediate repair is highly probable.

Answer the following questions about wound repairs to help code accurately:

- How many wounds were repaired?
- What was the anatomic site of the wound?
- What was the length of the wound?
- What type of repair was performed?
- Was an adhesive strip applied?
- Was chemical or electrocauterization employed?
- Does the documentation state simple, intermediate, or complex?
- Was debridement performed?
- Were blood vessels, tendons, or nerves repaired?
- Was the wound explored and were the vessels ligated?
- Was secondary wound repair performed?
- If multiple wounds were repaired with the same type of closure technique, were any of the wounds in the same anatomical grouping?

Key Documentation Terms

Documentation should indicate the complexity of the surgical procedure that was performed. Terms such as simple, intermediate, or layered and the anatomical location provide the guidance needed to ensure correct code assignment. Above all else, the documentation should support the medical necessity of the procedure. The documentation for these procedures should include the depth, length, and anatomical location of the wound and a narrative of the procedure performed. Documentation for open wounds for ICD-10-CM, will include laceration with or without foreign body, puncture with or without

> ### 📖 DEFINITIONS
>
> **dehiscence.** Complication of healing in which the surgical wound ruptures or bursts open, superficially or through multiple layers.

foreign body, open bite, and avulsion; also laterality is specified when appropriate. This requires that the provider's documentation clearly state where and exactly what the injury is, instead of stating just that it is an open wound.

Coding Tips

- Decontamination and debridement may be reported separately when documentation indicates that because the wound contained significant foreign material such as dirt, gravel, splinters, or required the removal of devitalized tissue. See codes 11010–11012 and 11042–11047 to select the appropriate code.

- A separately identifiable evaluation and management service may be reported, if necessary, to assess the patient for additional injuries that may have occurred with the wound.

Tissue Transfers, Skin Replacement Surgery, and Flaps (14000–14350, 15002–15278, 15570-15777)

In order to efficiently report codes in the skin replacement section, it is important to know the difference between adjacent tissue transfers/rearrangements, autografts, skin substitutes, flaps, and grafts.

Two of the most important terms that a coder must know when reporting these codes are defect and donor site. A defect is the actual area being repaired. It may be caused by an injury, removal of a lesion, or by a skin graft itself. A donor site is the area of the body from which the grafting tissue is obtained. When a defect created at the donor site requires a skin graft, it is considered an additional procedure and may be reported separately in some instances. Because codes for flaps and grafts may or may not include repair of the donor site, it is important to read **all** CPT® guidelines under the following subheadings before reporting the repair:

- Adjacent Tissue Transfer or Rearrangement (14000–14350)
- Skin Replacement Surgery and Skin Substitutes (15002–15278)
- Flaps (Skin and/or Deep Tissues) (15570–15738)
- Other Flaps and Grafts (15740–15777)

Procedure Differentiation

An adjacent tissue transfer (14000-14302) occurs when tissue from an adjacent area is relocated to the recipient area leaving a large portion of skin attached to the donor site to maintain vascularization of the skin graft. Undermining, separating the dermis from the fascia, may be necessary to facilitate the rearrangement of the skin to accomplish the repair. Undermining is considered an inherent component of adjacent tissue transfers. These procedures include such techniques as Z-plasty, W-plasty, V-Y plasty, or rotation flaps. These codes are chosen according to the size of the defect.

When an adjacent tissue transfer or rearrangement is performed in conjunction with excision of a lesion, the lesion excision is not reported separately.

Key Documentation

Documentation includes terms such as -plasty, W-plasty, V-Y plasty, or rotation flaps, as well as the anatomic location and size of the defect. These terms help provide the guidance needed to ensure correct code assignment.

Procedure Differentiation

Skin replacement surgery (15002–15278) is defined by size, recipient site (location of the defect), and type of graft (e.g., autograft, allograft, homograft, xenograft). Skin replacement surgery and skin substitutes should be reported separately as a secondary procedure when performed in conjunction with other procedures. Examples of procedures that might require skin replacement surgery at the time of the primary procedure include musculoskeletal deep tumor removal, neck dissection, and radical mastectomy.

When the recipient site is prepared to receive a free skin graft needed to close or repair a defect, these services are reported with 15002-15005. Skin, subcutaneous tissue, scars, burn eschar, and lesions are excised to provide a healthy, vascular tissue bed (where new vessels have been formed) onto which a skin graft will be placed. A physician may also choose to prepare tissue by incising or excising a scar contracture that is causing excessive tightening of the skin. Simple debridement of granulations or of recent avulsion is included in the procedure.

An autograft (15040-15157) is any tissue harvested from one anatomical site of a person and grafted to another anatomical site of the same person. Although there are various types of autografted tissues, such as blood vessels and bones, this section of the CPT book covers skin autografts. The procedure codes are reported based on percent of body area for infants and children under the age of 10 but are reported per 100 sq cm for adults and children age 10 and older. These codes include the application and/or harvesting of the autologous skin graft and removal of the current graft if applicable. If the donor site requires a skin graft or local flap, it is reported separately.

The following are a few different types of autografts:

- Epidermal autograft: contains only the epidermis
- Split thickness autograft: contains the epidermis and part of the dermis
- Dermal autograft: contains dermis
- Tissue cultured skin: skin that has been cultured in a laboratory from skin cells harvested from the patient and grown into sheets of graft material

A full thickness skin graft (15200–15261) is defined as complete excision of skin from one site for attachment or suture to a distant recipient site. It consists of the superficial and deeper layers of skin (epidermis and dermis). They are typically used for more visible locations such as the face, neck, and the ears because they preserve the appearance of the skin in color, texture, and thickness. These grafts tend to be small and are generally harvested from the nasolabial fold, pre- and postauricular areas, supraclavicular fossa, and upper eyelid. Common reasons for this type of graft are skin cancer, burns, or large wounds. Codes are defined by anatomical area and each 20 sq. cm treated.

If a repair of the donor site requiring skin grafting or local flaps is necessary, it should be reported separately with the appropriate code. Skin substitute grafts (15271–15278) are used as temporary wound closure for wounds of the trunk, arms, or legs. Skin substitutes may be temporary or permanent. When they are used as a temporary measure, they close wounds, protect against fluid loss, reduce pain, and promote healing of underlying tissues until a permanent graft can be applied. Permanent skin substitutes are used in the case of wounds (e.g., diabetic foot ulcers) or burn sites. Common skin substitutes include nonautologous human skin (e.g., dermal or epidermal, cellular and acellular), grafts (e.g., homograft, allograft), nonhuman skin substitute grafts usually from a pig (e.g., xenograft), and biological products that form a support for skin growth. These procedures are reported according to size and location of the defect (recipient site) and include the harvest and/or application of the autologous skin graft.

Codes 15271–15278 should not be reported for the application of injected skin substitutes or non-graft wound dressings. Removal of the current graft is included if applicable. Debridement is only reported separately when used to remove significant amounts of devitalized skin or the wound is grossly contaminated and requires prolonged cleansing.

Key Documentation

Documentation includes terms such as dermal, epidermal, nonautologous, permanent, temporary, and xenograft, as well as the anatomic location and size of the wound surface area. These terms help provide the guidance needed to ensure correct code assignment.

Procedure Differentiation

Flaps and grafts (15570–15777) are different than skin replacement and skin substitutes (15002–15278); they involve moving normal tissue (i.e., skin, skin and deep tissues, muscle, and composite tissue) from one site to another. The site where the tissue originates is referred to as the donor site, while the site where the tissue is being relocated is referred to as the recipient site. With these procedures, surgical preparation of the recipient site should be reported separately with 15002–15005. In this procedure, skin, subcutaneous tissue, scars, burn eschar, and lesions are excised to provide a healthy, vascular tissue bed (where new vessels have been formed) onto which a skin graft will be placed.

Flaps of skin and deep tissues (15570–15738) are defined by type of graft (i.e., direct, tube, delayed, intermediate, muscle, myocutaneous, and fasciocutaneous) and site. The site listed is the recipient site when the flap is being attached to the final site. However, when the flap is being formed for delayed transfer, the site refers to the donor site. Any extensive immobilization with casts or other devices is considered an additional procedure and should be reported separately. Repairs of the donor site with skin grafts or local flaps are reported separately.

Codes 15570–15576 involve using a pedicle flap. This is a piece of skin and subcutaneous tissue that is detached from its bed at one end and moved to another part of the body while one end (the pedicle) of the flap is still attached to its original blood supply at the donor site.

Codes 15600–15630 describe the delay of a flap. This is reported when the physician sections the direct or tubed pedicle flap several weeks following the reconstruction of a traumatic defect. Blood flow is now established in the recipient area. The unused portion of the flap is detached and prepared for reinsertion into its original anatomic site. Previous skin grafts are removed from the donor beds. The returned flap is sutured in layers to the harvest site. Any exposed subcutaneous tissue is closed primarily or covered with a split-thickness skin graft.

An intermediate transfer (15650) is when a previously placed pedicle flap has been in position long enough to receive a good blood supply from the recipient area. As an intermediate step, the physician releases the flap from its donor attachment and moves it to a new location. This same tissue may be moved further along the body in a similar manner at a later date. This is known as walking the flap or walk-up procedure.

A flap graft excises the tissue, either split or full thickness, from the donor site leaving a pedicle or portion of the graft still attached to provide vascularization. One key in determining if a tissue transfer or flap was performed is to determine the size of the tissue attachment. An adjacent tissue transfer leaves a large portion of skin attached, while a flap graft involves only a small attachment.

Codes 15730–15733 are used to report skin flap procedures performed of the midface and neck. Code 15730 is used to report a zygomatic flap with preservation of the vascular pedicle(s) of the midface, while 15731 reports an axial pattern or paramedian flap involving the forehead. The documentation for these procedures should describe the physician forming a vascular pedicle flap from the forehead to correct an adjacent defect of the nose, forehead, temple, or scalp. The physician determines the best site for supratrochlear or supraorbital artery via Doppler. A flap with an artery along its long axis is called an axial flap. A paramedian flap is an axial flap with origins along the midline of the forehead and is commonly used in nasal reconstructive surgery following excision of a malignancy. The physician cuts and undermines the skin and subcutaneous tissue, taking care to preserve vascular flow to the flap tissue. The thickness of the flap may be reduced, depending on the thickness of the defect at the recipient site. The flap is rotated or advanced to the defect site and secured with sutures. The donor site is closed directly.

Code 15733 utilizes muscle, muscle and skin, or a fasciocutaneous flap of the head and/or neck. These types of flaps are larger than those described by 15730–15731. The documentation for this procedure should state that the physician repairs a defect area using a muscle, muscle and skin, or a fasciocutaneous flap. The physician rotates the prepared flap from the donor area to the site needing repair, suturing the flap in place. The donor area is closed primarily with sutures. If a skin graft or flap is used to repair the donor site, it is considered an additional procedure and is reported separately.

Key Documentation
Documentation includes terms such as delay of a flap, intermediate transfer, split thickness, full thickness, from a donor site, and pedicle. Documentation specific to 15730 includes terms such as a zygomaticofacial flap, lateral canthotomy, and/or zygomaticofacial arteries. Documentation for 15731 includes terms such as a paramedian flap, vascular pedicle, or axial flap. Documentation for 15733 is usually based on the vascular pedicle specifically being performed, including terms such as buccinators, genioglossus, levator scapulae, masseter, sternocleidomastoid, and temporalis.

Procedure Differentiation
Other flaps and grafts (15740-15777) include island pedicle, free muscle, skin, or fascial flaps requiring microvascular anastomosis and composite grafts. An island pedicle is reported with 15740. This requires complete excision of the skin and tissue with only the artery or vein and sometimes the nerve remaining intact to vascularize and enervate the skin flap. This code also specifies that it requires an axial vessel to be identified and dissected.

A free muscle graft with anastomosis occurs when a muscle is completely excised from the donor site, preserving the vessel ends. Upon grafting, the muscle is attached to vessels at the donor site to provide blood supply to the graft. A myocutaneous graft involves muscle and overlying skin as the graft.

 © 2020 Optum360, LLC

A free skin flap or fascial flap with anastomosis occurs when the donor site is completely excised and upon transfer the vessels are attached to the surrounding vessels to provide blood supply to the graft.

The *CPT Assistant*, April 1997, page 4 provides additional guidance stating, "The word free indicates that the tissue is actually separated from its blood supply and transferred to a recipient site where it is reanastomosed to the recipient blood vessels. This is different from other flaps that remain attached to their blood supply. It should be noted that all of the free tissue transfer codes include transferring a portion of the fascia. The fascia is very important as it contains the vascular supply to the skin."

A composite graft (15760) includes different types of tissue, such as skin and cartilage. For example, the naris (nostril) edge or the external ear is a composite graft.

An autologous soft tissue graft, harvested by direct excision, is reported with 15769. In this procedure, the physician obtains a fat, dermis, or fascial graft. The physician incises the skin and retracts the skin flap to expose the underlying connective tissue. The tissue is incised to the required layer. The graft is lifted and implanted in the recipient site. Both donor and recipient sites are sutured. If the donor site repair requires skin graft or local flaps, it is reported separately.

A derma-fat-fascia graft (15770) may be a continuous piece of all three of these layers, individual sections done layer by layer, or graft pieces laid in the recipient bed as combinations, such as a fascia-fat layer, followed by a dermal layer. The graft is laid in the recipient area so as to fill and blend in pockets of defects to restore the surrounding area to normal positioning and to maintain the continuity of the local flesh. This code is reported only once per graft site.

Autologous fat grafts may also be harvested by liposuction (15771–15774). This type of graft may be utilized in many areas of soft tissue augmentation or reconstruction, including congenital defects, contouring of face or breasts, and scarring as a result of burns, radiation, surgical procedures, or trauma. The physician obtains an autologous fat graft by liposuction technique. After identifying the most suitable area of fat harvesting (commonly the abdomen, trochanteric region, or the insides of the thighs and/or knees), the physician makes small incisions in the skin overlying the harvest area. A liposuction cannula is inserted through the incision. The physician moves the cannula through the fat deposits, collecting parcels of fat. The fat graft is processed using a variety of techniques, most commonly sedimentation, filtering, washing, and centrifugation. The physician inserts the fat graft at the chosen anatomical region. A small incision is made, a cannula is inserted, and the fat graft is typically distributed in small portions at varying depths into the soft tissues. Donor and recipient incisions are closed. Report 15771 for grafting of 50 cc or less of the fat injectate to the trunk, breasts, scalp, arms, and/or legs, and 15772 for each additional 50 cc. Report 15773 for grafting of 25 cc or less of the fat injectate to the face, eyelids, mouth, neck, ears, orbits, genitalia, hands, and/or feet, and 15774 for each additional 25 cc.

A punch graft (15775) is obtained by using a skin punch to obtain a small circular graft into the dermis. The graft may be full or partial thickness. This technique is commonly used for hair transplants and scarring such as "ice-pick" acne scars. When used for hair transplants, the graft contains multiple hair follicles. Most payers consider a hair transplant or acne scar revision to be cosmetic and not a covered benefit. Code 15776 is reported when more than 15 punch grafts are obtained.

Key Documentation
Documentation includes terms such as composite grafts, derma-fat-fascia, free muscle, fascial flaps, island pedicle, microvascular anastomosis, punch, and skin flap. These terms help provide the guidance needed to ensure correct code assignment. Special care should be taken when reporting these codes. The coder needs to have complete documentation on the current procedure, as well as any staged procedures performed at the site, in order to make the appropriate code and modifier selection.

Coding Tips
- It is important to note that autograft codes (15040–15157) are reported by the size of the recipient area. For children 10 years of age or older and adults, 100 square centimeters of measurement should be used. For infants and children up to 9 years of age, each 1 percent of body surface should be reported. For multiple wounds of the same anatomical area, the surface areas are added together. If there are multiple wounds of different anatomical areas, add the anatomical areas that are grouped together, and report multiple codes within code range 15040–15157. For each subsequent code after the primary procedure, modifier 59 should be appended.

- The supply of skin substitute grafts is reported separately with 15271–15278, using the appropriate HCPCS Level II code.

- Repair of the donor site that requires a skin graft or local flaps is considered an additional, separate procedure and should be coded separately.

- Extensive immobilization and/or repair of the donor site is reported separately.

Destruction of Lesions (17000–17999)
The codes for destruction include ablation of benign, premalignant, or malignant tissue by any of the following methods used alone or in combination: electrosurgery, cryosurgery, laser, and chemical treatment.

Procedure Differentiation
Codes 17000–17111 report destruction of benign or premalignant lesions. Codes are differentiated by the type of lesion, the number of lesions, or the size of the lesion.

Medical Necessity
The following conditions may warrant these procedures (this list is not all inclusive):

- Acquired hyperkeratosis (keratoderma)
- Actinic keratosis
- Condyloma
- Herpetic lesions
- Milia
- Molluscum contagiosum
- Other benign (e.g., vascular proliferative) or premalignant lesions
- Papilloma

DEFINITIONS

condyloma. Infectious tumor-like growth caused by the human papilloma virus, with a branching connective tissue core and epithelial covering that occurs on the skin and mucous membranes of the perianal region and external genitalia.

milia. Tiny, round, white to yellow slightly elevated epidermal cysts containing keratin found on superficial skin in the hair follicles and sebaceous glands of all ages, even neonates.

papilloma. Benign skin neoplasm with small branchings from the epithelial surface.

- Sebaceous (epidermoid) cysts
- Seborrheic keratosis
- Warts

Procedure Differentiation

Codes 17260–17286 report destruction of malignant lesions.

Codes are differentiated by the size of the lesion and location.

Medical Necessity

The following conditions may warrant these procedures (this list is not all inclusive):

- Kaposi's sarcoma
- Malignant neoplasms
- Melanoma

Key Documentation Terms

The key terms should include benign, malignant, or premalignant. The documentation for these procedures should include the indications for the procedure, the narrative of the procedure that describes the destruction, including anatomical site, morphology (benign or malignant), and size of the lesion. Documentation of lesions under ICD-10-CM needs to be more specific and include the precise location of the lesion on the body, including which side of the body (e.g., left ear, right ear or unspecified ear).

Coding Tips

- Codes from this section should not be used when a more specific destruction code is listed under a specific anatomic site. For example, code 40820 should be used to report destruction of lesions of the vestibule of the mouth. Review all notes within this section that refer to other types of lesion treatment.

- As an "add-on" code, 17003 is not subject to multiple procedure rules. No reimbursement reduction or modifier 51 is applied. The following table provides additional information for these codes as found in the Medicare Physician Fee Schedule Database.

Parent Code	Add-On	GLOB DAYS	MULT PROC	BILAT SURG	ASST SURG	CO-SURG	TEAM SURG
17000		010	2	0	1	0	0
	17003	ZZZ	0	0	1	0	0

Mohs Surgery (17311–17315)

Mohs surgery is listed in the destruction subsection. This technique is performed on cutaneous malignancies that are ill-defined or complex in nature. In this surgical procedure a single physician performs both the surgical and pathological examinations of the specimen(s). The first service is surgical and involves the destruction of the lesion by a combination of chemosurgery and excision. The second service is that of a pathologist and includes mapping, color coding of specimens, microscopic examination of specimens, and complete histopathologic preparation.

The codes in this section should not be used if two physicians perform each function separately. Documentation should clearly reflect that both services were performed by a single physician and include results of the specimen examination. Code selection is based upon the lesion site, number of stages performed, and the number of specimens excised.

Medical Necessity

The following conditions may warrant these procedures (this list is not all inclusive):

- Adenocystic carcinoma of the skin
- Angiosarcoma of the skin
- Apocrine or eccrine carcinoma of the skin
- Atypical fibroxanthoma
- Basal cell carcinomas
- Basal cell nevus syndrome
- Basalosquamous cell carcinomas
- Bowenoid papulosis
- Dermatofibrosarcoma protuberans
- Erythroplasia of Queyrat
- Extramammary Paget's disease
- Keratoacanthoma
- Leiomyosarcoma or other spindle cell neoplasms of the skin
- Malignant fibrous histiocytoma
- Merkel cell carcinoma
- Microcystic adnexal carcinoma
- Sebaceous gland carcinoma
- Squamous cell carcinomas
- Verrucous carcinoma

Key Documentation Terms

Terms should include the anatomical location, a stage, bone, muscle, and tendon. These terms help provide the guidance needed to ensure correct code assignment. The documentation for these procedures should include the indications for the procedure, the narrative of the procedure including anatomical site, and the size of the lesion. The documentation should also clearly show that Mohs surgery was chosen because of the complexity (e.g., poorly defined clinical borders, possible deep invasion, prior irradiation) and size or location (e.g., maximum conservation of tumor-free tissue is important).

Coding Tip

- In the event that a lesion has not been previously biopsied, the biopsy may be reported separately. If it is performed on the same day as a Mohs procedure, codes 11102, 11104, and 11107 may be used to report the service in addition to 88331 (frozen section pathology). Note that modifier 59 should be appended to the biopsy and pathology procedures to distinguish that they are separate procedures.

- Repairs, grafts, and flaps are separately reportable with the Mohs micrographic surgery CPT codes.

DEFINITIONS

Merkel cell carcinoma. Rare form of skin cancer that typically presents on the face, head, or neck as a flesh-colored or bluish-red lesion. This neoplasm is fast growing and can metastasize quickly to other areas of the body. Risk factors include older patients with weakened immune systems and/or long-term exposure to the sun.

myositis. Inflammation of a muscle with voluntary movement.

Coding Trap
- Code 88314 should not be reported in addition to codes 17311-17315 unless a non-routine histochemical stain is performed on frozen tissue. In that case, modifier 59 should be appended to 88314.

Breast Biopsies, Localization, and Radiation Therapy Placement (19081–19101, 19281–19288, and 19294–19298)

Procedure Differentiation

Codes 19081–19086 describe percutaneous breast biopsies. Using image guidance, the physician places a metallic clip or pellet adjacent to a breast lesion to mark the site. A large gauge (e.g., 14 gauge), hollow core biopsy needle or the biopsy device is inserted through the skin of the breast and into the suspicious breast tissue. The physician takes multiple core tissue samples from a single lesion to obtain a sufficient amount of tissue for diagnosis. Codes are defined by the type of guidance used. Report code 19081 for the first lesion and 19082 for each additional lesion removed using stereotactic guidance. Report codes 19083–19084 if ultrasound guidance is used. Report codes 19085–19086 if magnetic resonance imaging (MRI) is used.

When a breast biopsy is performed via percutaneous needle core, the physician inserts a needle into the abnormal tissue and a plug of tissue is removed for microscopic examination. This procedure is performed without imaging guidance; report code 19100.

An open incisional breast biopsy is performed when only a portion of the lesion is removed and should be assigned to code 19101. This specimen is often examined immediately.

Codes 19281–19288 describe the procedure in which a breast localization device is placed prior to a breast biopsy. Documentation will indicate that imaging guidance is used and that the physician placed a metallic clip, pellet, wire, needle, or radioactive seed adjacent to a breast lesion to mark the site for an open breast biopsy or a percutaneous breast biopsy to be performed during the same or a different encounter. Codes are defined by the type of guidance used. Report code 19281 for the first lesion and 19282 for each additional lesion marked using mammographic guidance. Report code 19283–19284 if stereotactic guidance is used. Report codes 19285–19286 if ultrasound guidance is used. Report codes 19287–19288 if magnetic resonance imaging (MRI) is used.

Codes 19294-19297 are reported for placement of radiation therapy devices. In 19294, the surgeon prepares the tumor cavity and delivers intraoperative radiation therapy (IORT) at the same time as the patient is undergoing a lumpectomy or partial mastectomy. A miniature, low energy, isotope-free x-ray source delivers a precise and targeted dose of radiation directly to the lumpectomy cavity. The surgeon removes the malignant tumor and awaits the initial pathology report. Once the malignancy is confirmed, the physician prepares the tumor cavity for temporary insertion of a flexible balloon applicator. The radiation oncologist inserts the miniature x-ray source inside a balloon-shaped catheter device, and a single dose of radiation is directed at the tumor cavity while medical personnel remain behind a rolling shield. The process takes eight to 12 minutes. Once the treatment is complete, the catheter is withdrawn and the applicator is removed. The incision is closed. In 19267 and 19297, a remote single or multichannel afterloading expandable catheter for

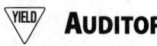

AUDITOR'S ALERT

When multiple biopsies are performed, an additional primary code may be reported if a different imaging modality is used.

interstitial radiotherapy treatment is placed in the breast following partial mastectomy. A catheter is placed at a later date, separate from the lumpectomy surgery in 19296 and concurrently with the lumpectomy in 19297. In 19298, remote afterloading catheters are placed into the breast for interstitial radiotherapy application at the time of a partial mastectomy, or subsequent to a partial mastectomy having been performed. The lumpectomy site is identified. A template with pre-drilled holes that function as coordinates for catheter placement around the surgical area may be applied for imaging. Brachytherapy needles are first inserted into the chosen coordinates. The brachytherapy catheters are fed into position through the needles, which are removed. Imaging guidance is included in this procedure.

Medical Necessity

The following conditions may warrant a breast biopsy (this list is not all inclusive):

- Abnormal findings on radiological exam (mammogram) of the breast
- Benign neoplasm
- Carcinoma in situ of breast
- Lump or breast mass
- Malignant neoplasm of female or male breast
- Neoplasm of unspecified nature

Key Documentation Terms

Documentation should indicate the surgical procedure that was performed. Terms such as type of imaging guidance, open, percutaneous, first or additional lesion provide the guidance needed to ensure correct code assignment. Documentation for these procedures should include the indications for the procedure, procedure performed, method, and the location of the breast abnormality.

Coding Tips

- As add-on codes, 19082, 19084, 19086, 19282, 19284, 19286, 19288, 19294, and 19297 are not subject to multiple procedure rules. No reimbursement reduction or modifier 51 is applied. Add-on codes describe additional intraservice work associated with the primary procedure. It is performed by the same provider on the same date of service as the primary service/procedure, and must never be reported as a stand-alone code. The following table provides additional information for these codes as found in the Medicare Physician Fee Schedule Database.

 DEFINITIONS

carcinoma in situ. Malignancy that arises from the cells of the vessel, gland, or organ of origin that remains confined to that site or has not invaded neighboring tissue.

gynecomastia. Condition in which the male mammary glands are abnormally large.

© 2020 Optum360, LLC

Parent Code	Add-On	GLOB DAYS	MULT PROC	BILAT SURG	ASST SURG	CO-SURG	TEAM SURG
19081		000	2	1	0	0	0
	19082	ZZZ	0	0	0	0	0
19083		000	2	1	0	0	0
	19084	ZZZ	0	0	0	0	0
19085		000	2	1	0	0	0
	19086	ZZZ	0	0	0	0	0
19281		000	2	1	0	0	0
	19282	ZZZ	0	0	0	0	0
19283		000	2	1	0	0	0
	19284	ZZZ	0	0	0	0	0
19285		000	2	1	0	0	0
	19286	ZZZ	0	0	0	0	0
19287		000	2	1	0	0	0
	19288	ZZZ	0	0	0	0	0
	19294	ZZZ	0	0	0	0	0
	19297	ZZZ	0	0	0	0	0
19301		090	2	1	0	0	0
19302		090	2	1	2	1	0

- The codes for breast procedures reflect unilateral procedures only. If a bilateral breast procedure is performed, append modifier 50.

- A biopsy performed at the time of another more extensive procedure (e.g., excision, removal) is reported separately under specific circumstances. If the biopsy is performed on a separate lesion, it is reported separately. This situation may be reported with anatomic modifiers or modifier 59.

- When multiple breast biopsies are performed on the same breast or the contralateral breast using the same modality, the add-on code for that modality should be reported.

- When more than one localization device is placed that employs a different imaging modality, an additional primary code may be reported.

- Placement of a percutaneous localization clip is reported separately, see 19281–19288.

- Fine needle aspiration is reported using a code from range 10004–10021.

- For a localization device identified only as soft tissue, see 10035–10036.

Mastectomies: Partial, Simple, Radical (19300–19307)

Many different mastectomy codes are included in this section. It is important to understand the differences when coding these procedures. This section contains codes for partial (19301-19302) and total (19303-19307) mastectomies.

In a partial mastectomy, the focus is to remove adequate surgical margins that surround the breast lesion or mass.

A total mastectomy includes the following:

- Complete mastectomy

- Modified radical mastectomy
- Radical mastectomy
- Simple mastectomy
- Subcutaneous mastectomy

Procedure Differentiation

A mastectomy for gynecomastia (19300) involves the removal of male breast tissue because of abnormal enlargement (without removing lymph nodes or muscles).

Medical Necessity

Coverage will be denied if a mastectomy for gynecomastia is performed for cosmetic reasons. Coverage generally is provided if it is documented that the tissue is primarily breast tissue and not just adipose (fatty tissue).

Key Documentation Terms

The key documentation term for this procedure is gynecomastia. The documentation for this procedure should include the indications for the procedure and the procedure performed. Preoperative photographs should be included in the patient's medical record. If this procedure is performed due to pain or tenderness in the breast tissue, the medical record should contain documentation of the clinically significant impact upon activities of daily living and that it has been refractory to a trial of analgesics or anti-inflammatory agents (for a reasonable time period adequate to assess therapeutic effects).

Procedure Differentiation

Partial mastectomy or segmental mastectomy (19301) involves the partial removal of the breast tissue, leaving the breast nearly intact (also called lumpectomy or tylectomy). A wedge of tissue that amounts to approximately one-fourth of the breast (including the overlying skin) is removed for a quadrantectomy.

Partial mastectomy with axillary lymphadenectomy (19302) involves the complete removal of axillary lymph nodes. This procedure is performed for a malignancy. ICD-10-CM code assignment should denote a malignant condition to substantiate medical necessity.

Simple complete mastectomy (19303) involves the removal of all subcutaneous breast tissue, with or without nipple and skin (without removing lymph nodes or muscle). When documentation indicates that a breast implant was immediately inserted, code 19340 should also be reported.

Radical mastectomy (19305–19307) is used when the patient has a malignant neoplasm with possible or confirmed invasion of other tissue and lymph nodes. There are three types of radical mastectomies:

- Code 19305 includes pectoral muscles and axillary lymph nodes.

- Code 19306 includes breast tissue, skin, pectoral muscles, all tissue within the parameters of the sternum, the rectus fascia, the latissimus dorsi muscle, the clavicle, and the axillary and internal mammary lymph nodes.

- Code 19307 reports a modified radical mastectomy. The procedure includes dissection of the axillary lymph nodes, with or without pectoralis minor muscle. The pectoralis major muscle is left intact.

Medical Necessity

The following conditions may warrant other types of mastectomies (excluding gynecomastia) (this list is not all inclusive):

- Carcinoma in situ of breast
- Family history of malignant neoplasm of breast
- Genetic susceptibility to malignant neoplasm of breast
- Malignant neoplasm of the breast
- Neoplasm of uncertain behavior of breast
- Personal history of malignant neoplasm of breast
- Secondary malignant neoplasm of breast

Key Documentation Terms

Terms such as lymphadenectomy, partial, modified, simple, subcutaneous, and radical provide the guidance needed to ensure correct code assignment. The documentation for this procedure should include the indications for the procedure and the procedure performed. Preoperative photographs should be included in the patient's medical record. If this procedure is performed due to pain or tenderness in the breast tissue, the medical record should contain documentation of the clinically significant impact upon activities of daily living and that it has been refractory to a trial of analgesics or antiinflammatory agents (for a reasonable time period adequate to assess therapeutic effects).

Coding Tips

- Chest wall tumors are reported with a code from range 21601–21603 depending on how invasive the malignancy is found to be.
- These are unilateral procedures. If performed bilaterally, some payers require that the service be reported twice with modifier 50 appended to the second code while others require identification of the service only once with modifier 50 appended. Check with individual payers. Modifier 50 identifies a procedure performed identically on the opposite side of the body (mirror image).
- If a mastectomy is performed as a staged procedure, modifier 58 would be appended to the mastectomy code. Example: A right breast biopsy (19100) is performed. As a result of the biopsy, a malignant tumor was diagnosed. One week later, (within the global period of the previous surgery), a modified radical mastectomy including axillary lymph nodes, with or without pectoralis minor muscle (19307) is performed. Modifier 58 should be appended to code 19307, since the mastectomy procedure was a more extensive procedure than the biopsy.
- Breast reconstruction should be reported separately.
- When breast tissue is removed that is not related to gynecomastia, as in breast-size reduction surgery, 19318 should be reported.
- Percutaneous image-guided placement of a localization device (19281–19288) may be reported separately when performed with 19101.
- For intraoperative margin assessment, at the time of partial mastectomy using real time, radiofrequency spectroscopy, report 0546T.

Coding Traps

- The intraoperative placement of clips should not be reported separately.

Plastic, Reconstructive, and Aesthetic Breast Procedures (19316–19396)

This section includes many breast procedures, which may be required because of tissue loss due to a medical condition needing surgical excision or a congenital condition. The procedures include insertion, replacement, or removal of breast implants, breast lifts, reductions, and augmentations.

Procedure Differentiation

Code 19316 describes a breast lift. In this procedure the physician performs mastopexy, relocating the nipple and areola to a higher position and removing excess skin below the nipple and above the lower breast crease. The physician makes a skin incision above the nipple, in the location to which the nipple will be elevated. Another skin incision is made around the circumference of the nipple. Two skin incisions are made from the circular cut above the nipple to the fold beneath the breast, one on either side of the nipple, forming a keyhole shaped skin incision. This skin is cut away from the breast tissue and removed. The physician elevates the breast to its new position and closes the incision, excising any redundant skin in the fold beneath the breast. The incision is repaired with layered closure.

Breast reductions are reported with code 19318. The documentation for this procedure would state that the physician reduces the size of the breast, removing wedges of skin and breast tissue from a female patient. The physician makes a circular skin incision above the nipple, in the position to which the nipple will be elevated. Another skin incision is made around the circumference of the nipple. Two incisions are made from the circular cut above the nipple to the fold beneath the breast, one on either side of the nipple, creating a keyhole shaped skin and breast incision. Wedges of skin and breast tissue are removed until the desired size is achieved. Bleeding vessels may be ligated or cauterized. The physician elevates the nipple and its pedicle of subcutaneous tissue to its new position and sutures the nipple pedicle with layered closure. The remaining incision is repaired with layered closure.

Medical Necessity

The following conditions may warrant a breast reduction (this list is not all inclusive):

- To reduce the size of the hypertrophic breast(s) and reduce or alleviate symptoms caused by the breast hypertrophy

- To reduce the size of a normal breast to bring it into symmetry with a breast reconstructed after breast cancer surgery

Non-surgical interventions preceding reduction mammoplasty should include as appropriate, but are not limited to, the following:

- Determining the macromastia is not due to an active endocrine or metabolic process

- Determining the symptoms are refractory to appropriately fitted supporting garments, or following unilateral mastectomy, persistent with an appropriately fitted prosthesis or reconstruction therapy at the site of the absent breast

- Determining that dermatologic signs and/or symptoms are refractory to, or recurrent following, a completed course of medical management

For Medicare purposes a mammoplasty may be indicated in the presence of significantly enlarged breasts and the presence of **at least two** of the following signs and/or symptoms when present for at least six months and have not responded to a reasonable non-surgical care program:

- Chronic breast pain due to the excessive weight of the breasts
- Headache (cephalgia) when same can be directly attributed to the excessive breast weight and its effect on the neck and/or shoulders and other reasonable causes of a headache have been addressed/ruled out
- Intertriginous maceration or infection of the inframammary skin refractory to usual dermatologic measures
- Shoulder grooving from supporting garment (bra strap)
- Significant thoracic kyphosis which is felt to be directly correlated to the breast hypertrophy
- Upper back, shoulder and/or neck pain that appears to be directly correlated to the macromastia
- Upper extremity paresthesia due to brachial plexus compressions syndrome secondary to the weight of the breasts being transferred to the shoulder strap area

Procedure Differentiation

A breast augmentation is performed in 19325. In this procedure, the physician increases the size of the breast by inserting an implant. The physician makes an incision in the fold under the breast and dissects the breast tissue and muscle layer free from the chest wall to accommodate an implant positioned under the muscle. As an alternative, the implant may also be positioned between the muscle and the existing breast tissue or skin. The incision is repaired with layered closure.

Medical Necessity

Coverage will be denied if this procedure is performed for cosmetic reasons.

Procedure Differentiation

Removal of breast implants are reported with codes 19328–19330. If the implant is intact (19328), the documentation will state that the physician makes an incision in the fold under the breast, around the nipple, or at the site of an existing mastectomy incision and dissects muscle, fat, and breast tissue from the existing implant. The intact implant is removed. Any infection is irrigated. The implant material is removed, including all implant contents such as saline or silicone gel. The surrounding tissue is checked closely for adhesions or deposits of the material that have infiltrated beyond the capsule. The implant material and any affected tissue are excised. Placement of a new implant during the same surgical setting is reported with 19342.

Medical Necessity

For a patient who has had an implant(s) placed for reconstructive or cosmetic purposes, Medicare considers treatment of any one or more of the following conditions to be medically necessary:

- Broken or failed implant
- Implant extrusion
- Infection
- Interference with diagnosis of breast cancer

 DEFINITIONS

kyphosis. Abnormal posterior convex curvature of the spine, usually in the thoracic region, resembling a hunchback.

paresthesia. Skin sensation produced by no obvious cause but typically involves disruption to a nerve.

- Painful capsular contracture with disfigurement
- Siliconoma or granuloma

Procedure Differentiation

Insertion of breast implants are reported with codes 19340–19342. Code selection is dependent upon when the breast implant was placed: immediate insertion is reported with 19340 and delayed insertion on a day different than the mastectomy with 19342.

Procedures performed on the nipples are reported with codes 19350–19355. In nipple reconstruction, the physician excises graft skin, usually from the inner thigh, behind the ear, or a section excised from the patient's existing areola. The donor site is repaired with sutures. To create a new nipple, the physician excises the lower section of tissue from the patient's existing nipple or removes tissue from the ear or labia. This donor site is repaired with sutures. A thin, circular layer of surface skin is removed from the breast at the site of the graft. The areola skin graft is positioned and sutured to the breast and the nipple graft is sutured to a small, circular incision in the areola's center. This procedure is reported with 19350 and includes local flaps, grafts, and tattooing. Inverted nipples are corrected in 19355. The documentation will state two or more radial incisions are made in the areola elevating the inverted nipple into an everted position. Ductal channels and fibrous bands may be transected to accomplish this. Tissue may be removed. The nipple is secured with sutures and incisions in the areola are closed.

The physician performs breast reconstruction with a tissue expander in code 19357. A breast tissue expander is an inflatable breast implant intended to stretch the skin and soft tissue to make room for a future implant. Using saline or carbon dioxide, the tissue expander is inflated, over time, until the skin and soft tissue are the required size for a permanent implant. Code 19357 reports the initial expander placement as well as subsequent expansions.

Flap breast reconstructions are reported with codes 19361–19369. In 19361, a latissimus dorsi flap is used to perform a breast reconstruction. The physician transfers skin and muscle from the patient's back to the breast area to correct defects created from a previous modified radical or radical mastectomy. The physician makes a skin incision in the back and dissects a portion of the latissimus muscle and the overlying skin from surrounding structures. The muscle-skin flap remains attached to a main artery. In preparation for the transfer, the mastectomy scar is excised. The muscle flap is rotated to the front of the chest through a tunnel under the armpit so that it extends through to the mastectomy incision. The incision in the back is repaired with layered closure. The physician adjusts the flap for the most aesthetic appearance and secures it with sutures to the chest wall, adjacent muscles, and skin.

In 19364, a free flap of skin, fat, and muscle is excised from another site on the patient for use in the reconstruction of the breast following a modified radical or radical mastectomy. The free flap is excised with careful dissection of vascular channels, commonly from the thigh or buttocks, and the operative wound is sutured in a layered repair. In preparation for the graft, the mastectomy scar is excised with blood vessels preserved. The free flap is transferred to the mastectomy site and microvascular anastomosis is done to provide the graft with a viable blood supply. The physician adjusts the flap for the most aesthetic appearance and secures it with sutures to the chest wall, adjacent muscles, and skin. If the free flap does not have enough fat, a breast implant may be required.

 AUDITOR'S ALERT

See Appendix 1 for the surgical auditing worksheet.

© 2020 Optum360, LLC

In 19366, the physician excises skin, fat, and/or muscle from another site on the patient for use in the reconstruction of the breast following a modified radical or radical mastectomy. The tissue is excised, and the operative wound is sutured in a layered repair. In preparation for the graft, any mastectomy scar is excised. The tissue is transferred to the mastectomy site. The physician adjusts the flap for the most aesthetic appearance and secures it with sutures to the chest wall, adjacent muscles, and skin. An operating microscope may be employed. If the tissue does not have sufficient bulk, a breast implant may be required.

Codes 19367–19369 use a rectus abdominis myocutaneous flap (TRAM) procedure for breast reconstruction. The physician first designs and then cuts a skin island flap on the lower abdominal wall. A superior skin and fat flap are elevated off the rectus abdominis muscle. A transverse incision is made in the rectus sheath and the muscle is divided and elevated, keeping the superior epigastric arteries intact for blood supply. Once the muscle is elevated, the physician makes an incision through the chest skin. This is also elevated, creating a pocket for the muscle flap. A connecting tunnel is made between the elevated chest skin and the inferiorly positioned flap. The flap is passed superiorly under the tunnel of tissue, placed into its new position, and sutured, after contouring a breast. The abdominal wall is closed by reapproximating the remaining anterior rectus muscle to the remaining lateral muscle and sheath. Skin edges are brought together and sutured in layers. Suction drains are also placed. Report 19368 if microvascular anastomosis for connecting blood vessels is used. Report 19369 if the muscle/skin complex has two pedicles or both sides of the rectus abdominis are elevated (bilateral or hemiflaps).

All of the flap reconstruction codes include flap harvesting, donor site closure, and flap insetting and shaping. If placement of a breast implant or a tissue expander is performed with flap reconstruction, it is reported separately.

Medical Necessity

The following conditions may warrant flap reconstruction (this list is not all inclusive). Reconstructive surgery is performed on abnormal structures of the body caused by:

- Congenital defects
- Developmental abnormalities
- Disease
- Infection
- Trauma
- Tumors

Procedure Differentiation

In 19370, the physician revises a peri-implant capsule of the breast by making an incision in the skin of the breast, at the site of a mastectomy scar, in the skin fold beneath the breast, or around the nipple. In a capsulotomy, the physician uses a cautery knife to cut into the area of fibrous scarring associated with a breast implant. Incisions are made into the scar (contracted capsule) to cut around its circumference and enlarge the pocket in which the implant is placed. Loosening the capsule relieves pain and tightness caused by the contracture. No tissue is removed. The incision is repaired with layered closure. A capsulorrhaphy reshapes or recontours the capsule while tightening and repositioning the capsule pocket so that the capsule fits back within the sutures surrounding the implant, while a capsulectomy removes a part of or the entire capsule. Code 19370 includes a partial capsulectomy. If a complete capsulectomy is performed, code 19371 is reported. In a complete procedure, the contracted capsule is excised from the breast tissue and the implant, along with all intracapsular contents.

Code 19380 reports a revision on a reconstructed breast, usually to correct a problem with asymmetry. This may require substantial tissue removal, reinsertion or readvancement of flaps in autologous reconstruction, or, in implant-based reconstruction, significant revision of the capsule in conjunction with soft tissue excision. The physician makes an incision in the breast skin along the areola or at the fold under the breast or in prior surgical incisions. Tissue therein may be rearranged or secured with sutures to revise the shape of the reconstructed breast. An existing breast implant may be replaced with an implant of a different configuration. Excess skin or tissue from the reconstructed breast may be removed. Once the breast has been revised to its desired shape, the physician repairs the incision with layered closure.

A breast moulage for a custom implant is reported with code 19396.

Key Documentation Terms
The key documentation terms for these procedures are augmentation, flap, implant, contracture, mastopexy, reduction, reconstruction, and removal. The documentation for this procedure should include the indications for the procedure and the procedure performed. Preoperative photographs should be included in the patient's medical record. If this procedure is performed due to pain or tenderness in the breast tissue, the medical record should contain documentation of the clinically significant impact upon activities of daily living and that it has been refractory to a trial of analgesics or anti-inflammatory agents (for a reasonable time period adequate to assess therapeutic effects).

Coding Tips
- To report fat grafting used at the time of a breast augmentation (19325), see 15771–15772.
- Removal of a tissue expander and placement of a breast implant is reported with 11970.
- Removal of a tissue expander without a replacement of a breast implant is reported with 11971.
- To report breast reconstruction using a latissimus dorsi flap with an immediate breast implant, see 19361 and 19340.
- All flap reconstruction codes include flap harvesting, donor site closure, and flap insetting and shaping. If placement of a breast implant or a tissue expander is performed with flap reconstruction, it is reported separately.

Procedures Performed on the Musculoskeletal System

Therapeutic Injection—Tendon and Trigger Points (20550–20553)

Injections of tendon sheaths, ligaments, trigger points, or aponeurosis are commonly performed.

Procedure Differentiation

Code selection for tendon and trigger point injection is determined by the anatomical site of injection, sheath, or origin.

Report the injection of a single tendon sheath, ligament, or aponeurosis with 20550 and each tendon insertion with 20551.

Medical Necessity

The following conditions may warrant these procedures (this list is not all inclusive):

- Adhesive capsulitis of shoulder
- Ankylosing spondylitis
- Bursitis
- Carpal or tarsal tunnel syndrome
- Epicondylitis
- Lesions of plantar nerve
- Sacroiliitis
- Spinal enthesopathy

Procedure Differentiation

Trigger points are reported according to number of muscles: 20552 for one or two and 20553 for three or more. Multiple trigger points may be injected in a single muscle.

Medical Necessity

The following conditions may warrant these procedures (this list is not all inclusive):

- Cervicalgia
- Fascitis
- Myalgia and myositis
- Muscle spasm
- Sciatica
- Tendinitis

Key Documentation Terms

The key term in this procedure is the number of muscles treated. Documentation should include details that support the medical necessity, in addition to the number of muscles treated and therapies tried prior to this procedure.

📖 DEFINITIONS

adhesive capsulitis. Excessive scar tissue in the shoulder, causing stiffness and pain.

bursitis. Inflammation of a bursa.

carpal tunnel syndrome. Swelling and inflammation in the tendons or bursa surrounding the median nerve caused by repetitive activity. The resulting compression on the nerve causes pain, numbness, and tingling especially to the palm, index, middle finger, and thumb.

cervicalgia. Pain localized to the cervical region, generally referring to the posterior or lateral regions of the neck.

enthesopathy. Disorders that occur at points where muscle, tendons, and ligaments attach to bones or joint capsules.

epicondylitis. Inflammation of the humeral epicondyle and the tissues adjoining it.

sciatica. Low back, buttock, and hip pain that radiates down the leg, sometimes accompanied by paresthesia and weakness, usually caused by a herniated disk in the lumbar spine or neuropathy affecting the sciatic nerve.

Documentation for ICD-10-CM will need to be more specific and include the precise location of the issue; for example, sciatica is broken down by left side, right side or unspecified side.

Coding Tips

- Moderate sedation is reported separately when required.

- Medications injected are reported separately with the appropriate HCPCS Level II codes.

- When multiple, separate tendon sheaths are injected in the same encounter, each injection is reported separately. Report 20550 and append modifier 59 for the second and subsequent sites.

- If imaging guidance is performed, see 76942, 77002, and 77021.

Coding Traps

- Codes 20550–20551 should not be reported with autologous protein solution (0481T) or platelet-rich plasma (0232T) injections.

- Note that codes 20560–20561 are reported for needle insertion in a muscle without an injection and should not be reported with 20552–20553 for the same muscle.

Aspiration and/or Injection of Joint (20600–20611)

Arthrocentesis is a puncture of the joint and includes aspiration and/or injection. The physician may aspirate fluid from the joint and/or inject a medication to control pain and inflammation. Only one service is reported per joint.

Procedure Differentiation

Code selection for arthrocentesis is based upon the size of the joint treated and whether or not it was performed under ultrasound guidance. Pathology exams are reported separately. Local anesthesia is not reported separately. If a drug is injected into the joint, identify the drug with the appropriate HCPCS Level II code (J code). Report 20600 or 20604 for a small joint or bursa (e.g., fingers, toes) with or without ultrasound guidance, 20605 or 20606 for an intermediate joint or bursa (e.g., temporomandibular, acromioclavicular, wrist, elbow, ankle, olecranon bursa) with or without ultrasound guidance, and 20610 or 20611 for a major joint or bursa (e.g., shoulder, hip, knees, subacromial bursa) with or without ultrasound guidance.

Medical Necessity

The following conditions may warrant these procedures (this list is not all inclusive):

- Adhesive capsulitis of shoulder
- Arthritis
- Derangements or tears of the lateral or medial meniscus
- Gout
- Joint effusion
- Osteoarthrosis
- Villonodular synovitis

Key Documentation Terms

Terms such as small, intermediate, major joint, ultrasound, or recording and report provide the guidance needed to ensure correct code assignment.

AUDITOR'S ALERT

See Appendix 1 for the audit worksheet for facet joint injections.

DEFINITIONS

arthritis. Inflammation of the joints often accompanied by swelling, stiffness, pain, and deformity.

chondrocalcinosis. Presence of calcium salt deposits within joint cartilage.

contracture. Shortening of muscle or connective tissue.

effusion. Escape of fluid from within a body cavity.

gout. Metabolic condition causing painful and inflamed joints.

osteoarthrosis. Most common form of a noninflammatory degenerative joint disease with degenerating articular cartilage, bone enlargement, and synovial membrane changes.

villonodular synovitis. Inflammation of the synovial membrane due to excessive synovial tissue formation, especially in the knee.

Documentation should include details that support the medical necessity, in addition to therapies tried prior to this procedure. Documentation for ICD-10-CM needs to be specific and include the precise location of the issue; for example, bursitis is broken down by left hip, right hip, or unspecified hip.

Coding Tips

- An E/M service performed on the same day may be separately reported with modifier 25 when considered to be a significant separate service from the biopsy.

- Arthrocentesis procedures (20600–20611) should not be reported separately with an open or arthroscopic joint procedure when performed on the same joint. However, if an arthrocentesis procedure is performed on one joint and an open or arthroscopic procedure is performed on a different joint, the arthrocentesis may be reported separately.

- When performed with fluoroscopic, CT, or MRI guidance, see the appropriate code form the radiology section (77002, 77012, or 77021).

Coding Trap

- When the services are performed under ultrasound guidance, do not report code 76942 separately.

Fracture Care

Fracture codes are packaged services and include percutaneous pinning and open or closed treatment of the fracture, application and removal of the initial cast or splint, and normal, uncomplicated follow-up care.

Several techniques apply to caring for bone injuries. Guidelines at the beginning of this subsection in CPT define terms unique to fracture care.

Exercise caution when coding fractures, especially when differentiating between the type of fracture and the type of treatment. A closed fracture may require closed or open treatment; whereas, an open fracture requires open treatment. Be sure to identify the site of the fracture, whether the fracture and treatment were open or closed, if manipulation was part of the treatment, and whether the procedure included internal or external skeletal fixation of the fracture or traction.

Initial treatment codes for fractures include application and removal of the cast or traction device.

While reduction of a fracture is a common term used in the medical community, the term reduction does not appear frequently in the CPT classification system. Instead, the term manipulation is used. Manipulation specifically means the attempted or successful reduction or restoration of a fracture or joint dislocation to its normal anatomic alignment by the use of manually applied forces.

Types of Fracture Treatment

The CPT book uses many terms to describe the different types of fracture treatment.

Procedure Differentiation

Closed Treatment

Closed treatment is defined as a realignment of a fracture without surgically opening the skin to reach the site.

 AUDITOR'S ALERT

See Appendix 1 for the fracture auditing worksheet.

- **Without manipulation:** This is the application of a cast, splint, bandage, or other traction, immobilization, or stabilization device, without fracture reduction. Such devices are usually applied to fractures of the long bones or back, because the bones of the fracture site remain aligned and there is no need for reduction or fixation. However, this can also be the case in smaller bones such as in the hands and feet.

- **With manipulation.** This is defined as skillful treatment by hand to reduce fractures and dislocations, or provide therapy through forceful passive movement of a joint beyond its active limit of motion.

- **Skin or skeletal traction.** This is the application of force to reinforce the stabilization as follows:

  - skin traction is the application of a pulling force to a limb accomplished by a device fixed to felt dressings or strappings applied to the body surface (skin).

  - skeletal traction applies a direct pulling force on the long axis of bones by inserted wires or pins and using weights and pulleys to keep the bone in proper alignment. Skeletal traction is often initially necessary with extensively comminuted fractures (broken or shattered into a number of small or large pieces) that are difficult to reduce and hold, or when an open procedure cannot be performed. Thus, open, closed, or percutaneous skeletal fixation treatment and the use of an external fixator is delayed.

Open Treatment

Open treatment is used when the fracture is surgically opened (exposed to the external environment). In this instance, the fracture (bone ends) is visualized, and internal fixation may be used. Uncomplicated soft tissue closure may involve closing an open fracture in which there is no damage to adjacent structures, such as the blood vessels, nerves, or lymphatic channels (i.e., a "clean break" in the bone). Two types of fixation—internal and external—are described in the CPT book.

Internal skeletal fixation involves wires, pins, screws, and plates placed through or within the fractured area to stabilize and immobilize the injury. This procedure is generally accomplished through an incision over the fracture site. It is commonly described as an open reduction with internal fixation (ORIF). Internal fixation may also be accomplished by percutaneous technique. Deep internal devices may be left in place even after the fracture has healed. If the hardware is removed, report 20670 or 20680. Use modifier 78 Return to the operating room, for a related procedure or modifier 58 Staged or related procedure by the same physician or other qualified healthcare professional during the postoperative period, if removal is performed during the initial hospital care or during the postoperative follow-up period. If the removal is performed after the postoperative follow-up period, report 20670 or 20680 without a modifier. The ICD-10-CM code is assigned according to the reason for the removal (e.g., pain, infection). Codes describing internal fixation are placed throughout the fracture care code section according to anatomic site.

External fixation (20690–20697) is hardware passing through bone and skin and held rigid by cross-braces outside the body. External fixation is always removed after the fracture has healed and removal is usually considered part of the global service. However, if the hardware is required to remain in place beyond the usual postoperative period, its removal should be reported (20694) when anesthesia is required. Removal of the external fixator performed without anesthesia is not a separately reported procedure.

Casting, bracing, or surgery may follow external fixation. The major indications for external fixation include limb fractures, major pelvic disruption, arthrodesis, osteotomy, and bone infection.

An external stabilization device is attached to internal pins, screws, etc., for the temporary or definitive treatment of bony disorders. These codes should only be used when the repair involves external fixation that is not included as part of a basic procedure.

Code 20690 is used when pins or wires are applied in one plane, unilaterally, as an external fixation device. This type of device consists of two or more pins. Code 20692 is used when a multiplane external fixation system is applied. Pins may be inserted at intervals through soft tissue and bone and mounted on rings that encircle the limb. Application of a multiplane system with subsequent adjustments is reported with 20696. Replacement of a strut in a multiplane system is reported with 20697.

Percutaneous Skeletal Fixation

Percutaneous skeletal fixation involves fracture treatment that is not described as open or closed (often the method of treatment for extra-articular fractures) and the injury site is not directly visualized. Fixation devices (pins, screws) are placed through the skin to stabilize the dislocation using x-ray guidance.

Key Documentation Terms

Documentation for fractures should include the type and location of fracture and the procedure performed to correct it, including percutaneous skeletal fixation if applicable. Terms such as open, closed, fixation pins, or wires provide the guidance needed to ensure correct code assignment.

ICD-10-CM requires specific information in order to correctly code fractures, such as the exact bone fractured, what part of the bone was fractured, whether the fracture was pathological or traumatic, and whether it is considered open or closed. The documentation must also state laterality and if there is a complication (e.g., delayed healing, malunion, or nonunion). If the fracture is classified as pathological, the underlying disease (e.g., osteoporosis, bone cyst) should be documented in the medical record.

Coding Tips

- Casting, splinting, or strapping may be reported when the service is performed either without musculoskeletal restoration treatment or as a replacement procedure performed during or after the postoperative period.

- In cases of multiple fractures, always list the most severe fracture as the primary diagnosis.

- If a fracture and dislocation must be reduced for a second time, consider using modifier 76 or 77 as appropriate to the circumstances.

- When medically necessary, report moderate (conscious) sedation provided by the performing physician or OQHCP with 99151–99153. When provided by another physician or other qualified health care professional, report 99155–99157.

DEFINITIONS

pathological fracture. Break in bone due to a disease process that weakens the bone structure, such as osteoporosis, osteomalacia, or neoplasia, and not traumatic injury.

- The application of external immobilization devices (casts, splints, strapping) at the time of a procedure includes the subsequent removal of the device when performed by the same physician or physician group.

- CPT codes for closed, open, or percutaneous treatment of fractures include the application of casts, splints, or strapping and should not be reported separately.

- If a closed reduction procedure fails and is converted to an open reduction procedure at the same patient encounter, only the more extensive open procedure should be reported.

Dislocations

This section of CPT is used to report the displacement of bones, especially joints.

Procedure Differentiation

Exercise caution when coding dislocations, especially differentiating between types of dislocation and types of treatment. Closed dislocations may require closed or open treatment, whereas open dislocations require open treatment. Make certain to identify:

- Site

- Dislocation type: open or closed

- Treatment type: open or closed

- Treatment

- Includes manipulation

- Procedure includes internal and external skeletal fixation of the dislocation

The use of CPT codes for dislocation treatment hinge upon whether anesthesia is administered. See dislocation in the CPT book index for a complete list of CPT codes by anatomic location.

Key Documentation Terms

Documentation for dislocation should include the type of dislocation and the procedure performed to correct it. Key terms will include open or closed and the anatomical location.

When assigning ICD-10-CM codes for dislocations, it is important to understand terminology. A subluxation is a partial or incomplete dislocation (separation) of a joint with misalignment but maintains some contact between the bones. A dislocation is a complete disruption of the joint. In ICD-10-CM, for most body sites the code selection is basic, being determined by site and laterality, but it is further divided by whether the injury is a subluxation or dislocation. For certain sites of dislocation or subluxation, code selection is further divided by degree or direction of separation. There is no subdivision in ICD-10-CM for open and closed joint dislocation or subluxation. Also, the ICD-10-CM codes for dislocation and subluxation include an instructional note indicating a separate code is assigned for any associated open wound.

Coding Tip
- CPT codes for closed, open, or percutaneous treatment of dislocations include the application of casts, splints, or strapping and should not be reported separately.

Casting, Splinting, and Strapping (29000–29799)

These codes are commonly used when a cast, splint, or strapping is replaced during the postoperative follow-up portion of a more complex service or procedure. It is also appropriate to assign a code from this heading when the provider applies a cast, splint, or strapping to immobilize an injury such as a sprain or before a more intense restorative procedure is performed. For example, the provider may elect to splint a fractured wrist until the patient can be seen by an orthopedist and more definitive fracture care can be provided. However, when all of the fracture care is provided the use of one of these codes is not reported separately as the application of the first cast, strap, or splint is included in the global package for fractures and dislocations.

Certain orthopedic problems are routinely treated with splints or splint-like devices. The following are considered medically necessary:

- Shoulder immobilizer
- Clavicle splint (also called a figure-eight splint)
- Acromioclavicular splint (also called a Zimmer splint)
- Finger splints
- Carpal tunnel splints

Casting material used in fracture care can be fiberglass or plaster. The choice of material is dictated by the individual situation and is left to the discretion of the treating provider.

Certain nondurable items (e.g., arm slings, Ace bandages, splints, foam cervical collars, etc.) may be eligible for payment in some circumstances even though they are not durable and do not fit within the definition of durable medical equipment. These nondurable items may be covered when charges are made by a hospital, surgical center, home health care agency, or provider for necessary medical and surgical supplies used in connection with treatment rendered at the time the supply is used. However, charges for take home supplies (e.g., extra bandages, cervical pillows, etc.) are not covered. Please check benefit plan descriptions for details.

Coding Tip
- An E/M service performed on the same day may be reported separately with modifier 25. All of the elements of the E/M service must be satisfied. This is generally not an issue because the patient is assessed for other injuries in addition to the fracture. Make sure that the ICD-10-CM codes support the medical necessity of the additional E/M service.
- To report orthotics management training, see 97760-97763.

Procedures Performed on the Spine (22010–22899)

Procedure codes used to report spine surgeries are found in two sections of the CPT book: the Musculoskeletal System and the Nervous System.

Procedure Differentiation

Excision, fracture/dislocation, spinal fusion/instrumentation, and treatment of scoliosis/kyphosis are reported with codes from the musculoskeletal section (22100–22899).

Two codes, 22010 and 22015, report the open incision and drainage of a deep spinal abscess. These codes are reported according to area of the spine.

 DEFINITIONS

durable medical equipment. Medical equipment that can withstand repeated use, is not disposable, is used to serve a medical purpose, is generally not useful to a person in the absence of a sickness or injury, and is appropriate for use in the home. Examples of durable medical equipment include hospital beds, wheelchairs, and oxygen equipment.

Excision codes are reported with 22100–22116.

Osteotomy codes (22206–22226) are reported by approach and the section of spine where the procedure is performed.

Spinal fractures and/or dislocations are reported with codes 22310–22328.

Pay close attention to add-on codes in each of the sections above as they denote each additional vertebral segment. Read each code description thoroughly before assigning a code.

Many spinal procedures are grouped into families of codes where there are separate primary procedure codes describing the procedure at a single vertebral level in the cervical, thoracic, or lumbar region of the spine. Within some families of codes there is an add-on code for reporting the same procedure at each additional level without specifying the spinal region for the add-on code. When multiple procedures from one of these families of codes are performed at contiguous vertebral levels, a physician should report only one primary code within the family of codes for one level and should report additional contiguous levels using the add-on code(s) in the family of codes. The reported primary code should be the one corresponding to the spinal region of the first procedure. If multiple procedures from one of these families of codes are performed at multiple vertebral levels that are not contiguous and in different regions of the spine, the physician may report one primary code for each noncontiguous region.

Percutaneous vertebroplasty and vertebral augmentation procedures are reported with the appropriate code from the 22510–22515 range. When a code for a percutaneous vertebroplasty is reported, the documentation should indicate that the provider, under imaging guidance, injected a cement material into the vertebral body in an effort to reinforce the structure. Augmentation is differentiated by documentation indicating that before the injection, the provider had to create a cavity into which to inject the material. Bone biopsies and imaging guidance are included and should not be reported separately. Code selection depends on the level (cervical, thoracic, lumbar) and the number of vertebral bodies the procedure is performed on. Sacral augmentation or sacroplasty is not reported with a code from this range. A Category III code (0200T–0201T) should be reported for sacral procedures.

Codes 22510–22512 represent a family of codes describing percutaneous vertebroplasty, and codes 22513–22515 represent a family of codes describing percutaneous vertebral augmentation. Within each of these families of codes, the physician may report only one primary procedure code and the add-on procedure code for each additional level(s) whether or not the additional level(s) are contiguous.

Percutaneous annuloplasty procedures are reported with codes from range 22526–22527. These codes represent annuloplasty procedures performed with intradiscal electrothermal therapy (IDET).

Arthrodesis of the spine is reported with codes from range 22532–22812. These codes are assigned based on technique and approach (anterior, posterior/posterolateral, or lateral). Codes 22532–22533, 22548, 22551, 22554–22558, 22586, 22590–22612, 22630, and 22633 are for single interspace arthrodesis—two adjacent vertebral segments. When the surgery is performed on more than one interspace, each additional interspace is reported with 22534,

22552, 22585, 22614, 22632, or 22634. These procedures are considered add-on services and are not reported alone or with modifier 51.

Some additional guidance is given in the January 2021 NCCI policy manual, chapter 4, regarding reporting within a family of codes. The family of codes 22532–22534 describe arthrodesis by lateral extracavitary technique. Code 22532 describes the procedure for a single thoracic vertebral segment, code 22533 describes the procedure for a single lumbar vertebral segment, and 22534 is an add-on code describing the procedure for each additional thoracic or lumbar vertebral segment. As an example of the family of codes mentioned above, if a physician performs arthrodesis by lateral extracavitary technique on contiguous vertebral segments such as T12 and L1, only one primary procedure code, the one for the first procedure, may be reported. The procedure on the second vertebral body may be reported with code 22534. If multiple procedures from one of these families of codes are performed at multiple vertebral levels that are not contiguous and in different regions of the spine, the physician may report one primary code for each noncontiguous region. For example, if a physician performs the procedure at T10 and L4 through separate skin incisions, the physician may report codes 22532 and 22533.

The procedures specific to scoliosis and kyphosis are 22800–22819; these codes also include arthrodesis procedures. The arthrodesis procedures in this section are different from other arthrodesis procedures as they involve different approaches and multiple vertebral segments. Codes are assigned based on the number of segments treated.

The use of bone grafts and bone marrow aspiration for bone grafting in addition to the fusion are reported separately with 20930, 20931, and 20936-20939.

Procedures of the spine with spinal cord involvement are reported with codes from the nervous system section (62263–63746). It is not unusual for procedures to require a procedure from the musculoskeletal section (arthrodesis, instrumentation) with a procedure from the nervous system section (laminectomy, hemilaminectomy, discectomy), and it is appropriate to report both procedures separately.

Spinal instrumentation (22840–22847) involves placement of rods, hooks, and wires to stabilize the fusion or fracture. Instrumentation codes are assigned based on the type of instrumentation (segmental, nonsegmental), the approach (anterior, posterior), and the number of vertebral segments involved. Instrumentation codes are reported in addition to a code for the definitive procedure. Biomechanical devices are another type of spinal instrumentation that may be used to fill a defect in an intervertebral disc or vertebral body. Examples of these devices are mesh or a synthetic cage, which may be anchored by screws or flanges, or methylmethacrylate which is used as a bone cement. They are reported with codes 22853–22854 and 22859.

The CPT book has offered additional guidelines to describe the types of spinal instrumentation. Segmental instrumentation is defined as fixation at each end of the instrumentation and at least one principal bony connection. This means that the instrumentation is attached at the beginning, end, and at least one extra site in between. Nonsegmental fixation is attached only at the top and bottom. This fixation may span several vertebral segments without attaching to multiple vertebrae between the ends. Harrington rods, for instance, may be considered segmental or nonsegmental, depending upon the sites of attachment.

 DEFINITIONS

bone graft. Bone that is removed from one part of the body and placed into another bone site without direct re-establishment of blood supply.

kyphosis. Abnormal posterior convex curvature of the spine, usually in the thoracic region, resembling a hunchback.

scoliosis. Congenital condition of lateral curvature of the spine, often associated with other spinal column defects, congenital heart disease, or genitourinary abnormalities. It may also be associated with spinal muscular atrophy, cerebral palsy, or muscular dystrophy.

Spinal instrumentation codes are always listed in addition to a code for the definitive treatment.

Code 22840 describes placement of nonsegmental instrumentation (a construct placed with fixation at either end only and not in the intervening levels). The physician makes a midline incision in the skin, fascia, and paravertebral muscles over the affected vertebrae. Upper and lower hooks or screws are introduced into the vertebral pedicles. A rod fashioned to fit the spinal contours is anchored to the screws or hooks. The minimal wiring inherent in this procedure should not be reported with 22841.

Code 22841 is reported when the physician documents that wiring of spinous process was performed. Code 22842 reports posterior segmental instrumentation with three to six vertebral segments; code 22843 reports seven to 12 vertebral segments, and code 22844 reports 13 or more vertebral segments.

Anterior instrumentation is described by codes 22845–22847. This type of instrumentation is reserved for flexible lumbar or thoracolumbar scoliotic curves. Several methods and types are available (e.g., Dwyer, Zielke, Scottish Rite) but all are based on a rod or cable fixated through large-headed, slotted, or cannulated screws. Code 22845 is reported when documentation indicates two to three vertebral segments, 22846 for four to seven vertebral segments, and 22847 for eight or more vertebral segments.

Code 22848, describes pelvic fixation. The rod is placed through the ilium and negates the need for anterior instrumentation. This procedure, usually called the "Galveston technique," often accompanies a procedure for scoliosis, myelomeningocele, or paralytic spinal defects where sacral fixation is not desirable.

Code 22849 describes the procedures used following failure of devices such as wires, screws, cables, plates, or rods used in spinal fixation. The spinal fixation is reinserted but in most cases, the device must be replaced.

Code 22850 describes when a patient's posterior spinal nonsegmental instrumentation is removed. Code 22852 is reported when posterior spinal segmental instrumentation is removed.

In 22853 the physician replaces an intervertebral disc resected due to destruction by disease, trauma, or other processes. Once the vertebral disc has been removed by a separately identifiable procedure, a hole is cored out of the vertebral bodies above and below the removed vertebrae to secure a biomechanical device (synthetic cage or mesh) into the resulting intervertebral disc space. The physician selects the biomechanical device best suited to the location and type of deformity being corrected. Screws, wires, or plates may be used to secure the device. Muscles are allowed to fall back into place and the wound is closed over a drain with layered sutures. This procedure is performed in conjunction with an interbody arthrodesis. Code 22854 is reported when a vertebral body or partial vertebral body is resected and replaced with a biomechanical device. This procedure is also performed in conjunction with an interbody arthrodesis. Code 22859 is reported when a biomechanical device, such as, mesh, methylmethacrylate, or a synthetic cage is inserted in an intervertebral disc space or vertebral body defect without an interbody arthrodesis being performed.

© 2020 Optum360, LLC

When auditing these procedures:

- Clarify whether segmental or nonsegmental instrumentation is performed.

- Count the number of segments, as codes that are assigned are dependent upon the number of segments.

- Remember that the placement of screws into the facet joint are reported with 22840.

- Report 22849 when documentation indicates nonunion exploration with replacement of instrumentation.

- Report code 22853, 22854, or 22859 for placement of biomechanical devices.

Medical Necessity

There are multiple indications for these services to be performed (this list is not all inclusive); however, please verify coverage with the payer:

- Degenerative disc disease
- Spinal debridement for infection
- Spinal deformity
- Spinal fracture
- Spinal tuberculosis
- Spondylolysis

Key Documentation Terms

Documentation should include details that support the medical necessity of the procedure, a narrative of the procedure, the vertebral segments involved, and use of any hardware if applicable. Terms such as abscess, corpectomy, dislocations, excision, fracture, kyphosis, methylmethacrylate, osteotomy, and scoliosis provide the guidance needed to ensure correct code assignment.

Coding Tips

- As "add-on" codes, 22103, 22116, 22208, 22216, 22226, 22328, 22512, 22515, 22527, 22534, 22552, 22585, 22614, 22632, 22634, 22840–22848, 22853–22854 and 22859 are not subject to multiple procedure rules. No reimbursement reduction or modifier 51 is applied. See the CPT book for the codes with which these add-on codes should be reported.

- Casting, splinting, or strapping may be reported when the service is performed either without musculoskeletal restoration treatment or as a replacement procedure performed during or after the postoperative period.

- In the event that two surgeons perform as primary surgeons on distinct parts of an excision procedure, modifier 62 may be appended to the CPT code.

- Bone allografts and autografts should be reported separately with 20930, 20931, and 20936-20939. These codes are considered add-on services and are not reported with modifier 51. They are reported in addition to the definitive procedure. Only one code from this section can be reported per operative session.

- If arthrodesis is performed in addition to another definitive procedure, append modifier 51.

- Instrumentation and bone graft procedures are reported in addition to arthrodesis codes without modifier 51.

Arthroscopic Procedures (29800–29999)

Arthroscopy is a surgical procedure orthopedic surgeons use to visualize, diagnose, and treat problems inside a joint. Diagnosing joint injuries and disease begins with a thorough medical history, physical examination, and usually x-rays. Additional tests, such as an MRI or CT scan, may also be needed. Through the arthroscope, a final diagnosis is made, which may be more accurate than through "open" surgery or from x-ray studies.

Note that all surgical arthroscopic services, regardless of site, include a diagnostic arthroscopy of the same site. When multiple surgical procedures are performed, read the descriptions carefully to determine what is included in each service to avoid unbundling. Debridement is included in more extensive procedures, particularly when performed in the same joint or joint space.

Procedure Differentiation

Below are a few of the more common arthroscopies.

Surgical Shoulder Arthroscopy

In addition to diagnostic services many procedures may be performed arthroscopically in the shoulder joint. Surgical repairs of the shoulder may include a combination of open and arthroscopic surgery to complete the procedure. It is important to have a basic understanding of shoulder anatomy to be able to identify the structures involved so that the appropriate codes may be selected. This includes the clavicle, acromioclavicular joint, acromion process, coracoid process, and humeral head. Notes in this section direct coders to open procedures and instruct the coder when two codes may be reported together if performed and documented.

Medical Necessity

There are multiple indications for shoulder arthroscopy to be performed (this list is not all inclusive, including:

- Frozen shoulder
- Impingement syndrome
- Infections
- Instability (recurrent dislocations)
- Removal of loose bodies
- Rotator cuff tears
- Rotator cuff tendonitis
- SLAP tears

Surgical Knee Arthroscopy

Knee arthroscopy procedures represent a major portion of outpatient surgical procedures on the musculoskeletal system. Note that a diagnostic knee arthroscopy (29870) is included in all of these procedures and, as such, does not warrant a separate code assignment. Also included are "integral procedures" that often are performed as part of the overall procedure and do not warrant separate code identification in the CPT book. The integral procedures documented are not intended to present a medical standard of care or practice parameter for the health care community.

 DEFINITIONS

acromioclavicular joint. Junction between the clavicle and the scapula. The acromion is the projection from the back of the scapula that forms the highest point of the shoulder and connects with the clavicle. Trauma or injury to the acromioclavicular joint is often referred to as a dislocation of the shoulder. This is not correct, however, as a dislocation of the shoulder is a disruption of the glenohumeral joint.

acromion process. Highest point and outer most projection of the shoulder joint, formed from a lateral projection of the spine of the scapula.

anterior cruciate ligament. Ligament composed of two parts: anteromedial and posterolateral bundle. It helps hold the tibia and femur together deep within the knee joint. When this tears or ruptures, it creates instability of the knee. Repair can be done open or arthroscopically.

clavicle. Bone located between the sternum and scapula, connecting the arm to the body.

coracoid process. Curved process arising from the upper neck of the scapula and overhanging the glenoid cavity.

meniscus. Crescent-shaped fibrous cartilage found within the knee, temporomandibular, acromioclavicular, and sternoclavicular intraarticular joint.

osteoarthritis. Most common form of a noninflammatory degenerative joint disease with degenerating articular cartilage, bone enlargement, and synovial membrane changes.

posterior cruciate ligament Ligament that attaches the posterior tibia to the front of the femur.

rotator cuff. Four muscles that originate on the scapula and form a single tendon that inserts on the head of the humerus. The supraspinatus, infraspinatus, subscapularis, and teres minor are the four muscles that come together to help lift and rotate the arm.

SLAP. Superior labral anteroposterior (lesion).

Loose bodies may be removed from the knee joint in 29874. This may be accomplished by suctioning or irrigating them from the joint. Larger loose bodies are grasped by a clamp and removed. Very large loose bodies may require enlargement of a portal or division with an arthroscopic scissor before removal.

Minor and major synovectomy procedures are described and the number of compartments of the knee that are entered define code selection (e.g., two or more compartments). The synovium is the lining of the joint compartment and is involved with making and containing joint fluids. A limited synovectomy is reported with 29875. A major synovectomy procedure (29876) involving multiple compartments may take several hours to perform. Report 29877 when motorized shaving of articular cartilage is performed. This is also reported as a "notch plasty" procedure. Articular cartilage is the white, rubbery cap on the end of bones of the major joints.

Codes 29874 and 29877 should not be reported with other knee arthroscopy codes (29866-29889). However, it is appropriate to report HCPCS Level II code G0289 (Surgical knee arthroscopy for removal of loose body, foreign body, debridement/shaving of articular cartilage at the time of other surgical knee arthroscopy in a different compartment of the same knee) with other knee arthroscopy codes. The descriptions of 29880 and 29881 indicate that debridement/shaving of articular cartilage of any compartment is included in the procedure; therefore, it would be inappropriate to report additional debridement procedures. HCPCS Level II code G0289 may be reported with CPT codes 29880 or 29881 only when the documentation indicates that removal of a loose body or foreign body from a different compartment of the same knee was performed. Append modifier 51 on subsequent procedures. This is per the Medicare NCCI policy so one would need to verify what other payer policies are on this section of codes.

A synovectomy to "clean up" a joint on which another more extensive procedure is performed is not reported separately. Code 29875 should never be reported with another arthroscopic knee procedure on the ipsilateral knee. Code 29876 may be reported for a medically reasonable and necessary synovectomy with another arthroscopic knee procedure on the ipsilateral knee if the synovectomy is performed in two compartments on which another arthroscopic procedure is not performed. For example, code 29876 should never be reported for a major synovectomy with code 29880 (knee arthroscopy, medial AND lateral meniscectomy) on the ipsilateral knee since knee arthroscopic procedures other than synovectomy are performed in two of the three knee compartments.

Medical Necessity

There are multiple indications for knee arthroscopy to be performed (this list is not all inclusive), including:

- Anterior cruciate ligament (ACL) tear
- Arthroscopic assisted fixation of tibial plateau fractures
- Articular cartilage injuries
- Derangement of lateral meniscus
- Infection (pyogenic arthritis, tuberculous arthritis)
- Joint derangement
- Loose body in knee
- Meniscal tear

- Osteoarthritis
- Posterior cruciate ligament (PCL) tear

Key Documentation Terms

Documentation should include details that support the medical necessity of the arthroscopy and a narrative of the procedure. If additional procedures are performed, they must also support the medical necessity. Terms such as limited, minor, major, open, or arthroscopic provide the guidance needed to ensure correct code assignment.

Documentation for ICD-10-CM needs to be specific and include the precise location of the issue; for example, ACL tears and joint derangements are broken down by specific site, such as left knee, right knee, or unspecified knee.

Coding Tips

- A diagnostic arthroscopy is not reported separately. If a diagnostic arthroscopy leads to a surgical arthroscopy at the same patient encounter, only the surgical arthroscopy may be reported.

- If the procedure code is unilateral, and the procedure performed was bilateral, some payers require that the service be reported twice with modifier 50 appended to the second code while others require identification of the service only once with modifier 50 appended. Check with individual payers for specific guidelines. Modifier 50 identifies a procedure performed identically on the opposite side of the body (mirror image).

- Arthroscopic removal of a loose or foreign body should be reported only when the loose/foreign body is at least the size of the diameter of the arthroscopic cannula that is being used for the procedure or larger. When removing the loose/foreign body, it must be performed through a cannula larger than the one being used for the actual procedure or a separate incision or a portal that is large enough to allow removal of the loose/foreign body.

- If an arthroscopic procedure is converted to an open procedure, only the open procedure may be reported. Neither a surgical arthroscopy nor a diagnostic arthroscopy code should be reported with the open procedure code when a surgical arthroscopic procedure is converted to an open procedure.

- If an arthroscopy is performed as a "scout" procedure to assess the surgical field or extent of disease, it is not separately reportable. If the findings of a diagnostic arthroscopy lead to the decision to perform an open procedure, the diagnostic arthroscopy may be separately reportable. Modifier 58 may be reported to indicate that the diagnostic arthroscopy and nonarthroscopic therapeutic procedures were staged or planned procedures. The medical record must indicate the medical necessity for the diagnostic arthroscopy.

- Arthroscopic debridement should not be reported separately with a surgical arthroscopy procedure when performed on the same joint at the same patient encounter.

Arthroplasty

Procedure Differentiation

Arthroplasty describes the repair of a joint usually involving replacement of part or the entire joint with an artificial joint. The prosthesis may be metal,

© 2020 Optum360, LLC

porcelain, or other material. Sometimes only part of the joint is replaced, such as the head of the femur. At other times the entire joint may be replaced as done when the head of the femur and the acetabulum are replaced in a total hip replacement procedure. Arthroplasty is performed as a result of injury, excessive wear, or erosion of the joint as in arthritis, osteomyelitis, and other diseases. The muscles may be attached to existing bone or the prosthesis to ensure full mobility after the procedure. There are also procedures for revision of a total joint replacement for some joints.

Abrasion arthroplasty (29879) involves removal of bone matter (usually dead). Another technique used to achieve the removal of dead bone may be drilling multiple holes or microfracture. Bilateral meniscus removal on a single knee is reported with 29880. Medial or lateral (unilateral) removal is reported with 29881. Repairs to a damaged meniscus (29882–29883) are usually attempted before removal is considered.

Codes 29885–29887 are specific to the treatment of osteochondritis dissecans, a bone disorder involving the epiphyseal growth tissues in young people or the bone/cartilage interface in adults. A separate code may be assigned if the bone graft is taken from the patient's hip (20900 or 20902) or obtained from a bone bank (20999).

Medical Necessity

The following conditions may warrant these procedures (this list is not all inclusive):

- Advanced joint disease
- Arthritis
- Excessive wear
- Failure of a previous osteotomy
- Infection
- Injury
- Instability of joint
- Malignancy of the joint involving the bones or soft tissues
- Osteochondritis dissecans
- Osteomyelitis
- Progressive or substantial bone loss
- Recurrent or irreducible dislocation

Key Documentation Terms

Documentation should include details that support the medical necessity, in addition to therapies tried prior to this procedure, and use of any hardware, if applicable. Terms such as bone grafting, drilling, microfracture, meniscectomy, osteochondritis dissecans, or repair provide the guidance needed to ensure correct code assignment.

 DEFINITIONS

dislocation. Displacement of a bone in relation to its neighboring tissue, especially a joint.

osteochondritis dissecans. Avascular necrosis caused by lack of blood flow to the bone and cartilage of a joint causing the bone to die. This can result in splinters or pieces of cartilage breaking off in the joint.

osteomyelitis. Inflammation of bone that may remain localized or spread to the marrow, cortex, or periosteum, in response to an infecting organism, usually bacterial and pyogenic.

osteotomy. Surgical cutting of a bone.

Procedures Performed on the Respiratory System

Rhinoplasty (30400–30462)

Rhinoplasty is a reconstructive, restorative, or cosmetic plastic surgery to reshape the external nose. Depending on the procedure performed, surgery on the nasal septum may or may not be necessary. Surgery may be performed to improve abnormal function caused by a hereditary condition or as the result of a trauma that produced an unacceptable function and/or appearance.

Procedure Differentiation

Code selection is dependent upon the intensity of and the reason for the procedure. Primary rhinoplasty procedures are reported with 30400–30420 and secondary rhinoplasty procedures are classified to 30430–30450.

In 30400–30410, surgery is not performed on the nasal septum. Report 30420 when documentation indicates that the physician reshaped a fractured or deformed septum.

Secondary rhinoplasty may be performed to revise a previous procedure where the outcome may not have been what was intended.

Rhinoplasty for nasal deformities that are due to a cleft lip and/or palate are reported with 30460–30462.

When auditing these procedures, the following questions should be answered before determining code assignment:

- Why was the procedure performed?
- Is the procedure primary, secondary, or due to congenital deformity?
- What was the complexity of the procedure (e.g., minor, intermediate, or major)?

Medical Necessity

Coverage will be denied if this procedure is performed for cosmetic reasons.

The following conditions may warrant this procedure (this list is not all inclusive):

- Acquired deformity of nose
- Benign neoplasm
- Cleft lip and/or palate
- Malignancy
- Nasal fracture
- Plastic surgery for unacceptable cosmetic appearance

Key Documentation Terms

Documentation should include details that support the medical necessity and the intent of the procedure. Preoperative photographs should be included in the patient's medical record. Terms such as primary, secondary, minor, major, or congenital provide the guidance needed to ensure correct code assignment.

 AUDITOR'S ALERT

Obtaining tissues for graft may be reported separately, see codes 15769, 20900–20924, and 21210.

Coding Tips

- Tissue grafts may be reported separately using codes 15769, 20900–20924, and 21210. However, local grafts from adjacent nasal bones and cartilage are not reported separately.

- Topical vasoconstrictive agents and local anesthesia are not reported separately.

Coding Trap

- When these procedures are performed for cosmetic reasons they will be deemed not medically necessary and denied coverage.

Sinusotomy (31020–31090)

In a sinusotomy, the sinus is entered, drained, and irrigated clean of any debris; polyps or other structural abnormalities are removed, but the mucous membrane of the sinus is left intact. In a sinusectomy, all of the sinus contents, including the mucous membrane, are removed.

Procedure Differentiation

Code selection is based upon the sinuses treated and the type of treatment performed. Some of the procedures also include reconstructive surgery to repair the resulting defect.

Code 31020 reports an intranasal maxillary sinusotomy. Codes 31030–31032 are differentiated by whether antrochoanal polyps are removed at the same time as the Caldwell-Luc procedure.

Code 31040 is specific to procedures performed on the pterygomaxillary fossa.

Codes 31050 and 31051 report sinusotomies of the sphenoid sinus differentiated by whether a biopsy is performed or mucosal stripping or polyps are removed.

Codes 31070–31087 report sinusotomies of the frontal sinus and are differentiated by additional procedures performed (e.g., osteoplastic [bone] flap) and the incision type (brow or coronal). In obliterative procedures (31080–31085), the sinus cavity is eliminated by filling it with autologous fat harvested from the abdomen or buttocks. In 31086-31087, the frontal bone is removed with the attached periosteum overlying the frontal sinus. No obliteration of the sinus is necessary.

Code 31090 Sinusotomy, unilateral, three or more paranasal sinuses (frontal, maxillary, ethmoid, and sphenoid), should be used in place of separate codes when surgical sinusotomy is performed in three or more of these areas.

Medical Necessity

The following conditions may warrant these procedures (this list is not all inclusive):

- Benign neoplasm
- Foreign body
- Malignancy
- Nasal polyps
- Sinusitis

 DEFINITIONS

autologous. Tissue, cells, or structure derived from the same individual.

Caldwell-Luc operation. Intraoral antrostomy approach into the maxillary sinus for the removal of tooth roots or tissue, or for packing the sinus to reduce zygomatic fractures by creating a window above the teeth in the canine fossa area.

polyp. Small growth on a stalk-like attachment projecting from a mucous membrane.

pterygomaxillary fossa. Wide depression on the external surface of the maxilla above and to the side of the canine tooth socket.

 AUDITOR'S ALERT

Code 31090 Sinusotomy, unilateral, three or more paranasal sinuses (frontal, maxillary, ethmoid, sphenoid), should be used in place of separate codes when surgical sinusotomy is performed in three or more of these areas.

Key Documentation Terms

Documentation should include details that support the medical necessity, which area of the sinus was involved, and a narrative summary of the procedure. Terms such as brow, coronal, osteoplastic flap, obliterative, nonobliterative, and polyp provide the guidance needed to ensure correct code assignment.

Coding Tips

- Topical vasoconstrictive agents and local anesthesia are not reported separately.

- These are unilateral procedures. If performed bilaterally, some payers require that the service be reported twice with modifier 50 appended to the second code, while others require identification of the service only once with modifier 50 appended. Check with individual payers. Modifier 50 identifies a procedure performed identically on the opposite side of the body (mirror image).

Nasal Endoscopy, Diagnostic or Surgical (31231–31298)

Nasal endoscopy is a commonly performed procedure. In order to correctly report these services it is important to understand the anatomy.

There are four pairs of paranasal sinuses named from the bones in which they are found: the frontal, maxillary, ethmoid, and sphenoid. Each sinus is an air-containing space lined by respiratory mucosa and produces secretions that drain into the nasal cavity.

The right and left frontal sinuses are above the eye sockets, and the maxillary sinuses are on each side of the nose. The sphenoid sinuses lie deeper, at the midline, and are close to the pituitary gland and the optic nerve. The ethmoid sinuses are collections of small air cells that open independently into the upper nasal cavity. The sinuses serve both to lighten the bones of the skull and to provide resonating chambers for speech.

When a nasal endoscopy is performed, an endoscope is placed into the nose and a thorough inspection of internal nasal structures is accomplished. Many other codes included in this section report procedures performed via a nasal endoscopy.

Procedure Differentiation

Code 31231 reports a diagnostic nasal endoscopy. Diagnostic evaluation refers to an inspection of the interior of the nasal cavity and the middle and superior meatus, the turbinates, and the sphenoethmoid recess. Any time a diagnostic evaluation is performed, all of these areas are inspected and a separate code is not reported for each area.

Codes 31233 and 31235 also describe diagnostic nasal endoscopy and include a maxillary or sphenoid sinusoscopy.

Surgical nasal/sinus endoscopies are reported with 31237–31298. These procedures are reported based on the anatomical structures visualized and any procedures that may be performed via the scope during the same operative session. Procedures include biopsy, excision of tissue/lesion, control of bleeding, decompression, and dilation. It is very important to thoroughly read the code descriptions when assigning a code for the service performed.

Codes 31254-31259 describe nasal endoscopies with ethmoidectomies. It is important to note that these codes are differentiated by whether a partial

DEFINITIONS

decompression. Release of pressure.

dilation. Artificial increase in the diameter of an opening or lumen made by medication or by instrumentation.

turbinates. Scroll or shell-shaped elevations from the wall of the nasal cavity, the inferior turbinate being a separate bone, while the superior and middle turbinates are of the ethmoid bone.

(anterior) or total (anterior and posterior) ethmoidectomy is performed, and if other services, such as removal of tissue from the frontal sinus (31253), sphenoidotomy (31257), or sphenoidotomy and removal of tissue from the sphenoid sinus (31259), are performed. In addition, many endoscopy procedures cannot be performed together when both procedures are done on the ipsilateral side (same side).

Medical Necessity

The following conditions may warrant nasal endoscopy (this list is not all inclusive):

- Chronic dacryocystitis
- Chronic or recurrent sinusitis
- Evaluation of a patient with atypical asthma refractory to usual treatment
- Evaluation of moderate to severe signs and/or symptoms of upper airway abnormalities:
  - anosmia
  - change in voice quality
  - dysphagia
  - facial pain
  - hyposmia
  - obstructive apnea
  - odynophagia
  - persistent hoarseness
  - recurrent epistaxis
  - serosanguineous nasal discharge
  - tightness in throat
- Nasal polyps
- Neoplasm of the upper airway
- Persistent nasal obstruction not due to septal deviation and not responding to standard medical therapy (e.g., decongestants, steroids)
- Sarcoidosis

Key Documentation Terms

In order to assign the most appropriate code, the medical record documentation must be reviewed to determine why the procedure was performed (i.e., biopsy, nasal hemorrhage, or resection, with antrostomy). Key terms may also include partial or total. Documentation must clearly support the medical necessity of the service being reported. It also must include the portion of the nose or sinus that is treated and the procedure(s) performed.

Coding Tips

- A sinusotomy and diagnostic endoscopy are considered integral parts of a surgical sinus endoscopic procedure, when appropriate. However, diagnostic endoscopy can be identified separately when performed at the same surgical session as an open procedure.
- Codes from range 31233–31298 report unilateral procedures unless otherwise specified.
- For multiple surgical endoscopic procedures performed during the same session, code the appropriate endoscopy of each anatomic site examined.

DEFINITIONS

anosmia. Decrease or loss of sense of smell.

dacryocystitis. Lacrimal sac inflammation.

dysphagia. Difficulty and pain upon swallowing.

epistaxis. Nosebleed; hemorrhaging from the nose.

hyposmia. Diminished sense of smell.

odynophagia. Pain during swallowing

sarcoidosis. Clustering of immune cells resulting in granuloma formation. Often affects the lungs and lymphatic system but can occur in other body sites.

- Control of bleeding is an integral part of endoscopic procedures and is not reported separately. For example, control of nasal hemorrhage (code 30901) is not reported separately or control of bleeding due to a nasal/sinus endoscopic procedure. If bleeding occurs in the postoperative period and requires a return to the operating room for treatment, a CPT code for control of the bleeding may be reported with modifier 78 indicating that the procedure was a complication of a prior procedure and required treatment in the operating room. However, control of postoperative bleeding not requiring return to the operating room is not reported separately.

- Topical vasoconstrictive agents and local anesthesia are not reported separately.

- If a biopsy is performed on a separate lesion, it is reported separately, with modifier 59 or XS appended to the CPT code for the second and subsequent lesion.

- To report stereotactic computer-assisted navigation performed in conjunction with endoscopic sinus surgery, see 61782.

- For endoscopic anterior and posterior ethmoidectomy (APE) with or without removal of polyp(s), including frontal sinus exploration, report 31255 and 31276; if the procedure includes antrostomy, report 31255, 31256, and 31276; if the procedure does not include frontal sinus exploration but antrostomy is performed, report 31255 and 31256.

- If endoscopic APE, with or without removal of polyps, includes antrostomy and removal of antral mucosal disease, report 31255 and 31267; if this procedure also includes frontal sinus exploration, report 31255, 31267, and 31276.

- For intranasal or extranasal ethmoidectomy without endoscopy, see 31200–31205.

Coding Trap

- There are many parenthetical notes in this section that instruct that certain procedures may not be performed on the ipsilateral side. Be sure to read all section guidelines thoroughly when reporting these codes to avoid denials.

Endoscopy of the Larynx (31505–31579)

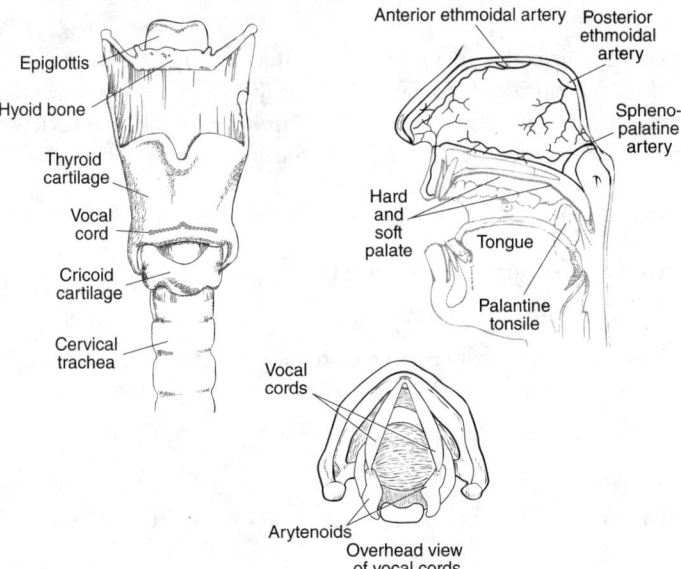

Very simply, a laryngoscopy visualizes the interior of the tongue base, larynx, and hypopharynx; it can be done for diagnostic purposes or surgical purposes. Within the structures examined, there are midline (single anatomic sites) and paired structures. When reporting procedures, if one side of a paired structure is involved then a unilateral code is reported. The structures are identified below.

Midline	Paired
Epiglottis	Arytenoids
Posterior pharyngeal wall	Aryepiglottic folds
Subglottis	False vocal cords
Tongue base	Pyriform sinuses
Vallecula	True vocal cords
	Ventricles

There are different approaches that may be used, including indirect, direct, and direct operative. Each is explained briefly below.

Procedure Differentiation

An indirect laryngoscopy involves the visualization of the larynx using a warm laryngeal mirror positioned at the back of the throat and a head mirror held in front of the mouth containing a light source. This method should be attempted prior to considering a flexible or rigid laryngoscopy.

Direct laryngoscopy involves the visualization of the tongue base, larynx, and hypopharynx by passing a rigid or flexible fiberoptic endoscope through the mouth and pharynx to the larynx. If the laryngoscopy was direct, ascertain whether the procedure was performed with an operating microscope (microsurgery), telescope, or flexible fiberoptic scope. A flexible laryngoscopy is often used when gagging limits the mirror used in an indirect exam, as well as to obtain a more clear view of laryngeal structures when the diagnostic need arises.

Operative direct laryngoscopy involves an examination of the tongue base, larynx, and hypopharynx by the passing of a rigid or fiberoptic endoscope

DEFINITIONS

abscess. Circumscribed collection of pus resulting from bacteria, frequently associated with swelling and other signs of inflammation.

aphasia. Partial or total loss of the ability to comprehend language or communicate through speaking, the written word, or sign language. Aphasia may result from stroke, injury, Alzheimer's disease, or other disorder. Common types of aphasia include expressive, receptive, anomic, global, and conduction.

goiter. Abnormal enlargement of the thyroid gland commonly caused by a deficiency of dietary iodine.

hemoptysis. Coughing up or spitting out blood or blood-streaked sputum.

operating microscope. Compound microscope with two or more lens systems or several grouped lenses in one unit that provides magnifying power to the surgeon up to 40X.

through the mouth and pharynx to the larynx with the patient under general anesthesia.

Separate endoscopic codes are provided for direct and indirect procedures; procedures on newborns; and diagnostic, biopsy, foreign body removal, and injection procedures. Review each code description carefully and review the provider's documentation before assigning the code.

When auditing laryngoscopy determine:

- Is it a diagnostic or surgical procedure?
- Is the procedure direct or indirect?
- If direct, is the procedure performed with an operating microscope (microsurgery) or flexible scope?
- Does the procedure include repair or reconstruction?

Medical Necessity
The following conditions may warrant nasal endoscopy (this list is not all inclusive):

- Aphasia
- Benign neoplasm
- Foreign body
- Goiter
- Hemoptysis
- Laryngitis
- Malignancy
- Paralysis of vocal cords
- Pharyngeal abscess
- Speech disturbance
- Tracheostomy complication

Key Documentation Terms
In order to assign the most appropriate code, the medical record documentation must be reviewed to determine why the procedure was performed (e.g., for removal of a foreign body, removal of a lesion, biopsy, or injection) and if the procedure was unilateral or bilateral. Documentation must clearly support the medical necessity of the service being reported. It also must include the procedure(s) performed in addition to the laryngoscopy. If a direct laryngoscopy was performed, a provider must document that a supporting diagnostic concern existed, and why the mirror examination failed to provide enough information.

Coding Tip
- If medically reasonable and necessary endoscopic procedures are performed on two regions of the respiratory system with different types of endoscopes, both procedures may be reported separately. For example, if a patient requires diagnostic bronchoscopy for a lung mass with a fiberoptic bronchoscope and a separate laryngoscopy for a laryngeal mass with a fiberoptic laryngoscope at the same patient encounter, CPT codes for both procedures may be reported separately.

Endoscopy of the Lung (31622–31654)

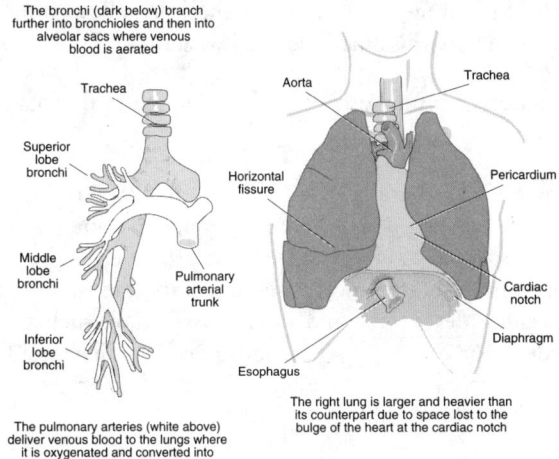

A bronchoscopy is a visual inspection of the bronchus. Many codes are contained in this section as there are many different anatomical locations within the bronchus. It is of the utmost importance to read the entire code description before assigning a code to a procedure. In order to accurately report these services it is important to know some anatomy.

The trachea and bronchi with their many branches resemble an inverted tree trunk and its branches and are commonly referred to as the bronchial tree.

The trachea, or windpipe, extends from the larynx in the neck to the branches of the primary bronchi in the thorax. It is usually about 11 centimeters long by 2.5 centimeters in diameter. It is a flexible, tubular structure formed by approximately 20 C-shaped rings of cartilage that are embedded in smooth muscle. The trachea is lined with specialized epithelium tissue that produces and moves mucus up and out of the respiratory tract, keeping the lungs and air passages free.

The trachea divides at its lower end into two primary bronchi. The right bronchus is slightly larger and more vertical than the left (accounting for aspirated objects lodging more frequently in the right bronchus). As each bronchus enters the lung, it divides into smaller branches called secondary bronchi; these continue to further branch into tertiary bronchi and small bronchioles. The structure of the primary bronchi is similar to the trachea; however, the cartilaginous rings become complete, versus C-shaped, as the bronchi enter the lungs. The bronchi are lined with ciliated mucosa, similarly to the trachea.

Procedure Differentiation
A bronchoscopy may be performed with a rigid or flexible bronchoscope. Surgical endoscopy includes a diagnostic endoscopy; however, diagnostic endoscopy can be identified separately when performed at the same surgical session as an open procedure. A bronchoscopy may be the approach used to perform a surgical procedure such as a biopsy, lavage, stent placement, removal of a foreign body, or stent placement as an example.

Code 31622 reports a bronchoscopy that is diagnostic in nature. The provider may also perform cell washing.

Bronchoscopy with protected brushing (31623) is the collection of lung material using a catheter through which a brush is advanced, often using fluoroscopic guidance. Bronchial lavage (31624) is a method that allows lung tissue to be sampled by irrigating with saline followed by suctioning the fluid.

Code 31626 reports a bronchoscopy with placement of fiducial markers used with radiation.

Many codes within this section include biopsy (31625, 31628, 31629, 31632, and 31633). When coding a biopsy, read the operative and pathology reports to determine if the specimen was taken from the bronchus or the lung since both sites have upper, middle, and lower lobes. It is important to note the anatomical location in the code description and special instructions such as single or multiple. Codes 31632 and 31633 are add-on codes. They should only be reported once regardless of how many transbronchial biopsies are performed in the trachea or the additional lobe.

Dilation or closed fracture reduction of the trachea or bronchus is reported with 31630. In this procedure, the physician uses the views obtained through the bronchoscope to identify any narrowing or fracture of the trachea or bronchus. A wire is introduced through the narrowed or fractured part of the airway and removes the bronchoscope. A series of dilators or stents are passed over the wire to open the airway until sufficient dilation or closed reduction of the stricture or fracture is accomplished. This procedure may be done with or without fluoroscopic guidance.

Bronchopleural fistula (BPF) is treated with a bronchoscopic balloon occlusion with 31634. BPF is often a serious postoperative complication of thoracic surgery, although it can also occur as a complication in a diseased lung or a previously normal lung. This procedure may use fluoroscopy to assist with navigation of the bronchoscope tip to the area of the air leak, which is then assessed. A balloon catheter is placed at the site of the leak and inflated until the leak is occluded. Keeping the inflated catheter in this position, an appropriate sealant (e.g., fibrin) may be injected.

Stent procedures (31631, 31636, 31637, and 31638) include dilation. Again pay close attention to the anatomical location and whether it is the initial stent or subsequent.

Foreign body removal is reported with 31635. This procedure may use a snare, basket, or biopsy forceps through a channel in the bronchoscope to aid in the removal of the foreign body.

Tumor excision/destruction is reported with 31640–31641.

In 31643 a catheter is inserted through the bronchoscope into a lung cavity and is placed at the site where intracavitary radioelements are applied. This code includes the use of fluoroscopic guidance, when performed.

Therapeutic aspirations of the trachobronchial tree via a bronchoscopy are reported with 31645 or 31646, dependent upon whether it is the initial or subsequent aspiration.

Codes 31647 and 31651 describe insertion of one or more bronchial valves using a bronchoscopic approach. Typically a bronchial valve is inserted to control leaks within the bronchus due to lung disease (e.g., emphysema). Codes 31648 and 31649 describe removal of one or more previously placed bronchial valves using a bronchoscopic approach. Codes 31649 and 31651 are add-on codes that identify each additional lobe.

Codes 31652–31654 describe procedures using endobronchial ultrasound (EBUS). EBUS is a minimally invasive technique utilizing ultrasound in conjunction with bronchoscopy to view the airway wall and adjacent structures. The physician performs a transbronchial needle aspiration (TBNA) biopsy on lymph nodes via a thin flexible instrument (bronchoscope) fitted with an ultrasound processor, as well as a fine-gauge aspiration needle guided through the patient's mouth and trachea, permitting real-time imaging of the airways, blood vessels, lungs and lymph nodes. The physician is able to view hard-to-reach areas and gain greater access to biopsy smaller lymph nodes than would be possible via conventional mediastinoscopy. A pathologist in the operating room with the surgeon is able to immediately process the biopsy samples and/or request additional samples as necessary leading to a quicker diagnosis of cancer, infections, or other inflammatory diseases of the lungs as well as to assist in staging lung cancer. There are two types of EBUS: Radial probe EBUS and linear probe EBUS. The radial probe EBUS has a rotating mechanical transducer with very good image quality that permits the airway layers to be identified but TBNA is not possible with this device; the linear probe EBUS is a fixed array of electronic transducer aligned in a curvilinear pattern and permits real-time guidance for mediastinal lesion sampling. EBUS procedures may be performed under general anesthesia or with moderate conscious sedation and typically allow for patients to go home the same day as the procedure.

Report code 31652 for one or two mediastinal and/or hilar lymph node stations or structures; code 31653 for three or more stations or structures. Add-on code 31654 should be reported when EBUS is performed during diagnostic or therapeutic bronchoscopy for peripheral lesions. These codes should be reported only one time per encounter.

Code 31627 is an add-on code used in conjunction with certain bronchoscopy codes (listed below) that denotes the service was performed with computer-assisted, image-guided navigation. This add-on service may be necessary for diagnosis and possible placement of fiducial markers in patients with a confirmed or suspected malignancy.

When auditing bronchoscopy procedures, determine:

- Whether the bronchoscopy is diagnostic or if it is performed in conjunction with another procedure, such as destruction of a tumor or a biopsy.
- Whether the biopsy or lesion removal is performed on the lung or the bronchus.
- If fluoroscopy was reported separately. Fluoroscopic guidance is an integral part of the procedure and should not be reported separately.
- If the procedure involved ultrasound.
- If tracheal or bronchial stents were placed or revised.

Medical Necessity

The following conditions may warrant bronchoscopy (this list is not all inclusive):

- Benign neoplasm

DEFINITIONS

bronchiolitis. Inflammation of the finer subbranches of the bronchial tree due to infectious agents or irritants. Most commonly a disease of children, symptoms include cough with differing productions of sputum, fever, and lung rales.

empyema. Accumulation of pus within the respiratory, or pleural, cavity.

pleural effusion. Collection of lymph and other fluid within the pleural space.

pneumothorax. Collapsed lung due to air or gas trapped in the pleural space formed by the membrane that encloses the lungs and lines the thoracic cavity.

- Congenital anomalies
- Cystic fibrosis
- Emphysema
- Empyema with fistula
- Foreign body
- Malignancy
- Pleural effusion
- Pneumonia
- Pneumothorax
- Pulmonary fibrosis
- Respiratory bronchiolitis interstitial lung disease
- Respiratory failure

Key Documentation Terms

Documentation for these procedures must clearly support the medical necessity of the service being reported. It also must include the procedure(s) performed in addition to the bronchoscopy. If computer assisted, image-guided navigation, or endobronchial ultrasound was used, the provider must document why the use was warranted. Terms such as aspiration, biopsy, computer-assisted, image-guided navigation, initial lobe, each additional lobe, and stent provide the guidance needed to ensure correct code assignment.

Coding Tips

- Note that 31622, a separate procedure by definition, is usually a component of a more complex service and is not identified separately. When performed alone or with other unrelated procedures/services, it may be reported. If performed alone, list the code; if performed with other procedures/services, list the code and append modifier 59.

- Fluoroscopic guidance is included in codes 31622–31651, 31660, and 31661.

- As "add-on" codes, 31627, 31632, 31633, 31637, 31649, 31651, and 31654 are not subject to multiple procedure rules. No reimbursement reduction or modifier 51 is applied. The following table provides additional information for these codes as found in the Medicare Physician Fee Schedule Database

Parent Code	Add-On	GLOB DAYS	MULT PROC	BILAT SURG	ASST SURG	CO-SURG	TEAM SURG
31615		000	2	0	1	0	0
31622		000	2	0	1	0	0
31623		000	3	0	1	0	0
31624		000	3	0	1	0	0
31625		000	3	0	1	0	0
31626		000	2	0	0	0	0
	31627	ZZZ	0	0	0	0	0
31628		000	3	0	1	0	0
31629		000	3	0	1	0	0
31630		000	3	0	1	0	0

Parent Code	Add-On	GLOB DAYS	MULT PROC	BILAT SURG	ASST SURG	CO-SURG	TEAM SURG
31631		000	3	0	1	0	0
	31632	ZZZ	0	0	1	0	0
	31633	ZZZ	0	0	1	0	0
31635		000	3	0	1	0	0
31636		000	3	0	1	0	0
	31637	ZZZ	0	0	1	0	0
31638		000	3	0	1	0	0
31640		000	3	0	1	0	0
31641		000	3	0	1	0	0
31643		000	2	0	1	0	0
31645		000	3	0	1	0	0
31646		000	2	0	1	0	0
31647		000	3	0	1	0	0
31648		000	3	0	1	0	0
	31649	ZZZ	0	0	1	0	0
	31651	ZZZ	0	0	1	0	0
	31654	ZZZ	0	0	1	0	0

Thoracotomy (32096–32160)

A thoracotomy is an incision into the thorax. Code selection is based upon the extent of the procedure and concurrent services performed. Thoracotomy codes include procedures for control of hemorrhage, cyst removal, resection, and cardiac massage, just to name a few.

Procedure Differentiation

There are three codes used when a thoracotomy is performed with a biopsy: of lung infiltrates, report 32096; for lung nodules or masses, report 32097; of the pleura, report 32098.

Code 32100 is reported for a diagnostic thoracotomy.

In 32110, a thoracotomy is performed and the site of the hemorrhage or lung tear is identified and repaired.

Code 32120 is a thoracotomy that is specifically performed to identify any thoracic postoperative complications.

In 32124, the surgeon manually divides the tissues attaching the lung to the wall of the chest cavity, to permit collapse of the lung. This procedure is used to treat tuberculosis.

Code 32140 is used to report the removal of one or more lung cysts. In order to perform this procedure, the pleural surface may require an operative procedure such as pneumonolysis (separation of the surface of the lung that has become adherent to the inside surface of the chest cavity). The pneumonolysis is not reported separately.

Code 32141 is used to report removal of one or more lung bullae (large nonfunctional air sacs).

DEFINITIONS

emphysematous bleb. Formation of blisters or vesicles greater than 1.0 mm within an emphysematous lung, containing serum or blood.

fibrin. Main fibrous composition of blood clots.

foreign body. Any object or substance found in an organ and tissue that does not belong under normal circumstances.

hemothorax. Blood collecting in the pleural cavity.

Kaposi's sarcoma. Malignant neoplasm caused by vascular proliferation of cutaneous tumors characterized by channels lined with endothelial tissue containing vascular space.

pleura. Thin membrane covering the lungs and lining the inside of the chest wall.

There are two codes that describe foreign body removal. Code 32150 reports intrapleural removal of not only foreign bodies but also fibrin deposits. Code 32151is reported for intrapulmonary foreign bodies.

In 32160, the chest cavity is opened to perform manual cardiac massage in the case of cardiac arrest.

Medical Necessity
The following conditions may warrant thoracotomy (this list is not all inclusive):

- Abscess
- Benign neoplasm
- Emphysematous bleb
- Foreign body
- Hemothorax
- Kaposi's sarcoma
- Lung contusion/laceration
- Malignancy
- Pneumonia
- Pneumothorax
- Respiratory bronchiolitis interstitial lung disease

Key Documentation Terms
In order to assign the most appropriate code, the medical record documentation must be reviewed to determine why the procedure was performed (e.g., biopsy, control of hemorrhage, removal of a foreign body, repair, or resection). Documentation for these procedures must clearly support the medical necessity of the service being reported. It also must include the procedure(s) performed in addition to the thoracotomy. When documenting for ICD-10-CM, specificity is crucial. The provider must be specific in documenting the types of pneumonia, tuberculosis, and many other infections. ICD-10-CM has broken these down, making them very specific.

Coding Tips
- These are unilateral procedures, if performed bilaterally append modifier 50 to the second procedure.
- Codes 32096–32097 should not be reported more than one time per lung.
- For percutaneous drainage of a lung abscess or cyst, see 49405.

Thoracic Surgery: Video-Assisted (VATS) (32601–32674)
A thoracoscopy is the examination of the inside of the chest cavity through a rigid or flexible fiberoptic endoscope. The procedure can be done under local or general anesthesia. The contents of the chest cavity are examined by direct visualization and/or the use of a video camera. Still photographs may be taken as part of the procedure.

Procedure Differentiation
Thoracoscopies can be done for diagnostic purposes or surgical purposes. The diagnostic thoracoscopies all include biopsies except for 32601, which is an exploration of the chest cavity by direct visualization and/or the use of a video camera only. Pay close attention to the anatomical location of each procedure.

As with other scope procedures, a diagnostic procedure is always included in a surgical thoracoscopy.

Surgical thoracoscopic procedures in this section are differentiated by the procedure that was performed (e.g., decortication, pleurodesis, pneumonolysis, removal of foreign body, control of hemorrhage, or excision of a portion of the lung) and by the anatomical location. It is important to read each code description carefully.

It is also important to note if the decortication was partial or total and whether the cyst was removed from the pericardium or mediastinum.

In the event that these procedures are performed in conjunction with a lobectomy, the resection may only be reported if it is performed on a different lobe or on the contralateral lung. Make sure to identify what was removed, such as a single lobe (lobectomy), a segment (segmentectomy), two lobes (bilobectomy), or the total lung (pneumonectomy).

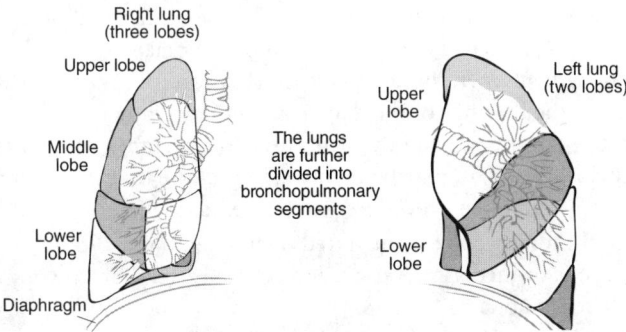

Thoracoscopy with diagnostic wedge resection followed by a resection (32668) or removal of a lung lobe is reported with codes from range 32669–32671. When a resection is performed for lung volume reduction, report 32672. This is generally performed for patients with severe emphysema in order to allow the remaining compressed lung to expand, and thus, improve respiratory function.

If performed with resection of thymus, report 32673; with mediastinal and regional lymphadenectomy, report 32674.

Medical Necessity

The following conditions may warrant these procedures (this list is not all inclusive):

- Abscess
- Benign neoplasm
- Cystic fibrosis
- Emphysematous bleb
- Empyema
- Kaposi's sarcoma
- Malignancy
- Pneumothorax
- Pulmonary fibrosis

 DEFINITIONS

contralateral. Located on, or affecting, the opposite side of the body, usually as it relates to a bilateral body part.

decortication of lung. Removal of a constricting membrane or layer of pleural tissue from a portion of the lung surface to allow for lung expansion.

pleurodesis. Injection of a sclerosing agent into the pleural space for creating adhesions between the parietal and the visceral pleura to treat a collapsed lung caused by air trapped in the pleural cavity, or severe cases of pleural effusion.

pneumonectomy. Surgical removal of a lung or lung tissue.

segmentectomy. Removal of a segment of a gland or an organ.

VATS. Video-assisted thoracic surgery. Less invasive technique than open thoracic surgery for various procedures on the heart and lungs. The surgeon typically gains access to the chest cavity using trocars (slender tube-like instruments), through which an endoscope and the surgical instruments are passed. The patient's internal organs can then be viewed intraoperatively on a monitor.

Key Documentation Terms

Terms such as bilobectomy, decortication, lobectomy, mediastinal, pericardial, pleura, pleurectomy, pneumonolysis, or segment provide the guidance needed to ensure correct code assignment. Documentation for these procedures must clearly support the medical necessity of the service being reported and a narrative of all procedures performed.

Coding Tips

- Thoracoscopy codes 32601–32606 are separate procedures, by definition, and are usually a component of a more complex service and not identified separately. When performed alone or with other unrelated procedures/services, it may be reported. If performed alone, list the code; if performed with other procedures/services, list the code and append modifier 59.
- A diagnostic thoracoscopy is considered an integral part of a surgical thoracoscopic VATS procedure.
- Codes 32607–32608 should not be reported more than one time per lung.
- A diagnostic thoracoscopy to assess the surgical field or extent of disease prior to an open thoracotomy, thoracostomy, or mediastinal procedure is not reported separately. However, a diagnostic thoracoscopy is reported separately with an open thoracotomy, thoracostomy, or mediastinal procedure if the findings of the diagnostic thoracoscopy lead to the decision to perform an open thoracotomy, thoracostomy, or mediastinal procedure. Modifier 58 may be reported to indicate that the diagnostic thoracoscopy and open procedure were staged or planned.
- If a surgical thoracoscopy is converted to an open thoracotomy, thoracostomy, or mediastinal procedure, the surgical thoracoscopy is not separately reportable.
- As "add-on" codes, 32667, 32668, and 32674 are not subject to multiple procedure rules. No reimbursement reduction or modifier 51 is applied. Please see the CPT book for the codes these add-on codes should be reported with.

Ablation of Pulmonary Tumors (32994 and 32998)

The ablation of pulmonary tumors is used in the treatment of lung malignancy to destroy or debulk the tumors for either radical cure or palliative care. Correct code assignment is dependent upon the instrumentation used, either radiofrequency (32998) or cryoablation (32994).

Procedure Differentiation

Both procedures are minimally invasive. Code 32998 will indicate that the physician uses the heat created from high-frequency radiowaves to destroy one or more tumors in the lung, pleura, or chest wall. Treatment with the heat probe usually takes several minutes and may include repositioning the probe within the lesion so that overlapping ablations treat the entire tumor. This process may be repeated for multiple lesions within the same lung. In 32994 the procedure is performed using cryoablation. Imaging guidance is included in these procedures, when performed.

Coding Tips

- These procedures are unilateral services. If performed bilaterally, some payers require that the service be reported twice with modifier 50 appended to the second code, while others require identification of the service only once with modifier 50 appended. Check with individual payers.

Procedures Performed on the Cardiovascular System

Circulatory System: Arterial

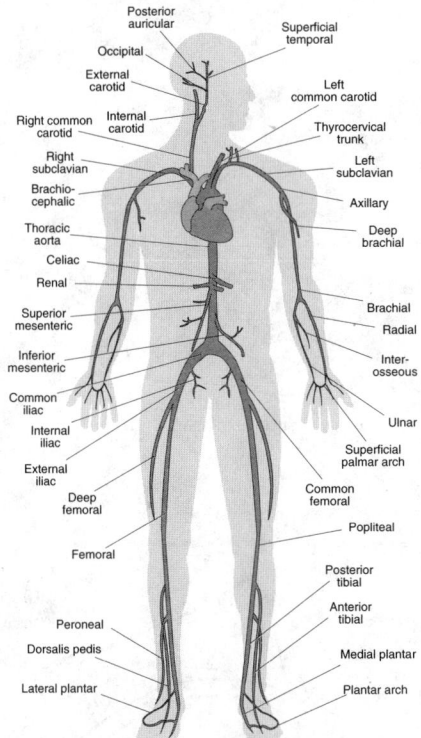

Circulatory System: Venous

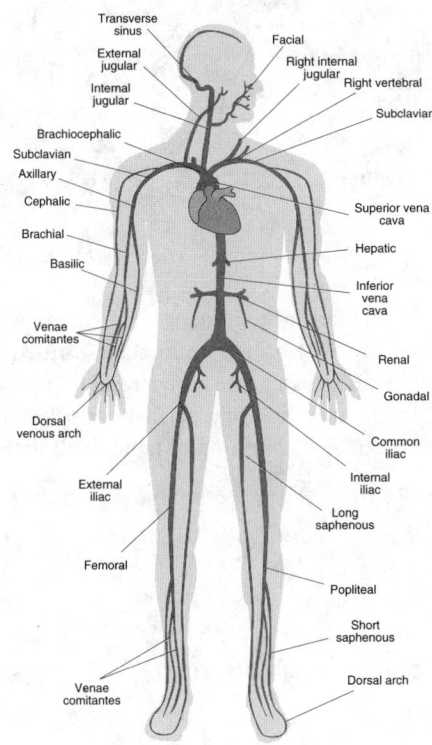

Pacemakers/Implantable Defibrillators (33202–33249, 33262–33264, and 33270–33275)

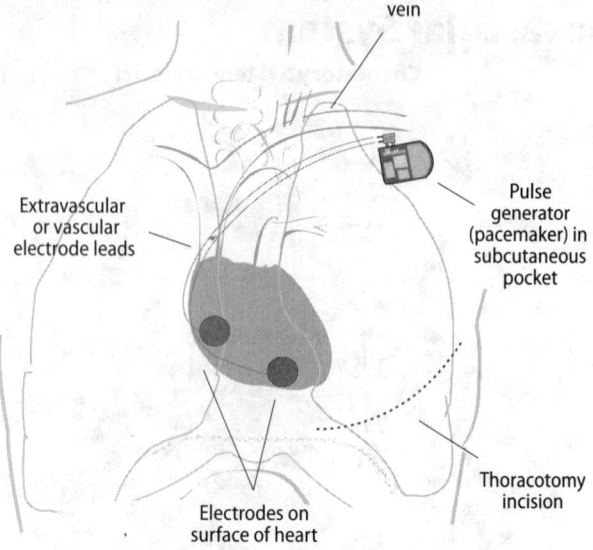

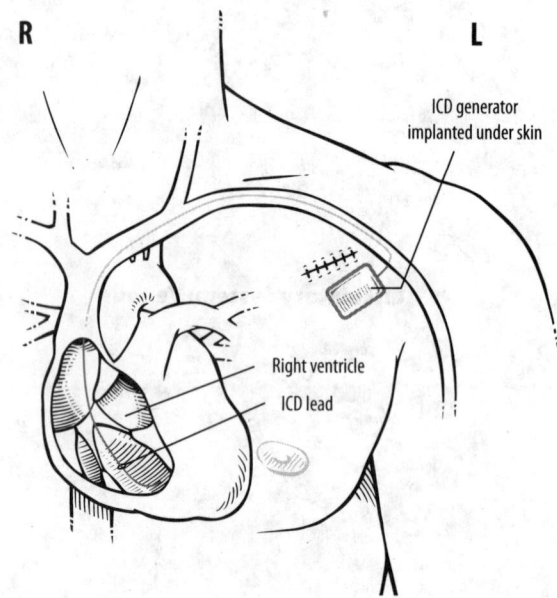

DEFINITIONS

defibrillator system. System that includes a pulse generator and electrodes, implanted in the same manner as the pacemaker systems.

dual chamber system. System that includes a pulse generator with one electrode inserted into the right atrium and one into the right ventricle.

multiple-lead device. Implantable cardiac device (pacemaker or implantable cardioverter-defibrillator [ICD]) in which pacing and sensing components are placed in three or more chambers of the heart.

pacemaker. Implantable cardiac device that controls the heart's rhythm and maintains regular beats by artificial electric discharges. This device consists of the pulse generator with a battery and the electrodes, or leads, which are placed in single or dual chambers of the heart, usually transvenously.

A pacemaker may be permanent or temporary. A permanent pacemaker is used to maintain cardiac stability. A temporary pacemaker is used to treat transient bradycardias that may be due to an acute myocardial infarction or drug toxicity, and may be followed by the insertion of a permanent pacemaker. Below are the major components of pacemakers and implantable defibrillators:

Operating system

- Pacemaker
  - pulse generator (battery and electronics)
  - electrodes (leads)
- Implantable defibrillator (subcutaneous)
  - pulse generator
  - subcutaneous electrode (leads)

- pacemakers are placed subcutaneously within a pocket in either subclavicular area of chest (most common) or above the abdominal muscles that are found below the rib cage
- the operating system IS NOT implanted in incidences of temporary pacemakers
- implantable defibrillators are placed subcutaneously within a pocket in either the abdomen, axillary, or infraclavicular area

- Electrodes

  - pacemaker
    - leads may be inserted through a vein (transvenous), placed on the surface of the heart (epicardial), or placed in the subcutaneous space near the heart. Epicardial placement of electrodes requires a thoracotomy for electrode insertion.
    - single chamber
      - one electrode placed in atrium OR ventricle OR a subcutaneous electrode
    - dual chamber
      - two electrodes one placed in atrium AND one placed in the right ventricle
      - in some instances, a third electrode may be placed in the left ventricle (biventricular pacing)
    - multiple-lead
      - the system may have electrodes in the right atrium and ventricle and the coronary sinus for left ventricular pacing
  - Implantable Defibrillator System—transvenous (ICD)
    - single chamber (pacing in the ventricle)
    - dual chambers (pacing in the atrium and ventricle)
    - biventricular system (pacing in the left and right ventricles), whereas the
  - Implantable Defibrillator System—subcutaneous (S-ICD)
    - single lead subcutaneous lead that rests near the heart but not within it

- Biventricular pacing may be necessary to achieve pacing of the left ventricle. An additional electrode placed:
  - transvenous electrode lead placement, placed into the coronary sinus (33224 or 33225)
  - epicardial electrode lead placement, placed on the left ventricular epicardium, (33202–33203)

Both types of devices commonly require removal and replacement of the pulse generator, which has an average life span of five to eight years. Repair, repositioning, removal, and replacement of electrodes may be necessary over the period of time that the patient has the device.

Temporary pacemakers (33210–33211) are used to treat transient bradycardias that may be due to an acute myocardial infarction or drug toxicity, or prior to insertion of a permanent pacemaker. A temporary pacemaker does not include an internally placed pulse generator. It is an external pacemaker and can be a transvenous single or dual chamber cardiac electrode.

Permanent pacemakers consist of a pulse generator, a battery, and one (single chamber) or two or more electrodes (dual chamber). The pulse generator is

 AUDITOR'S ALERT

Codes 33206–33249, 33262–33264 and 33270–33273 include the revision of the skin pocket. However, when incision and drainage of an abscess or seroma or hematoma or debridement due to complex wound infection is performed these may be reported separately.

placed in a "pocket" just under the skin in either the subclavicular or abdominal areas. The electrodes may be placed transvenously or on the epicardium. When placed on the epicardium, documentation will indicate that a thoracotomy was performed.

As with pacemakers, there a two types of implantable defibrillator systems that can be placed: a transvenous implantable pacing cardioverter-defibrillator (ICD) or a subcutaneous implantable defibrillator (S-ICD).

Codes 33202 and 33203 are used to report the insertion of epicardial electrodes through either an incision or endoscopic approach. Report 33202 or 33203 when an epicardial lead is placed by the same physician during the same session as the insertion of a pulse generator; report 33212, 33213, or 33221 for a pacemaker; and report 33230, 33231, or 33240 for implantable defibrillator.

Codes 33206–33208 report a global service that includes subcutaneous placement of a pacemaker with transvenous placement of the electrode. These procedures include any repositioning or replacement, as well as fluoroscopic guidance. For removal and replacement of a pacemaker pulse generator and transvenous electrodes, report 33233 in conjunction with 33234 or 33235 and 33206, 33207, or 33208. When this procedure is performed on an implantable defibrillator, report 33241, 33244, and 33249. In some cases, a pacing electrode is also placed with these procedures, which is reported with 33225.

Temporary pacemaker procedures are reported with codes 33210–33211. The documentation will indicate that the access to the central caval veins was obtained through the subclavian or jugular vein. The vein is penetrated with a large needle, and a wire is passed through it. A fluoroscope is used to guide the wire into the right atrium and/or right ventricle. The wire is connected to a generator that is not implanted but temporarily placed outside the body. Report 33210 when a single-chamber temporary transvenous electrode or pacemaker catheter is placed (atrial or ventricular) and 33211 when dual-chamber electrodes or catheters are placed (atrial and ventricular). Fluoroscopy is included in these procedures and is not reported separately.

Codes 33212–33213 and 33221 report the insertion of a single- or dual-chamber pacemaker pulse generator, which is then connected to previously placed, existing leads. If this is an initial insertion, a pocket for the pacemaker generator is created subcutaneously in the subclavicular region or underneath the abdominal muscles just below the ribcage. The generator is inserted into the pocket, and the pocket is closed. Report 33212 for insertion of a single-chamber (atrial or ventricular) pacemaker pulse generator, 33213 for a dual-chamber (atrial and ventricular) pacemaker pulse generator, or 33221 for a pulse generator with multiple existing leads. Fluoroscopy is included in these procedures and is not reported separately.

When a removal and replacement of a pacemaker pulse generator is performed, the global codes (33227–33229) should be reported instead of individual codes for removal of pulse generator (33233) and replacement (33212, 33213, 33221). Report 33227 for removal and replacement of a single-lead system generator, 33228 for a dual-lead system generator, and 33229 for a multiple-lead system generator.

When a single-chamber system is converted to a dual-chamber system, code 33214 is reported. The documentation should indicate that the existing pacemaker generator pocket is opened and the single-chamber generator removed. The dual-chamber generator is placed into the existing pocket. The existing pacer wire is tested and connected to the generator, and then a second lead is placed and tested. The pocket is closed. Do not report additional codes for the insertion of electrodes (33216–33217) or removal and replacement of a pacemaker pulse generator (33227–33229) since code 33214 includes those services.

Code 33215 describes the repositioning of a previously placed transvenous pacemaker or implantable defibrillator right atrial or ventricular electrode. Repositioning is done when the system does not function due to improper placement of the electrode wire itself. The generator is removed, and the wire is tested to ensure that the wire is not defective but simply in the wrong place. It is reattached to the generator in its new position and tested again. Code 33216 describes the insertion of a single transvenous electrode and 33217 describes the insertion of two transvenous electrodes in a permanent pacemaker or implantable defibrillator. The generator is removed, and the wire is tested. When the wire is found defective, another transvenous electrode is inserted. Access to the central caval veins is obtained through the subclavian or jugular vein. The vein is penetrated with a large needle, and a wire is passed through it. Fluoroscopy is used to guide the wire into position. The wire is connected to the generator, and testing is done again. Imaging guidance is included in these procedures and not separately reported.

Codes 33218 and 33220 report repair of permanent pacemaker or implantable defibrillator electrodes. Code 33218 is reported when the pocket is opened and the generator is removed. The electrode wire is then tested, and the single electrode is repaired. The wire is then retested and reconnected to the generator, which is placed back in its pocket, and the pocket is closed. Report 33220 if two electrodes are repaired.

Codes 33222 and 33223 indicate the relocation of the pacemaker or defibrillator skin pocket. This could be necessary due to infection, erosion, or complications from the original generator placement. The procedure involves opening the pocket, removing the generator, and forming a new pocket in the subcutaneous tissue within reach of the already present electrodes. The electrodes are brought through a new subcutaneous tunnel into the new pocket, and the old pocket is closed. The existing or new generator is placed in the new pocket, and the electrodes are connected. The pocket is closed. Report 33222 when a permanent pacemaker pocket is relocated and 33223 when an implantable defibrillator pocket is relocated.

Code 33224 reports the insertion of an electrode on a previously placed permanent pacemaker or implantable defibrillator for left ventricular pacing. This procedure is done under local anesthesia. A fluoroscope may be used for guidance, and a pacing electrode is inserted in the left ventricular chamber of the heart, usually in the coronary sinus tributary. The electrode is connected to the pulse generator, and the pocket is closed. The generator pocket may be revised and/or the existing generator removed, inserted, or replaced. In rare cases, when transvenous approach cannot be used, the device is implanted in the pocket underneath the skin in the lower abdomen (epicardial approach). Implantation using this approach is done under general anesthesia. For epicardial electrode placement at the time of insertion of a pacing electrode in the cardiac venous system, report 33202 or 33203 in addition to 33224.

Code 33225 reports the insertion of a pacing electrode for left ventricular pacing and applies to either an implantable defibrillator or pacemaker pulse generator.

If biventricular pacing is required, an additional electrode is placed in the left ventricle. During insertion of an implantable defibrillator or pacemaker pulse generator, the physician gains access transvenously through the subclavian or jugular vein. A fluoroscope may be used for guidance, and a pacing electrode is inserted in the left ventricular chamber of the heart, usually in the coronary sinus tributary. The generator is upgraded to a dual-chamber system. The electrode is connected to the generator, and the generator pocket is closed. Fluoroscopy is included in 33225 and is not reported separately. Report 33225 with 33222 when a pacemaker generator pocket is relocated and 33223 when an implantable defibrillator pocket is relocated.

Code 33226 reports the repositioning of an electrode in a previously placed implantable defibrillator or pacemaker pulse generator for left ventricular pacing. Fluoroscopy is included and is not reported separately.

Codes 33227–33229 describe removal and replacement of a permanent pacemaker pulse generator. The existing generator is disconnected from the wire or wires and removed. The wire or wires are left in place in the pocket, and a new permanent pacemaker pulse generator is inserted. The existing pacer wire or wires are tested and connected to the generator. Report 33227 for removal and replacement of a single-lead system generator, 33228 for a dual-lead system generator, and 33229 for a multiple-lead system generator.

Procedure code 33233 reports removal of the pacemaker pulse generator only. This procedure involves disconnecting the generator from the wire or wires and removing it. The wires are left in place in the pocket, and the pocket is closed.

Codes 33234 and 33235 indicate removal of pacemaker leads without concurrent replacement. Documentation for code 33234 states that the generator pocket is opened and the wire is disconnected from the generator. The wire is dissected from the scar tissue that has formed around it. Once the wire is completely freed, it is twisted in a direction opposite to that used for insertion (counter clockwise). The wire is then withdrawn. Bleeding from the tracts leading to the vein is controlled with sutures. A new wire may be placed but is reported separately. Report 33235 for a dual-lead system (removal of two wires).

Codes 33236 and 33237 indicate removal of the epicardial pacemaker and electrodes. Code 33236 describes the opening of the old pacemaker pocket removal of the generator. The old wires are cut, and the incision is closed. The old chest incision is then opened, and the wires are pulled into the chest and followed onto the heart surface. The electrodes are then detached from the heart, and the chest incision is closed. Report 33237 if a dual-lead epicardial system is being removed.

Code 33238 reports removal of transvenous electrode(s) by thoracotomy. The documentation should indicate that before this procedure, the pacemaker pocket was opened, the generator removed, and the wires cut. The right chest is opened, and the superior caval vein is dissected out. Tourniquets are placed around the vein above and below the planned site of opening. The tourniquets are tightened, and a hole is made in the caval vein. The cut ends of the wires are pulled out through the hole in the caval vein. The ends of the wires that are still in the heart are twisted counterclockwise until they are free and are withdrawn through the caval vein. The hole in the caval vein is closed and the tourniquets released. The chest is then closed.

Codes 33230, 33231, and 33240 are used to report the insertion of an implantable defibrillator pulse generator when the patient has had leads placed previously. The code section is determined by the number of leads. Report 33240 when there is an existing single-lead (electrode); 33230 when there are existing dual leads (electrodes); and 33231 when there are existing multiple leads (electrodes). Epicardial lead placement codes (33202, 33203) could be reported in addition to 33230, 33231, and 33240 when the placement is performed by the same physician during the same operative session.

Code 33241 is reported when documentation indicates that the physician removes only the implantable defibrillator pulse generator. The subcutaneous generator pocket is opened, and the generator is removed. The electrodes are detached from the generator, and the electrodes are placed in the pocket. Fluoroscopy is included and should not be reported separately.

Removal of both the pulse generator and electrodes for an implantable defibrillator system requires reporting multiple codes. For removal of an electrode by thoracotomy and removal of the pulse generator, report 33243 in conjunction with 33241. For removal of an electrode by transvenous extraction and removal of the pulse generator, report 33244 in conjunction with 33241. A transvenous extraction is normally attempted initially, but if it is unsuccessful a thoracotomy is performed. Removal and reinsertion of a new implantable defibrillator generator and electrodes also requires reporting of multiple codes. Report 33241, and 33243 or 33244 for the removal portion of the procedure. Report 33249 for insertion of the new system when a transvenous lead is placed; when placed subcutaneously report codes 33270 and 33272.

When a removal and replacement of an implantable defibrillator pulse generator is performed, the global codes (33262–33264) should be reported instead of individual codes for removal of the pulse generator (33241) and replacement (33230, 33231, 33240). Report 33262 for removal and replacement of a single-lead system generator; 33263 for a dual-lead system generator; and 33264 for a multiple-lead system generator.

Codes 33270–33273 are used to report procedures related to subcutaneous implantable defibrillators. Code 33270 indicates the initial insertion or replacement of a subcutaneous implantable defibrillator (S-ICD) system, including the pulse generator and lead. The pulse generator is placed in a subcutaneous pocket on the left side of the chest next to the ribs. Two small incisions are made above the sternum, and the lead wire is threaded through and sutured into place. The lead is then connected to the pulse generator. The physician records cardiac electrical signals from the leads and paces the heart through the leads to determine pacing threshold. The physician uses the S-ICD pulse generator to pace the heart into an arrhythmia, such as ventricular tachycardia or fibrillation. The S-ICD detects and terminates the arrhythmia using pacing or shocking the heart through the lead. The physician may reprogram the treatment parameters to optimize the device function to best treat the patient's arrhythmia. The incisions are closed. Report 33271 for insertion of the lead only. These codes should not be reported in conjunction with codes used to report implantable defibrillator services (33240, 33462, 33270) or programming or evaluation of implantable defibrillators (93260–93261, or 93644).

Code 33272 represents the removal of the subcutaneous implantable defibrillator lead only. An incision is made in the area above the sternum where the lead is located. The lead is disconnected from the pulse generator, pulled through, and removed. Code 33273 reports the repositioning of a previously placed implanted subcutaneous defibrillator lead (electrode). This procedure is performed when the system does not function due to improper placement of the lead. An incision is made over the previous subcutaneous pocket on the left side of the chest next to the ribs. The lead is disconnected from the pulse generator, and the generator is removed and the lead tested for proper function. It is then reattached to the generator in the new position and retested. These services should not be reported with codes indicating the programming of implantable defibrillators (93260–93261).

Medical Necessity

The following conditions may warrant implantable defibrillators (per Medicare):

- Patients with a personal history of sustained ventricular tachyarrhythmia (VT) or cardiac arrest due to ventricular fibrillation (VF). Patients must have demonstrated:

  - an episode of sustained VT, spontaneous or induced by an electrophysiology (EP) study, not associated with an acute myocardial infarction (MI), and not due to a transient or reversible cause

  - an episode of cardiac arrest due to VF, not due to a transient or reversible cause

- Patients with a prior MI and a measured left ventricular ejection fraction (LVEF) ≤ 30 percent. Patients must not have:

  - New York Heart Association (NYHA) classification IV heart failure

  - had a coronary artery bypass graft (CABG) or percutaneous coronary intervention (PCI) with angioplasty and/or stenting within the past three (3) months

  - had an MI within the past 40 days

  - clinical symptoms and findings that would make them a candidate for coronary revascularization

  - for patients identified in B2, a formal shared decision making encounter must occur between the patient and a physician (as defined in Section 1861(r)(1) of the Social Security Act (the Act)) or qualified non-physician practitioner (meaning a physician assistant, nurse practitioner, or clinical nurse specialist as defined in §1861(aa)(5) of the Act) using an evidence-based decision tool on ICDs prior to initial ICD implantation. The shared decision making encounter may occur at a separate visit

- Patients who have severe, non-ischemic, dilated cardiomyopathy but no personal history of sustained VT or cardiac arrest due to VF, and have NYHA Class II or III heart failure, LVEF ≤ 35 percent. Additionally, patients must not have:

  - had a CABG or PCI with angioplasty and/or stenting within the past three (3) months

  - had an MI within the past 40 days

  - clinical symptoms and findings that would make them a candidate for coronary revascularization

  - for patients identified in B3, a formal shared decision making encounter must occur between the patient and a physician (as defined in Section 1861(r)(1) of the Act) or qualified non-physician practitioner (meaning a physician assistant, nurse practitioner, or clinical nurse specialist as defined in §1861(aa)(5) of the Act) using an evidence-based decision tool on ICDs prior to initial ICD implantation. The shared decision making encounter may occur at a separate visit

- Patients with documented, familial or genetic disorders with a high risk of life-threatening tachyarrhythmias (sustained VT or VF, to include, but not limited to, long QT syndrome or hypertrophic cardiomyopathy).

- For these patients identified in B5, a formal shared decision making encounter must occur between the patient and a physician (as defined in Section 1861(r)(1) of the Act) or qualified non-physician practitioner (meaning a physician assistant, nurse practitioner, or clinical nurse specialist as defined in §1861(aa)(5) of the Act) using an evidence-based decision tool on ICDs prior to initial ICD implantation. The shared decision making encounter may occur at a separate visit.

- Patients with an existing ICD may receive an ICD replacement if it is required due to the end of battery life, Elective Replacement Indicator (ERI), or device/lead malfunction.

For each of the six (6) covered indications above, the following additional criteria must also be met:

- patients must be clinically stable (e.g., not in shock, from any etiology);
- LVEF must be measured by echocardiography, radionuclide (nuclear medicine) imaging, cardiac Magnetic Resonance Imaging (MRI), or catheter angiography;
- patients must not have:
  - significant, irreversible brain damage; or,
  - any disease, other than cardiac disease (e.g., cancer, renal failure, liver failure) associated with a likelihood of survival less than one (1) year; or,
  - supraventricular tachycardia such as atrial fibrillation with a poorly controlled ventricular rate

Exceptions to waiting periods for patients that have had a CABG, or PCI with angioplasty and/or stenting, within the past three (3) months, or had an MI within the past 40 days:

- Cardiac Pacemakers: Patients who meet all CMS coverage requirements for cardiac pacemakers, and who meet the criteria in this national coverage determination for an ICD, may receive the combined devices in one procedure, at the time the pacemaker is clinically indicated;
- Replacement of ICDs: Patients with an existing ICD may receive an ICD replacement if it is required due to the end of battery life, ERI, or device/lead malfunction.

The following conditions may warrant cardiac pacemaker (this list is not all inclusive) (per Medicare):

- Documented nonreversible symptomatic bradycardia due to second degree and/or third degree atrioventricular block

- Documented nonreversible symptomatic bradycardia due to sinus node dysfunction

The following indications are **noncovered** for implanted permanent single chamber or dual chamber cardiac pacemakers (per Medicare):

 DEFINITIONS

arrhythmia. Irregular heartbeat.

atrial fibrillation. Cardiac arrhythmia caused by small areas of muscle fibers becoming erratically and spontaneously activated through multiple circuits in uncoordinated phases of depolarization and repolarization.

bradycardia. Slowed heartbeat, usually defined as a rate fewer than 60 beats per minute. Heart rhythm may be slow as a result of a congenital defect or an acquired problem.

carotid sinus syndrome. Stimulation of an overactive carotid sinus, causing a marked drop in blood pressure, which, in turn, may stop the heart.

sinus node. Group of cells located on the wall of the right atrium, close to the superior vena cava, that naturally discharge electrical impulses initiating heart contracture. For this reason, it is often referred to as the "physiologic pacemaker."

syncope. Light-headedness or fainting caused by insufficient blood supply to the brain.

tachycardia. Excessively rapid beating action of the heart, defined as more than 100 beats per minute for an adult, that is usually defined by its origin (atrial or ventricular) and whether the onset and cessation occurs in sudden attacks (paroxysmal) or in a slow pattern (nonparoxysmal).

- A clinical condition in which pacing takes place only intermittently and briefly, and which is not associated with a reasonable likelihood that pacing needs will become prolonged

- Asymptomatic bradycardia in postmyocardial infarction patients about to initiate long-term beta-blocker drug therapy

- Asymptomatic first degree atrioventricular block

- Asymptomatic second degree atrioventricular block of Mobitz Type I unless the QRS complexes are prolonged or electrophysiological studies have demonstrated that the block is at or beyond the level of the His Bundle (a component of the electrical conduction system of the heart).

- Asymptomatic sinoatrial block or asymptomatic sinus arrest

- Asymptomatic sinus bradycardia

- Bradycardia during sleep

- Frequent or persistent supraventricular tachycardias, except where the pacemaker is specifically for the control of tachycardia

- Ineffective atrial contractions (e.g., chronic atrial fibrillation or flutter or giant left atrium) without symptomatic bradycardia

- Reversible causes of bradycardia such as electrolyte abnormalities, medications or drugs, and hypothermia

- Right bundle branch block with left axis deviation (and other forms of fascicular or bundle branch block) without syncope or other symptoms of intermittent atrioventricular block

- Syncope of undetermined cause

Key Documentation Terms

Documentation for these procedures must clearly support the medical necessity of the service being reported and a narrative of all procedures performed. Terms such as single-chamber, dual-chamber, insertion, removal, or replacement provide the guidance needed to ensure correct code assignment. Documentation should also state the decision to use a dual-chamber rather than a single-chamber system. All procedures should be clearly identified.

Coding Tips

- Note that codes 33210–33211, separate procedures by definition, are usually components of a more complex service and are not identified separately. When performed alone or with other unrelated procedures/services, however, they may be reported. If performed alone, list the code; if performed with other procedures/services, list the code and append modifier 59 or the appropriate X{EPSU} modifier.

- Do not report device evaluation codes (93260–93261 or 93279–93298) in addition to pulse generator and lead insertion/revision codes.

- Revision of a skin pocket is included in 33206–33249, 33262–33264, and 33270–33273 and should not reported separately.

- For insertion and replacement of a cardiac venous system electrode, see 33224 and 33225.

- For removal and replacement of an implantable defibrillator pulse generator and electrodes, report 33243 or 33244 and 33249 for transvenous electrodes or 33270 and 33272 for subcutaneous electrodes in conjunction with 33241.

- For procedures performed on leadless and pocketless pacemaker systems see codes 33274–33275.

- For insertion or replacement of a permanent implantable defibrillator system with a substernal electrode, see Category III code 0571T.

- For insertion of a substernal lead only, see Category III code 0572T.

- For removal and replacement of a sternal implantable pulse generator, see Category II code 0614T.

- For the removal of a generator only, in an implantable defibrillator with a substernal lead, see Category III code 0580T.

- There are many instructional notes throughout the pacemaker and implantable defibrillator section, including those on what codes should not be reported with other codes. An example is do not report 33216–33217 with 33206–33208, 33212–33214, 33221, 33227–33231, 33240, 33249, or 33262–33264. Please see the CPT book for the instructional notes. The list is too extensive to document here.

- As an "add-on" code, 33225 is not subject to multiple procedure rules. No reimbursement reduction or modifier 51 is applied. The following table provides additional information for these codes as found in the Medicare Physician Fee Schedule Database.

Parent Code	Add-On	GLOB DAYS	MULTI PROC	BILAT SURG	ASST SURG	CO-SURG	TEAM SURG
33206		090	2	0	1	2	0
33207		090	2	0	1	2	0
33208		090	2	0	1	2	0
33212		090	2	0	1	0	0
33213		090	2	0	1	0	0
33214		090	2	0	0	2	0
33216		090	2	0	1	0	0
33217		090	2	0	1	0	0
33221		090	2	0	1	0	0
33223		090	2	0	0	0	0
	33225	ZZZ	0	0	1	0	0
33228		090	2	0	1	0	0
33229		090	2	0	1	0	0
33230		090	2	0	1	0	0
33231		090	2	0	1	0	0
33233		090	2	0	1	0	0
33234		090	2	0	1	0	0
33235		090	2	0	1	0	0
33240		090	2	0	1	0	0
33249		090	2	0	1	1	0
33263		090	2	0	1	0	0
33264		090	2	0	1	0	0

Coding Trap
- Incision and drainage of abscesses or seromas, debridement, and complex wound closure of the initial skin pocket are all inclusive in the relocation

of skin pocket procedures (33222–33223) and should not be reported separately.

Leadless Pacemakers (33274–33275)

There are two codes specific to leadless pacemakers (33274–33275). Wireless pacemakers are small self-contained devices that are inserted directly into the right ventricle. It does not require leads, generator, or creation of the pacemaker pocket. Leadless pacemakers are inserted using a cardiac catheterization. Code 33274 is reported for the insertion or replacement of the leadless pacemaker, and 33275 reports the removal of the leadless pacemaker using imaging guidance.

Medical Necessity

The Food and Drug Administration has approved leadless pacemakers only for patients who have bradycardia and need only single-chamber pacing.

Coding Tips

- Do not report the insertion and removal for the same surgical session.
- These procedures should not be reported with femoral venography (75820), fluoroscopy (76000, 77002), right ventriculography (93566), or ultrasound guidance for vascular access [76937].
- Codes 93451, 93453, 93456, 93457, 93460, 93461, and 93530–93533 should not be reported separately unless the complete right heart catheterization is performed for a diagnosis separate from the insertion or removal of a leadless pacemaker procedure.
- To report subsequent device evaluation for leadless pacemakers, see 93279, 93286, 93288, 93294, or 93296.
- To report procedures for pacemaker systems with leads, see 33202–33273.

Electrophysiologic Operative Procedures (33250–33261 and 33265–33266)

Operative electrophysiologic (EPS) procedures describe the treatment of arrhythmia by surgical methods including ablation, disruption, incision, ligation, or reconstruction.

Procedure Differentiation

Ablation of supraventricular focus or pathway (Wolff-Parkinson-White syndrome) is reported with 33250–33251, while ablation of ventricular arrhythmogenic focus is reported with 33261. Open operative tissue ablation and reconstruction of atria is reported with 33254–33259. For a limited operative ablation and reconstruction (33254), also referred to as a modified maze procedure, an incision is made into the left or right atrium. A combination of surgical incision and/or energy sources such as heat, microwave, laser, ultrasound, or cryoprobe is used to create lesions that will heal into scars that disrupt conduction. In 33255 and 33256, an extensive operative ablation and reconstruction is performed. In an extensive procedure, the right and/or left atrial tissue and/or atrial septum is treated as described in 33254, and additional operative ablation involving the atrioventricular annulus is performed. In any of these procedures, the left atrial appendage may be excised or isolated. In 33256, lines are placed for cardiopulmonary bypass. When cardiopulmonary bypass is achieved, an extensive ablation and reconstruction procedure is performed. Codes 33257-33259 are add-on codes to be used concurrently with other cardiac procedures. For a limited operative tissue ablation and reconstruction of atria (33257), also referred to as a modified maze procedure, an incision is made into the left or right atrium. A combination of surgical incision and/or energy sources, such as heat, microwave, laser, ultrasound, or cryoprobe, is used to create lesions that will heal into scars that disrupt conduction. In 33258 and 33259, an extensive operative tissue ablation and reconstruction of the atria is performed. In these extensive procedures, the right and/or left atrial tissue and/or atrial septum is treated as described in 33257, and additional operative ablation involving the atrioventricular annulus is performed. In any of these procedures, the left atrial appendage may be excised or isolated. In 33259, lines are placed for cardiopulmonary bypass. When cardiopulmonary bypass is achieved, an extensive tissue ablation and atria reconstruction procedure is performed. Endoscopic operative tissue ablation and reconstruction of atria is reported with 33265–33266. Pay close attention to code descriptions; procedures are differentiated by with or without cardiopulmonary bypass.

Medical Necessity

The following conditions may warrant cardiac ablation (this list is not all inclusive):

- Atrial tachyarrhythmias
- Atrial tachycardia, flutter, and fibrillation
- Atrioventricular nodal reentrant tachycardia (AVNRT)
- Multifocal atrial tachycardia (MAT)
- Ventricular tachycardia (VT)

Key Documentation Terms

There are two main terms used in this section: limited and extensive.

Limited is described as surgically isolating the trigger of supraventricular dysrhythmias by surgical ablation of the pulmonary veins or other triggers in the left or right atrium of the heart.

Extensive is described as including the service in limited in addition to ablation of atrial tissue to remove supraventricular dysrhythmias. This surgical ablation must include one of the following: the atrial septum, left atrium, or the right atrium.

Documentation for these procedures must clearly support the medical necessity of the service being reported and a narrative of all procedures performed.

Coding Tips

- Codes 33250–33266 include cardioversion as an integral component of the procedures. Codes 92960 or 92961 should not be reported separately with these codes unless an elective cardioversion is performed at a separate patient encounter on the same date of service.
- As "add-on" codes, 33257–33259 are not subject to multiple procedure rules. No reimbursement reduction or modifier 51 is applied. Please see the CPT book for the codes that these add-on codes should be reported with.
- If an electrophysiologic study with pacing and recording is performed during these procedures, it is integral to the procedure and should not be reported separately with code 93624.

📖 **DEFINITIONS**

cardiac arrest. Sudden, unexpected cessation of cardiac action, including absence of heart sounds and/or blood pressure.

Coronary Bypass: Arterial, Venous, and Arterial-Venous Grafts (33510–33536)

Procedure Differentiation

Coronary Artery Bypass: Venous Grafts (33510–33516)

Codes 33510–33516 are used to report venous-only grafts used for coronary artery bypass graft (CABG) procedures and not for bypass procedures that use arterial grafts only or a combination of arterial and venous grafts during the same operative session. Code selection is based on the number of bypass grafts performed, which is determined by counting the number of grafted veins or arteries sutured to the diseased coronary arteries.

Coronary Artery Bypass: Venous AND Arterial Grafts (33517–33530)

This series of codes is reported when coronary artery bypass procedures are performed that use both venous and arterial grafts during the same operative session. Coronary artery bypass grafts (CABG) are coded by type of graft. When reporting these services it is required that two codes are assigned. The first reports the arterial-venous grafting that is performed. A code from the range 33517–33523 is used for this procedure. A second code representing the arterial grafting (33533–33536) is also required to represent a complete arterial-venous procedure.

Venous grafting alone is reported with 33510–33516. Arterial grafting alone is reported with 33533–33536.

Add-on codes 33517–33523 are used for coding procedures involving both arterial and venous grafts and may not be used alone. These codes specifically state that they are to be used in conjunction with code range 33533–33536. Code selection is based on the number of venous grafts performed, which is determined by counting the number of grafted veins or arteries sutured to the diseased coronary arteries.

For reoperation performed more than one month after the original procedure, report add-on code 33530 in addition to the code for CABG procedure. Included in these procedures is that portion of the operative angiogram performed by the surgeon.

> *Example*
> Coronary artery bypass using venous (saphenous) and arterial grafts for a single artery and two veins is reported with 33533 and add-on code 33518.

Coronary Artery Bypass: Arterial Grafts (33533–33536)

Codes from range 33533–33536 are reported for coronary artery bypass procedures using only arterial grafts, or a combination of arterial grafts and venous grafts. Obtaining arterial grafts excluding upper extremity (35600) may be reported separately. However, other sites such as epigastric, internal mammary, gastroepiploic, and others are included in these procedures.

Medical Necessity

The following conditions may warrant arterial/venous grafting (this list is not all inclusive):

- Aneurysm of coronary vessels
- Congenital coronary artery/vein anomaly

- Coronary atherosclerosis
- Coronary occlusion
- Dissection of coronary artery
- Myocardial infarction

Key Documentation Terms for Coronary Artery/Venous Bypass Grafts

Terms such as arterial, venous, and the number of grafts used provide the guidance needed to ensure correct code assignment. Documentation for these procedures must clearly support the medical necessity of the service being reported and a narrative of all procedures performed. Documentation should also include the number of grafts performed and the location of where the vein was harvested. With implementation of ICD-10-CM, documentation has changed for most of the diagnoses listed above. For example, in patients with atherosclerosis, the provider will need to document what type of graft (e.g., autologous, nonautologous biological) has the atherosclerosis. In addition, documentation will have to note whether the patient has other conditions such as angina and whether such conditions are unstable, with spasm, or unspecified. So again, documenting to the highest specificity will be crucial.

Coding Tips

- These codes include obtaining a saphenous vein graft, which is not reported separately.

- During venous or combined arterial venous coronary artery bypass grafting procedures (codes 33510–33523), it is occasionally necessary to perform epiaortic ultrasound. This procedure may be reported with 76998 (ultrasonic guidance, intraoperative) with modifier 59 or XS appended to it. Code 76998 should not be reported for ultrasound guidance utilized to procure the vascular graft.

- If a surgical assistant harvests the vein/artery graft, modifier 80 is added to codes from range 33510–33523 and 33533–33536, as appropriate.

- When a procedure is performed to obtain a femoropopliteal vein graft (35572), an upper extremity vein graft (35500), or an upper extremity artery graft (35600), it may be reported separately.

- As "add-on" codes, 33517–33530 are not subject to multiple procedure rules. No reimbursement reduction or modifier 51 is applied. The following table provides additional information for these codes as found in the Medicare physician fee schedule database.

Parent Code	Add-On	GLOB DAYS	MULT PROC	BILAT SURG	ASST SURG	CO-SURG	TEAM SURG
	33517	ZZZ	0	0	2	0	0
	33518	ZZZ	0	0	2	0	0
	33519	ZZZ	0	0	2	0	0
	33521	ZZZ	0	0	2	0	0
	33522	ZZZ	0	0	2	0	0
	33523	ZZZ	0	0	2	0	0
33533		090	2	0	2	0	0
33534		090	2	0	2	0	0
33535		090	2	0	2	0	0
33536		090	2	0	2	0	0

DEFINITIONS

artery. Vessel through which oxygenated blood passes away from the heart to any part of the body.

atherosclerosis. Buildup of yellowish plaques composed of cholesterol and lipoid material within the arteries.

graft. Tissue implant from another part of the body or another person.

myocardial infarction. Obstruction of circulation to the heart, resulting in necrosis.

occlusion. Constriction, closure, or blockage of a passage.

venous. Relating to the veins.

Please see the CPT book for the codes that add-on code 33530 should be reported with. The list is too extensive to document here.

Surgical Revascularization: Veins and Arteries (34001–34490)

Codes under this subheading describe blood clots or other foreign material that are removed from various vessels. The codes are differentiated by arterial and venous procedures, as well as by the specific vessel affected. The physician component of the operative arteriogram and sympathectomy are integral in these procedures along with ensuring that the vein/artery has an inflow and outflow.

Medical Necessity

The following conditions may warrant these procedures (this list is not all inclusive):

- Atheroembolism
- Atherosclerosis
- Occlusion
- Steal syndrome
- Stenosis
- Vessel injury

Key Documentation Terms

Terms such as anatomical location, embolectomy, or thrombectomy provide the guidance needed to ensure correct code assignment. Documentation for these procedures must clearly support the medical necessity of the service being reported and a narrative of all procedures performed.

Coding Tips

- See codes 35875–35876 for thrombectomy and revision of an arterial or venous graft.

Endovascular Stent Grafting for Aorta and Iliac Arteries (34701–34834)

These codes repair a number of different conditions, such as aneurysms (circumscribed dilation or outpouching of an artery wall, often containing blood clots connecting directly with the lumen of the artery), pseudoaneurysms (false aneurysms produced by a dilated vessel wall or a ruptured blood vessel that has formed a clot that pulsates, mimicking a true aneurysm), and arteriovenous malformation (an abnormal connection between arteries and veins).

Procedure Differentiation

These procedures include:

- Sizing and device selection prior to the procedure
- All nonselective catheterizations
- Radiological supervision and interpretation
- All angioplasty or stenting
  - codes 34701–34702 go to the level of the renal arteries to the aortic bifurcation
  - codes 34703–34706 go to the level of the renal arteries to the iliac bifurcation

DEFINITIONS

angioscopy. Visualization of capillary blood vessels with a microscope, or the inside of a blood vessel with a fiberoptic-equipped catheter.

arteriogram. Radiograph of arteries.

embolectomy. Surgical excision of a blood clot or other foreign material that broke away from its original source and traveled in the blood stream, becoming lodged in a blood vessel and blocking circulation.

steal. Diversion of blood to another channel.

sympathectomy. Surgical interruption or transection of a sympathetic nervous system pathway.

thrombectomy. Removal of a clot (thrombus) from a blood vessel utilizing various methods.

- – codes 34707–34708 and 34717–34718 go to the treatment zone only
- Endograft extensions placed in the aorta
  - – note that the codes have different routes
    - codes 34701–34702 go to the level of the renal arteries to the aortic bifurcation
    - codes 34703–34706 go to the level of the renal arteries to the iliac bifurcation
    - codes 34707–34708 go proximally to the aorta bifurcation and distally to the iliac bifurcation
- Endograft extensions placed in the iliac
  - – codes 34717–34718 are proximally to the aortic bifurcation and distally in the internal iliac, external iliac, and common femoral arteries

There are numerous definitions and guidelines that precede the codes in this section. Carefully review is necessary before reporting services in this section.

Codes 34701 and 34702 describe introduction, positioning, and deployment of an endograft to treat abdominal aortic conditions, with or without rupture, such as an aneurysm, pseudoaneurysm, dissection, penetrating ulcer, or traumatic disruption, located in the infrarenal abdominal aorta that may or may not extend into the iliac arteries. The infrarenal aortic endograft may be an aortic tube device, a bifurcated unibody device, a modular bifurcated docking system with docking limbs, or an aorto-uni-iliac device. The abdominal aortic treatment zone is defined as the infrarenal aorta. This procedure requires a vascular surgeon and a radiologist. In 34701, a catheter with a stent-transporting tip is advanced over the guidewire into the vessel. The catheter carries the aortic tube prosthesis, approximately 6 inches long and contained inside a holding capsule, through the arterial tree to the site of the aortic infrarenal aneurysm. Once the stent is in proper position, the holding capsule is removed and the stent is deployed, expanding like a spring to anchor itself to normal walls of the aorta above and below the aneurysm. The device serves as a substitute channel for blood flow. If full expansion of the prosthesis does not occur, or leaks are present, a balloon catheter is threaded to the graft site and inflated within the prosthesis until full expansion is achieved and leaking is stopped. The catheter/guidewire is removed and the arteriotomy site is closed. The aneurysm, excluded from the blood flow, typically shrinks over time. The treatment zone for endograft procedures is defined by those vessels that contain an endograft (main body, docking limbs, and/or extensions) deployed during that operative session. Code 34702 is reported when this procedure is performed on a ruptured aneurysm in the aorta or iliac.

Codes 34703, 34704, 34705, and 34706 describe introduction, positioning, and deployment of an endograft to treat abdominal aortic conditions, with or without rupture, located in the infrarenal abdominal aorta that may or may not extend into the iliac arteries. The infrarenal aortic endograft may be an aortic tube device, a bifurcated unibody device, a modular bifurcated docking system with docking limb(s), or an aorto-uni-iliac device. In 34703 and 34704, the abdominal aortic treatment zone is typically defined as the infrarenal aorta and ipsilateral common iliac artery. In 34705 and 34706, the abdominal aortic treatment zone is typically defined as the infrarenal aorta and both common iliac arteries. These procedures require a vascular surgeon and a radiologist. In 34703, under general anesthesia, a small incision is made in the groin over one femoral artery or both femoral arteries through which the endovascular devices are inserted. If contralateral femoral access is necessary, a percutaneous sheath may be placed. An aorta-uni-iliac prosthetic graft device contained inside a plastic holding capsule is threaded through the arteries to the site of the infrarenal aneurysm. The endograft is deployed by slowly removing the holding capsule away from the endograft, with continual monitoring of the exact positioning. Once the prosthesis is in place, the holding capsule is removed. Balloon angioplasty is performed at the ends of the prosthesis to expand and seat the graft. Stents are also deployed within the body of the endograft to maintain expansion forces. The aorta-uni-iliac prosthetic endograft is supported along its length by a series of metal rings sutured to the graft and is held in place by the radial force applied by the rings to the patient's aorta. Once in place, the arteriotomy site is closed. Code 34705 should be reported for simultaneous bilateral iliac artery aneurysm repairs with aorto-bi-iliac endograft. Codes 34704 and 34706 should be reported when endovascular repair is performed on a ruptured aneurysm in the aorta or iliac arteries. Rupture is defined as clinical and/or radiographic evidence of acute hemorrhage. A chronic, contained rupture is considered a pseudoaneurysm, and its endovascular treatment is reported with 34703 or 34705. Nonselective catheterization is included in 34703, 34704, 34705, and 34706. Balloon angioplasty and/or stenting at the sealing zone of an endograft is an integral part of the procedure. Fluoroscopic guidance and radiological supervision and interpretation in conjunction with endograft repair is not separately reported, and includes all intraprocedural imaging (e.g., angiography, rotational CT) of the aorta and its branches prior to deployment of the endovascular device, fluoroscopic guidance and roadmapping used in the delivery of the endovascular components, and intraprocedural and completion angiography (e.g., confirm position, detect endoleak, evaluate runoff) performed at the time of the endovascular infrarenal aorta and/or iliac repair.

Code 34707 and 34708 describe introduction, positioning, and deployment of an ilio-iliac endograft for treatment of isolated arterial pathology (with or without rupture), such as an aneurysm, pseudoaneurysm, dissection, arteriovenous malformation, or trauma involving the iliac artery. The treatment zone is defined as the portion of the iliac artery (e.g., common, internal, external iliac arteries) involved. The procedure requires a vascular surgeon and a radiologist. The patient receives medication (Heparin) to help prevent blood clots prior to the procedure. In 34707, under general anesthesia, the physician makes a small incision near the patient's hipbone area to enter the iliac artery. A proprietary device is used which is comprised of two main components: a trunk component and a contralateral leg component. The endoprosthesis, contained inside a holding device, is introduced into the artery under fluoroscopy and positioned at the target zone area of repair by threading guidewires and catheters. Nonselective catheterization is included. Report 34708 when an endovascular repair is performed on a ruptured aneurysm in the iliac artery. Rupture is defined as clinical and/or radiographic evidence of acute hemorrhage. A chronic, contained rupture is considered a pseudoaneurysm, and its endovascular treatment is reported with 34707. Balloon angioplasty and/or stenting at the treatment zone of an endograft is an integral part of the procedure. Fluoroscopic guidance and radiological supervision and interpretation, in conjunction with endograft repair, are not reported separately. Included are all intraprocedural imaging (e.g., angiography, rotational CT) of the iliac artery prior to deployment of the endovascular device, fluoroscopic guidance and roadmapping used in the delivery of the endovascular components, and intraprocedural and completion angiography (e.g., confirm position, detect endoleak, evaluate runoff) performed at the time of the endovascular iliac repair.

© 2020 Optum360, LLC

In 34709, the physician places an extension prosthesis distal to the common iliac artery or proximal to the renal artery for endovascular repair of an infrarenal abdominal aortic or iliac aneurysm, pseudoaneurysm, dissection, penetrating ulcer, endoleak, or endograft migration that terminates in the internal iliac, external iliac, or common femoral arteries or in the abdominal aorta proximal to the renal arteries. Using aortography, the target site is identified. The proper extension prosthesis is selected. Under fluoroscopy, the extension prosthesis, contained inside a long plastic holding capsule, is threaded through the arteries to the leak site. Once the extension prosthesis is in place, the holding capsule is removed. The extension prosthesis, activated by heat, expands like a spring and becomes anchored to the artery wall at the site of the endoleak. If full expansion of the prosthesis does not occur automatically, a balloon catheter is threaded to the graft site and inflated within the endovascular prosthesis until full expansion is achieved. The catheter is removed and the arteriotomy site is closed. Code 34709 should be reported once per vessel treated.

In 34710, a leak may occur at fixation sites of a grafted aneurysm through the body of the graft or from patent arteries within the aneurysm sac and may require endovascular reparation. This code describes delayed endovascular placement of a distal or proximal extension prosthesis to repair an infrarenal abdominal aortic or iliac aneurysm, pseudoaneurysm, dissection, endoleak, or endograft migration. Using separately reportable aortography, the target site is identified. The proper extension prosthesis is selected. Under separately reportable fluoroscopy, the extension prosthesis, contained inside a long plastic holding capsule, is threaded through the arteries to the site of the leak. Once the extension prosthesis is in place, the holding capsule is removed. The extension prosthesis, activated by heat, expands like a spring and becomes anchored to the artery wall at the site of the endoleak. If full expansion of the prosthesis does not occur automatically, a balloon catheter is threaded to the graft site and inflated within the endovascular prosthesis until full expansion is achieved. The catheter is removed and the arteriotomy site is closed. All nonselective catheterizations, sizing and device selection prior to the procedure, radiological supervision and interpretation, and treatment zone angioplasty or stenting is included in this procedure, when performed. Codes 34710 and 34711 may only be reported once per vessel treated (i.e., multiple endograft extensions placed in a single vessel may only be reported once). Report 34710 for placement of an extension prosthesis in the initial vessel and 34711 for placement of an extension prosthesis in each additional vessel.

Code 34712 reports the delivery of an enhanced fixation device, commonly referred to as a bioprosthesis. This procedure is used for patients with abdominal aortic and/or iliac artery conditions, such as an aneurysm with complex anatomies or for patients who are experiencing an endoleak. Proprietary devices ensure a safe and effective treatment solution for these types of repairs. They enhance durability to the level of a surgical anastomosis and address concerns for future complications. They are used to improve fixation and sealing of an endovascular graft, either in primary cases or to fix endoleaks and stent migration. The devices lock the endograft to the abdominal aorta and/or iliac artery to secure the patient's future and maximize outcomes in challenging patients. The fixation devices quickly identify, aim, and activate a sealing mechanism to close up endoleaks. EndoAnchors are used to repair an endovascular graft in cases where the original graft has moved away from the implant site and developed endoleaks. In such cases, augmented fixation and/or sealing is required to regain or maintain effective aneurysm exclusion. These devices can be placed during the initial endoprosthesis placement procedure or

DEFINITIONS

aneurysm. Circumscribed dilation or outpouching of an artery wall, often containing blood clots and connecting directly with the lumen of the artery.

aortic dissection. Pathologic process characterized by splitting of the wall of the aorta, caused by blood entering a tear in the vessel intima or an interstitial hemorrhage, leading to formation of a dissecting aneurysm.

balloon angioplasty. Procedure for treating blockages and plaque build-up within blood vessels. A small balloon-tip catheter is inflated inside an artery to open clogged or narrowed areas, stretching the intima and breaking up the plaque deposit.

ectasia. Pathological expansion, dilation, or distension of a hollow or tubular anatomic organ or structure.

embolization. Placement of a clotting agent, such as a coil, plastic particles, gel, foam, etc., into an area of hemorrhage to stop the bleeding or to block blood flow to a problem area, such as an aneurysm or a tumor.

endoprosthesis. Intravascular device in the form of a hollow stent placed within a duct or artery to provide passage through an obstructed area, such as in a bile duct, or to act as a replacement for damaged arterial walls, as in treating an aneurysm.

stent. Tube to provide support in a body cavity or lumen.

for a subsequent repair procedure. Percutaneous access using a sheath smaller than 12 French is included in 34712 and is not reported separately. Radiologic supervision and interpretation are included in this procedure.

Code 34717 reports a procedure where at the time of aorto-iliac artery endograft placement, the physician repairs a unilateral iliac artery rupture, aneurysm, pseudoaneurysm, arteriovenous (AV) malformation, dissection, penetrating ulcer, or traumatic disruption by placing an iliac branched endograft. The endograft, contained inside a holding device, is introduced into the artery under fluoroscopy and positioned at the target zone area of repair. This may require open access exposure of the artery or may be accomplished by threading guidewires and catheters through to the site. Once the endoprosthesis is in place, it is deployed within the artery at the targeted site. The position of the endoprosthesis is confirmed, any endoleaks are identified, and the status of runoff vessels is evaluated for any related stenosis, dissection, thrombosis, or embolism. All selective ipsilateral catheterization(s) necessary for device placement, device selection and preprocedural sizing, endograft extension(s), angioplasty or stenting within the treatment zone, as well as radiological supervision and interpretation, are included in this procedure. Code 34717 should be reported once per side in addition to the code for the primary procedure. When this procedure is not performed in the same operative session as an aorto-iliac artery endograft, 34718 should be reported.

In 34713, the femoral artery may be accessed percutaneously or by open incision. For percutaneous access, the femoral artery is identified using ultrasound guidance, and the guide catheter is percutaneously inserted with subsequent insertion of a large arterial sheath (e.g., 12 French or larger). Closure may involve the use of an arterial closure device (ACD). Several types of ACDs may be used for closure including a small balloon that ensures sealant coverage of the arteriotomy, four needles that anchor and close suture material upon removal, or a collagen sponge with polymer that forms a self-tightening suture seal. Alternately, the femoral artery may be examined via an open technique. With the patient in the supine position, the physician exposes the femoral artery through an incision in the groin area revealing the femoral artery on one side while underlying subcutaneous layers and muscles incised to reach the artery are placed out of the way as hemostasis is achieved in preparation for delivery of the endograft, endovascular prosthesis, or creation of a conduit. Closure may be by direct suture. Report 34713 for percutaneous access and closure of a femoral arteriotomy for delivery of an endovascular prosthesis. Ultrasound guidance is included. Report 34812 for open femoral artery exposure with delivery of an endovascular prosthesis and repair and closure of the femoral artery. Report 34714 for open femoral artery exposure with endovascular device delivery or establishment of cardiopulmonary bypass that requires creation of a prosthetic conduit utilizing a femoral artery.

In 34715, the axillary or subclavian artery is exposed for delivery of an endovascular prosthesis and performs closure of the artery with an arterial closure device (ACD). In one method, an ACD is inserted through the existing procedural sheath. A small balloon is inflated within the artery and pulled back to the arterial wall, serving as an anchor to ensure proper placement, and is inflated. The balloon is deflated and removed through the tract, leaving behind only the expanded sealant, which seals the arteriotomy. In an alternate method, an ACD utilizes four needles (two sutures) directed outward from within the arterial lumen. It is advanced over a guidewire until blood return indicates proper placement. When the physician pulls the device handle, the needles are deployed and pulled through the arterial wall. The needles remain contained

© 2020 Optum360, LLC

within the device shaft and are removed by pulling them up through the device shaft, leaving behind the suture ends which are then tied, and the device is removed. Yet another method uses an ACD composed of collagen sponge and polymer anchor joined together with a self-tightening suture that seals and sandwiches the arteriotomy for a more complete closure. The device stops the flow of blood mechanically, which is supported by the platelet-inducing properties of the collagen. Report 34715 for delivery of an endovascular prosthesis by axillary or subclavian exposure through an infraclavicular or supraclavicular or sternotomy incision during endovascular aneurysm repair. The patient is placed in supine position and open incision is made. Hemostasis of vessels is achieved. The underlying subcutaneous layers and muscles are incised to reach the artery and reflected out of the way. The axillary or subclavian artery is exposed in preparation for delivery of the endovascular prosthesis and its sheath is opened with tape placed about it. Report 34716 for endovascular device delivery or establishment of cardiopulmonary bypass that requires creation of a prosthetic conduit utilizing axillary or subclavian artery exposure through an infraclavicular or supraclavicular or sternotomy incision during endovascular aneurysm repair or cardiac procedures requiring cardiopulmonary bypass.

Code 34820 reports when an abdominal or retroperitoneal incision is made to expose the iliac artery on one side to facilitate the delivery of an endovascular prosthesis or to perform temporary iliac artery occlusion during a procedure for endovascular therapy. The patient is placed supine and the buttocks are elevated. An incision is made parallel with and just above the inguinal ligament. The incision is in the middle third of a proximally curved line extending from the anterior superior iliac spine to the pubic symphysis. Hemostasis of vessels is achieved, and the aponeuroses of the external and internal oblique and the transversus muscles are incised parallel to the inguinal ligament. The structures are reflected upward and medially, the transversalis fascia is opened, and the retroperitoneal space is entered. The iliac artery is exposed in preparation for delivering an endovascular prosthesis and its sheath is opened with tape placed about it. If the artery has been exposed for the purpose of placing a temporary occlusion device, the clamp is placed.

In 34833, a conduit is created for the delivery of an endovascular prosthesis or for the establishment of cardiopulmonary bypass via transabdominal or retroperitoneal incision. A skin incision is made parallel with and just above the inguinal ligament. The skin is incised, and the retroperitoneal space is entered to access the iliac artery. Bowels, blood vessels, and other soft tissue are mobilized from the area to give clear access to the iliac artery. With adequate exposure, loops are passed around the vessel proximally and distally. Anticoagulation is achieved and vascular clamps are applied. An arteriotomy is made for creation of the conduit, which is formed by placing a tubular piece of bypass graft material that has been fashioned into the right size onto the iliac artery and suturing it together. The conduit is clamped, and the vascular clamps are removed from the iliac artery. Additional sutures are placed as needed. Through the newly created conduit, endovascular repair by deployment of a prosthesis may be undertaken. After the repair is complete, the conduit may be closed in one of two ways. The open end of the conduit may be sewn to the distal external iliac artery, and thereby left in place as a channel for external iliac bypass graft, or it may be cut close to the iliac artery and simply oversewn with sutures. This code reports the creation of the conduit, not the endovascular repair. In 34834, open brachial artery exposure is done for delivery of an endovascular prosthesis. An incision is made in the skin of the upper arm and nerves, blood vessels, and other soft tissues are mobilized from the area to give clear access to the brachial artery. With adequate exposure, loops are passed around the vessel proximally and distally. Anticoagulation is achieved and vascular clamps are alternately applied and removed as needed for introduction of guidewires, sheaths, and catheters through the brachial artery for accomplishing deployment of an aortic or iliac endovascular prosthesis. After the endovascular repair is complete, the opening remaining in the brachial artery is closed with fine sutures after irrigation and trimming of the edges has been done. Hemostasis is achieved and the wound is irrigated and closed. This code reports the open brachial artery exposure, not the endovascular repair.

There are times when the service cannot be completed endovascularly. The CPT book includes three codes that specifically describe a conversion to open aortic aneurysm repair following an unsuccessful endovascular repair (34830, 34831, and 34832). These codes identify dissection of the affected vessels, repair of associated arterial trauma and placement of a traditional "sewn-in" graft to repair the aneurysm.

Medical Necessity
The following conditions may warrant these procedures (this list is not all inclusive):

- Abdominal aneurysm
- Aneurysm of renal or iliac artery
- Aortic dissection
- Aortic ectasia
- Arteriovenous malformation
- Atherosclerosis
- Injury to abdominal aorta
- Penetrating ulcer
- Saddle embolus of abdominal aorta
- Traumatic disruption

Key Documentation Terms
Terms such as bifurcation, common iliac, distal, iliac, infrarenal aorta, open, other than rupture, percutaneous, proximal, rupture, and transcatheter provide the guidance needed to ensure correct code assignment. Documentation for these procedures must clearly support the medical necessity of the service being reported and a narrative of all procedures performed. In addition, any procedures performed, such as intravascular ultrasound, should also be documented.

Coding Tips
- As "add-on" codes, 34709, 34711, 34713–34718, 34808, 34812, 34813, 34820, 34833, and 34834 are not subject to multiple procedure rules. No reimbursement reduction or modifier 51 is applied. Report these codes with the appropriate procedure codes as outlined in the CPT book.

- Codes 34713–34717, 34812, 34820, 34833, and 34834 should be reported twice when performed bilaterally. Do not report with modifier 50.

- A decompression laparotomy (49000) may be reported separately with 37202, 37204, 37206, and 37208.

- Endovascular repair of the iliac bifurcation with a bifurcated endograft may be reported separately with code 34717 or 34718.

- Intravascular ultrasound may be reported separately when performed in conjunction with an endovascular aneurysm, see 37252–37253.

- Extension prostheses of the abdominal aorta (proximal) that conclude in the aorta below the renal artery are an inherent component of the procedure and should not be reported separately when performed in conjunction with 37401–37406.

- If more than one endograft extension is placed in a single vessel, it may only be reported one time.

- For placement of an iliac branched endograft in the same operative session as an aorto-iliac endograft placement, see 34717. If performed in a separate operative session, see 34718.

Endovascular Repairs of The Infrarenal Abdominal Aorta and Visceral Aorta (34839–34848)

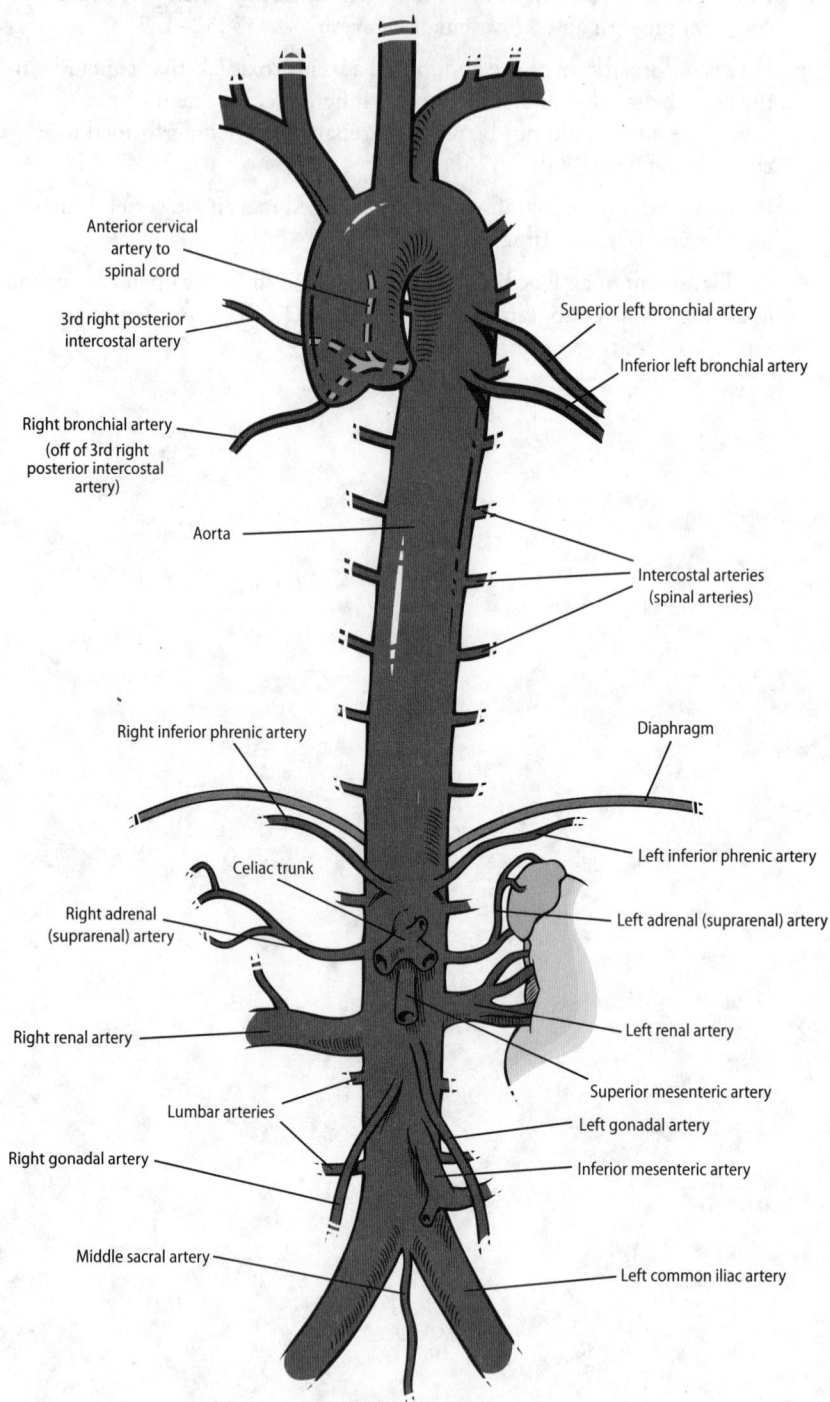

Anterior cervical artery to spinal cord

3rd right posterior intercostal artery

Superior left bronchial artery

Inferior left bronchial artery

Right bronchial artery (off of 3rd right posterior intercostal artery)

Aorta

Intercostal arteries (spinal arteries)

Right inferior phrenic artery

Diaphragm

Celiac trunk

Left inferior phrenic artery

Right adrenal (suprarenal) artery

Left adrenal (suprarenal) artery

Right renal artery

Left renal artery

Superior mesenteric artery

Lumbar arteries

Left gonadal artery

Right gonadal artery

Inferior mesenteric artery

Middle sacral artery

Left common iliac artery

There is also a section of codes for endovascular repair of an abdominal aortic aneurysm, pseudoaneurysm, or dissection involving visceral branches of the aorta (superior mesenteric, celiac, and renal arteries) and infrarenal abdominal aorta. These procedures require the skills of a vascular surgeon and a radiologist.

Procedure Differentiation

Under fluoroscopic guidance, the physician inserts an aortic component through one femoral artery. These are contained inside a plastic holding capsule that is threaded through the arteries to the site of the aneurysm. The physician places the necessary extension prostheses and cuts fenestrations (holes) at each visceral artery orifice to allow side branch perfusion of these vessels. Next, catheters are used to place overlapping stents at each fenestration and vessel orifice to secure the junction. Once the graft components and stents are in place, the holding capsule and catheters are removed and the arteriotomy site is closed. Report 34841 when one visceral artery is included, 34842 for two, 34843 for three, and 34844 for four or more arteries. Codes 34841-34844 do not enter the common iliac artery.

In 34845-34848, report procedures for repair including the visceral aorta and infrarenal abdominal aorta. These procedures are also performed using fluoroscopic guidance. The physician inserts the aortic component and one iliac limb through one femoral artery. These are contained inside a plastic holding capsule that is threaded through the arteries to the site of the aneurysm. Next, the physician inserts the opposite iliac limb by contralateral femoral artery access. The physician mates the aortic and iliac limb inserted into the first femoral artery to the opposite iliac limb inserted by contralateral femoral artery access. Since this repair extends above the visceral vessels, a visceral extension prosthesis is required. The physician places the extension prosthesis and cuts fenestrations (holes) at each visceral artery orifice to allow side branch perfusion of these vessels. Catheters are used to place overlapping stents at each fenestration and vessel orifice to secure the junction. Once the graft components and stents are in place, the holding capsule and catheters are removed and the arteriotomy site is closed. Report 34845 when one visceral artery is included, 34846 for two, 34847 for three, and 34848 for four or more arteries. These codes should not be reported in addition to planning services (34839) performed the day of or the day before the procedure.

Very precise imaging of the patient's anatomy is required prior to delivery of an endovascular prosthesis as the device must be exactly the correct diameter and length to make a secure seal that will exclude the arterial blood flow from the aneurysm. Imaging is performed with digital computerized reconstruction arteriography, computerized tomography (radiographic and/or magnetic resonance) that allows multiple projections to fully appreciate the three dimensional configuration of the arterial tree. The arterial lumen may be imaged with intravascular ultrasound. Arterial embolization may be required to occlude side branches communicating with the aneurysm. Angioplasty may be used to enlarge the iliac arteries to permit delivery of the graft components.

Code 34839 describes the planning required for these procedures,. The documentation for this service should indicate that the physician spends at least 90 minutes planning for the placement of a fenestrated visceral aortic endograft, which requires detailed planning before implantation. The planning includes review of radiological imaging enhanced by computer software to help create the device. Before placement, the physician needs to determine the size parameters of the graft that will conform to the branches of the aorta. These dimensions allow the physician to cut holes (fenestrations) in the device at each visceral artery orifice to allow side-branch perfusion of these vessels. Precise planning has to allow for adequate blood flow upon completion of placement. The physician must document at least 90 minutes of planning in the medical record to report this service.

Medical Necessity

The following conditions may warrant these procedures (this list is not all inclusive):

- Aneurysm
- Dissection
- Intramural hematomas
- Penetrating ulcer
- Pseudoaneurysm
- Recurrent congestive heart failure, pulmonary edema, or coronary ischemia due to stenosis of the renal artery
- Renal artery stenosis of > 50 percent in a transplanted kidney
- Renal insufficiency due to atherosclerotic stenosis

Key Documentation

Terms such as visceral aorta or visceral aorta and infrarenal abdominal aorta provide the guidance needed to ensure correct code assignment. Documentation for these procedures must clearly state the number of visceral artery repaired during the procedure.

Coding Tips

- The introduction of catheters and guidewires into the aorta and visceral and or renal arteries should not be reported separately when reporting these procedures.
- Balloon angioplasty within the target zone of the endograft is not reported separately, whether prior to or after graft deployment.
- Fluoroscopic guidance in conjunction with these procedures is considered an integral component and is not reported separately.
- Catheterization of the hypogastric arteries, arterial families outside of the treatment zone of the graft, exposure of the access vessels, extensive repair of the access artery, and other separate interventional procedures outside of the target treatment zone performed at the time of this service may be reported separately.
- Exposure access to a vessel may be reported separately with codes 34713-34716, 34812, 34820, 34833, and 34834.
- For simultaneous endovascular repair of the thoracic aorta (descending), report 33880-33886 and transcatheter therapy (75956-75959) with 34841-34848.

Repair Aneurysm, False Aneurysm, Related Arterial Disease (35001–35152)

Procedure Differentiation

These procedures include all the steps necessary to prepare the artery for anastomosis, as well as endarterectomy, which is not reported separately. The physician component of the operative arteriogram is integral in these procedures along with ensuring that the vein/artery has an inflow and outflow. Correct code selection is determined by the specific vessel affected and whether it is a ruptured aneurysm or an aneurysm, pseudoaneurysm, and associated occlusive disease.

 DEFINITIONS

anastomosis. Surgically created connection between ducts, blood vessels, or bowel segments to allow flow from one to the other.

occlusive disease. Vascular disease causing constriction, closure, or blockage of an artery or vein due to stenosis, deposits of fatty or hardened plaque, or blood clots. This would be coded according to the specific type of occlusion and the vessel involved.

pseudoaneurysm. False aneurysm produced by a dilated vessel wall, or a ruptured blood vessel that has formed a clot that pulsates, mimicking a true aneurysm. For coding classification purposes, pseudoaneurysm is coded as an aneurysm to the site and/or type. The index entry directs the coder to aneurysm, for which "false" is a nonessential modifier.

stenosis. Narrowing or constriction of a passage.

Medical Necessity

The following conditions may warrant these procedures (this list is not all inclusive):

- Aneurysm of artery
- Artery injury
- Dissection of artery
- Occlusion
- Rupture of artery
- Steal syndrome
- Stenosis

Key Documentation Terms

Documentation should indicate the surgical procedure that was performed. Terms such as aneurysm, pseudoaneurysm, ruptured aneurysm, incision type (arm, neck, or thoracic), and vessels involved (iliac, visceral) provide the guidance needed to ensure correct code assignment. Above all else, the documentation should support the medical necessity of the procedure.

Coding Tips

- When these codes are performed with another separately identifiable procedure, the highest dollar value code is listed as the primary procedure and subsequent procedures are appended with modifier 51.

- Harvested vein or synthetic material may be used for the graft, but the harvest of the graft is not reported separately.

- Angioscopy performed during therapeutic intervention should be reported in addition to the code for the primary procedure; see 35400.

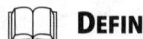

DEFINITIONS

claudication. Lameness, pain, and weakness occurring in the arms or legs during exercise due to muscles not receiving the needed oxygen and nutrients.

percutaneous. Through the skin.

vascular insufficiency. Inadequate blood flow and oxygenation.

Vascular Injection: Arterial, Aortic, Venous, and Central Venous Access (36000–36598)

This broad subsection of codes includes all vascular injection procedures: venous, arterial, aortic, and central venous access procedures. These procedures include local anesthesia, the introduction of needles and catheters, the injection of contrast media (which may be performed with or without automatic power injection), and all care related to the procedure. The drugs, contrast media, and catheters are not included in the code and should be reported separately.

Procedure Differentiation

Below is a brief explanation of the services within the vascular injection procedures category (36000–36598).

Procedures Preformed Intravenously (36000–36015)

The codes under this subheading are often incorrectly coded to report the placement of a routine IV catheter. See code 36005 if the catheter is inserted for venography or code 36000 if the catheter is inserted for another purpose.

Selective vascular catheterization is coded as such to include the introduction and all of the lesser order selective vessels used in the approach. Additional second and third order catheterizations that are within the same vascular family and supplied by a single first order vessel are reported using 36012, 36218, or 36248, as appropriate. When additional first order or higher catheterization is performed in a vascular family that is different from the initial vascular family, these procedures are reported separately using the same guidelines. For instance, a first order branch from the vena cava (36011) is any initial vessel draining directly into the vena cava (e.g., renal vein or jugular vein). A second order branch of the vena cava (36012) is any vein draining into a first order branch (e.g., left adrenal, petrosal sinus).

Medical Necessity

There are multiple indications for each of these procedures. It would be wise to verify coverage with payers.

Key Documentation Terms

In order to assign the most appropriate vascular injection procedure code, the medical record documentation must be reviewed to determine why the procedure was performed (i.e., injection, introduction, or selective catheter placement).

Coding Tips

- Imaging may be reported separately when performed at the time of an injection procedure (36002). See codes 76942, 77002, 77012, or 77021.

- Imaging performed in conjunction with extremity venography (36005) may be reported separately. See codes 75820 and 75822.

- Insertion of a flow directed catheter, such as a Swan-Ganz, is reported separately.

Refer to the table provided to determine the order of the vessels catheterized. The starting point of the catheterization would be the aorta in this example.

© 2020 Optum360, LLC

First Order (Aorta)	Second Order (Selective Vessel Order)	Third Order	Beyond Third Order Branches
Innominate	common carotid (right)	internal carotid (right)	ophthalmic (right) posterior communicating (right) middle cerebral (right) cerebral (right, anterior)
		external carotid (right)	superior thyroid (right) ascending pharyngeal (right) facial (right) lingual (right) occipital (right) posterior aurical (right) superficial temporal (right) internal maxillary (right) middle meningeal (right)
	subclavian and axillary (right)	vertebral (right)	basilar
		internal mammary (right)	
		thyrocervical trunk (right)	inferior thyroid (right) suprascapular (right) transverse cervical (right)
		costocervical trunk (right)	highest intercostal (right) deep cervical (right)
		lateral thoracic (right) thoracoacromial (right) humeral circumflex (right)	
		subscapular (right)	circumflex scapular (right)
		brachial (right)	
		brachial, deep (right)	ulnar (right) radial (right) interosseous (right) deep palmar arch (right) superficial palmar arch (right) metacarpals and digitals (right)
Common carotid (left)	internal carotid (left)	ophthalmic (left) posterior communicating (left) middle cerebral (left) anterior cerebral (left)	
	external carotid (left)	superior thyroid (left) ascending pharyngeal (left) facial (left) lingual (left) occipital (left) posterior auricular (left) superficial temporal (left)	
	internal maxillary (left)		middle meningeal (left)
Subclavian & axillary (left)	vertebral (left) internal mammary (left)		
	thyrocervical trunk (left)	inferior thyroid (left) supracapular (left) transverse cervical (left)	
	costocervical trunk (left)	highest intercostal (left) cervical, deep (left)	
	lateral thoracic (left) thoracoacromial (left) humeral circumflex (left) subscapular (left) brachial, (left)	circumflex scapular (left)	
	deep brachial (left)	radial (left), ulnar (left)	
		interosseous (left)	deep palmar arch (left) superficial palmar arch (left) metacarpals and digitals (left)

First Order (Aorta)	Second Order (Selective Vessel Order)	Third Order	Beyond Third Order Branches
Intercostal			
Bronchials			
Esophageal (recurrent)			
Phrenic (inferior)	suprarenal (superior)		
Celiac trunk	gastric (left)	esophageal branch	
	splenic	pancreatic, dorsal pancreatic, great pancreatic, caudal gastroepiploic short gastrics	transverse pancreatic, inferior

	common hepatic	gastroduodenal	posterior superior
			  pancreaticoduodenal
			anterior superior
			  pancreaticoduodenal

		proper hepatic	hepatic (left) hepatic (right) cystic gastroepiploic supraduodenal intermediate hepatic
Middle suprarenal			
Superior mesenteric artery	colic (middle)		

	pancreaticoduodenal (inferior)	posterior inferior
		  pancreaticoduodenal
		anterior inferior
		  pancreaticoduodenal	

	jejunal ileocolic appendicular posterior cecal anterior cecal marginal colic (right)		
Renal	inferior suprarenal		
Testicular/ovarian			
Lumbar			
Inferior mesenteric artery	colic (left)		
	sigmoid	rectosigmoid superior rectal	

© 2020 Optum360, LLC

First Order (Aorta)	Second Order (Selective Vessel Order)	Third Order	Beyond Third Order Branches
Middle sacral			
Common iliac	internal iliac	iliolumbar lateral sacral superior gluteal umbilical superior vesical obturator inferior vesical rectal, middle inferior rectal inferior pudental inferior gluteal	
	external iliac	inferior epigastric	cremasteric pubic
		circumflex iliac, deep	deep circumflex liliac, ascending
	common femoral	profunda femoris	medial descending perforating branches lateral descending lateral circumflex
		pudendal, deep, external pudendal, superficial, external circumflex femoral, ascending, lateral circumflex femoral, descending, lateral circumflex femoral, transverse, lateral	
		superficial femoral	geniculate popliteal anterior tibial peroneal posterior tibial
Main pulmonary arteries, (right/left)			

Intra-arterial, Intra-aortic (36100–36299)

Selective vascular catheterization is coded as such to include the introduction and all of the lesser order selective vessels used in the approach. Additional second and third order catheterizations that are within the same vascular family and supplied by a single first order vessel are reported using 36012, 36218, or 36248, as appropriate. When additional first order or higher catheterization is performed in a vascular family that is different from the initial vascular family, the procedure is reported separately using the same guidelines.

Diagnostic studies may be performed using selective or nonselective catheter placement and are reported with codes 36221–36228. These studies include the following:

- Accessing the vessel
- Arterial contrast injection that includes arterial, capillary, and venous phase imaging, when performed
- Arteriotomy closure (pressure or closure device)
- Catheter placement
- Fluoroscopy
- Radiologic supervision and interpretation

Reporting of selective catheter placement is based on intensity of services. Things to keep in mind when reporting these services include:

- Report the most intensive code first
- When reporting ipsilateral carotid territory, only one code should be reported from the 36222–36224 range
  - Listed in order of intensity 36224>36223>36222
- When reporting ipsilateral vertebral territory, only one code should be reported from the 36225–36226 range
  - Listed in order of intensity 36226>36225

The following procedures are excluded and may be reported separately:

- 3D rendering when performed (76376–76377)
- Interventional procedures
- Ultrasound guidance (76937)
- Diagnostic angiography of upper extremities/other vascular beds of the neck and/or shoulder girdle during the same session, if performed (75774)

In a selective catheter placement, the physician passes a needle into the skin into an extremity artery, usually in the upper thigh. A guidewire is threaded through the needle into the vessel. The needle is removed. The wire is threaded into the aorta and up to the thoracic aorta where it is manipulated into a branch off the aortic arch. A catheter follows the wire into a first order thoracic or brachiocephalic artery. The wire is removed. The catheter may pass through the first order vessel into a second order thoracic or brachiocephalic artery. Contrast material for arteriography is injected into the catheter that has been guided to an area upstream of the site under investigation. In 36215, the catheter remains in a first order artery. In 36216, the catheter travels farther to a second order artery. Upon completion, the catheter is removed and pressure applied to stop bleeding at the puncture site.

In 36217, the physician punctures the skin and underlying artery with a needle and threads a guidance wire through the needle into the artery. The needle is removed. The guidewire is manipulated into the specific artery. A catheter follows the wire into a first order thoracic or brachiocephalic artery. The catheter passes through the first order vessel into the second order thoracic or brachiocephalic artery. The catheter continues to a third order vessel. Contrast material for arteriography is injected into the catheter that has been guided to the site under investigation. Once the procedure is complete, the catheter is removed and pressure applied to stop bleeding at the injection site. Code 36218 should be reported for an additional second order, third order, and beyond, thoracic or brachiocephalic branch, within a vascular family.

Report the code for the highest order vessel cannulated, but not for any lesser order vessels cannulated in the approach.

Please carefully review the CPT guidelines prior to coding services in this section.

Medical Necessity
There are multiple indications for each of these procedures. It would be wise to verify coverage with payers.

Key Documentation Terms
In order to assign the most appropriate vascular injection procedure code, the medical record documentation must be reviewed to determine why the procedure was performed (e.g., introduction, selective or superselective catheter placement, revision, or removal).

Coding Tips
- Introduction of a needle or intracatheter into the carotid or vertebral artery (36100) is a unilateral procedure. If performed bilaterally, append modifier 50 according to payer guidelines.

- As "add-on" codes, 36218, 36227, 36228, and 36248 are not subject to multiple procedure rules. No reimbursement reduction or modifier 51 is applied. Report these codes with the appropriate procedure codes as outlined in the CPT book.

Miscellaneous Venous Procedures (36400–36522)
The codes under this subheading are for a wide range of services including routine venipuncture, transfusions, therapeutic apheresis, endovenous ablation therapy, and an injection of sclerosing solution into veins. Criteria for code selection includes the procedure performed, the age of the patient, and the specific number of veins treated.

Transfusions are reported according to the type of transfusion (e.g., exchange, intrauterine, partial exchange, or push) or substance (e.g., blood, plasma, or crystalloid) and the age of the patient. Code 36430 describes blood or blood components being transfused to a patient. Code 36440 is reported when the documentation states a push transfusion was performed on a child 2-years-old and under. The physician calculates the amount of blood to be transfused and slowly injects it into the patient using a needle or existing catheter.

An exchange transfusion (36450–36455) is a procedure where the patient's blood is removed and replaced simultaneously to maintain blood pressure. A partial exchange transfusion (36456) is the commonly accepted method of treatment in newborns. This condition is sometimes associated with babies who

 DEFINITIONS

ablation. Removal or destruction of a body part or tissue or its function. Ablation may be performed by surgical means, hormones, drugs, radiofrequency, heat, chemical application, or other methods.

apheresis. Process of extracting blood from a donor, centrifuging or separating the desired part of the blood, and transfusing the remainder back into the donor.

laser. Concentrated light used to cut or seal tissue.

radiofrequency ablation. To destroy by electromagnetic wave frequencies.

sclerotherapy. Injection of a chemical agent that will irritate, inflame, and cause fibrosis in a vein, eventually obliterating hemorrhoids or varicose veins.

are post-term, small for gestational age (SGA) or with /intrauterine growth restriction (IUGR), identical twins with twin-to-twin transfusion, babies of diabetic mothers, or in babies with chromosomal abnormalities. In this procedure, blood is slowly removed from the newborn replacing it with fluids that assist in the dilution of the red blood cell concentration, usually normal saline (crystalloid), blood, or plasma. The amount of blood to be exchanged is based on the observed and desired hematocrit, which is usually 55 percent. This procedure may be performed in cases of severe, chronic anemia or polycythemia with or without hyperviscosity of newborns typically in the neonatal intensive care unit.

Code 36460 reports an intrauterine blood transfusion to a fetus. The physician uses separately reportable ultrasound guidance to locate the umbilical vein. A needle is directed through the abdominal wall into the amniotic cavity. The umbilical vein is pierced and fetal blood is exchanged with transfused blood. The needle is withdrawn and the fetus is observed under separately reportable ultrasound.

Codes 36465–36471 are used to report the injection of sclerosant substances into veins. Sclerotherapy irritates the lining of the vein and causes the vessel to collapse. Correct code assignment is dependent upon the vessel being injected and the type of sclerosant being injected. Codes 36465–36466 are reported when the provider injects a noncompounded foam sclerosant into incompetent lower-extremity veins. Ultrasound-guided outflow compression maneuvers are also performed during the session. Code 36468 is specific to spider veins of the limb or trunk. It should only be reported once per extremity per session. Codes 36470–36471 are reported when a compounded sclerosant foam is injected for treatment of an incompetent extremity truncal vein, other than telangiectasias (spider veins). Ultrasound imaging guidance provided with codes 36468–36471 may be reported using 76942 when performed.

Endovenous ablation therapy (36473–36479 and 36482–36483) is included in the venous section. This procedure is destruction or ablation of incompetent veins. These services include the imaging guidance and all procedural monitoring. When the services are performed in an office setting, supplies and equipment are an integral part of the procedure and may not be reported separately. When mechanochemical endovenous ablation (MOCA) is used, report 36473 for the first vein and 36474 for the subsequent veins treated through separate access sites. This method employs a rotating wire in conjunction with an infused sclerosing agent to damage the wall of the vein. This procedure is performed under local anesthesia. The most common site of treatment is the greater saphenous vein. When radiofrequency is used, report 36475 for the first vein and 36476 for the subsequent veins treated through separate access sites. If laser is used for the ablation, report 36478 for the first vein and 36479 for the subsequent veins treated through separate access sites. When duplex ultrasound is used to create a detailed outline or mapping of the veins in the lower legs to identify all vein abnormalities, along with additional nearby structures to include deep veins and arteries, report 36482 for the first vein and 36483 for subsequent veins treated through separate access sites.

CPT codes 36474, 36476, 36479, and 36483 should be reported only once per extremity regardless of how many veins are treated in the encounter.

Medical Necessity

There are multiple indications for each of these procedures. It would be wise to verify coverage with payers.

Key Documentation Terms

In order to assign the most appropriate vascular injection procedure code, the medical record documentation must be reviewed to determine why the procedure was performed (e.g., ablation therapy, injection, transfusion, or venipuncture).

Coding Tip

- As "add-on" codes, 36474, 36476, 36479, and 36483 are not subject to multiple procedure rules. No reimbursement reduction or modifier 51 is applied. The following table provides additional information for these codes as found in the Medicare physician fee schedule database.

Parent Code	Add-On	GLOB DAYS	MULT PROC	BILAT SURG	ASST SURG	CO-SURG	TEAM SURG
36473		XXX	2	1	1	0	0
	36474	ZZZ	0	1	1	0	0
36475		000	2	1	1	0	0
	36476	ZZZ	0	1	1	0	0
36478		000	2	1	1	0	0
	36479	ZZZ	0	1	1	0	0
36482		000	2	1	1	0	0
	36483	ZZZ	0	1	1	0	0

Services Performed on Central Venous Access Catheters or Devices (36555–36598)

The following must be true to meet the criteria of a central venous access catheter or device:

- Devices that are inserted via cutdown or percutaneous access, either centrally (e.g., femoral, jugular, subclavian veins, or inferior vena cava) or peripherally (e.g., basilic, cephalic, or saphenous vein)
- Devices that terminate in the brachiocephalic (innominate), iliac, or subclavian veins, vena cava, or right atrium

Once in place, the devices may be accessed by a subcutaneous port or pump, or by an exposed catheter.

Procedure Differentiation

The CPT codes for these devices are further differentiated by whether the device is inserted centrally in the jugular, femoral, subclavian vein, or the inferior vena cava or inserted peripherally.

These procedures are categorized as:

- Insertion of device or catheter through new venous access
- Repair device without replacement of device or catheter, nonmechanical or pharmacologic
- Replacement of catheter component of device
- Replacement of catheter and device through same access
- Removal of device and catheter

 DEFINITIONS

cutdown. Small, incised opening in the skin to expose a blood vessel, especially over a vein (venous cutdown) to allow venipuncture and permit a needle or cannula to be inserted for the withdrawal of blood or administration of fluids.

peripheral. Outside of a structure or organ.

subcutaneous. Below the skin.

venotomy. Incision or puncture of a vein.

These codes are also separated according to whether the insertion of the device involves the creation of a subcutaneous tunnel from the chest wall to the site of the venotomy with the catheter passing through the tunnel (tunneled) or the direct insertion of the device into the venotomy site (nontunneled).

Each of these types of service is listed as a subcategory in the CPT book. Understanding the type of procedure performed helps in determining which set of codes should be used to report the services provided by the provider. When removing an existing device and inserting a new device in a new venous system, through separate venous access sites, more than one subcategory of codes is used to report the services appropriately.

Patient age is used to define code selection to reflect the work required in patients older than age 5 years and those younger than age 5. Use modifier 63 as appropriate for neonates and infants up to 4 kg current weight. Physician work is also defined by determination of tunneled versus nontunneled insertion.

For removal of a central venous catheter that requires removing only skin sutures holding it in place, such as nontunneled, the appropriate level of evaluation and management (E/M) service (see codes 99202–99499) should be assigned.

Tunneled catheter removal is reported with 36589 or 36590.

Types of central venous catheters and devices include but are not limited to:

- Arrow multilumen
- Button Port
- Dual Port
- Groshong
- Hickman
- Infuse-a-Port
- Macro Port
- Medtronic CAP
- Micro Port
- Port-A-Cath
- Q-Port
- Rauf dual-lumen
- Rauf triple-lumen
- Tesio

Medical Necessity

The following conditions may warrant these procedures (this list is not all inclusive):

- Aneurysm of upper or lower extremity
- Arteriovenous fistula acquired
- Atherosclerosis of bypass graft
- Embolism and thrombosis of upper or lower extremity
- Infection and inflammatory reaction due to vascular device
- Mechanical complication of vascular device

- Complications due to renal dialysis device, implant, or graft
- Stricture of artery
- Vein compression

Key Documentation Terms

Documentation should indicate the surgical procedure that was performed. Terms such as insertion, complete or partial replacement, removal, or repair provide the guidance needed to ensure correct code assignment. Above all else, the documentation should support the medical necessity of the procedure. Be sure to also include use of imaging guidance or ultrasound guidance in documentation, if applicable.

Coding Tips

- Radiologic guidance is reported using 76937 or 77001.
- Codes 36572-36573 and 36584 include all imaging, venography (performed through the same venous puncture), necessary to complete the procedure and assure that the final position of the catheter is correct.
- A chest x-ray (71045-71048) should not be used as verification of catheter position on the same date of service as 36572-36573 and 36584. This service is an integral component of the catheter placement codes.
- Midline catheter placements, which terminate in the peripheral venous system, should be reported with 36400, 36406, and 36410.

Hemodialysis Access, Cannulation, Arteriovenous Fistula (36800–36909 and 37607)

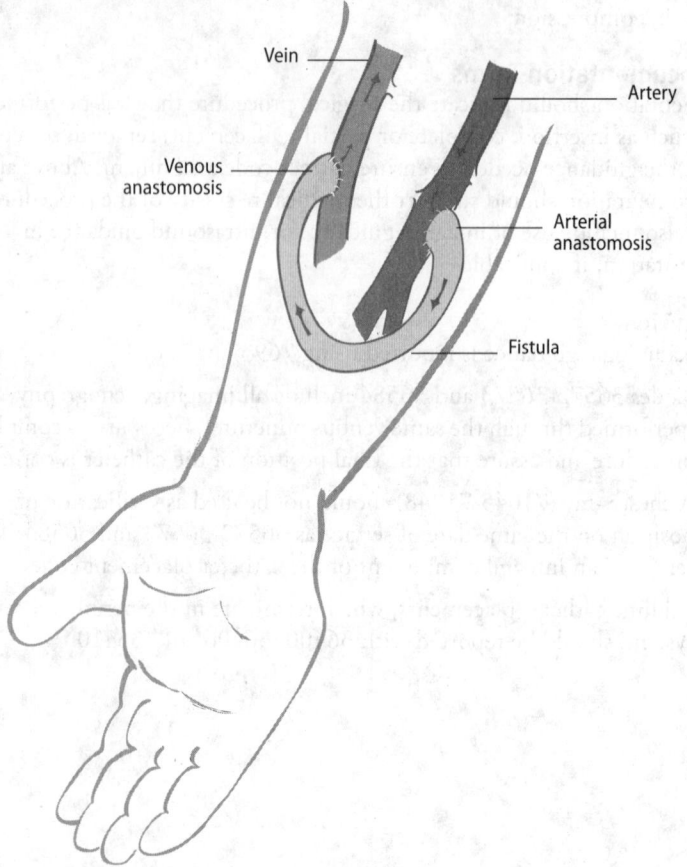

The codes listed under this subheading report procedures involving hemodialysis access, intravascular cannulation for extracorporeal circulation, or the insertion of a shunt.

Procedure Differentiation

Before selecting a procedure code describing a surgically created arteriovenous (AV) fistula, check the documentation to see which procedure was performed:

In 36818–36819, a connection between an artery and a vein is created for a vascular access site in patients with end stage renal disease who require hemodialysis. In 36819, the surgeon dissects down to the basilic vein on the medial side of the upper arm and mobilizes the vein. A subcutaneous tunnel on the anterior side of the arm is created, and the mobilized basilic vein is transposed to this tunnel and anastomosed to the brachial artery. Report 36818 if a similar arteriovenous connection is made in the upper arm by anastomosing the cephalic vein to the brachial artery.

In 36820, a connection between an artery or vein is created using a forearm vein in the arm inverted end-to-end. The physician dissects down to the vein and artery. The subfascial plane is identified and elevated laterally to the flexor carpi radialis (FCR) and medially to the brachioradialis (BR). The plane between the BR and FCR is dissected, and the perforating vessels are identified and cauterized. The pedicle is followed to the antecubital fossa. The tourniquet is released, and the vessels are further cleaned of their adventitia under loupe visualization. Using microvascular techniques, a suture for the arterial anastomosis is performed and closure is completed. Suction drains are placed in the neck. If a Doppler is to be used for postoperative assessment, a suture is placed to mark the pedicle site. A splint is fabricated and secured to the arm with an elastic bandage.

Code 36821 Direct arteriovenous anastomosis, any site, describes the connection of a vein directly to an artery without an interposing graft (i.e., two adjacent vessels are connected). This is usually possible when the artery and vein are very close to each other.

Code 36823 Insertion of arterial and venous cannula(s) for isolated extracorporeal circulation, describes the insertion of arterial and venous cannula(s) for isolated extracorporeal circulation to an extremity to provide regional perfusion chemotherapy (RPC) with or without hyperthermia. The external iliac, common femoral, or subclavian artery and vein are isolated depending on the site of the tumor. A cannula is inserted into the selected artery and vein to isolate blood flow to and from the extremity. The blood flow from the isolated extremity is connected to a perfusion pump where the blood is oxygenated. The blood may be heated to between 40° and 40.5° C (104° to 105° F). One or more high-dose chemotherapy agents are injected and perfused over an hour or more with flow rates monitored and adjusted to minimize leakage into the systemic circulation. The combination of heat and the chemotherapy agent act to destroy the cancer cells. After completion of the perfusion procedure, the cannulas are removed and the artery and vein repaired.

Code 36825 Creation of autogenous arteriovenous fistula by other than direct arteriovenous anastomosis, describes arteriovenous anastomosis between two vessels using an interposing graft made of the patient's natural vein (autogenous). This is usually performed for chronic hemodialysis administration.

Code 36830 Creation of nonautogenous arteriovenous fistula by other than direct arteriovenous anastomosis, describes the arteriovenous anastomosis between two vessels using a synthetic material as an interposing graft (nonautogenous). A nonautogenous AV fistula is a tube made from Gore-Tex, polytetrafluoroethylene (PTFE), or similar biocompatible material. The artery and vein are far enough apart that they cannot be directly anastomosed, so graft material must be used to connect them.

Code 36831 Thrombectomy, arteriovenous fistula; without revision, autogenous or nonautogenous dialysis graft, describes a thrombectomy without revision of the AV fistula.

Code 36832 Revision open, arteriovenous fistula, without thrombectomy, autogenous or nonautogenous, dialysis graft, describes revision (opening the AV fistula in order to straighten a kink) and may require creating a new anastomosis with a graft obtained from a separate site or created with synthetic material.

Code 36833 Revision, open, arteriovenous fistula; with thrombectomy, autogenous or nonautogenous dialysis graft, should be reported when a thrombectomy (removal of a blood clot) at the fistula site is performed in addition to revising the existing arteriovenous fistula.

Codes 36860-36861 External cannula declotting with or without balloon catheter, describe a thrombectomy procedure performed externally. The cannula is injected with a solution containing enzymes to dissolve the clot (36860) or, after injecting a solution, a balloon catheter is inserted (36861) into the cannula to retrieve a clot.

Code 37607 Ligation or banding of angioaccess arteriovenous fistula, describes ligation (occluding the lumen of a vessel by application of a suture ligature to cut off the flow of the vessel and cause it to clot) and banding (wrapping the AV fistula, usually with synthetic material, in order to reduce blood flow from any outside source).

If the hemodialysis procedure is done intraoperatively and is a standard and necessary part of the main procedure during the same surgical session, the cannula insertion should not be reported separately.

A Thomas shunt is reported with 36835. This type of shunt is infrequently used; verify this is the correct code by obtaining a copy of the shunt label from the medical record.

Procedures performed on the dialysis circuit are reported with 36901-36909. These codes are built on progressive hierarchies, meaning the more-intensive procedures include the less-intensive procedures that may be identified by separate codes within this section, but only the most intensive procedure performed should be reported. There are numerous definitions and guidelines that precede the codes in this section. Please carefully review them prior to reporting services in this section.

This section of codes has many procedures that are integral components of the main code.

A diagnostic examination of the dialysis circuit is reported with code 36901. The physician inserts a needle or catheter into a dialysis circuit via a puncture in the skin overlying the circuit of a dialysis patient. The catheter is guided into the circuit and vessel to an area upstream of the site under investigation, and contrast material is injected into it. Report 36901 for the initial access, including shunt access, contrast injections, and all fluoroscopic imaging deemed necessary from the arterial anastomosis and adjacent artery through the entire venous outflow (inferior and superior vena cava included). In 36902, a transluminal balloon angioplasty is performed. In this procedure a catheter with a balloon attached is inserted into the peripheral dialysis segment and fed into the narrowed portion where its balloon may be inflated several times in order to stretch the diameter, allowing a more normal flow of blood through the area. In 36903, documentation should state that a catheter with a stent-transporting tip is threaded over the guidewire into the peripheral dialysis segment, and the wire is extracted. The catheter travels to the point where the vessel needs additional support. The compressed stent is passed from the catheter into the vessel where it deploys, expanding to support the vessel walls.

Codes 36904–36906 report procedures performed for occlusions in the dialysis circuit by means of a mechanical thrombectomy and/or thrombolysis infusion. In 36904 the devices used for mechanical thrombectomy include those that fragment the thrombus with or without removal of the clot, as well as those that come into contact with the vessel wall. The dialysis circuit is cannulated to gain access, and 5,000 units of heparin are administered. Angiography is performed to confirm the occluded segment. A hydrophilic wire is passed across the occlusion, followed by passing of the Trellis device over a stiff exchange length wire. The distal and proximal balloons are inflated in the segment on either side of a treatment zone containing infusion to isolate the treatment zone and to sustain the fluid concentration that is infused. One milligram of tissue

DEFINITIONS

arteriovenous fistula. Connecting passage between an artery and a vein.

hemodialysis. Cleansing of wastes and contaminating elements from the blood by virtue of different diffusion rates through a semipermeable membrane, which separates blood from a filtration solution that diffuses other elements out of the blood.

ligation. Tying off a blood vessel or duct with a suture or a soft, thin wire.

lumen. Space inside an intestine, artery, vein, duct, or tube.

thrombectomy. Removal of a clot (thrombus) from a blood vessel utilizing various methods.

plasminogen activator (TPA) is infused into the treatment zone. The Turbo Trellis is run at 4,000 rpm for five minutes. After the proximal balloon is deflated, small clots are removed via the integral aspiration port to prevent embolization. Thrombolysis infusion may be performed with a catheter threaded over the wire for pharmaceutical administration directly within the thrombosis. When the procedure is complete, the instruments are removed and pressure is applied over the puncture site to stop the bleeding. This procedure includes imaging guidance, diagnostic angiography, catheter placement, and intraprocedural pharmacological thrombolytic injections. Report 36905 when the peripheral dialysis segment is treated with balloon angioplasty. A catheter with a balloon attached is inserted into the segment and fed into the narrowed portion, where its balloon may be inflated several times in order to stretch the diameter allowing a more normal flow of blood through the area. Report 36906 when the peripheral dialysis segment is treated with an intravascular stent. A catheter with a stent-transporting tip is threaded over the guidewire into the vessel, and the wire is extracted. The catheter travels to the point where the vessel needs additional support. The compressed stent is passed from the catheter into the vessel where it deploys, expanding to support the vessel walls. Once the procedure is complete, the catheter is removed and pressure is applied over the puncture site.

Codes 36907–36908 describe procedures performed on the central dialysis segment. In 36907, a catheter with a balloon attached is inserted into the central dialysis segment and fed into the narrowed portion, where its balloon may be inflated several times in order to stretch the diameter, allowing a more normal flow of blood through the area. In 36908, a catheter with a stent-transporting tip is threaded over the guidewire into the central dialysis segment, and the wire is extracted. The catheter travels to the point where the vessel needs additional support. The compressed stent is passed from the catheter out into the vessel where it deploys, expanding to support the vessel walls. Once the procedure is complete, the catheter is removed and pressure is applied over the puncture site. All imaging radiological supervision and interpretation is included.

Code 36909 is an add-on code for embolization or occlusion of a dialysis circuit (main circuit or any accessory vein). This may be due to complications or to assist in circuit maturity and/or patency. A needle is inserted through the skin and into a blood vessel. A guidewire is threaded through the needle into the vessel. The needle is removed. A catheter is threaded into the vessel and the wire is extracted. The catheter travels to the appropriate blood vessel and beads, coils, or another vessel-blocking device are released. The beads or other device block the vessel. The catheter is removed, and pressure is applied over the puncture site to stop bleeding.

Medical Necessity

The following conditions may warrant these services (this is not an all-inclusive list).

Arterial inflow impediment clinical findings include:

- diminished intra-access flow
- ischemic changes of the extremity (steal syndrome)
- low pressure in graft even when outflow is manually occluded

Venous outflow impediment clinical findings include:

- abnormal physical findings, specifically pulsatile graft/fistula or loss of thrill
- development of large superficial collateral venous channels
- development of pseudoaneurysm(s)
- elevated venous/arterial ratio (static venous pressure ratio — above 40%)
- elevated venous pressure in the AV dialysis access
- inefficient dialysis
- loss of "machine-like" bruit, i.e., short sharp bruit
- prolonged bleeding following needle removal
- recirculation percentage greater than 10–15%
- swelling of the extremity, face, or neck

Key Documentation Terms

Documentation should indicate the surgical procedure that was performed. Terms such as creation, revision, thrombectomy, central, peripheral, or autogenous or nonautogenous graft provide the guidance needed to ensure correct code assignment. Above all else, the documentation should support the medical necessity of the procedure.

Coding Tips

- As add-on codes, 36907–36909 are not subject to multiple procedure rules. No reimbursement reduction or modifier 51 is applied. Add-on codes describe additional intraservice work associated with the primary procedure. It is performed by the same provider on the same date of service as the primary service/procedure, and must never be reported as a stand-alone code.

  The following table provides additional information for these codes as found in the Medicare physician fee schedule database.

Parent Code	Add-on	GLOB DAYS	MULT PROC	BILAT SURG	ASST SURG	CO-SURG	TEAM SURG
36818		090	2	0	2	1	0
36919		090	2	0	2	1	0
36820		090	2	1	2	1	0
36821		090	2	0	2	1	0
36823		090	2	0	1	0	0
36825		090	2	0	2	1	0
36830		090	2	0	2	1	0
36832		090	2	0	2	1	0
36833		090	2	0	2	1	0
	36901	000	2	0	1	0	0
	36902	000	2	0	1	0	0
	36903	000	2	0	1	0	0
	36904	000	2	0	1	1	0
	36905	000	2	0	1	1	0
	36906	000	2	0	1	1	0

- Code 36907 should only be reported once for all central dialysis segment angioplasties performed.

- Code 36908 should only be reported once for all central dialysis segment stenting.

- Code 36909 should only be reported once per date of service.

- Ultrasound guidance (76937) may be reported separately with 36901–36906 if necessary for immature or failing AV fistulas.

- For open creation, revision, and/or thrombectomy of the dialysis circuit, see 36818–36833.

- For open ligation/occlusion of a dialysis access, see 37607.

- Chemotherapy perfusion supported by a membrane oxygenator/perfusion pump is an integral part of code 36823.

- Many procedures in the code range of 36800–36861 are separate procedures. A separate procedure by definition is usually a component of a more complex service and is not identified separately. When performed alone or with other unrelated procedures/services, it may be reported. If performed alone, list the code; if performed with other unrelated procedures/services, list the code and append modifier 59.

Transluminal Angioplasty, Percutaneous (37246–37249)

Transluminal angioplasty is a procedure where a balloon-tipped catheter is placed within a narrowed artery or vein, and the balloon is inflated to stretch the vessel to a larger diameter for increased blood flow. This procedure is done open or percutaneously.

Procedure Differentiation

The procedures are differentiated by the area of the occlusion. Codes 37246–37247 report procedures performed in an artery but exclude the following areas: central nervous system, coronary, lower limbs if performed for occlusive disease, intracranial, pulmonary, and dialysis circuit. Codes 37248–37249 report procedures in a vein but exclude the dialysis circuit. These codes include all radiological imaging within the same artery.

Medical Necessity

The following conditions may warrant these services (this is not an all-inclusive list).

Arterial inflow impediment clinical findings include:

- diminished intra-access flow

- ischemic changes of the extremity (steal syndrome)

- low pressure in graft even when outflow is manually occluded

Venous outflow impediment clinical findings include:

- abnormal physical findings, specifically pulsatile graft/fistula or loss of thrill

- development of large superficial collateral venous channels

- development of pseudoaneurysm(s)

- elevated venous/arterial ratio (static venous pressure ratio — above 40%)

- elevated venous pressure in the AV dialysis access

- inefficient dialysis

- loss of "machine-like" bruit, i.e., short sharp bruit
- prolonged bleeding following needle removal
- recirculation percentage greater than 10–15%
- swelling of the extremity, face, or neck

Key Documentation Terms

Documentation should indicate the surgical procedure that was performed.

Terms such as anatomical locations, artery, vein, initial, or subsequent provide the guidance needed to ensure correct code assignment. Above all else, the documentation should support the medical necessity of the procedure.

Coding Tips

- As add-on codes, 37247 and 37249 are not subject to multiple procedure rules. No reimbursement reduction or modifier 51 is applied. Add-on codes describe additional intraservice work associated with the primary procedure. It is performed by the same provider on the same date of service as the primary service/procedure and must never be reported as a stand-alone code.
- The following table provides additional information for these codes as found in the Medicare Physician Fee Schedule Database.

Parent Code	Add-On	GLOB DAYS	MULT PROC	BILAT SURG	ASST SURG	CO-SURG	TEAM SURG
37246		000	2	1	1	0	0
	37247	ZZZ	0	1	1	0	0
37248		000	2	1	1	0	0
	37249	ZZZ	0	1	1	0	0

- When multiple angioplasties are performed in a single artery/vein, regardless of the number of lesions, only one code is reported.
- Intravascular ultrasound may be reported separately with codes 37252–37253.
- Mechanical thrombectomy and/or thrombolytic therapy may be reported separately with codes 37184–37188 and 37211–37214.

Coding Traps

- Only one code should be reported if a lesion involves two vessels but can be treated with one therapy.

© 2020 Optum360, LLC

Procedures Performed on the Digestive System

Codes within this section of the CPT book describe open and endoscopic procedures performed on the digestive system, including the mouth and related oral structures, the pharynx, adenoids and tonsils, esophagus, stomach, intestines, appendix, rectum, anus, liver, biliary tract, and pancreas.

Resection and Repair Procedures of the Lips (40490–40799)

There are two classifications of procedures performed on this lips: excisions and repairs.

Cheiloplasty (40700–40761)

A cleft lip or palate is the failure for the muscle and/or bone to fuse leaving an opening in the anatomical structure. This occurs in the 8th through 12th week of gestation. In order to code appropriately for cleft palate and cleft lip, the type of cleft must be identified.

Cleft lip occurs when there is an opening or cleft in the lip. A small cleft may be referred to as partial or incomplete and a large cleft, which continues into the nose, is sometimes referred to as a complete cleft lip. This can occur unilaterally (one side of the mouth), bilaterally (both sides of the mouth), or median (middle or directly under the nose). A cleft in the lip does not mean that there is a cleft in the palate and vice versa. A patient can have one or the other, or both. The repair of a cleft lip, also known as a cheiloplasty, may involve other reconstructive procedures that are reported using the appropriate codes from the integumentary subsection.

 AUDITOR'S ALERT

Nasal deformities repaired at the same time as a cleft lip are included in the cleft lip repair.

Procedure differentiation

Repair of a cleft lip is also known as cheiloplasty. Code 40700 involves the surgical correction if unilateral cleft lip. Any nasal deformity often caused by the cleft lip may also be repaired during the surgical encounter. The cleft margins are incised on either side from the mouth toward the nostril and through the full-thickness layers of mucosa, muscle, and skin. The vermilion border of the cleft lip is turned downward to restore the normal shape of the lip and the muscle and skin are brought together to close the cleft separation and preserve muscle function. The physician closes the prepared margins in layers from the intraoral mucosa through the muscle with final closure of the skin.

Codes 40701 and 40702 report the surgical correction of a bilateral developmental cleft lip deformity. Code 40701 is reported when the repair is done in one stage. Report 40702 when documentation indicates that one stage of a two stage repair is performed. Typically, the cleft lip is repaired first and nasal deformities are repaired in a second surgical session.

When documentation indicates that the physician recreates the cleft defect and then makes the repair, 40720 is reported. This is most frequently performed when the previous correction has an unfavorable result, such as scar contracture (permanent shortening), wound dehiscence (splitting), or infection. The cleft margins are recreated to define clean edges for the defect through full-thickness layers of mucosa, muscle, and skin. The prepared margins are again closed in layers from the intraoral mucosa through muscle with final closure of the skin.

 DEFINITIONS

bilateral cleft lip. Two congenital fissures or openings in the upper lip that occur on both the left and right of the philtrum (indentation in the center of the lip).

complete cleft lip. Congenital fissure or opening in the upper lip that extends to the nose.

partial cleft lip. Congenital fissure or opening in the upper lip that does not extend to the nose.

unilateral cleft lip. Congenital fissure or opening in the upper lip on one side of the philtrum (indentation in the center of the lip).

Complicated repairs using a pedicle flap from the lower lip are reported with 40761. Documentation must indicate that in addition to the repair usually performed to correct the cleft defect, a pedicle flap was designed from the lower lip based on blood supply. The flap is created with a full-thickness incision and rotated on its pedicle to the desired location. The flap is sutured in layers to the recipient tissue location.

The table below may be used to help determine which code is appropriate for the procedure performed.

Cheiloplasty

	40700	40701	40702	40720	40761
Unilateral	X			X*	
Bilateral		X	X		
One stage procedure		X			
One stage of a two stage procedure			X		
Primary repair	X	X	X		
Secondary repair				X	
With pedicle flap					X

*When performed bilaterally modifier 50 should be appended to 40720.

Key Documentation Terms
The medical record documentation must indicate the following:

- Unilateral or bilateral
- Primary or secondary
- With or without flap

Coding Tips
- To report the performance of a rhinoplasty to correct a nasal deformity that is secondary to a congenital cleft lip, see 30460–30462.
- Two codes are necessary when both a cleft lip and a cleft palate are repaired.

Coding Trap
The following procedures are excluded from this section of codes and may be reported separately:

- Cleft palate repair (42200–42225)
- Other reconstructive procedures (14060, 14061, 15120–15261, 15574, 15576, 15630)

Procedures Performed on the Tongue and Floor of Mouth (41000–41599)
Codes within this subsection are used to report procedures such as the incision and drainage of abscesses or cysts, the excision of lesions or structures within the mouth, and the repair of lacerations.

Surgical Incision of Floor of Mouth or Tongue (41000–41018)
This subheading contains codes that are used to report procedures that require incision into the structures within the floor of the mouth and/or the tongue,

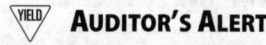

AUDITOR'S ALERT

The mouth has mucocutaneous margins. If a procedure is performed on a lesion at or near a mucocutaneous margin, report only the CPT code that best describes the procedure reported. For example, when a tissue transfer is performed and a code from the digestive system includes a tissue transfer service, that code and not one from the integumentary section should be reported.

such as intraoral abscesses, cysts, or hematomas. Documentation must indicate that the physician made a small intraoral incision through the mucosa of the tongue or floor of the mouth overlying an abscess, cyst, or hematoma, and drained the fluid.

Procedure Differentiation

In 41000, the incision and drainage site of the cyst, hematoma, or abscess is on the tongue (lingual). In 41005, the lesion is located superficially under the tongue (sublingual). In 41006, the sublingual lesion is deep into the supramylohyoid muscle. In 41007, the physician dissects through the anterior floor of the mouth into the supramylohyoid muscle to drain an abscess in the submental space. In 41008, the physician incises through the mucosa of the floor of the mouth to the supramylohyoid muscle and carries the dissection deeper into the tissue to reach the submandibular space. In 41009, dissection is carried out down through the mouth and into the masticator space, containing the ramus, the posterior portion of the mandible, and the masticator muscles to drain the abscess. If the abscess, cyst, or hematoma is extraoral, see 41015–41018.

Resection and Repair of the Tongue (41100–41599)

This subheading contains codes that are used to report procedures that require excision of a lesion of the structures within the floor of the mouth and/or the tongue. Other procedures include ablation, fixation, frenoplasty, and suspension.

Procedure Differentiation

Excision services include biopsy of the tongue based upon the part of the tongue (41100–41105) and the floor of the mouth (41108). Lesion excision of the tongue is reported with 41112–41114 according to the part of the tongue treated and the extent of the wound closure; without wound closure 41110. When a frenectomy is performed, it is reported with code 41115. Use 41116 for excision of a lesion of the floor of the mouth.

Repairs of the tongue and floor of the mouth lacerations, if performed, are reported with 41250–41252. The size of the laceration and the location are used to select the specific code.

Other procedures on the tongue include suturing the tongue to the lip to treat micrognathia, congenital hypoplasia, or abnormal smallness of the maxilla or mandible and is reported with 41510. There are two procedures specific for treatment of sleep apnea. Code 41512 reports tongue-base suspension using a wire attached to the mandible, and 41530 is used for ablation of the tongue base. Code 41520 is reported when a frenoplasty is performed. The frenum tissue is surgically altered, usually with a Z-plasty technique. An incision in the shape of a "Z" is made through the frenum and the tissues are then reapproximated in a different position and sutured.

Coding Tip

- When performing a glossectomy (41120–41155), specific code selection is based upon the amount of the tongue excised, as well as other surrounding structures that are included in the surgical procedure.

 DEFINITIONS

glossectomy. Excision of all or a portion of the tongue.

lingual. Surface of the tooth closest to the tongue or relating to the tongue and its surrounding areas.

micrognathia. Congenital hypoplasia or abnormal smallness of the maxilla or mandible. The alveolar tissue of the upper or lower jaw may be incomplete or underdeveloped in micrognathia.

sleep apnea. Intermittent cessation of breathing during sleep that may cause hypoxemia and pulmonary arterial hypertension.

Definitions

cleft lip. Congenital fissure or opening in the upper lip due to failure of embryonic cells to fuse completely.

cleft palate. Congenital fissure or defect of the roof of the mouth opening to the nasal cavity due to failure of embryonic cells to fuse completely. A cleft palate can be unilateral (left or right of the midline of the mouth) or bilateral (on both the left and right of the midline of the mouth) and complete (extending to nose) or incomplete (does not involve the nose).

Procedures Performed on the Palate and Uvula (42000–42281)

The palate is divided into two parts: the soft palate, which is the soft tissue located at the back of the mouth that is responsible for closing off the nasal passages during swallowing, and the hard palate, which is the bony structure at the roof of the mouth.

Suturing of the Palate (42180–42281)

Codes within this section are used to report repairs made to the palate including those due to trauma or congenital defects.

Procedure differentiation

The repair of a cleft palate or palatoplasty is reported using the appropriate code from range 42200–42225. Code selection is dependent upon the anatomical structures involved, the type of revision, and any additional procedures such as lengthening the palate or use of a pharyngeal flap. The cleft size and location dictates the type of repair to be performed. The benefits of palatal closure include restoration of swallowing and speech functions. When only the soft and/or hard palate are repaired, report 42200. For palatoplasty with closure of the alveolar ridge, see 42205–42210. For palatoplasty for cleft palate, major revision, see 42215; for a secondary lengthening procedure, see 42220; for attachment of the pharyngeal flap, see 42225.

Key Documentation Terms

When coding for cleft palate, documentation must indicate:

- Soft or hard palate
- Involvement of alveolar ridge when applicable
- Bone graft when used to repair alveolar ridge
- If a major revision was performed
- Attachment of a pharyngeal flap

Coding Tip

- When a major revision palatoplasty is performed, the defect dictates the type of repair. Typically, the documentation indicates that incisions are made in the palatal mucosa adjacent to the alveolar (tooth-bearing) bone. The mucosa is elevated and loosened from the bony palate and the previous midline incisions are excised and dissected to develop mucosal and muscular layers.

Procedures Performed on the Salivary Gland and Ducts (42300–42699)

Salivary glands are found in and around the mouth and throat and secret saliva, which moistens the mouth, initiates digestion, and helps to prevent tooth decay. There are three major salivary glands: the parotid, submandibular, and sublingual glands.

The saliva produced by these glands drains into the mouth by means of tubes called ducts. The parotid gland duct is located near the upper teeth, the submandibular ducts are under the tongue, and the sublingual ducts are located on the floor of the mouth. Besides these glands, there are many tiny glands called minor salivary glands located in the lips, inner cheek area (buccal mucosa), and extensively in other linings of the mouth and throat.

Surgical Incision of Salivary Gland and Ducts (42300–42340)

Procedure Differentiation

Abscess procedures are reported with 42300–42320, with code selection based upon the site and extent of the drainage. Sialolithotomy, incision in the submandibular, sublingual, or parotid ducts to remove a calculus or stone from within a salivary duct, is reported with 42330–42340.

Resection: Salivary Gland (42400–42450)

Procedure Differentiation

Biopsy of the salivary gland can be performed by a number of methods. If the medical record documentation states that a needle was inserted through the skin overlying a salivary gland to obtain a tissue sample, report 42400.

For an incisional biopsy, an incision is made in the skin overlying the salivary gland. Blunt and sharp dissection is carried out to the gland. An incision is made in the tissue of the gland and a small piece of gland is removed. Suture closure is required. Use 42405 to report this procedure.

Removal of salivary cysts are reported using 42408.

In marsupialization of a sublingual salivary cyst, the physician incises and removes the mucosa overlying a cyst on the floor of the mouth. The roof of the cyst is removed and the remaining sides of the cyst wall are sutured to the mucosa, creating a pouch. The saliva then drains through the pouch. The pouch shrinks in size to a small opening in the floor of the mouth. Saliva from the sublingual gland then flows through this opening. This procedure is reported with 42409.

Parotid tumors or parotid gland excision are reported with 42410–42426. Code selection is dependent upon whether a lobe is removed or a total excision is performed.

In 42410, the main trunk of the facial nerve is visualized and the lateral (superficial) lobe of the parotid gland is freed and excised. In 42415, the facial nerve is identified and the lateral lobe is lifted off the branches of the nerve using dissection. In 42420, the facial nerve is identified and the lateral lobe is lifted off the branches of the nerve using dissection. The nerve is retracted so the deep parotid gland can be removed without damaging the facial nerve. In 42425, the physician removes the gland without capsule disruption, sacrificing the facial nerve. In 42426, the physician removes the gland without capsule disruption, sacrificing the facial nerve. The incision is extended inferiorly to dissect the unilateral neck for lymph node excision.

Coding Tips

- If documentation states that a fine-gauge (22- or 25-gauge) needle attached to a syringe to obtain fluid or a cluster of cells was used, see 10004–10021 (fine-needle aspiration).

- It is appropriate to report radiological supervision and interpretation when performed, see 76942, 77002, 77012, and 77021.

 AUDITOR'S ALERT

It should be noted that HCPCS Level II code D7980 is usually required by dental payers when reporting a sialolithotomy.

 DEFINITIONS

cricoid. Circular cartilage around the trachea.

myotomy. Surgical cutting of a muscle to gain access to underlying tissues or for therapeutic reasons.

sialography. Radiographic examination of the ductal system of a salivary gland by instilling radiographic dye into a major duct and taking x-ray pictures.

sialolithotomy. Incision in the submandibular, sublingual, or parotid ducts to remove a calculus or stone from within a salivary duct. If the stone is large, a portion of the surrounding tissue may also be removed.

Procedures Performed on the Pharynx, Adenoids, and Tonsils (42700–42999)

Tonsillectomy and Adenoidectomy (42820–42836)

These codes describe the removal of the tonsils, with or without removal of the adenoids, and removal of the adenoids alone.

Procedure Differentiation

The physician uses an intraoral approach to access the tonsils and adenoids. The physician removes the tonsils by grasping the tonsil with a tonsil clamp. The capsule of the tonsil is dissected. The tonsil is removed. Bleeding vessels are clamped and tied. Bleeding may also be controlled using silver nitrate and gauze packing.

To remove the adenoids, the physician uses a mirror or nasopharyngoscope for visualization and employs an adenotome or a curette and basket punch to excise the adenoids. Alternate surgical techniques for a tonsillectomy and adenoidectomy include electrocautery, laser surgery, and cryogenic surgery.

Coding Tip

- The appropriate code is selected according to the patient's age.

Coding Trap

- These codes represent bilateral procedures. Do not append modifier 50 to these codes.

Procedures Performed on the Esophagus (43020–43499)

Surgical Incision of the Esophagus (43020–43045)

Procedure Differentiation

The incision codes in this subsection are for the esophagus (esophagotomy) by way of a cervical approach (43020) and thoracic approach (43045). Removal of a foreign body is also included in these services. In addition, code 43030 is used to report a cricopharyngeal myotomy, or incision into the pharynx through the muscle and cricoid.

Resection of the Esophagus (43100–43135)

 AUDITOR'S ALERT

CPT codes 39000 and 39010 should not be reported separately for exploration of the mediastinum when performed with an esophageal procedure.

Procedure Differentiation

This section begins with lesions of the esophagus, including primary repair with cervical approach (43100) and thoracic or abdominal approach (43101). Esophagectomy, removal of the esophagus, is reported with 43107–43124. Codes describe partial (43116–43123) and total or near total (43107–43113) excision. Codes are further defined by approach and the extent of the repair.

In 43124, the esophagus is removed with no attempt to reconstruct the esophagus. The physician first creates a permanent tracheoplasty. The affected portion of the esophagus is resected and sutured to the cervical incision, creating a connection from the exterior of the neck to the esophageal lumen to provide drainage of saliva and mucus. This usually is performed for malignancy.

Diverticulectomy or excision of diverticula (pouch or sac in the wall of the esophagus) is reported with 43130 for a cervical approach and 43135 for a thoracic approach.

© 2020 Optum360, LLC

Coding Tip

- When a biopsy is performed on a lesion at the time that a more extensive procedure is performed on a different lesion, the biopsy may be reported separately with modifier 59 or XS appended.

- For laparoscopic esophagectomies, see 43286-43288.

Coding Trap

- When a biopsy is performed on a lesion that a more extensive procedure is also performed on, the biopsy is reported separately only when used for immediate pathologic diagnosis and the decision to perform the more extensive procedure is based on the diagnosis established by the biopsy.

Endoscopic Procedures on the Esophagus and Stomach (43180–43278)

Procedure Differentiation

An esophagoscopy is the direct visualization of the esophagus with a rigid or flexible fiberoptic endoscope. In these procedures, the physician uses an esophagoscope to view the esophagus. For 43180–43196 the physician introduces a rigid esophagoscope through the patient's mouth or nose and into the esophagus under general anesthesia. The physician views the esophagus (from the cricopharyngeus muscle to the gastroesophageal junction, which is also included) with or without taking a specimen collection of cells by brushing or washing the esophageal lining with saline, followed by aspiration. Within this section, codes are further divided by the procedures performed (e.g., diverticulectomy, biopsy, injection, removal of foreign body, and removal of tumor). Esophagoscopies can also be performed with a flexible fiberoptic endoscope (43200–43232) or with a flexible scope inserted through the nose (transnasal) and is reported with codes 43197–43198.

When documentation indicates that in addition to the esophagus, the stomach, duodenum, and/or jejunum are visualized, an esophagoduodenoscopy (EGD) is performed and codes 43210 and 43235–43259 are reported. It may be necessary to append modifier 52 or 53 to an EGD that cannot be completed due to patients that have surgically altered anatomy that prevents the provider from performing a safe examination of the duodenum. Per the CPT book, modifier 52 should be used when a repeat EGD is not planned and modifier 53 should be used when a repeat EGD is planned in the future. Verify payer policies in these circumstances.

 AUDITOR'S ALERT

See Appendix 1 for the audit worksheet for upper endoscopy.

Esophagoscopy/EGD Crosswalk

Procedure	Esophagus Only	EGD
Band ligation varices	43205	43244
Biopsy	43193, 43198, 43202	43239
Brushing and washings	43191, 43197, 43200	43235
Control of bleeding	43227	43255
Dilation		
any method		43245
balloon greater than 30 mm	43214	43233
balloon less than 30 mm	43195, 43220	43249
balloon or dilator, retrograde	43213	
over guidewire	43196, 43226	43248
Diverticulectomy	43180	
Drainage of pseudocyst		43240
Foreign body removal	43194, 43215	43247
Fundoplasty, esophagogastric, partial or complete		43210
Injection		
submucosal	43192, 43201	43236
varices	43204	43243
Insertion		
intraluminal tube or catheter		43241
percutaneous gastrostomy tube		43246
tube or stent	43212	43266
Lesion removal or destruction		
ablation	43229	43270
hot biopsy or bipolar	43216	43250
snare	43217	43251
Mucosal resection	43211	43254
Optical endomicroscopy	43206	43252
Thermal energy for gastroesophageal reflux		43257
Ultrasound examination		
esophagus only	43231	
esophagus, stomach or duodenum, and adjacent structures		43237
esophagus, stomach and either duodenum or jejunum distal to anastomosis of surgical altered stomach		43259
intramural or transmural fine needle aspiration/biopsy	43232	43238, 43242
transmural injection of diagnostic or therapeutic substance		43253

DEFINITIONS

fine needle aspiration biopsy.
Insertion of a fine-gauge needle attached to a syringe into a tissue mass for the suctioned withdrawal of cells used for diagnostic study.

AUDITOR'S ALERT

When 43206 or 43252 (optimal endomicroscopy) is performed, the interpretation and report are an integral component of the procedure and are not reported separately.

Endoscopic retrograde cholangiopancreatography (ERCP) (43260–43278) is the examination of the gastrointestinal tract, including the biliary tree and gallbladder, with an endoscope and fluoroscopy for diagnostic or therapeutic reasons. Documentation must indicate that the physician passed the endoscope through the patient's oropharynx, esophagus, and stomach. The scope is then advanced into the small bowel. The ampulla of Vater is cannulated and filled with contrast. Documentation may indicate that the physician was unable to insert the catheter through the ampulla of Vater. In these instances, report 43260 with the reduced service modifier 52. An ERCP is considered complete if one or more ductal systems (pancreatic or biliary) are visualized. The biliary ductal system includes the common bile duct, right/left hepatic duct, and the cystic duct/gallbladder. The pancreatic ductal system includes the minor and major ducts.

The procedures that may be performed using an ERCP are very similar to those performed with an esophagoscopy or EGD and include biopsy (43261), ablation of tumors (43278), destruction of calculi (43265), and removal of calculi/debris (43264).

Code 43262 describes an ERCP with sphincterotomy/papillotomy. Code 43263 is reported if documentation states a pressure measurement of sphincter of Oddi was performed. Stent procedures are reported with 43274–43276.

In 43277, the physician performs an ERCP. The common bile duct and the whole biliary tract, including the gallbladder, are visualized. A stricture or obstruction is visualized. A sphincterotomy may be performed to reach the area to be treated with the balloon dilator. Once the balloon is in place, it is expanded multiple times until the desired outcome is achieved. The endoscope and all surgical instruments are removed. This code should be reported for each biliary duct and ampulla dilated with modifier 59 appended to each additional site.

In the event that an ERCP is performed and the physician also performs an endoscopic cannulation of the papilla of the pancreatic and/or common bile duct(s), add-on code 43273 is reported. Documentation will state that a catheter or papillotome is inserted through the channel of the ERCP scope. With or without the use of a guidewire, the pancreatic and/or common bile duct are located and visually inspected.

Medical Necessity

The following conditions may warrant upper endoscopy procedures:

- Barrett's esophagus
- Chronic diarrhea
- Dysphagia or odynophagia
- Esophageal, gastric, or stomal ulcers
- Esophageal or proximal gastric varices
- Esophageal reflux
- Foreign body removal
- Gastric polyps
- Gastrointestinal bleeding
- Persistent vomiting
- Strictures of the esophagus
- Suspected neoplastic lesion

Generally, ERCP procedures are performed for:

- Biliary calculus
- Biliary fistula
- Cholangitis

DEFINITIONS

calculus. Abnormal, stone-like concretion of calcium, cholesterol, mineral salts, or other substances that forms in any part of the body.

cautery. Destruction or burning of tissue by means of a hot instrument, an electric current, or a caustic chemical, such as silver nitrate.

duodenum. First portion of the small intestine connected to the stomach at the pylorus and extending to the jejunum.

hot biopsy. Using forceps technique, the physician simultaneously excises and fulgurates polyps; avoids the bleeding associated with cold-forceps biopsy; and preserves the specimen for histologic examination (in contrast, a simple fulguration of the polyp destroys it).

jejunum. Highly vascular upper two-fifths of the small intestine, extending from the duodenum to the ileum.

snare. Wire used as a loop to excise a polyp or lesion.

- Malignancies of the biliary tract
- Pancreatitis
- Spasm of sphincter of Oddi

Key Documentation Terms

Within this area of procedures it is important to make sure that the documentation clearly identifies what was examined and the procedure(s) performed. Codes within this section are further classified by the procedures performed (e.g., biopsy, injection, removal of foreign body, and removal of tumor).

When reporting procedures within this family of codes, each procedure must be clearly documented. For instance, when performing code 43250 Esophagogastroduodenoscopy, flexible, transoral; with removal of tumor(s), polyp(s), or other lesion(s) by hot biopsy forceps, at the minimum the documentation should include what was removed and the key term "hot biopsy forceps." Code 43251 Esophagogastroduodenoscopy, flexible, transoral; with removal of tumor(s), polyp(s), or other lesion(s) by snare technique, should include what was removed and the key terms "removal of " and "snare technique" in the documentation for the procedure.

Coding Tips

- As an add-on code, 43273 is not subject to multiple procedure rules. No reimbursement reduction or modifier 51 is applied. Add-on codes describe additional intraservice work associated with the primary procedure. They are performed by the same provider on the same date of service as the primary service/procedure, and must never be reported as a stand-alone code. The following table provides additional information for these codes as found in the Medicare Physician Fee Schedule Database

Parent Code	Add-On	GLOB DAYS	MULT PROC	BILAT SURG	ASST SURG	CO-SURG	TEAM SURG
43260		000	2	0	1	0	0
43261		000	3	0	1	0	0
43262		000	3	0	1	0	0
43263		000	3	0	1	0	0
43264		000	3	0	1	0	0
43265		000	3	0	1	0	0
	43273	ZZZ	0	0	0	0	0
43274		000	3	0	1	0	0
43275		000	3	0	1	0	0
43276		000	3	0	1	0	0
43277		000	3	0	1	0	0
43278		000	3	0	1	0	0

- A diagnostic endoscopy includes the collection of specimens. A diagnostic esophagoscopy is designated as a separate procedure.

- A diagnostic endoscopy is not reported separately.

- If the larynx is viewed through an esophagoscope during esophagoscopy, a laryngoscopy CPT code cannot be reported separately. However, if the laryngoscopy is performed with a separate laryngoscope, the laryngoscopy and esophagoscopy codes may be reported with Correct Coding Initiative (CCI) associated modifiers.

- Control of bleeding that is the result of a surgical procedure is not reported separately. In the case of endoscopy, if it is necessary to repeat the endoscopy at a later time during the same day to control bleeding, a procedure code for endoscopic control of bleeding may be reported with modifier 78, indicating that this service represents a return to the endoscopy suite or operating room for a related procedure during the postoperative period. In the case of open surgical services, the appropriate complication codes may be reported if a return to the operating room is necessary, but the complication code should not be reported if the complication described by the CPT code occurred during the same operative session.

- When biopsy of a lesion is performed followed by excision or destruction of the same lesion, the biopsy is not reported separately.

- When endoscopic esophageal dilation is performed, the appropriate endoscopic esophageal dilation code is reported. Codes 43450 and 43453 (dilation of esophagus) are not used in addition (even if attempted unsuccessfully prior to endoscopic dilation); in such a case, modifier 22 could be used to indicate an unusual endoscopic dilation procedure.

- When two distinct endoscopic procedures are performed, such as an esophagogastroduodenoscopy (EGD) and a colonoscopy, both procedures should be reported with modifier 51 appended to the lesser of the two.

- Appropriate ERCP code assignment is based upon associated procedures performed, such as biopsy, sphincterotomy/papillotomy, removal of stones, insertion of stent, removal of a foreign body, dilation of ducts, and ablation of tumors.

- For a rigid esophagoscopy performed for injection of varices, report 43499.

Coding Traps

- Esophageal washings for cytology are described as part of an esophagoscopy and, therefore, should not be reported separately.

- If the same surgical endoscopy service is performed repeatedly (e.g., multiple polyps are removed through the scope), the service is reported only once.

- For codes that state "when performed" in the code description, such as code 43266 Esophagogastroduodenoscopy, flexible, transoral; with placement of endoscopic stent (includes pre- and post-dilation and guide wire passage, *when performed*), it is inappropriate to append modifier 52 to the procedure when all of the listed procedures are not performed.

- Services such as venous access (36000), infusions and injections (e.g., codes 96360–96379), noninvasive oximetry (94760 and 94761), and anesthesia provided by the surgeon are considered an integral part of the esophagoscopy and should not be reported individually.

- Only the more extensive endoscopic procedure is reported for a session. For example, if an esophagoscopy is completed and the physician performs an esophagogastroduodenoscopy (EGD) during the same session, only the EGD is reported.

DEFINITIONS

ablation. Removal or destruction of a body part or tissue or its function. Ablation may be performed by surgical means, hormones, drugs, radiofrequency, heat, chemical application, or other methods.

dilation. Artificial increase in the diameter of an opening or lumen made by medication or by instrumentation.

sphincterotomy. Incision into the ring-like band of muscle that surrounds a bodily opening, constricting and relaxing as required for normal physiological functioning.

Billing and Payment Issues

Endoscopies are paid for under the Medicare fee schedule's global surgery policy. When multiple surgical endoscopies are performed, the base endoscopy is paid only once.

It is acceptable to bill for multiple services provided during an endoscopic procedure (with the exception of treating bleeding induced by the procedure) when performed during the same operative session. For example, if an esophagoscopy with biopsy is performed, and the physician injects esophageal varices, then 43202 and 43204 may be reported. These services are reimbursed under the payer's multiple endoscopic payment rules.

Diagnostic endoscopy procedures can be reported with open or incisional procedures.

Regulatory Issues: Indications

The medical necessity of these procedures can only be allowed if abnormal signs or symptoms or known disease are present. The following conditions are generally accepted as indication(s) for the performance of an EGD(s).

- Upper abdominal distress that persists despite therapeutic interventions
- Upper abdominal distress associated with signs and symptoms including abdominal pain or weight loss, which suggests serious organic disease
- Dysphagia or odynophagia
- Esophageal reflux symptoms that are persistent or recurrent despite therapeutic interventions
- Persistent vomiting of unknown cause
- Other systemic diseases in which the presence of upper GI pathology might modify other planned management. Examples include patients with a history of GI bleeding who are scheduled for organ transplantation, long-term anticoagulation, and chronic nonsteroidal therapy for arthritis
- Radiologic findings of:
  - a suspected neoplastic lesion
  - gastric or esophageal ulcer
  - evidence of upper gastrointestinal tract stricture or obstruction
- When there is evidence of gastrointestinal bleeding, EGDs are generally considered medically necessary when:
  - the bleed is active
  - surgical therapy is being considered
  - re-bleeding occurs after acute self-limited blood loss
  - portal hypertension or aortoenteric fistula is suspected
  - a colonoscopy is negative; however, the patient is being treated for chronic blood loss and for iron deficiency anemia of other unknown origin
- When sampling of duodenal or jejunal tissue or fluid is indicated
- To assess acute injury
- Intraoperative EGD when necessary to clarify location or pathology of a lesion

© 2020 Optum360, LLC

Indications that support EGDs for therapeutic purposes include:

- Treatment of bleeding from lesions such as ulcers, tumors, or vascular malformations (e.g., electrocoagulation, heater probe, laser photocoagulation, or injection therapy)

- Sclerotherapy of esophageal or proximal gastric varices and/or banding of varices

- Foreign body removal

- Removal of selected polypoid lesions

- Placement of feeding (oral, percutaneous endoscopic gastrostomy, percutaneous endoscopic jejunostomy)

- Dilation of stenotic lesions (e.g., with transendoscopic balloon dilators or dilating systems employing guidewires)

- Palliative therapy of stenosing neoplasms (e.g., laser, bipolar electrocoagulation, stent placement)

Sequential or periodic diagnostic EGD may be indicated for:

- Follow-up of selected esophageal, gastric, or stomal ulcers to demonstrate healing (frequency of follow-up EGD is variable, but every two to four months until healing is demonstrated is reasonable)

- Follow-up in patients with prior adenomatous gastric polyps (approximate frequency of follow-up EGDs would be every one to four years depending on the clinical circumstance, with occasional patients with sessile polyps requiring every six-month surveillance initially)

- Follow-up for adequacy of prior sclerotherapy and/or band ligation of esophageal varices (approximate frequency of follow-up EGDs is variable depending on the state of the patient, but every six to 24 months is reasonable after the initial sclerotherapy and/or band ligation sessions are completed)

- For follow-up of Barrett's esophagus (approximate frequency of follow-up EGDs is one to two years with biopsies, unless dysplasia or atypia is demonstrated, in which case a repeat biopsy in two to three months might be indicated)

- Follow-up in patients with familial adenomatous polyposis (approximate frequency of follow-up EGDs would be every two to four years, but might be more frequent, such as every six to 12 months, if gastric adenomas or adenomas of the duodenum were demonstrated)

The endoscopic retrograde cholangiopancreatography (ERCP) procedure is generally indicated for certain biliary and pancreatic conditions.

Indications for ERCP procedures include (this list is not all-inclusive):

- It is generally not indicated for the diagnosis of pancreatitis except for gallstone pancreatitis.

- It is not usually indicated in early stages or in acute pancreatitis and could possibly exacerbate the pancreatitis.

- ERCP may be useful in traumatic pancreatitis to accurately localize the injury and provide endoscopic drainage.

- ERCP may be useful in pancreatic duct stricture evaluation.

- ERCP may be useful for the extraction of bile duct stones in severe gallstone induced pancreatitis.

 DEFINITIONS

Barrett's esophagus. Complication of gastroesophageal reflux disease causing peptic ulcer and stricture in the lower part of the esophagus due to columnar epithelial cells from the lining of the stomach and intestine replacing the natural esophageal lining made of normal squamous cell epithelium. Barrett's esophagus is linked to an elevated risk of esophageal cancer, and is sometimes followed by esophageal adenocarcinoma.

varices. Enlarged, dilated, or twisted, turning veins.

- ERCP may be useful in detecting pancreatic ductal changes in chronic pancreatitis and also the presence of calcified stones in the ductal system. A pancreatogram may be performed and is likely to be abnormal in chronic alcoholic pancreatitis but less so in nonalcoholic induced types.

- ERCP may be useful in detecting gallstones in symptomatic patients whose oral cholecystogram and gallbladder ultrasonograms are normal.

- ERCP may be indicated in patients with radiologic imaging suggestive of common bile duct stones or other potential pathology.

Laparoscopic Esophagectomy (43286–43288)

These procedures to be performed using laparoscopic and thorascopic techniques to remove either a significant portion or the entire esophagus. These procedures are commonly performed for conditions such as esophageal cancer and/or Barrett's esophagus. In Barrett's esophagus, a complication resulting from chronic gastroesophageal reflux (GERD), the normal tissue lining the esophagus transforms into the tissue lining the intestine, which can develop into esophageal precancer or cancer. Laparoscopic esophagectomy is also used to treat patients who have damaged their esophagus by ingesting a caustic or burning substance or for patients with achalasia.

Procedure Differentiation

In 43286, a total or near total transhiatal esophagectomy involving two incisions is performed. The physician removes the entire or near total esophagus through the abdomen then reattaches the stomach to the remaining esophagus (anastomosis) through a left neck incision. Of the three procedures being described, the transhiatal esophagectomy is considered the least invasive.

In 43287, an esophagectomy, also referred to as the Ivor Lewis esophagectomy, is performed. The physician removes the distal two-thirds including the tumor via an incision in the abdomen and performs an anastomosis through a right thoracotomy. In 43288, all or almost all of the esophagus is removed via a three-incision procedure. This is also referred to as a McKeown esophagectomy. The physician removes the tumor via incisions made in the abdomen, chest, and neck and performs anastomosis through the neck incision. Pyloric drainage is included in all three techniques, when performed.

Key Documentation Terms

To assign the most appropriate code, the medical record documentation must be reviewed to determine the extent of the procedure (e.g., total, near total). Terms such as distal two-thirds, open cervical pharyngogastrostomy, thorascopic mobilization, and tri-incisional provide the guidance needed to ensure correct code assignment.

Coding Tips

- Do not report a right tube thoracostomy (32551) in addition to 43287 and 43288. However, when the documentation indicates that a left tube thoracostomy was performed, code 32551 may be reported separately. Modifier 59 or XS may be required by payers.

Open Esophageal Repair Procedures (43300–43425)

Repair codes include esophagoplasty procedures for fistula using a cervical approach (43300–43305), a thoracic approach (43310–43312), and due to congenital defects (43313-43314).

Procedure Differentiation

Codes 43300–43305 indicate that the physician made an incision in the neck while 43310–43312 state that the incision was made further down in the upper chest. Codes 43313-43314 are reported for repairs required due to congenital defects.

Fundoplasty is a repair of the esophagus by wrapping with the fundus, or lowest part of the stomach. Report 43327 when the physician performs a partial or complete fundoplasty through an abdominal incision or 43328 when the incision is through the chest cavity.

Paraesophageal Hernias

For repair of paraesophageal hernias, see 43332–43337. A paraesophageal hernia occurs when a portion of the stomach passes through the hiatus and rests in the chest next to the esophagus. Correct code selection is dependent upon the approach used to correct the repair. Once the incision is made, the physician pulls the stomach back down and into the correct position and sutures it to the rectus sheath. The diaphragm is often sutured and the hiatus is sutured along the gastroesophageal junction. Fundoplication is performed to prevent the stomach from moving out of position again. The table below can be used to select the appropriate code based upon approach and the use of mesh.

Paraesophageal Hernias

	Incision site	Without Mesh	With Mesh
Via laparotomy	Abdomen	43332	43333
Via thoracotomy	Chest wall	43334	43335
Via thoracoabdominal incision	Chest wall and abdomen	43336	43337

Medical Necessity

Esophagoplasties are most frequently performed for strictures, foreign bodies, and esophageal injuries. Codes within range 43332–43337 are considered medically necessary when performed for treatment of paraesophageal hernias.

Key Documentation Terms

A paraesophageal hernia may also be documented as a hiatal hernia. Paraesophageal hernias can be further classified as:

- **Type I:** This is the most common type of paraesophageal hernias. In this type of hernia, the gastroesophageal junction herniates into the chest cavity. It may also be documented as a sliding hiatal hernia.

- **Type II:** The stomach herniates through the diaphragmatic esophageal hiatus alongside the esophagus. The gastroesophageal junction remains below the hiatus and the stomach rotates in front of the esophagus and herniates into the chest. When more than 30 percent of the stomach herniates into the chest, this condition may be referred to as a giant paraesophageal hernia.

 DEFINITIONS

hiatal hernia. Protrusion of an abdominal organ, usually the stomach, through the esophageal opening within the diaphragm and occurring in two types: the sliding hiatal hernia and the paraesophageal hernia.

laparotomy. Incision through the flank or abdomen for therapeutic or diagnostic purposes.

thoracotomy. Surgical procedure for opening the chest wall in order to access the lungs, esophagus, trachea, aorta, heart, and diaphragm.

- **Type III:** This hiatal hernia is a combined hernia in that the gastroesophageal junction is herniated above the diaphragm and the stomach is herniated alongside the esophagus.

- **Type IV:** In this type of hernia, organs other than the stomach including the colon, small intestine, or spleen herniate into the chest.

Documentation must indicate that an incision is made into the chest or abdomen. When documentation indicates that multiple small incisions were made, the procedure is more than likely performed laparoscopically and would not be reported using one of the open procedure codes.

Coding Tips
- Hiatal hernias are more frequently repaired using a laparoscopic approach.

- For other types of hernias, see 49491–49659.

- Paraesophageal hiatal hernia repairs performed on neonates should be reported with code 39503, for diaphragmatic hernia repair.

Coding Traps
- Do not use modifier 22 when reporting the implantation of mesh or other prosthetic materials at the time of a paraesophageal hernia repair. Instead, report the codes that include the placement of the mesh (43333, 43335, 43337).

- An exploratory laparotomy is not separately reportable with an open abdominal procedure.

Esophageal Dilation (43450–43453)
Esophageal dilation is performed for treatment of esophageal strictures and stenosis. The procedure may be accomplished by a number of methods (balloon, bougie dilator, or sound dilator) and without visualization (by guidewire), under direct supervision (endoscopically), or under radiologic guidance.

Review documentation to determine:

- Type of dilator used:
  - bougie
  - sound
  - over guide wire
- Method of visualization if any:
  - none
  - fluoroscopy
  - endoscopy
  - esophagoscopy
  - esophagogastroduodenoscopy (EGD)

The codes in this range are not to be used when the dilation is performed under direct visualization, see 43180–43278.

The following table may be used to determine if an esophageal dilation has been coded correctly.

AUDITOR'S ALERT

When a paraesophageal hernia repair is performed on a neonate, see 39503.

DEFINITIONS

bougie. Probe used to dilate or calibrate a body part.

Esophageal Dilation Endoscopic vs. Nonendoscopic

Type of Dilator	Endoscopic	Nonendoscopic
Balloon, greater than 30 mm in diameter	43214 (esophagoscopy) 43233 (esophagogastroduodenoscopy)	
Balloon, less than 30 mm in diameter	43195, 43220 (esophagoscopy) 43249 (esophagogastroduodenoscopy)	
Dilators, retrograde	43213 (esophagoscopy)	
Insertion of guidewire followed by dilation over guidewire	43196, 43226 (esophagoscopy) 43248 (esophagogastroduodenoscopy)	43453
Unguided bougie, or sound single or multiple passes		43450

Key Documentation Terms:

The medical record documentation must be carefully reviewed to determine the type of dilator the physician used, as well as whether the dilation was performed with direct visualization. Also determine if other procedures were performed during the same operative session as these may be separately reportable.

Coding Tips

- When the dilatation is performed endoscopically, see the appropriate endoscopy code.

- Codes from this range are not used in addition to endoscopic codes, even if attempted unsuccessfully prior to endoscopic dilation; in such a case, modifier 22 could be used to indicate an unusual endoscopic dilation procedure.

- To report dilation of the esophagus by unguided sound or bougie, see 43450

- When appropriate, an esophagogram may be reported separately with code 74220.

- When performing esophageal dilation procedures, radiological supervision and interpretation may be reported separately with code 74360.

Coding Traps

- Code 43450 is reported once per session even when the sound or bougie size is increased due to the fact that the description includes multiple passes.

- When the bougie is passed over a guidewire that is placed via an endoscope during the same surgical session, code 43196, 43226, or 43248 is reported. No additional codes are reported.

- When the balloon is inserted via the endoscope, report 43195, 43214, 43220, 43233, or 43249.

Procedures Performed on the Stomach (43500–43999)

Gastrotomy (43500–43510)

A gastrotomy is the surgical opening of the stomach. Documentation must indicate that the physician made a midline epigastric incision and retracted the skin and underlying tissues laterally and that the stomach was incised and explored.

Procedure Differentiation

In 43500, a foreign body is removed. In 43501, a bleeding ulcer is identified and bleeding is controlled with electrocautery or ligation of vessels, and the mucosa is drawn over the ulcer and sutured. In 43502, an esophagogastric laceration is identified and bleeding is controlled with electrocautery or ligation of vessels, and the mucosa is drawn over the defect and sutured. In 43510, the physician introduces dilators into the esophagus from the stomach to increase the diameter of the esophagus. When dilation is complete, a stent is placed and secured with sutures to maintain patency. After exploration or repair, the stomach is closed in sutured layers, the soft tissues are returned to anatomical position, and the operative incision is closed in sutured layers.

Medical Necessity

The medical necessity of the procedure is dependent upon why the procedure was performed.

Key Documentation Terms

In order to assign the most appropriate code, the medical record documentation must be reviewed to determine why the procedure was performed (e.g., for removal of a foreign body, repair of a bleeding ulcer, suture of a preexisting esophagogastric laceration, or dilation and insertion of a stent into the lower esophagus).

Pyloromyotomy (43520)

When a pyloromyotomy is performed, the pyloric muscle is incised. The physician makes a small subcostal incision over the pyloric olive. The peritoneum is incised, the tissues are retracted, and the pylorus is identified. The serosa is incised, and the tension of the pyloric muscle is released with longitudinal incisions. The peritoneum is sutured closed, and the operative site is closed in sutured layers. This procedure is sometimes referred to as the Fredet-Ramstedt operation.

Medical Necessity

The procedure is performed for malignant neoplasms, pylorospasm, angiodysplasia, and congenital hypertrophic pyloric stenosis.

Coding Tip

- For an incision into the esophagus for removal of a foreign body, see 43020 for a cervical approach or 43045 for a thoracic approach.

Coding Traps

- Vagotomy and pyloroplasty are included in 43502 and should not be reported separately.

- Modifier 63 should not be reported with 43520.

DEFINITIONS

Mallory-Weiss syndrome. Tear in the esophagus following several hours or days of vomiting, marked by vomiting of blood.

stent. Tube to provide support in a body cavity or lumen.

Gastrectomy (43620–43634)

Procedure Differentiation
A gastrectomy is the partial or total removal of the stomach. When selecting a code for gastrectomy procedures, the following must be determined:

- Was only a portion of the stomach removed or the entire stomach?
- What type of reconstruction was performed?
- Was a vagotomy also performed?
- Was a pyloroplasty performed?

Total Gastrectomy (43620–43622)
When a total gastrectomy is performed, documentation must indicate that the entire stomach was removed and that a limb of small bowel was approximated to the esophagus by performing an esophagoenterostomy (43620), a Roux-en-Y reconstruction (43621), or that an intestinal pouch was created (43622). In 43620, the operative report should indicate that the remaining duodenal end of the intestine was mobilized up to the end of the esophagus and connected. In 43621, documentation must indicate that the upper jejunum was divided and that the distal portion (or the limb in continuity with the ileum) is anastomosed to the esophagus. The operative report should also indicate that the proximal end of the divided jejunum (the segment containing the duodenum) is connected back into the limb of small bowel farther down from the esophageal anastomosis.

In 43622, documentation must indicate that the proximal jejunum was divided and the distal end of bowel was folded upon itself and approximated in such a way as to form a pouch. The pouch is connected to the esophagus. The divided proximal jejunum is connected to the limb of small bowel distal to the esophageal anastomosis to restore intestinal continuity.

Partial Gastrectomy (43631–43634)
A partial gastrectomy is the removal of a portion of the stomach. In 43631, documentation must indicate that the distal portion of the stomach (antrum) was removed and the proximal portion was approximated to duodenum. In 43632, an anastomosis is made between the proximal stomach and the jejunum with staples or sutures. If documentation indicates that a Roux-en-Y anastomosis is performed, report 43633. Documentation supporting this code assignment must indicate that the proximal jejunum was divided and the distal limb connected to the proximal stomach while the proximal jejunum was connected to the limb of jejunum distal to the gastrojejunostomy to restore intestinal continuity. The physician may also elect to create an intestinal pouch (43634). If this is performed, documentation must indicate that the antrum was removed, the proximal jejunum was divided, and the distal end folded upon itself and approximated in such a way as to form a pouch. The pouch is then connected to the proximal stomach and the proximal end of the divided jejunum is connected to the jejunal limb distal to the pouch anastomosis re-establishing intestinal continuity.

If the documentation indicates that the physician severed both right and left vagus nerves just below the diaphragm, then a vagotomy was performed. In these instances, it is appropriate to report add-on code 43635 in addition to 43631–43634.

 DEFINITIONS

antrum. Chamber or cavity, typically with a small opening.

roux-en-Y anastomosis. Y-shaped attachment of the distal end of a divided small intestine segment to the stomach, esophagus, biliary tract, or other structure with anastomosis of the proximal end to the side of the small intestine further down for reflux-free drainage.

vagotomy. Division of the vagus nerves, interrupting impulses resulting in lower gastric acid production and hastening gastric emptying.

Medical Necessity

The following conditions may warrant a gastrectomy (this list is not all inclusive):

- Bleeding
- Gastric ulcers
- Inflammation
- Malignant lesions
- Nonmalignant lesions
- Polyps

Key Documentation Terms

To assign the most appropriate code, the medical record documentation must be reviewed to determine the extent of the procedure (e.g., partial, total). Terms such as Roux-en-Y, intestinal pouch, gastrojejunostomy, and vagotomy provide the guidance needed to ensure correct code assignment.

Coding Tips

- When documentation indicates that the stomach was incised (gastrostomy) and a suture repair of a bleeding ulcer was performed, see 43501.
- For a vagotomy performed with a partial, distal gastrectomy, report 43635 in addition to the gastrectomy code.
- As an "add-on" code, 43635 is not subject to multiple procedure rules. No reimbursement reduction or modifier 51 is applied. The following table provides additional information for these codes as found in the Medicare Physician Fee Schedule Database.

Parent Code	Add-On	GLOB DAYS	MULT PROC	BILAT SURG	ASST SURG	CO-SURG	TEAM SURG
43631		090	2	0	2	1	0
43632		090	2	0	2	1	0
43633		090	2	0	2	1	0
43634		090	2	0	2	1	0
	43635	ZZZ	0	0	2	1	0

Coding Traps

- An excisional biopsy is not reported separately when a therapeutic excision is performed during the same surgical session.
- Laparotomy, celiotomy (49000) is included in these procedures and should not be reported separately.

Laparoscopic Gastric Bypass, Neurostimulators, and Other Gastric Procedures (43644–43659)

Many digestive system procedures can be performed by open or laparoscopic approach. The CPT book classifies procedures done laparoscopically in a different heading within each section.

Procedure Differentiation

Laparoscopy procedures in this section are divided into four major types:

Gastric restrictive procedures: In 43644, a laparoscopic gastric bypass is performed for morbid obesity by partitioning the stomach and performing a small bowel division with anastomosis to the proximal stomach (Roux-en-Y gastroenterostomy). This bypasses the majority of the stomach. A short limb of the proximal small bowel (150 cm or less) is divided and the distal end of the short intestinal limb is brought up and anastomosed to the proximal gastric pouch. The other end of the divided bowel is then connected back into the small bowel distal to the short limb's gastric anastomosis to restore intestinal continuity.

In 43645, a laparoscopic gastric bypass is performed with small intestine reconstruction to limit absorption. This procedure is done to combine gastric restriction of intake with limited intestinal absorption. In one method used, the physician places a trocar though an incision above the umbilicus and insufflates the abdominal cavity. The laparoscope and additional trocars are placed through small portal incisions. The stomach is mobilized and the distal half is resected along a line from the lesser to greater curvature, leaving a "pouch" of stomach, which is connected directly to the final, distal section of small intestine. The bypassed duodenum, jejunum, and upper part of the divided ileum—the segment in connection with the gallbladder and pancreas, or the biliopancreatic loop—is anastomosed back to the common distal segment of the small intestine. This leaves a short common channel where food coming through the shortened alimentary tract combines with digestive juices from the much longer biliary tract before entering the colon.

Implantation or replacement of gastric neurostimulator electrodes in the antrum: Gastric neurostimulators, also known as a gastric pacemaker, are used to provide stimulation to the nerves in the lower stomach, which encourages the stomach to contract and helps relieve nausea and vomiting. Using the laparoscopic techniques, the antrum of the stomach is identified and the physician secures two electrodes into the muscle of the pyloric antrum. The electrodes are connected to a neurostimulator that has been secured in a subcutaneous pocket in the abdomen in a separately reportable procedure. Code 43647 is reported if electrodes are placed or if existing electrodes are removed and replaced with new ones. Report 43648 for the revision or removal of the electrodes.

Transection of vagus nerves: The vagus nerve, or 10th cranial nerve, splits into branches that go to different areas of the stomach. These branches stimulate the production of acid. A vagotomy is performed to reduce acid secretion in the stomach. Code 43651 describes the physician removing a small segment of each nerve, also referred to as a truncal vagotomy. Using laparoscopic techniques, the fascia anterior to the esophagus is incised and the distal esophagus is mobilized. The anterior and posterior vagal nerve trunks are identified and divided. In 43652, a selective or highly selective vagotomy is performed. The main nerve trunks are followed down onto the stomach and the branches from the nerves to the proximal half of the stomach are divided.

Gastrostomy without construction of gastric tube: In 43653, a temporary or permanent gastrostomy is created for feeding using laparoscopic techniques. An additional trocar is inserted through the abdominal wall into the intraabdominal cavity and a gastrostomy tube is pulled through the trocar from outside the abdomen into the intraabdominal cavity. The physician identifies the stomach and introduces instruments to open the organ and create a viable receptacle for the tube. The tip of the gastrostomy tube is inserted into the stomach, and the tube is clamped off on the outside of the body and sutured into place on the stomach. Additional sutures are placed in the abdominal wall to hold the gastrostomy tube in place and to secure the tube.

Coding Tips

- A diagnostic laparoscopy is not reported separately.

- If an unsuccessful laparoscopic procedure is converted to an open procedure, report only the open procedure.

- When a laparoscopic procedure is performed for bariatric surgery, see 43770–43775.

- If vagus nerve neurostimulators are inserted, revised, or removed laparoscopically, see 0312T-0317T.

- In the event that an esophagogastroduodenoscopy (EGD) is performed for a separately identifiable diagnosis, it may be reported with modifier 59.

- A gastric restrictive procedure with a roux limb greater than 150 cm is reported with 43645.

- Gastric neurostimulator procedures of lesser curvature, such as insertion, removal, or revision may be reported with unlisted procedure code 43659.

- For insertion of a gastric neurostimulator pulse generator, see 64590; revision or removal, see 64595. Gastric neurostimulator may require electronic analysis and programming; these services may be reported with 95980–95982.

- Code 43653 is a separate procedure by definition and is usually a component of a more complex service and is not identified separately. When performed alone or with other unrelated procedures/services it may be reported. If performed alone, list the code; if performed with other procedures/services, list the code and append modifier 59 or appropriate X modifier.

Coding Trap

- Do not report a laparoscopic gastric restrictive procedure (43644) in conjunction with 43846 or 49320.

Nonsurgical Gastric Tube Procedures (43752–43763)

Procedure Differentiation

Gastric tubes provide nutrition to patients who may not be able to swallow or tolerate solid or liquid nutrients. Placement of a gastric feeding tube through the nose or the mouth by the physician is reported with 43752. Fluoroscopic guidance is included in this procedure and is not reported separately. If gastric intubation and aspiration are performed with lavage, see 43753. If these services are provided concurrently with critical care, they are not reported separately and are considered part of the greater service provided.

Diagnostic gastric intubation is reported with codes from range 43754–43757. Gastric intubation and aspiration with collection of specimen(s) is reported with codes from range 43754–43755, depending upon single or multiple specimens. Additionally, code 43755 includes drug administration, gastric stimulation, and gastric secretory study. Duodenal intubation and aspiration, both single (43756) and multiple specimen (43757), include image guidance. Code 43757 also includes drug administration, gallbladder or pancreas stimulation, and gastric secretory study. Changing of a percutaneous gastrostomy tube without imaging or endoscopic guidance and not including a revision of the gastrostomy tract is reported with 43762; with revision of the gastrostomy tract is reported with 43763. If fluoroscopic guidance is required, report 49450; if endoscopically placed, report 43246. If a naso- or orogastric feeding tube is repositioned through the duodenum for enteric nutrition, report 43761. If endoscopy is used to convert the gastrostomy tube to a jejunostomy tube, report 44373. Report 44500 if a long gastrointestinal tube is placed into the duodenum.

Laparoscopic Bariatric Procedures (43770–43775)

Procedure Differentiation

Included here are codes for laparoscopic gastric banding procedures that are performed to treat morbid obesity. This procedure is an alternative to the more invasive gastric bypass surgery. During this procedure, an adjustable silicone band is placed around the upper stomach just below the gastroesophageal junction and attached to an access port secured to the abdominal wall. Saline liquid is injected into the band expanding a balloon that compresses the stomach and results in appetite suppression.

In 43770, an adjustable gastric device is placed. Revision of the device is reported with 43771; removal of device only 43772; removal and replacement 43773; and removal of device and subcutaneous ports 43774.

In a laparoscopic sleeve gastrectomy, the documentation must state that the physician placed a trocar though an incision, generally above the umbilicus, and insufflated the abdominal cavity. The laparoscope and additional trocars are placed through small portal incisions. The physician divides the greater curvature of the stomach from the left crus of the diaphragm to a point distal to the pylorus. The short gastric vessels are coagulated and gastric staplers are used. A gastric tube (sleeve) is formed and the remaining 80 percent of the stomach is excised. The instruments are removed and the incisions are closed. This procedure is reported with 43775.

Medical Necessity

Certain criterion needs to be met before a payer will cover a bariatric procedure. The following are the conditions that need to be met in order for Medicare to cover the procedure. Other payer policies may vary.

 DEFINITIONS

morbid obesity. Accumulation of excess fat in the subcutaneous connective tissue with increased weight beyond the limits of skeletal requirements, defined as 125 percent or more over the ideal body weight. It is often associated with serious conditions that can become life threatening, such as diabetes, hypertension, and arteriosclerosis.

- The patient meets the definition of morbid obesity, which is defined as a body mass index (BMI) ≥ 35, and comorbid conditions exist (e.g., hypertensive cardiovascular disease, pulmonary/respiratory disease, diabetes, sleep apnea, or degenerative arthritis of weight-bearing joints). Documentation of the level of severity of the comorbid existing condition must be included in the patient's medical record

- The patient has been previously unsuccessful with medical treatment for obesity

- Treatable metabolic causes for obesity (e.g., adrenal or thyroid disorders) have been ruled out or have been clinically treated if present

Key Documentation Terms

Documentation should indicate the surgical procedure that was performed. Terms such as adjustable gastric device, gastric sleeve, revision, removal, replacement, or subcutaneous ports provide the guidance needed to ensure correct code assignment. Above all else, the documentation should support the medical necessity of the procedure. Documentation for these procedures must include a history and physical containing evidence of comorbid conditions, an operative report containing a detailed procedure note, and office/progress notes documenting unsuccessful medical treatment for obesity.

Coding Tips

- For open gastric restrictive procedures, see 43842–43848.

- Band adjustment (injection or removal of saline through the subcutaneous port) is included in the global surgical package and should not be reported with this code.

- When reporting individual component placement, modifier 52 should be appended to code 43770.

Other Procedures Performed on the Stomach (43800–43999)

These codes are used for procedures that are not classified elsewhere, including pyloroplasty (when not performed at the time of a vagotomy), repair of the stomach (gastrorrhaphy), and open gastric restrictive procedures.

Pyloroplasty (43800)

Procedure Differentiation

A pyloroplasty is a surgical procedure to open the lower part of the stomach so that food may pass more easily from the stomach and into the small intestine.

Medical Necessity

A pyloroplasty is commonly performed in infants for a thickened pylorus. It is also performed on patients who are diagnosed with pyloric stenosis or for pyloric ulcers.

Key Documentation Terms

Documentation must indicate that the physician incised the pylorus and then closed the incision horizontally to keep the pylorus open and allow food to empty.

Coding Trap

- A pyloroplasty is often performed at the same time as a vagotomy. When this occurs, only code 43640 should be reported.

Open Bariatric Procedures for Morbid Obesity (43842–43848)

Gastric restrictive procedures are performed as a method of treating morbid obesity. Unlike the codes contained in the bariatric surgery heading, these codes are open procedures.

The documentation for code 43842 must indicate that the physician altered the stomach's size to help stem morbid obesity. The physician exposes the lesser curvature of the stomach via a midline abdominal incision through skin, fascia, and muscles. In 43842, a double row of staples is placed in the upper portion of the stomach to create a small stoma. A small strip of mesh or a Silastic ring is wrapped around the stoma and stapled to itself. Report 43843 if the technique used is other than the vertical-banded gastroplasty, and allows for staples restricting other parts of the stomach.

Code 43845 describes a biliopancreatic diversion with duodenal switch. Documentation must indicate that the stomach was resected leaving the pyloric valve intact with the remaining stomach that maintains its functionality. The duodenum is divided near the pyloric valve. The small intestine is also divided. The distal end of the small intestine in continuity with the large intestine is brought up and anastomosed to the short duodenal segment on the stomach. The other end of the small intestine (the duodenal segment in connection with the gallbladder and pancreas, or the biliopancreatic loop) is attached to the newly anastomosed other limb further down near the large intestine. This forms a 75 to 100 cm "common loop" where the contents of both of these segments channel together before dumping into the large intestine.

Code 43846 describes the construction of a small proximal gastric pouch, which is divided from the stomach with a short Roux-en-Y gastrojejunostomy.

Documentation for 43847 should indicate that the physician partitioned the stomach and performed a small intestine anastomosis to the proximal stomach (Roux-en-Y gastrojejunostomy) in order to bypass the majority of the stomach. The small intestine is reconstructed so that it is partially bypassed to limit the amount of area available for absorption of nutrients.

Code 43848 is used to report a revision performed for a failed gastric restrictive procedure for morbid obesity. Indications for revision include stomal stenosis, stomal dilation, nonemptying gastric pouch, gastroesophageal reflux, staple dehiscence, intragastric foreign body, gastric fistula, gastroesophageal fistula, failure to maintain weight loss, breakdown of staple continuity, and restored gastric continuity. It would be inappropriate to report this code for a revision of an adjustable gastric restrictive device. Revision techniques vary depending on the technique used in the initial gastric restrictive procedure (i.e., gastroplasty, partial gastrectomy, gastric bypass) and the nature of the gastric restrictive failure. Types of revision include gastroplasty, conversion of a gastroplasty to a gastric bypass, and revision of a gastric bypass.

Medical Necessity

Certain criterion needs to be met before a payer will cover a gastric restrictive procedure. The following are the conditions that need to be met in order for Medicare to cover the procedure. Other payer policies may vary.

- The patient meets the definition of morbid obesity, which is defined as a body mass index (BMI) ≥ 35, and comorbid conditions exist (e.g., hypertensive cardiovascular disease, pulmonary/respiratory disease, diabetes, sleep apnea, or degenerative arthritis of weight-bearing joints).

Documentation of the level of severity of the comorbid existing condition must be included in the patient's medical record

- The patient has been previously unsuccessful with medical treatment for obesity
- Treatable metabolic causes for obesity (e.g., adrenal or thyroid disorders) have been ruled out or have been clinically treated if present

Key Documentation Terms
In order to assign the most appropriate code, the medical record documentation must be reviewed to determine why the procedure was performed (i.e., for the initial procedure or a revision of the gastric procedure).

Terms such as vertical banded gastroplasty, biliopancreatic diversion, duodenoileostomy, ileoileostomy, partial gastrectomy, or revision provide the guidance needed to ensure correct code assignment. Above all else, the documentation should support the medical necessity of the procedure. Documentation for these procedures must include a history and physical containing evidence of comorbid conditions, an operative report containing a detailed procedure note, and office/progress notes documenting unsuccessful medical treatment for obesity.

Coding Trap
- Gastric restrictive procedures performed laparoscopically are reported with 43644–43645.

Procedures Performed on the Intestines (Excluding the Rectum) (44005–44799)

Excisional Procedures of the Intestine (44100–44160)

Procedure Differentiation
These procedures encompass the removal of tissue from the intestine (biopsies), partial removal of the intestine (partial colectomies), and removal of an entire section of the intestine.

Codes 44110–44111 describe an excision of one or more lesions. The codes are further differentiated by whether a single enterotomy or multiple enterotomies are performed.

Enterectomies are reported with 44120–44128. In 44120, the physician resects a single segment of small intestine and performs an anastomosis between the remaining bowel ends. Next, the selected segment of small bowel is isolated and divided proximally and distally to the remaining bowel and removed. The remaining bowel ends are reapproximated using staples or sutures. Report 44121 for each additional resection and anastomosis; an enterostomy performed with this procedure is reported with 44125.

Codes 44126–44128 are enterectomies specific to congenital atresia. In these procedures, the physician resects a segment of small intestine and may perform tapering to fit the area of anastomosis. The physician makes an abdominal incision. The selected segment of small intestine is isolated and divided proximally and distally to the remaining bowel and removed. An end-to-end anastomosis of the proximal rectum to the distal and canal is performed. The remaining bowel ends are reapproximated using staples or sutures. The incision is closed. Report 44126 for a single resection and anastomosis. Report 44127 when tapering (gradually narrowing toward one end) of the bowel is performed

 DEFINITIONS

anastomosis. Surgically created connection between ducts, blood vessels, or bowel segments to allow flow from one to the other.

atresia. Congenital closure or absence of a tubular organ or an opening to the body surface.

colostomy. Artificial surgical opening anywhere along the length of the colon to the skin surface for the diversion of feces.

enterostomy. Surgically created opening into the intestine through the abdominal wall.

ileostomy. Artificial surgical opening that brings the end of the ileum out through the abdominal wall to the skin surface for the diversion of feces through a stoma.

proctectomy. Surgical resection of the rectum.

resection. Surgical removal of a part or all of an organ or body part.

with the resection and anastomosis. Report 44128 for each additional resection and anastomosis beyond the first one.

An enteroenterostomy is reported with code 44130. Documentation must state that the physician performed a small bowel anastomosis, bringing one end of small bowel through the abdominal wall onto the skin as a stoma. A segment of small bowel may be resected and a small bowel anastomosis is performed with staples or sutures. An end or loop of small bowel may be brought through a separate incision in the abdominal wall onto the skin as a stoma.

Codes 44132–44137 describe services related to intestinal transplantation.

Codes 44140–44160 report colectomies. Codes 44140–44147 and 44160 are reported for partial colectomies and 44150–44158 are reported for total colectomies. Each of these procedures is further differentiated by the procedures performed in conjunction with the colectomy. Please read each code description thoroughly.

Key Documentation Terms

Documentation should indicate the surgical procedure that was performed. Terms such as anastomosis, cecostomy, with colostomy or ileostomy, enteroenterostomy, proctectomy, partial, or total provide the guidance needed to ensure correct code assignment. Above all else, the documentation should support the medical necessity of the procedure.

Coding Tips

- Intraoperative colonic lavage performed in conjunction with 44140 is reported separately, see add-on code 44701.

- Mobilization (take-down) of splenic flexure performed in conjunction with partial colectomy is reported separately, see add-on code 44139.

- As "add-on" codes, 44121, 44128, and 44139 are not subject to multiple procedure rules. No reimbursement reduction or modifier 51 is applied. The following table provides additional information for these codes as found in the Medicare Physician Fee Schedule Database.

Parent Code	Add-On	GLOB DAYS	MULT PROC	BILAT SURG	ASST SURG	CO-SURG	TEAM SURG
44120		090	2	0	2	1	0
	44121	ZZZ	0	0	2	1	0
44126		090	2	0	2	1	0
44127		090	2	0	2	1	0
	44128	ZZZ	0	0	2	1	0
	44139	ZZZ	0	0	2	1	0
44140		090	2	0	2	1	0
44141		090	2	0	2	1	0
44143		090	2	0	2	1	0
44144		090	2	0	2	1	0
44145		090	2	0	2	1	0
44146		090	2	0	2	1	0
44147		090	2	0	2	1	0

Laparoscopic Enterolysis and Enterostomy Procedures (44180–44238)

Procedure Differentiation

Many of the procedures performed on the digestive system can be performed through an open or laparoscopic approach. The CPT book classifies those procedures done laparoscopically in a different heading within each section.

Code 44180 describes a surgical laparoscopy in which enterolysis is performed. In this procedure, the documentation should indicate that intestinal adhesions were identified and instruments were passed through to dissect and remove the adhesions. This code is a separate procedure by definition and is usually a component of a more complex service and is not identified separately. When performed with other unrelated procedures, list the code and append modifier 59.

In 44186, the physician constructs a jejunostomy for decompression or feeding. The physician identifies the jejunum and resects it, rerouting it to an opening created in the skin. An ostomy is created in the skin. In 44187, a nontube ileostomy or jejunostomy is constructed. The selected segment of jejunum or ileum is isolated. A loop or end of the selected segment of bowel is located and grasped. The skin and fat are excised, the fascia is opened, and the loop is exteriorized through a previously defined ileostomy or jejunostomy site. The trocars are removed and the incisions are closed with sutures.

Code 44188 is used to report a laparoscopically created colostomy or skin level cecostomy.

Codes 44202–44213 describe excision procedures performed laparoscopically. Codes 44202–44203 report enterectomies. Partial colectomies are reported with 44204–44208 and total colectomies are reported with 44210–44212. Add-on code 44213 is used to report mobilization of the splenic flexure via a laparoscopic approach that is performed in conjunction with a separately reportable partial colon resection.

Closure of an enterostomy is reported with 44227.

Key Documentation Terms

Documentation should indicate the surgical procedure that was performed. Terms such as anastomosis, enterolysis, with cecostomy, colostomy, enterostomy, ileostomy, jejunostomy, partial, or total provide the guidance needed to ensure correct code assignment. The documentation should support the medical necessity of the procedure.

Coding Tips

- A diagnostic laparoscopy is not reported separately.
- If an unsuccessful laparoscopic procedure is converted to an open procedure, report only the open procedure.
- As "add-on" codes, 44203 and 44213 are not subject to multiple procedure rules. No reimbursement reduction or modifier 51 is applied. The following table provides additional information for these codes as found in the Medicare Physician Fee Schedule Database.

Parent Code	Add-On	GLOB DAYS	MULT PROC	BILAT SURG	ASST SURG	CO-SURG	TEAM SURG
44202		090	2	0	2	1	0
	44203	ZZZ	0	0	2	1	0
44204		090	2	0	2	1	0
44205		090	2	0	2	1	0
44206		090	2	0	2	1	0
44207		090	2	0	2	1	0
44208		090	2	0	2	1	0
	44213	ZZZ	0	0	2	1	0

Endoscopy, Small Intestine and Stomal (44360–44408)

Procedure Differentiation

The physician examines the small intestine to determine if bleeding, tumors, erosions, ulcers, or other abnormalities are present. In 44360, documentation must indicate that the physician performed an endoscopy of the proximal small bowel and obtained brushings or washings. The physician places an endoscope through the mouth and advances it into the small intestine beyond the second portion of the duodenum, but not including the ileum. An abdominal incision may be made to mobilize the small bowel and assist in running the bowel over the endoscope. The lumen of the small bowel is examined and brushings or washings may be obtained of suspicious areas. The endoscope is withdrawn at the completion of the procedure. If an incision was made, it is closed.

Within this section, codes are further divided by the procedures performed (e.g., biopsy, injection, removal of foreign body, and tumor removal). Codes 44360-44379 report endoscopies of the small intestine. Codes 44360-44373 do not include the examination of the ileum; codes 44376-44379 do include the ileum.

In this section there are also codes for endoscopies performed through a stoma or intestinal pouch. Codes 44380-44384 report ileoscopy via a stoma. In 44380, the documentation will state that the physician places the endoscope into the ileostomy and advances the endoscope into the small intestine. The small bowel lumen is visualized and brushings or washings may be obtained. Report 44382 when biopsies are obtained. Code 44381 is reported when the documentation states that the physician performs endoscopy through an ileostomy and dilates strictures by balloon catheter. The physician places the endoscope into the ileostomy and advances it into the small intestine. The lumen of the ileum, the last part of the small intestine, is visualized, areas of stenosis are identified, and a balloon catheter is passed to the point of constriction and a little beyond. The balloon is inflated to the appropriate diameter and gradually withdrawn through the stenosed area, stretching the walls of the bowel at the strictured area. The endoscope is withdrawn at the completion of the procedure.

Code 44384 is reported when a stent is placed at the site of an obstruction or stricture. This procedure involves placement of the endoscope at the site of an obstruction or stricture and determination of the necessary stent length. The stent (endoprosthesis) is introduced into the site of the obstruction and, using a commercial delivery system, a plastic covering over the stent is removed and the stent self-deploys, shoring-up the walls at a specific site in the ileum. When necessary, a balloon catheter is placed into the stent and gently inflated to more

DEFINITIONS

stoma. Opening created in the abdominal wall from an internal organ or structure for diversion of waste elimination, drainage, and access.

fully deploy the stent. The delivery system and endoscope are then removed. This code includes dilation before and after stent placement, as well as guidewire passage, when performed.

Codes 44385-44386 report an endoscopy of an intestinal pouch. The endoscope is placed into the pouch, through the anus or abdominal wall stoma. The lumen of the pouch is visualized and brushings or washings may be obtained (44385). Report 44386 when biopsies are obtained.

Codes 44388-44408 report colonoscopies performed through an abdominal wall stoma (colostomy). In 44388, a colonoscopy is performed through an abdominal wall colostomy and brushings or washings may be obtained. The physician places the endoscope into the colostomy and advances the endoscope into the colon. The lumen of the colon is visualized and brushings or washings may be obtained. The endoscope is withdrawn at the completion of the procedure.

This section of codes is further divided by the procedures performed (e.g., biopsy, removal of foreign body, ablation or removal of tumor, etc.). The same guidelines for assigning colonoscopy codes applies to these codes.

Medical Necessity

The following conditions may warrant a small intestine endoscopy (this list is not all inclusive and may vary by payer):

- Abnormalities found during imaging
- Acute, chronic, or occult intestinal bleeding without an etiology
- Crohn's disease of small bowel
- Foreign bodies
- Lymphoma
- Neoplasm (benign or malignant)
- Polyps
- Strictures
- Ulcers

Information regarding medical necessity of colonoscopies may be found later in the chapter under the heading Endoscopy of the Large Intestines and Anus (45300–45398, 46600–46615).

Endoscopy-Specific Documentation Recommendations

Endoscopy documentation varies from all other specialties in the basic requirements. The basic information that should be readily available from the endoscopy record includes:

- Preoperative diagnosis
- Postoperative diagnosis
- Procedure performed
- Endoscopy physician name
- Indications for procedure
- Informed consent for the procedure
- Anesthesia used
  - medications given for anesthesia

- Preparation (was bowel prep successful)
- Detailed description of the endoscopy service performed
  - actual process and events of how procedures were approached and performed
  - when a procedure is attempted but unsuccessfully completed, the provider should document the reason for the failure as well as to what degree the procedure was completed
  - precise anatomic terminology and names of structures observed or studied
  - instruments used
  - biopsies, if taken
  - pictures, if taken
- Findings
- Complications
- Estimated blood loss
- Specimens sent to pathology
- Patient's status at discharge
- Impression
  - comparisons with previous studies where applicable
  - precise diagnosis if possible
- Recommendations
- Postop orders
- Patient instructions

Patient demographic and other pertinent information should be contained in the procedure report format, such as patient name, facility name, patient account number, patient date of birth, referring physician name, date and time procedure dictated, as well as the date and time the report was transcribed.

The preendoscopy examination and evaluation should include a review of the patient's past medical history, medications, family history, social history, current lab work, and adverse reactions to previous anesthesia.

Key Documentation Terms
Documentation should indicate the surgical procedure that was performed during the encounter. Terms such as ablation, biopsy, colonoscopy, decompression, injection, removal, resection, stent placement, stoma, and ultrasound indicate the correct code assignment. The approach is also necessary to determine correct code assignment. For example, medical records should be carefully reviewed to determine if the scope was inserted via a stoma or the mouth.

Coding Tips
- It is acceptable to bill separately for multiple services provided during an endoscopic encounter (with the exception of treating bleeding induced by the procedure) when performed during the same operative session.
- Diagnostic endoscopy procedures can be reported with open or incisional procedures.
- When two distinct endoscopic procedures are performed, such as an EGD and a colonoscopy, both procedures should be reported with modifier 59 appended to the lesser of the two.

Coding Traps

- If an endoscopy or enteroscopy is performed as a common standard of practice when performing another service, the endoscopy or enteroscopy is not reported separately. For example, if a small intestinal endoscopy or enteroscopy is performed during the creation or revision of an enterostomy, the small intestinal endoscopy or enteroscopy is not reported separately.

- Control of bleeding that is the result of a surgical procedure is not reported separately. In the case of endoscopy, if it is necessary to repeat the endoscopy at a later time during the same day to control bleeding, a procedure code for endoscopic control of bleeding may be reported with modifier 78, indicating that this service represents a return to the endoscopy suite or operating room for a related procedure during the postoperative period.

- When biopsy of a lesion is performed followed by excision or destruction of the same lesion, the biopsy is not reported separately.

- If the same surgical endoscopy service is performed repeatedly (e.g., multiple polyps are removed through the scope), the service is reported only once.

- Services such as venous access (36000), infusions and injections (96360–96379), noninvasive oximetry (94760–94761), and anesthesia provided by the surgeon are considered an integral part of the endoscopy and should not be billed separately.

- When a surgical colonoscopy is performed, the diagnostic colonoscopy should not be reported separately.

Endoscopy of the Large Intestines and Anus (45300–45398, 46600–46615)

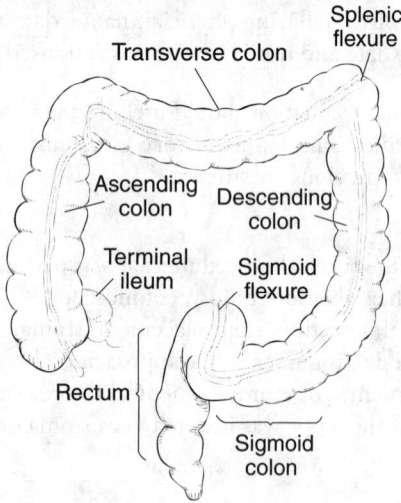

Procedure Differentiation

Proctosigmoidoscopy performed with a rigid scope is reported with 45300–45327. Code selection is based on the specific surgical treatment performed. Sigmoidoscopy performed with a flexible scope is reported with 45330–45350. Specific codes in this range identify the surgical procedures performed. Colonoscopy using a flexible scope is reported with 45378–45398. As with the other endoscopy procedures, the anatomical structures examined as well as any surgical service determine the actual code reported.

Colonoscopy is an examination from the rectum to the cecum, or the entire colon. It may also include the terminal ileum. Sigmoidoscopy examines the entire sigmoid colon and the entire rectum and may also include the descending colon. A proctosigmoidoscopy examines the rectum and a portion of the sigmoid colon. These are performed to determine if blood, tumors, erosions, ulcers, or other abnormalities are present.

The CPT book has guidelines at the beginning of this endoscopy section for patients with altered anatomy due to prior surgical procedures. Below is a brief description of the guidelines:

For a patient with colon resection proximal to sigmoid with an anastomosis (ileo-sigmoid or ileo-rectal), report codes 45330–45347.

For a patient with colon resection with an anastomosis (ileo-anal or J-pouch), report codes 45385–45386.

For a patient with segmental colon resection, report codes 45378–45398.

Some endoscopic procedures are performed through an existing stoma or opening. The first step in choosing a code is to determine the access used to perform the procedure. The most common procedures are colostomies (44388-44408).

Anoscopies are reported with 46600-46615. In 46600, a diagnostic anoscopy is performed. The physician inserts the anoscope into the anus and advances the scope. The anal canal and distal rectal mucosa are visualized and brushings or washings may be obtained. Within this section, codes are further divided by the procedures performed (e.g., biopsy, dilation, removal of foreign body, and removal of tumor). Anoscopies may also be performed with high resolution magnification (HRA) as in codes 46601 and 46607.

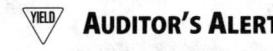

> **AUDITOR'S ALERT**
>
> See Appendix 1 for the audit worksheet for lower endoscopy.

Colorectal Cancer Screening

Regulatory Issues
Colorectal cancer is the third leading cause of cancer deaths in the United States. These types of cancers primarily affect people age 50 or older, with the risk of developing the disease increasing with age.

Colorectal cancers rarely display any symptoms, and the cancer can progress undiagnosed until it becomes fatal. The most common symptom of colorectal cancer is bleeding from the rectum. Other symptoms include cramping, abdominal pain, intestinal obstruction, or a change in bowel habits.

Colorectal cancer is largely preventable through screening since this allows a physician to identify and remove precancerous polyps. Screening can also detect malignancies early allowing for a good treatment outcome.

The Balanced Budget Act (BBA) of 1997 legislated Medicare coverage of colorectal screening. Under the BBA various types of colorectal cancer screening examinations became a covered service effective January 1, 1998. There are specific coverage, frequency, and payment limitations and these coverage guidelines may vary depending on the type of colorectal screening performed and/or the level of risk to the patient. Many non-Medicare payers also have strict guidelines regarding the coverage, frequency, and payment of colorectal cancer screening.

Medicare provides coverage of the following colorectal cancer screening services for the early detection of colorectal cancer.

Fecal occult blood test (FOBT). This test determines if there is any occult (hidden) blood in the stool. There are two methods of performing this test. The first is a guaiac-based test for peroxidase activity. In this method, the patient is provided a kit and advised to obtain three consecutive stool specimens following the instructions on the kit. The second method is immunoassay fecal occult blood testing. Patient instructions are the same as for the stool guaiac testing; however, the methodology used to determine the presence of occult blood is different.

Flexible sigmoidoscopy. A flexible sigmoidoscopy is a procedure where the physician inserts a flexible fiberoptic endoscopy into the patient's rectum and advances the endoscopy visualizing the lower one third of the colon. During this procedure, if the physician encounters polyps or other lesions, a biopsy may be performed or the polyp can be removed.

Colonoscopy. This test is performed in the same manner as the flexible sigmoidoscopy; however, a colonoscope is used and the entire colon (including the cecum) is visualized. As with a flexible sigmoidoscopy, the physician may obtain biopsies or perform a polypectomy during this procedure when necessary.

Barium enema (as an alternative to a covered screening flexible sigmoidoscopy or a screening colonoscopy). Following an enema of barium, x-rays of the entire colon, including the rectum, are obtained.

Cologuard—a Multitarget Stool DNA (sDNA) Test. Cologuard is a noninvasive screening test for colorectal cancer that analyzes both stool DNA and blood biomarkers. This test can detect altered DNA associated with colorectal cancer in a patient's stool. The colon wall along with polyps within the colon shed cells that end up in the stool stream and release DNA as they degenerate. Some of these cells contain altered DNA reflecting mutations associated with colorectal cancer. This altered DNA can be identified by an sDNA test. In a clinical study, Cologuard was able to detect 92 percent of colon cancers. Per CMS, CPT code 81528 should be reported when billing for the Cologuard™ test. **Note:** Only laboratories authorized by the manufacturer to perform the Cologuard test may bill for it.

Coverage Information

Most third-party payers who provide coverage for colorectal screening cover the following tests:

- Screening fecal occult blood test (FOBT)
- Screening flexible sigmoidoscopy
- Screening colonoscopy
- Screening barium enema (as an alternative to a covered screening flexible sigmoidoscopy or screening colonoscopy)

More detailed information defining each of these procedures may be found above.

Coverage may be affected by whether or not the patient is at high risk for colorectal cancer. For Medicare purposes, CMS has defined high-risk patients as those who have one or more of the following:

- A close family member who has had colorectal cancer or adenomatous polyps
- A family history of familial adenomatous polyposis
- A family history of hereditary nonpolyposis colorectal cancer
- A personal history of adenomatous polyps
- A personal history of colorectal cancer
- A personal history of inflammatory bowel disease, including Crohn's disease and ulcerative colitis

Most payers have strict age restrictions for the coverage of colorectal screening services. However, these age restrictions may be reduced or eliminated if the patient is high risk as defined above.

Cologuard—a Multitarget Stool DNA (sDNA) Test:
Medicare provides coverage for all Medicare beneficiaries ages 50 to 85 years once every three years. The beneficiaries may be asymptomatic and at average risk of developing colorectal cancer.

FOBT
Medicare provides coverage of a screening FOBT once every year (at least 11 months must have passed following the month in which the test is performed). Patients must be 50 years of age or older.

Screening Flexible Sigmoidoscopy
Medicare provides coverage of a screening flexible sigmoidoscopy for beneficiaries age 50 or older. A screening flexible sigmoidoscopy must be performed by a doctor of medicine or osteopathy, or by a physician assistant, nurse practitioner, or clinical nurse specialist.

Beneficiaries at high risk for developing colorectal cancer: Medicare provides coverage of a screening flexible sigmoidoscopy once every four years (i.e., at least 47 months have passed following the month in which the last covered screening flexible sigmoidoscopy was performed) for beneficiaries at high risk for colorectal cancer.

Beneficiaries not at high risk for developing colorectal cancer: Medicare provides coverage of a screening flexible sigmoidoscopy once every four years (i.e., at least 47 months have passed following the month in which the last covered screening flexible sigmoidoscopy was performed) for beneficiaries age 50 or older unless the beneficiary does not meet the high risk criteria for developing colorectal cancer and the beneficiary has had a screening colonoscopy within the preceding 10 years, then the next screening flexible sigmoidoscopy will be covered only after at least 119 months have passed following the month in which the last covered screening colonoscopy was performed.

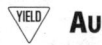

AUDITOR'S ALERT

For multitargets, DNA tests should be reported with ICD-10-CM codes Z12.11 and Z12.12.

Screening Colonoscopy

Medicare provides coverage of a screening colonoscopy for all beneficiaries without regard to age. A doctor of medicine or osteopathy must perform this screening. All Medicare beneficiaries age 50 or older are covered; however, when an individual is at high risk, there is no minimum age required to receive a screening colonoscopy.

Beneficiaries at high risk for developing colorectal cancer: Medicare provides coverage of a screening colonoscopy once every two years for beneficiaries at high risk for colorectal cancer. At least 23 months have passed following the month in which the last screening colonoscopy was performed. If a screening flexible sigmoidoscopy has been performed, Medicare covers a screening colonoscopy after at least 47 months has passed.

Beneficiaries not at high risk for developing colorectal cancer: Medicare provides coverage of a screening colonoscopy once every 10 years but not within 47 months of a previous screening sigmoidoscopy.

Screening Barium Enema

For Medicare patients, a screening barium enema may be performed as an alternative to a high risk screening colonoscopy or a high risk flexible sigmoidoscopy.

Beneficiaries at high risk for developing colorectal cancer: Medicare provides coverage of a screening barium enema as an alternative to a screening colonoscopy once every two years for high-risk patients. At least 23 months must have passed since the month in which the last covered screening barium enema was performed. Since the patient is at high risk, there are no age requirements that must be met.

Beneficiaries not at high risk for developing colorectal cancer: Medicare provides coverage of a screening barium enema as an alternative to a screening flexible sigmoidoscopy once every four years. In this scenario, at least 47 months must have passed following the month in which the last covered screening barium enema was performed and the patient must be age 50 or older.

According to CMS, it is preferable that a double contrast barium enema be ordered in writing. In situations where the patient cannot withstand a double contrast barium enema, a single contrast barium enema may be ordered. The attending physician must determine that the estimated screening potential for the barium enema is equal to or greater than the estimated screening potential for a screening flexible sigmoidoscopy, or for a screening colonoscopy, as appropriate, for the same individual.

Key Documentation Terms

It is essential to determine the type of lower GI endoscopy by examining the endoscopy report and identifying the anatomical structures that were visualized. The report should also be reviewed to determine what if any surgical services were performed during the encounter.

As with any service or procedure, the documentation must support the procedure being billed. In the case of screening colorectal cancer services:

- Documentation should include any risk factors identified.
- When a procedure is attempted but unsuccessfully completed, the provider should document the reason for the failure as well as to what degree the procedure was completed.

- When a screening barium enema is provided, the documentation must indicate the procedure for which the screening barium enema is being performed:
  - alternative to a screening flexible sigmoidoscopy
  - alternative to a screening colonoscopy
  - the reason(s) the screening barium enema was performed in lieu of one of the above

Coding Tips

- An anoscopy is always included with more extensive exams, such as colonoscopy, sigmoidoscopy, and proctosigmoidoscopy. Anoscopy alone is reported with 46600–46615. Code selection is based upon the surgical procedure performed.

- It is acceptable to bill for multiple services provided during an endoscopic procedure (with the exception of treating bleeding induced by the procedure) when performed during the same operative session. For example, if a colonoscopy with biopsy is performed, and the physician also removes a separate lesion by snare technique, then 45380 and 45385 may be reported. These services are reimbursed under the payer's multiple endoscopic payment rules for gastrointestinal endoscopy.

- Diagnostic endoscopy procedures can be reported with open or incisional procedures.

- When two distinct endoscopic procedures are performed, such as an EGD and a colonoscopy, both procedures should be reported with modifier 59 appended to the lesser of the two.

- Only the more extensive endoscopic procedure is reported for a session. For example, if the sigmoid and ascending colon are examined, only the colonoscopy code is reported.

- To report an endoscopy on a patient who has had a previous colectomy and now has a defunctionalized rectum or colon (distal) report the appropriate colonoscopy or ileoscopy code for the procedure performed via a stoma (44388–44408 or 44380–44384) in addition to the appropriate code for the proctosigmoidoscopy, sigmoidoscopy, or anoscopy.

- There are many instructional notes throughout the endoscopy section, including those discussing which codes should not be reported with other codes (for example, code 44388 should not be reported with 44389–44408). Please see the CPT book for the instructional notes, as the list is too extensive to document here.

Coding Traps

- Control of bleeding that is the result of a surgical procedure is not reported separately. In the case of endoscopy, if it is necessary to repeat the endoscopy at a later time during the same day to control bleeding, a procedure code for endoscopic control of bleeding may be reported with modifier 78, indicating that this service represents a return to the endoscopy suite or operating room for a related procedure during the postoperative period. In the case of open surgical services, the appropriate complication codes may be reported if a return to the operating room is necessary, but the complication code should not be reported if the complication described by the CPT code occurred during the same operative session.

- When biopsy of a lesion is performed followed by excision or destruction of the same lesion, the biopsy is not reported separately.

- Brushing and/or washings obtained for cytologic examination are described as part of a diagnostic endoscopy and, therefore, should not be separately reported.

- If the same surgical endoscopy service is performed repeatedly (e.g., multiple polyps are removed through the scope), the service is reported only once.

- Services such as venous access (36000), infusions and injections (96360–96379), noninvasive oximetry (94760–94761), and anesthesia provided by the surgeon are considered an integral part of the endoscopy and should not be reported separately.

- When submitting claims for colorectal cancer screening services it is important that the claim form be completed accurately and completely. This includes reporting the most appropriate HCPCS Level II and ICD-10-CM procedure codes.

Billing and Payment Issues

The table below can be used to determine the correct HCPCS Level II code for the colorectal screening procedure performed.

HCPCS/CPT Code	Code Descriptor
G0104	Colorectal cancer screening; flexible sigmoidoscopy
G0105	Colorectal cancer screening; colonoscopy on individual at high risk
G0106	Colorectal cancer screening; alternative to G0104, screening sigmoidoscopy, barium enema
G0120	Colorectal cancer screening; alternative to G0105, screening colonoscopy, barium enema
G0121	Colorectal cancer screening; colonoscopy on individual not meeting criteria for high risk
G0328	Colorectal cancer screening; fecal occult blood test, immunoassay,1-3 simultaneous determinations
00812	Anesthesia for lower intestinal endoscopic procedures, endoscope introduced distal to duodenum; screening colonoscopy
81528	Oncology (colorectal) screening, quantitative real-time target and signal amplification of 10 DNA markers (KRAS mutations, promoter methylation of NDRG4 and BMP3) and fecal hemoglobin, utilizing stool, algorithm reported as a positive or negative result
82270	Blood, occult, by peroxidase activity (eg, guaiac), qualitative; feces, consecutive collected specimens with single determination, for colorectal neoplasm screening (ie, patient was provided 3 cards or single triple card for consecutive collection)

Because this is a screening service, the patient does not have to have any signs or symptoms in order for the service to be covered. However, to prevent unnecessary claim delays or denials, inappropriate payment by the insurer, or increased patient responsibility for the service it is important that the most appropriate ICD-10-CM code be reported. Code Z12.11 Encounter for screening for malignant neoplasm of colon, should be reported on all claims, even those for patients at high risk.

For patients who are at high risk, an additional diagnosis code must be assigned to report the nature of the condition that places the patient at high risk. The table below provides a list of those codes most frequently used to report the conditions placing the patient at high risk. This list is not all inclusive and if the provider documents another condition, the appropriate code for that condition should be reported.

Polypectomy Performed During Screening Endoscopy

Because of confusion regarding the coding of the removal of a lesion found during a routine screening colonoscopy, the CMS Internet Only Manual (IOM), Pub.100-04, chapter 18, section 60.2 states:

> "If during the course of the screening colonoscopy, a lesion or growth is detected which results in a biopsy or removal of the growth, the appropriate diagnostic procedure classified as a colonoscopy with biopsy or removal along with modifier -PT should be billed and paid rather than HCPCS G0105."

When a colorectal cancer screening test becomes a diagnostic service, the Part B deductible is waived, and the appropriate diagnostic procedure code reported and paid rather than the screening code. Modifier PT should be appended to surgical procedure.

Furthermore, the initial diagnosis should be the appropriate Z code for the screening service since that is the primary reason why the encounter was performed. A second ICD-10-CM code indicating the finding should also be reported.

It should be noted that when a screening colonoscopy becomes a diagnostic colonoscopy, anesthesia services are reported with CPT code 00811 Anesthesia for lower intestinal endoscopic procedures, endoscope introduced distal to duodenum; not otherwise specified, and with modifier PT; only the deductible is waived.

If a screening flexible sigmoidoscopy is performed in the outpatient department of a hospital or in an ambulatory surgical center, the patient is responsible for 25 percent of the Medicare approved amount.

The following table can be used to determine the reimbursement for colorectal cancer screening procedures and the patient's responsibilities.

Type of Colorectal Screening	HCPCS Code(s)	Type of Payment	Deductible/Coinsurance
Cologuard	81528	Clinical Laboratory Fee Schedule (Medicare pays 100% of the Clinical Laboratory Fee Schedule amount or the provider's actual charge, whichever is lower.)	Deductible and coinsurance do not apply for this type of screening.
Fecal Occult Blood Tests	82270, G0328	Clinical Laboratory Fee Schedule (Medicare pays 100% of the Clinical Laboratory Fee Schedule amount or the provider's actual charge, whichever is lower.)	Deductible and coinsurance do not apply for this type of screening.

 AUDITOR'S ALERT

Anesthesia services furnished with a screening colonoscopy are reported with CPT code 00812, and the coinsurance and deductible are waived.

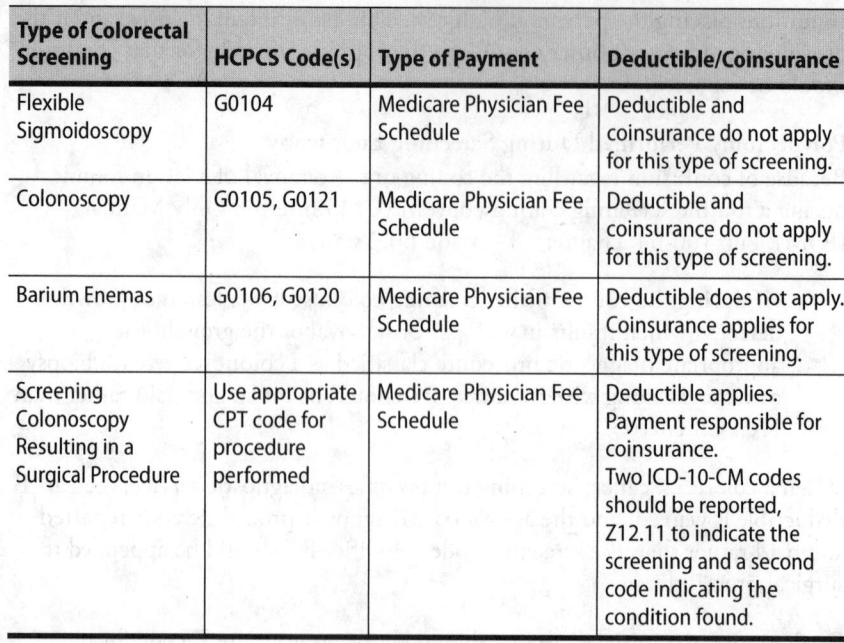

Type of Colorectal Screening	HCPCS Code(s)	Type of Payment	Deductible/Coinsurance
Flexible Sigmoidoscopy	G0104	Medicare Physician Fee Schedule	Deductible and coinsurance do not apply for this type of screening.
Colonoscopy	G0105, G0121	Medicare Physician Fee Schedule	Deductible and coinsurance do not apply for this type of screening.
Barium Enemas	G0106, G0120	Medicare Physician Fee Schedule	Deductible does not apply. Coinsurance applies for this type of screening.
Screening Colonoscopy Resulting in a Surgical Procedure	Use appropriate CPT code for procedure performed	Medicare Physician Fee Schedule	Deductible applies. Payment responsible for coinsurance. Two ICD-10-CM codes should be reported, Z12.11 to indicate the screening and a second code indicating the condition found.

DENIAL ALERT

When screening colonoscopy procedures are performed, be certain that the appropriate ICD-10-CM screening code is reported.

Most Common Reasons for Claim Denial

The following are the most common reasons for colorectal cancer screening claim denials:

- The patient does not meet the age requirements.

- The patient has exceeded the payer's frequency requirements.

- The patient does not meet the criteria for being at risk and therefore the procedure is noncovered because of the patient's age or the frequency of the service.

- Procedure code and diagnosis code do not match (i.e., diagnosis indicates a screening examination; however, procedure code indicates a diagnostic examination)

- Provider does not indicate that the procedure is screening by reporting Z12.11.

Procedures Performed on the Anus (46020–46999)

Surgical Incision of the Anus (46020–46083)

Incision codes include placement of a seton (46020). The physician makes an incision in the anal opening. A suture is passed and the seton is securely tied using a rubber band, or similar technique. A nylon suture is threaded around the sphincter and tied loosely. An elastic band is secured to the suture and a safety pin is attached. The pin is taped to the patient's thigh and the patient is instructed to adjust the amount of pull to produce minimal discomfort until the seton cuts through. Code 46030 reports the removal of a seton.

Treatment of an abscess by incision and drainage is reported with 46040–46060 according to the site and extent of the repair. Incision into the anal sphincter (sphincterotomy) is reported with 46080. In this procedure, the physician divides the anal sphincter. The patient is placed in jackknife or lithotomy position. The physician performs digital and instrumental dilation of the anus with exposure of the patient's anal canal. A small incision is made between the

DEFINITIONS

seton. Finely spun thread or other fine material for leading the passage of wider instruments through a fistula, canal, or sinus tract.

sphincter. Ring-like band of muscle that surrounds a bodily opening, constricting and relaxing as required for normal physiological functioning.

thrombosed hemorrhoid. Dilated, varicose vein in the anal region that has clotted blood within it.

muscle layers of the anus and internal muscle is divided without opening the lining of the anus.

Incision into an external hemorrhoid that is thrombosed is reported with 46083. Documentation must indicate that an incision was made in the skin over the hemorrhoid and the thrombus was removed. The incision is left open for continued drainage.

Key Documentation Terms

Documentation should indicate the surgical procedure that was performed. Terms such as placement, removal, perirectal, ischiorectal, intramural, intramuscular, submucosal or superficial provide the guidance needed to ensure correct code assignment. Above all else, the documentation should support the medical necessity of the procedure.

Coding Tips

- Code 46083 may be reported for each external thrombosed hemorrhoid that is excised.

Hemorrhoidectomy/Papilla Procedures (46220–46262, 46320, 46500, 46930, and 46945–46948)

With such a common condition as hemorrhoids, one might think coding the diagnosis and treatment is simple. However, because of several treatment methods and various conditions and complications that may occur with hemorrhoids, coding is not straightforward.

Understanding the terminology documented in the medical record and how to translate it into appropriate codes is essential. Not fully understanding ICD-10-CM and CPT code descriptions can lead to incorrect code assignments.

Procedure Differentiation

Knowing the different types of hemorrhoids, the various complications that may occur, and the related treatments is key to assigning the correct CPT codes.

In its simplest form, a hemorrhoid is a varicose vein of the superior or inferior hemorrhoidal plexus. There are three different types:

- Internal (the varicosity is in the superior vein)
- External (varicose dilation of the vein at the outer side of the external sphincter)
- Combined or mixed (both the superior and inferior portions of the vein are dilated)

Complications may affect not only the hemorrhoid but also the anus and the surrounding tissue. Complications to the anus may include a fistula (an opening in the cutaneous tissue near the anus, which may or may not communicate with the rectum) or a fissure (a painful linear groove of the anus).

Correct code assignment is determined by several factors, including:

- Type of hemorrhoid (internal, external, combined)
- Complication (e.g., thrombosis or ulceration)
- Other condition (e.g., as fissure or fistula)
- Method of treatment (excision, ligation, transanal dearterialization, destruction, injection)

AUDITOR'S ALERT

Codes 46040 and 46080 are separate procedures by definition and are usually a component of a more complex service and are not identified separately. When performed alone or with other unrelated procedures or services it may be reported. If performed alone, list the code; if performed with other procedures or services, list the code and append modifier 59.

Internal hemorrhoids may be removed using rubber band ligation (46221). The documentation must indicate that the physician performed hemorrhoidectomy by tying off (ligating) an internal hemorrhoid. The hemorrhoid is ligated at its base with a rubber band. The hemorrhoid tissue is allowed to slough over time.

Other types of internal hemorrhoid ligation are reported with 46945–46946. Report 46945 for ligation of a single hemorrhoid column or group and 46946 for ligation of two or more columns or groups. These procedures are performed without imaging guidance.

Prolapsing internal hemorrhoids may be treated by stapled hemorrhoidopexy (46947). In this procedure, a circular anal dilator is inserted that reduces the prolapsed anal tissue. The center obturator piece is removed and the prolapsed mucosa falls into the dilator lumen. An anoscope is inserted through the dilator that pushes the mucosa back against the rectal wall for 270 degrees of rotation. The other tissue protrudes through a window in the scope through which a purse string suture is made, containing only mucous membrane. The anoscope is rotated until a purse-string suture is completed around the anal circumference. A circular stapler is positioned proximal to the suture. The ends are tied externally. With traction on the purse string suture, the prolapsed mucosa is brought into the casing of the circular stapler, which is fired to release two staggered rows of staples while a circular knife removes a column of redundant mucosa from the upper anal canal. The staple line is examined and instruments are removed.

A transanal dearterialization of two or more hemorrhoid groups or columns may be performed as an alternative to an excisional hemorrhoidectomy or a stapled hemorrhoidopexy. With the patient under general anesthesia or IV sedation with infiltration of local anesthetic, the physician identifies the arteries supplying blood to the hemorrhoids utilizing a proctoscope coupled with a Doppler transducer. In order to interrupt the blood supply to the hemorrhoid, each selected artery is tied off (ligated) using a 2-0 absorbable suture. Mucopexy, or lifting and suturing of prolapsed mucosal membranes, may also be performed in cases of redundant prolapse. This procedure should be reported with 46948. If a single hemorrhoid column/group is dearterialized, report 46999.

Excision of external anal papillae or tags is reported with 46220 (single) and 46230 (multiple). The documentation for these procedures must indicate that the physician performed excision of external anal papillae or skin tags. The physician identifies the anal skin tags or papillae, which is usually associated with the external edge of a fissure or fistula. An incision is made around the skin tag or papilla and the lesion is dissected from the underlying sphincter muscle and removed. The incision is closed with sutures or may be left partially open to drain.

External thrombosed hemorrhoids are excised in 46320. The documentation must describe an external hemorrhoid that has become clotted with blood (thrombosed). The physician exposes the thrombosed external hemorrhoid and completely excises it with a scalpel. The site of the excision may be closed or left open to allow continued drainage.

External hemorrhoids are excised in 46250. Documentation must indicate that incisions are made around the hemorrhoids and the lesions are dissected from the underlying sphincter muscle and removed. The incisions are closed with sutures.

Hemorrhoidectomies for both internal and external, single column/groups are reported with 46255–46258. Code selection is dependant upon the additional procedures performed. Documentation for 46255 must indicate that the physician performed an excision of a single column or group of internal and external hemorrhoids. The physician explores the anal canal and identifies the hemorrhoid column. An incision is made in the rectal mucosa around the hemorrhoids and the lesions are dissected from the underlying sphincter muscles and removed. The incisions are closed with sutures. In 46257, hemorrhoidectomy with an associated fissure is performed. An incision is made around the fissure and the fissure is dissected from the underlying sphincter muscles and excised. In 46258, hemorrhoidectomy with associated fistulectomy and a possible fissurectomy is performed. If the fistula is in the same plane as the hemorrhoid, a single incision is made in the mucosa around the lesions and the lesions are dissected from the underlying sphincter muscles and removed. If the lesions are in different planes, separate incisions are used to excise the lesions. If a fissure is present it may be excised in a similar manner. The incisions are closed with sutures.

Hemorrhoidectomies for both internal and external, two or more column/groups are reported with 46260–46262. Documentation for 46260 must indicate that the physician performed excision of two or more columns or groups of internal and external hemorrhoids. The physician explores the anal canal and identifies the hemorrhoid columns. Incisions are made in the rectal mucosa around the hemorrhoid columns. The lesions are dissected from the underlying sphincter muscles and removed. The incisions are closed with sutures. In 46261, hemorrhoidectomy is performed as described above and an associated fissure is excised. In 46262, an associated fistulectomy and a possible fissurectomy are performed in addition to the hemorrhoidectomy.

Documentation for 46500 should indicate that the physician performed sclerotherapy of internal hemorrhoids. The physician explores the anal canal and identifies the hemorrhoid columns. Sclerosing solution is injected into the submucosa of the rectal wall under the hemorrhoid columns.

Removal of internal hemorrhoids by means of destruction (e.g., cautery, radiofrequency, infrared coagulation) is reported with 46930.

Key Documentation Terms
Documentation should indicate the surgical procedure that was performed. Terms such as external, internal, fissure, fistula, thrombosed, excision, ligation, or injection provide the guidance needed to ensure correct code assignment. Above all else, the documentation should support the medical necessity of the procedure.

Destruction Procedures: Anus (46900–46942)
These codes are intended for the destruction of anal lesions such as condylomas, papillomas, molluscum contagiosum, and herpetic vesicles.

Procedure Differentiation
Simple destruction of lesions (46900–46922) is reported according to the type of destruction performed. The documentation must indicate that the physician performed the destruction of anal lesions using chemicals in 46900. In 46910, the physician performs destruction of anal lesions with electrodesiccation. In 46916, the physician performs destruction of anal lesions with cryosurgery. The lesions are frozen and destroyed, usually with liquid nitrogen. The physician performs destruction of anal lesions with laser therapy in 46917. In 46922, anal

DEFINITIONS

chemosurgery. Application of chemical agents to destroy tissue, originally referring to the in situ chemical fixation of premalignant or malignant lesions to facilitate surgical excision.

condyloma. Infectious tumor-like growth caused by the human papilloma virus, with a branching connective tissue core and epithelial covering that occurs on the skin and mucous membranes of the perianal region and external genitalia.

cryosurgery. Application of intense cold, usually produced using liquid nitrogen, to locally freeze diseased or unwanted tissue and induce tissue necrosis without causing harm to adjacent tissue.

electrosurgery. Use of electric currents to generate heat in performing surgery.

fissure. Deep furrow, groove, or cleft in tissue structures.

molluscum contagiosum. Common, benign, viral skin infection, usually self-limiting, that appears as a gray or flesh-colored umbilicated lesion by itself or in groups, and later becomes white with an expulsable core containing the replication bodies. It is often transmitted sexually in adults, by autoinoculation, or close contact in children.

papilloma. Benign skin neoplasm with small branchings from the epithelial surface.

lesions are destroyed by excision. The perianal skin is exposed and the lesions are identified and surgically excised. The incisions are closed.

In 46924, destruction of extensive anal lesions is performed by various methods, such as laser surgery, electrosurgery, cryosurgery, or chemosurgery.

Treatment of an anal fissure with cautery or curettage is reported with 46940–46942, initial or subsequent. The documentation for this procedure must indicate that the physician performed an initial (46940) or subsequent (46942) curettage or cautery of an anal fissure with dilation of the anal sphincter. The physician exposes the perianal area and identifies the fissure. The fissure is debrided with curettage or cautery. The anal sphincter is manually dilated.

Key Documentation Terms
Documentation should indicate the surgical procedure that was performed. Terms such as fissure, laser surgery, cryosurgery, chemosurgery, electrosurgery, or excision provide the guidance needed to ensure correct code assignment. Above all else, the documentation should support the medical necessity of the procedure.

Liver Biopsy (47000–47001, 47100)
These codes describe needle and wedge biopsies performed on the liver.

Procedure Differentiation
Biopsy of the liver by percutaneous needle is reported with 47000 and 47001 if performed concurrent to another open surgical procedure. The documentation must indicate that the physician took tissue from the liver for examination. In 47000, the physician uses separately reportable ultrasound guidance to place a hollow bore needle between the ribs on the patient's right side. The liver biopsy is sent for pathology for separately reportable activity. Report 47001 when the liver biopsy is performed incidental to another major procedure.

Biopsy of the liver using a wedge excision is reported with 47100. The documentation must indicate that the physician took a wedge-shaped section of liver tissue for biopsy. The physician exposes the abdomen via an upper abdominal incision through skin, fascia, and muscle. Interrupted mattress sutures are placed on the edge of the liver lobe. A pie-shaped wedge of the liver is resected and sent for pathology in a separately reportable activity. Electrocautery is used to obtain hemostasis of the liver edge. The abdominal incision is closed with layered sutures.

Key Documentation Terms
Documentation should indicate the surgical procedure that was performed. Terms such as percutaneous needle, wedge excision or if performed concurrently with another major surgical procedure, provide the guidance needed to ensure correct code assignment. Above all else, the documentation should support the medical necessity of the procedure.

Coding Tips
- As an "add-on" code, 47001 is not subject to multiple procedure rules. No reimbursement reduction or modifier 51 is applied.
- When performing a liver biopsy, imaging guidance may be reported separately with codes 76942, 77002, 77012, or 77021.

 AUDITOR'S ALERT

Codes 46940 and 46942 are separate procedures by definition and are usually a component of a more complex service and are not identified separately. When performed alone or with other unrelated procedures or services it may be reported. If performed alone, list the code; if performed with other procedures or services, list the code and append modifier 59.

Cholecystectomy (47562–47564, 47600–47620)

A cholecystectomy is the surgical removal of the gallbladder and its contents. Cholecystectomy may be performed by an open incision into the abdominal cavity or laparoscopically via instruments inserted through small incisions into the peritoneum for video-controlled imaging.

Procedure Differentiation

The gallbladder may be removed laparoscopically or by incision. Code selection is based upon the excision of the gallbladder and concurrent procedures, such as exploration of the common duct.

When using a laparoscopic approach (47562–47564), documentation for 47562 must indicate that the physician made a 1.0-centimeter infraumbilical incision through which a trocar was inserted. Pneumoperitoneum is achieved by insufflating the abdominal cavity with carbon dioxide. A fiberoptic laparoscope fitted with a camera and light source is inserted through the trocar. Other incisions are made on the right side of the abdomen and in the subxiphoid area to allow other instruments or an additional light source to be passed into the abdomen. The tip of the gallbladder is mobilized and placed in traction. The Hartmann's pouch (junction of the cystic duct and gallbladder neck) is identified. Tissue is dissected free from around the area for exposure of Calot's triangle (formed by the cystic artery, and cystic and common bile ducts). Clips are applied to the proximal area of the cystic duct and artery (close to the gallbladder) and the cystic duct and artery are cut. In 47563, a contrast study is also obtained through the cystic duct. In 47564, exploration of the common bile duct is explored with a small choledochoscope through the cystic duct or a separate incision in the common bile duct. Stones may be extracted from the duct with a variety of instruments. If an incision was made in the common bile duct, this is usually closed with sutures over a T-tube that is brought out through the abdominal wall. The gallbladder is dissected from the liver bed and removed through a trocar site. Any loose stones that have dropped into the abdominal cavity are retrieved with forceps. The intraabdominal cavity is irrigated. The trocars are removed and the incisions are closed.

Open cholecystectomies are classified with 47600–47620. Code selection is dependant upon what other procedures are performed at the same time as the cholecystectomy.

A cholecystectomy performed with or without a cholangiography is reported with 47600 or 47605. Documentation must indicate that the physician removed the gallbladder. The physician exposes the liver and gallbladder via a right subcostal incision. The cystic duct and cystic artery are ligated and the gallbladder is removed using electrocautery. The incision is closed with layered sutures. Report 47605 if this is performed with a cholangiography.

Cholecystectomies that include common bile duct exploration, choledochoenterostomy, cholangiography, or transduodenal sphincterotomy or sphincteroplasty are reported with 47610–47620. Documentation for 47610 must indicate that the physician removed the gallbladder and explored the common duct. The physician exposes the liver and gallbladder via a right subcostal incision. The cystic duct and cystic artery are ligated and the gallbladder removed using electrocautery. The common bile duct is exposed in the portal triad, incised, and the stones removed. The common bile duct is closed and the abdominal incision is closed with sutures. Report 47612 if this procedure is performed with a choledochoenterostomy, the establishment of communication between the intestine and the common bile duct. Report 47620 if this procedure is performed with transduodenal sphincterotomy or sphincteroplasty, with or without cholangiography.

Key Documentation Terms

Documentation should indicate the surgical procedure that was performed. Terms such as laparoscopic, open, common bile duct exploration, choledochoenterostomy, cholangiography, sphincterotomy, or sphincteroplasty provide the guidance needed to ensure correct code assignment. Above all else, the documentation should support the medical necessity of the procedure.

Coding Tips

- An open cholecystectomy (47600–47620) includes examination of the abdomen through the abdominal wall incision. If this examination is performed laparoscopically, it is not reported separately.

- Laparoscopic procedures performed in place of an open procedure are subject to the standard surgical practice guidelines. A diagnostic laparoscopy is not reported separately. If an unsuccessful laparoscopic procedure is converted to an open procedure, only the open procedure may be reported.

Coding Traps

- A cholecystectomy should not be reported separately when performed during hepatectomy procedures (e.g., codes 47120–47130, 47133–47142).

- A cholecystectomy is an integral component of a Whipple type pancreatectomy (48150–48154) and should not be reported separately.

- If a laparoscopic cholecystectomy is converted to an open cholecystectomy, only the open procedure may be reported.

Laparoscopic Procedures of the Abdomen/Peritoneum/Omentum (49320–49329)

Many codes are available for laparoscopic procedures performed on the digestive system. They include biopsy, aspiration, drainage, and revisions.

When a diagnostic laparoscopy of the abdomen, peritoneum, and omentum is performed, code 49320 is reported. In this procedure, the physician makes a 1.0-centimeter incision in the umbilicus through which the abdomen is inflated and a fiberoptic laparoscope is inserted. Other incisions are also made through which trocars can be passed into the abdominal cavity to deliver instruments, a video camera, and, when needed, an additional light source. The physician manipulates the tools so that the pelvic organs, peritoneum, abdomen, and omentum can be viewed through the laparoscope and/or video monitor. Biopsy from any or all of the areas observed is obtained by brushing the surface and collecting the cells or by washing (bathing) the area with a saline solution, and suctioning out the cell rich solution. When the procedure is complete, the laparoscope, instruments, and light source are removed and the incisions are closed with sutures. If biopsy of pelvic organs is performed, the physician may also insert an instrument through the vagina to grasp the cervix and pass another instrument through the cervix, into the uterus to manipulate the uterus.

Codes 49321–49325 describe surgical laparoscopy procedures. Documentation for 49321 must indicate that a biopsy from any or all of the areas observed were obtained by grasping a sample with a biopsy forceps that is capable of "biting off" small pieces of tissue.

DENIAL ALERT

When a laparoscopic cholecystectomy (47562–47564) and open cholecystectomy (47600–47620) are both reported for the same date of service, the laparoscopic procedure will be denied.

In 49322, the physician makes a 1.0-centimeter incision in the umbilicus through which the abdomen is inflated and a fiberoptic laparoscope is inserted. A second incision is made directly below the umbilicus, just above the pubic hairline, through which a trocar can be passed into the abdominal cavity to deliver instruments. The physician manipulates the tools to view the pelvic organs through the laparoscope. An additional incision may be needed for a second light source. Once the biopsy site is viewed through the laparoscope, a 5.0-centimeter incision is made just above the site. Through this incision, the physician uses an aspirating probe to aspirate a cavity or cyst or to collect fluid for culture.

In 49323, drainage of a lymphocele to the peritoneal cavity is performed. Documentation must indicate that the physician places a trocar at the umbilicus into the abdominal or retroperineal space and insufflates the abdominal cavity. The physician places a laparoscope through the umbilical incision and additional trocars are placed into the abdomen. The lymphocele is identified and instruments are passed through to open and drain the lymphocele.

Insertion of a tunneled intraperitoneal catheter is reported with 49324. In this procedure, a permanent intraperitoneal catheter is inserted laparoscopically using a tunneling technique. The physician makes a 1 cm incision in the umbilicus through which the abdomen is inflated and a fiberoptic laparoscope is inserted. Other incisions are also made through which trocars can be passed into the abdominal cavity to deliver additional instruments. The physician manipulates the tools so that the pelvic organs, peritoneum, abdomen, and omentum can be viewed through the laparoscope and/or video monitor. Using various tunneling techniques, the physician inserts the intraperitoneal catheter, positioning the tip inside the peritoneal cavity. A separately reportable subcutaneous extension of the catheter with a remote chest exit site may also be performed. If the physician is revising an intraperitoneal catheter, the catheter is inspected and freed of occlusion or blockage. When either procedure is complete, the laparoscope and other instruments are removed and the incisions are closed with sutures. Report 49324 for the tunneled insertion of an intraperitoneal cannula or catheter and 49325 for its revision.

An omentopexy performed in addition to insertion or revision of an intraperitoneal catheter is reported with 49326. The documentation must indicate that the physician isolated the omentum at the stomach and intestine and cut, sutured, or plicated omental tissue to achieve the desired effect. When the procedure is complete, the laparoscope, instruments, and light source are removed and the incisions are closed with sutures.

Code 49327 is reported when interstitial devices for radiation are placed in conjunction with other laparoscopic abdominal, pelvic, or retroperitoneal procedures. Documentation must indicate that the physician placed one or more interstitial devices such as gold seeds (fiducial markers) for radiation therapy guidance or a dosimeter to gauge the amount of radiation received into the targeted soft tissue tumor. Allowing for precision in targeting radiation and/or for measuring the radiation doses received, a fiducial marker is visible by ultrasound and fluoroscopy and permits accurate triangulation of the tissue to be treated. A capsule dosimeter relays radiation dose information so that the clinical team can monitor for any deviation between the radiation plan and the actual radiation received.

Key Documentation Terms

Documentation should indicate the surgical procedure that was performed. Terms such as aspiration, biopsy, drainage, interstitial devices, omentopexy, placement, or revision provide the guidance needed to ensure correct code assignment. Above all else, the documentation should support the medical necessity of the procedure.

Coding Tips

- A diagnostic laparoscopy is not reported separately.

- As "add-on" codes, 49326–49327 are not subject to multiple procedure rules. No reimbursement reduction or modifier 51 is applied. The following table provides additional information for these codes as found in the Medicare Physician Fee Schedule Database.

Parent Code	Add-On	GLOB DAYS	MULT PROC	BILAT SURG	ASST SURG	CO-SURG	TEAM SURG
49324		010	3	0	2	2	0
49325		010	3	0	2	2	0
	49326	ZZZ	0	0	2	1	0

- Report 49327 in addition to a laparoscopic abdominal, pelvic, or retroperitoneal procedures, when performed at the same operative session.

Drainage of Fluid Collection, Image Guided (49405-49407)

Codes are available to report image guided percutaneous drainage of fluid collections within the body. These fluid collections may be hematomas, seromas, abscesses, lymphoceles, or cysts. Code selection is based upon anatomical location and the approach used to perform the procedure.

In 49405, a fluid collection in the visceral organs (kidney, liver, spleen, lung, mediastinum, etc.) is drained using a catheter. The area over the affected organ is cleansed and local anesthesia is administered. Imaging is performed to assist in the insertion of a needle or guidewire into the fluid collection. Small tissue samples may be collected from the site for pathological examination. A catheter is inserted to drain and collect the fluid for analysis. The catheter is removed. More imaging may be performed to ensure hemostasis. In 49406, a fluid collection in the peritoneum or retroperitoneum is drained using a catheter.

In 49407, a fluid collection in the peritoneum or retroperitoneum is drained via a vaginal or rectal approach. An intracavitary probe is used to create access through the rectal or vaginal wall. Imaging is performed to assist in the insertion of a needle or guidewire into the fluid collection. Small tissue samples may be collected from the site for pathological examination. A catheter is inserted to drain and collect the fluid for analysis and is then removed. In some cases, the catheter may be attached to a bag to allow for further drainage over the course of days.

Coding Tips

- These codes should be reported for each individual collection drained using a separate catheter. Append modifier 51 to subsequent procedures.

- For percutaneous, image guided drainage of soft tissue, see 10030.

- For diagnostic or therapeutic abdominal/peritoneal paracentesis or lavage, see 49082-49084.

▽YIELD AUDITOR'S ALERT

For drainage of a fluid collection, each collection drained using a separate catheter is reported. For multiple fluid collections/catheters, append a modifier 51 on subsequent procedures.

© 2020 Optum360, LLC

- The appropriate code for the open drainage of an abscess may be located by turning to the main term "Drainage," subterms "abscess" and the anatomical site (i.e., appendix, prostate, etc.) in the CPT index.

- To report percutaneous placement of a tunneled intraperitoneal catheter without a subcutaneous port, see 49418.

- To report percutaneous cholecystostomy, see 47490.

- Do not report 49405-49407 in conjunction with 75989, 76942, 77002-77003, 77012, or 77021.

Hernia Repair Open/Laparoscopic (49491–49590 and 49650–49659)

The codes used to report open surgical hernia repair are found in range 49491–49590. The codes for laparoscopic hernia repair are found in range 49650–49659. The intent of the surgical repair is to permanently close off the orifice through which the organs protrude.

Procedure Differentiation

Herniorrhaphy, herniotomy, and hernioplasty should be coded according to the type of hernia as follows:

- **Inguinal (49491–49525, 49650–49651):** Distinguish between recurrent, reducible, sliding, incarcerated, and strangulated. When none of these exists, choose the correct code based on the patient's age (younger than 5 years old or 5 years of age or older).

- **Lumbar (49540):** Lumbar hernias occur in the lateral abdominal wall. Lateral wall hernias are relatively uncommon, particularly those that occur naturally. Some protrude along old incisions made to access the kidney.

- **Femoral (49550–49557):** A femoral hernia is identified by whether it is recurrent, reducible, incarcerated, or strangulated.

- **Incisional or ventral (49560–49566, 49652–49657):** An incisional or ventral hernia is identified by whether it is recurrent, reducible, incarcerated, or strangulated.

- **Epigastric (49570–49572, 49652–49653):** An epigastric hernia is distinguished between reducible, incarcerated, and strangulated.

- **Umbilical (49580–49587, 49652–49653):** Umbilical hernias are distinguished by the patient's age (younger than 5 years old or 5 years of age or older), reducible, incarcerated, or strangulated.

- **Spigelian (49590, 49652–49653):** Spigelian hernias generally occur along the potentially weak lateral border of the rectus abdominis muscle.

When performing a hernia repair laparoscopically, some of the codes have been combined. For example, codes 49652–49653 describe epigastric, spigelian, umbilical, and ventral hernia repairs. Code selection is dependent upon whether the hernia is reducible (49652) or incarcerated or strangulated (49653). These codes also include mesh implantation.

Hernias can be defined as initial or recurrent, reducible, incarcerated, strangulated, or sliding.

A reducible hernia is one that may be manually returned to the correct anatomical position. Incarcerated or strangulated hernias result in a compromised blood supply to that area.

Incisional and ventral hernias may sometimes require a mesh implant (49568). Documentation for this procedure will state that the incision is closed with mesh or some other prosthetic material.

Coding Tip

- As an "add-on" code, 49568 is not subject to multiple procedure rules. No reimbursement reduction or modifier 51 is applied. The following table provides additional information for these codes as found in the Medicare Physician Fee Schedule Database.

Parent Code	Add-On	GLOB DAYS	MULT PROC	BILAT SURG	ASST SURG	CO-SURG	TEAM SURG
49560		090	2	1	2	1	0
49561		090	2	1	2	1	0
49565		090	2	1	2	1	0
49566		090	2	1	2	1	0
	49568	ZZZ	0	0	2	1	0

- When 49568 is performed bilaterally, it should be reported twice. Modifier 50 does not apply to add-on codes.

- Codes 49491–49561 are considered unilateral procedures. When open procedures 49491–49566, 49570–49590, and laparoscopic procedures 49650–49651 are performed bilaterally, modifier 50 should be appended to the procedure code.

DENIAL ALERT

If a hernia repair is performed at the site of an incision for an open or laparoscopic abdominal procedure, the hernia repair is not reported separately. An incidental hernia repair is not medically reasonable and necessary and will be denied by most payers.

Procedures Performed on the Urinary System

This subsection of the surgery section of the CPT book contains codes that are used to report procedures performed on the kidneys, ureter, bladder and urethra. Also included in this subsection are codes to report vesical neck and prostate procedures performed through a cystoscope (transurethral).

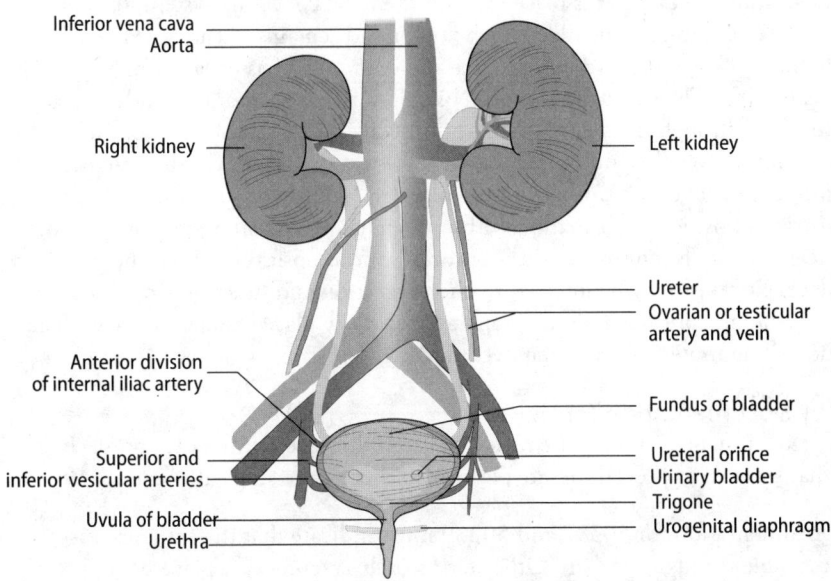

Labels on figure:
- Inferior vena cava
- Aorta
- Right kidney
- Left kidney
- Ureter
- Ovarian or testicular artery and vein
- Anterior division of internal iliac artery
- Fundus of bladder
- Superior and inferior vesicular arteries
- Ureteral orifice
- Urinary bladder
- Trigone
- Uvula of bladder
- Urethra
- Urogenital diaphragm

Kidney (50010–50593)

Codes within this range include drainage of renal abscess, nephrolithotomy procedures, biopsy and/or excision of lesions from the tumor, transplantation codes, renal catheter procedures, repair of injuries to the kidney, and laparoscopic and endoscopic procedures performed on the kidney.

Ureteral Stent Procedures (50382–50389)

Procedure Differentiation

Ureteral catheters are used to divert urine internally to the bladder or externally into a collection system. Renal pelvis catheter procedure code choice is determined by the following factors:

- Anatomical location of the stent
- If the stent is indwelling or externally accessible
- If replacement is performed
- Approach

Codes 50382–50386 are used to report internal dwelling procedures. In these procedures the stent is ureteral. Code 50384 is for removal only. Code 50382 is for removal and replacement of the ureteral stent. These procedures are performed percutaneously. When the approach is through the urethra, report 50385–50386. For these codes the documentation states that the physician removes (50386), or removes and replaces (50385) an internally dwelling

AUDITOR'S ALERT

Code 50382 is reported when the documentation indicates an internal double-J stent.

ureteral stent (a thin, flexible tube that is inserted into the ureter to help drain urine from the kidney). In one method, under appropriate sedation and sonographic guidance, a rigid biopsy forceps is introduced through the urethra and advanced to the urinary bladder, and the stent is grasped and removed. These codes are appropriate only when the procedure is performed via a transurethral approach, without the use of cystoscopy. Radiological supervision and interpretation is included and should not be reported separately.

Code 50387 reports removal and replacement of an externally accessible nephroureteral catheter, also referred to as an internal/external stent. A nephroureteral catheter is placed within the renal collecting system, through the renal pelvis and into the bladder; the other end remains outside the body for drainage. Contrast may be injected at the entry site to assess anatomy and positioning. The suture holding the pigtail in place is cut and a guidewire is threaded through the stent lumen until it exits the distal end. The original stent is removed over the guidewire. The new stent is threaded over the guidewire until the distal end forms within the bladder. Fluoroscopy is used to assess the proximal position of formation within the renal pelvis. After position is verified, the guidewire is removed and the suture is put in position to hold the pigtail in place. Contrast may be injected to check position and function. In 50389, an indwelling nephrostomy tube that was previously placed concurrently with an indwelling ureteral stent is removed under fluoroscopic guidance.

Key Documentation Terms
The documentation must be reviewed carefully to determine the approach and what services or procedures are performed during the surgical encounter.

Documentation for 50387 and 50389 must indicate that the catheter was accessible through the skin. Other terms such as removal, replacement, percutaneous, transnephric, or transurethral provide the guidance needed to ensure correct code assignment.

Coding Tips
- Codes 50382–50387 are unilateral procedures. If performed bilaterally, some payers require that the service be reported twice with modifier 50 appended to the second code while others require identification of the service only once with modifier 50 appended. Check with individual payers. Modifier 50 identifies a procedure performed identically on the opposite side of the body (mirror image).
- For externally accessible ureteral stent removal, report a code from the evaluation and management section if fluoroscopy is not required.
- Ureteral endoscopy is coded first, according to whether the procedure was performed through an established ureterostomy or through a ureterotomy. Additional codes are available when the ureteral endoscopy is performed in conjunction with another procedure, such as a ureteral catheterization, fulguration, or removal of calculus.

Coding Traps
- In the event that an externally accessible ureteral stent is removed and replaced through an ileal conduit or a ureterostomy, code 50688 should be reported.
- Removal of a nephrostomy tube without fluoroscopic guidance is considered part of an evaluation and management service and is not reported separately.

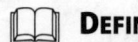

DEFINITIONS

nephr-. Relating to the kidney.

stent. Tube to provide support in a body cavity or lumen.

ureter. Tube leading from the kidney to the urinary bladder made up of three layers of tissue: the mucous lining of the inner layer; the smooth, muscular middle layer that propels the urine from the kidney to the bladder by peristalsis; and the outer layer made of fibrous connective tissue. Each ureter leaves the kidney from the hilum, a concave notch on the middle surface, and enters the bladder through a narrow valve-like orifice that prevents the backflow of urine to the kidney.

Endoscopic Procedures of Kidney via Nephrotomy/Pyelotomy Access (50551–50580)

Procedure Differentiation

Renal endoscopy code choice is determined by the following factors:

- Whether through established stoma or via an incision

- Other procedures performed during the endoscopy, including:
    - ureteral catheterization
    - biopsy and fulguration
    - removal of foreign body or calculus
    - insertion of radioactive substance
    - endopyelotomy
    - resection of tumor

Documentation should be reviewed to determine if the endoscope was passed through an established opening (50551–50562) or through an incision (50570–50580). Procedures are performed endoscopically when the documentation clearly states that an endoscope was passed through an established opening between the skin and kidney (nephrostomy) or renal pelvis (pyelostomy). Documentation for 50551 must state that the physician examined the kidney and ureter with an endoscope passed through an established opening between the skin and kidney (nephrostomy) or renal pelvis (pyelostomy). After inserting a guidewire, the physician removes the nephrostomy or pyelostomy tube and passes the endoscope through the opening into the kidney or renal pelvis. To better view renal and ureteric structures, the physician may flush (irrigate) or introduce by drops (instillate) a sterile saline solution. The physician may introduce contrast medium for radiologic study of the renal pelvis and ureter (ureteropyelogram). The physician removes the endoscope and guidewire and reinserts the nephrostomy tube or allows the surgical passageway to seal on its own. In 50553, documentation must indicate that a thin tube was passed through the endoscope into the ureter and when dilation is performed that a balloon catheter was inserted and inflated to dilate a ureteral constriction. In 50555, documentation must indicate that a cutting instrument was passed through the endoscope into the suspect renal tissue and excised (biopsied). However, when the documentation states that renal lesions were removed by electric current or by incision, report 50557. Documentation for 50561 must state that the removal of a foreign body or stone occurred through the scope. Documentation indicating the resection of a tumor (50562) must state that the tumor was removed by cold-cup biopsy forceps with the bulk of the tumor being grasped and then removed in piecemeal fashion until the base is reached. A cutting loop is used to remove the tumor at its base or the tumor may be ablated using a YAG laser.

Documentation indicating that the scope was passed through an incision must state that an incision in the skin of the flank was made and that the endoscope was guided through the incision. To better view renal and ureteric structures, the physician may flush (irrigate) or introduce by drops (instillate) a sterile saline solution or contrast medium (50570). In 50572, supporting documentation must indicate that a thin tube was passed through the endoscope into the ureter, and may or may not indicate that the physician inserted a balloon catheter to dilate a ureteral constriction. In 50574, documentation must state that the physician passed a cutting instrument through the endoscope into the suspect renal tissue and took a biopsy specimen. For endopyelotomy (50575),

 DEFINITIONS

nephrostomy. Placement of a stent, tube, or catheter that forms a passage from the exterior of the body into the renal pelvis or calyx, often for drainage of urine or an abscess, for exploration, or calculus extraction.

pyelostomy. Surgical creation of an opening through the abdominal wall into the renal pelvis.

ureterostomy. Placement of a stent, tube, or catheter into the ureter, forming a passageway from the exterior of the body to the ureter.

ureterotomy. Incision made into the ureter for accomplishing a variety of procedures such as exploration, drainage, instillation, ureteropyelography, catheterization, dilation, biopsy, or foreign body removal.

documentation must indicate that the physician placed an endoscope through the ureter and/or pelvis, incised the pelvis, enlarged the ureteropelvic junction, and sutured the junction as in a Y-V pyeloplasty. The physician inserts the stent through the renal pelvis into the junction, sutures the incisions, inserts a drain tube, and performs a layered closure.

Documentation for 50576 and 57580 are similar to that of 50557 and 50561, only documentation must indicate that the scope was passed through an incision.

Key Documentation Terms

Documentation should indicate the surgical procedure that was performed. Terms such as instillation, ureteral catheterization, dilation, biopsy, fulguration, foreign body, calculus, or tumor provide the guidance needed to ensure correct code assignment. Above all else, the documentation should support the medical necessity of the procedure.

Coding Tips

- If the nephrotomy or pyelotomy is done for an additional, significantly identifiable endoscopic service, report both the appropriate endoscopic procedure code (50570–50580) and 50045 or 50120.

- If the renal endoscopy is performed through a ureterotomy, nephrotomy, or pyelotomy, an additional code may be used for the ureterotomy, nephrotomy, or pyelotomy when these procedures provide a significant identifiable service.

- Renal endoscopy with endopyelotomy (50575) includes cystoscopy, ureteroscopy, dilation of pelvic junction and ureter, incision of ureteral pelvic junction, and insertion of endopyelotomy stent.

- Radiological services performed with endoscopies (50551–50580) are reported separately.

Procedures Performed on the Bladder (51020–52700)

Uroflowmetric Evaluations (51725–51798)

The urodynamics section includes procedures that can be provided separately or in combination with other procedures. Read the operative report carefully before assigning codes.

Procedure Differentiation

Cystometrogram (CMG) is reported with 51725–51729 according to the type of procedure (simple or complex) and the other services included in the code descriptor. A simple CMG is reported with 51725; complex, see 51726. Documentation for code 51725 must indicate that a pressure catheter was inserted into the bladder and connected to a manometer line filled with fluid to measure pressure and flow. When the documentation indicates that a transurethral catheter was inserted, that the bladder was filled with water or gas simultaneously obtaining rectal pressure, report 51726.

Codes 51727–51729 describe a complex cystometrogram (i.e., calibrated electronic equipment) with urethral pressure profile studies, voiding pressure studies, or a combination of voiding and urethral pressure studies, any method, respectively.

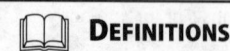
DEFINITIONS

cystometrogram. Recorded measurement of bladder pressure from multiple volume amounts.

nephrotomy. Incision into the body of the kidney.

pyelotomy. Incision or opening made into the renal pelvis. Pyelotomies are performed to accomplish other procedures such as exploration, drainage, removal of a kidney stone, instill medication, or perform ureteropyelography or renal endoscopy. The pyelotomy is included as part of the procedure or method of access.

ureterotomy. Incision made into the ureter for accomplishing a variety of procedures such as exploration, drainage, instillation, ureteropyelography, catheterization, dilation, biopsy, or foreign body removal.

urethral pressure profile. Measures urethral pressure by pulling a transducer through the urethra and noting pressure change.

Documentation supporting 51727 must state that the complex cystometrogram was performed in conjunction with a study measuring urethral pressure while the patient performed instructions, such as coughing or the Valsalva maneuver.

Voiding studies (51728) documentation must indicate that a transducer was placed into the bladder and the patient was instructed to attempt to void upon feeling bladder fullness. Recordings are taken of the bladder sensation and volume at specific intervals. In 51729, documentation must indicate that the cystometrogram was performed in conjunction with the voiding pressure and urethral pressure profile studies.

Voiding pressure studies performed intra-abdominally are reported with add-on code 51797 for use with 51728–51729.

Uroflowmetry (UFR) is reported with 51736–51741, depending on mechanical or electronic monitoring. Documentation for a simple flowmetry procedure (51736) must indicate that the service was performed without automated equipment. When the documentation indicates that calibrated electronic equipment was used, code 51741 is supported.

EMG studies are reported with 51784–51785, depending on needle use. In 51784, documentation must indicate that electrodes were placed in the anal or urethral sphincter to study the electrical activity. However, when needles are placed, report 51785.

Stimulus evoked response is reported with 51792. Documentation must indicate that the physician electrically stimulates the head of the penis. The physician measures the delay time for travel of stimulation through the pelvic nerves to the pudendal nerve.

Postvoiding residual urine measurement is reported with 51798. Documentation must indicate that residual urine and/or bladder capacity was measured by ultrasound after the patient had voided. A portable ultrasound scanner is used for this purpose. Operation of the scanner is done simply by directing the scanning head over the suprapubic area while the patient is lying down in the supine position. The software built in to the scanner calculates the postvoid residual urine volume immediately and also does calculations for the bladder capacity based on the individual's bladder shape and not on fixed geometric formulas.

Medical Necessity

These procedures are commonly performed to assist in the diagnosis of urologic dysfunction. These tests are generally a covered benefit when the following apply:

- Uncertain diagnosis and inability to develop an appropriate treatment plan based on the basic diagnostic evaluation above.

- Failure to respond to an adequate therapeutic trial.

- Consideration of urologic surgical intervention, particularly if previous surgery failed or if the patient is a high surgical risk.

- Presence of other comorbid conditions such as:

    - abnormal postvoid residual urinalysis

    - asymmetry or other suspicion of prostate cancer

    - history of previous anti-incontinence surgery or radical pelvic surgery

DEFINITIONS

transducer. Apparatus that transfers or translates one type of energy into another, such as converting pressure to an electrical signal.

DENIAL ALERT

Code 51784 or 51785 should not be reported unless a significant, separately identifiable diagnostic EMG service is provided. If either 51784 or 51785 is reported for a diagnostic electromyogram, a separate report must be in the medical record to indicate that the service was performed for diagnostic purposes, or it may result in a denial. Payers may require modifier 59.

- incontinence associated with recurrent symptomatic urinary tract infection
- neurological conditions affecting voiding function such as multiple sclerosis and spinal cord lesions or injury
- persistent symptoms of difficult bladder emptying
- prostate nodule
- symptomatic pelvic prolapse
- Urinary incontinence

Key Documentation Terms

Documentation should indicate the surgical procedure that was performed. Terms such as cystometrogram/CMG, electromyography/EMG, uroflowmetry/UFR, voiding pressure studies, simple, or complex provide the guidance needed to ensure correct code assignment. Above all else, the documentation should support the medical necessity of the procedure.

Coding Tip

- As an "add-on" code, 51797 is not subject to multiple procedure rules. No reimbursement reduction or modifier 51 is applied. The following table provides additional information for these codes as found in the Medicare Physician Fee Schedule Database.

Parent Code	Add-On	GLOB DAYS	MULT PROC	BILAT SURG	ASST SURG	CO-SURG	TEAM SURG
51728		000	2	0	0	0	0
51729		000	2	0	0	0	0
	51797	ZZZ	0	0	0	0	0

Billing and Payment Issues

When multiple procedures are performed, report secondary procedures with modifier 51.

This subset of CPT codes includes the technical, as well as the professional components. If the physician performs the procedure or the interpretation only, without all of the supplies, the service should be reported with modifier 26.

Urinary Endoscopic Procedures (52000–52010)

Codes for cystoscopy and urethroscopy are combined under the term "cystourethroscopy." The CPT coding system provides a code for cystourethroscopy when the procedure is performed alone (i.e., a separate procedure). However, since cystourethroscopy is often performed with other surgical procedures (ureteral catheterization, biopsy, resection of bladder tumors, etc.), the coder must choose carefully among the many codes available to describe the purpose and site of the cystourethroscopy. Careful selection is necessary when reporting cystoscopy procedures since the cystourethroscope is employed to perform procedures on the urethra, bladder, ureter, pelvis, vesical neck, and prostate. The anatomical structures as well as the condition all play major factors in correct code assignment.

Procedure Differentiation

A cystoscopy is the visual examination of the urethra, bladder, and ureteric openings into the bladder through an endoscope. Correct code assignment is dependent upon whether the procedure is diagnostic (52000) or surgical and, if surgical, what surgical procedures are performed.

Surgical Service	Code
Irrigation	52001
Evacuation of clots	52001
Ureteral catheterization	52005
Brush biopsy	52007
Catheterization ejaculatory duct	52010

Key Documentation Terms

The table below identifies key terms that may support the code identified.

Term	Procedure Code
Irrigated, suction, laser guide, evacuate, obstructing clots	52001
Introduction contrast dye, insertion of catheter into ureter, pyelogram, retrograde pyelogram	52005
Renal pelvis, ureter, brush biopsy	52007
Catheterization, ejaculatory duct, introduction contrast dye, insertion catheter ejaculatory duct	52010

Transurethral Surgery (52204–52356)

Transurethral surgical procedures also enlist the cystourethroscope to accomplish the procedure. This heading is divided into two sections: urethra and bladder and ureter and pelvis.

Procedure Differentiation

The operative report should be carefully reviewed to determine what surgical procedures were performed during the operative session. The table below assists in assigning the correct code for cystourethroscopy procedures.

Procedure	Code
Biopsy	
Urethra and bladder	52204
Ureter or renal pelvic	52354
Dilation	
Bladder	52260–52265
Intrarenal	52343, 52346
Ureteral	52341, 52344
Urethral	52281, 52285
Ureteropelvic	52342, 52345
Diverticulum	
Bladder	52305
Excision	
Urethra and bladder	
Minor lesions	52224
Small bladder tumor	52234
Medium bladder tumor	52235
Large bladder tumor	52240
Ureteral or renal pelvic	52355

 DENIAL ALERT

Cystourethroscopy with biopsy(s) (52204) includes all the biopsies performed in the same operative session and will be denied unless it has a unit of "1."

Procedure	Code
Fulguration	
Bladder neck	52214
Ureteral or renal pelvis	52354
Lesions	
Bladder and urethra	52214–52240, 52285
Ureter	52300, 52301
Periurethral glands	52214
Prostatic fossa	52214
Trigone	52214
Urethra	52214
Injection	
Chemodenervation, bladder	52287
Radiocontrast, radiologic study, bladder	52281
Into urethral/bladder stricture	52283
Subureteric implant material	52327
Insertion	
Guidewire	52334
Stent	
Urethra	52282
Ureter	52332
Lithotripsy	
Ureter and Pelvis	52353, 52356
Manipulation	
Ureteral calculus	52330, 52352
Nephrostomy tube (percutaneous)	52334
Pyeloscopy	52351
Radioactive substance	52250
Removal	
Calculus	
Urethra or bladder	52310–52315
Ureter and pelvis	52320–52325, 52352
By litholapaxy	52317–52318
Foreign Body	52310–52315
Stent	
Ureteral	52310–52315, 52356
Sphincterotomy	52277
Ureter Surgery	
Meatotomy	52281, 52290
Ureterocele	52300–52301
Urethral syndrome	52285
Ureteroscopy	52351
Urethrotomy	52270–52276

Key Documentation Terms

In order to assign the most appropriate code, the medical record documentation must be reviewed to determine why the procedure was performed (e.g., for removal of a foreign body, biopsy, excision of tumor, lithotripsy, dilation, or insertion of stent into the urethra, bladder, ureter, or renal pelvis).

Coding Tips

- When endoscopic visualization of the urinary system involves several regions (e.g., kidney, renal pelvis, calyx, and ureter), the approach (e.g., nephrostomy, pyelostomy, ureterostomy, etc.) is used to determine appropriate code assignment.

- In the event that multiple endoscopic approaches are necessary (e.g., renal endoscopy through a nephrostomy and cystourethroscopy) during the same surgical session to perform different surgical procedures, report the services separately using the appropriate CPT code and append modifier 51 to the less extensive procedure codes. However, it should be noted that when multiple endoscopic approaches are utilized to attempt the same procedure, only the completed approach is reported.

- When radiological supervision and interpretation is performed during the same encounter as 52010, report with code 74440.

- Report 52351 when documentation indicates that a diagnostic cystourethroscopy and ureteroscopy and/or pyeloscopy was performed during the same surgical session.

- Cystourethroscopy with biopsy(s) (52204) includes all biopsies during the procedure and should be reported with one unit of service.

- When a diagnostic endoscopy results in the performance of a laparoscopic or open procedure, the diagnostic endoscopy may be reported separately with modifier 58 appended.

- When an endoscopic procedure is converted to an open procedure, report only the appropriate code describing the open procedure.

- Code 52332 Cystourethroscopy, with insertion of indwelling ureteral stent, should not be used to report a temporary ureteral stent inserted and removed during a diagnostic or therapeutic cystourethroscopy with ureteroscopy and/or pyeloscopy (codes 52320–52330, 52334–52355). Do not report 52005 or 52007 with these procedures.

- Code 52353 should be reported with only one unit of service (UOS) per ureter. If the procedure is performed on bilateral ureters, it may be reported with one UOS and modifier 50. This code should not be reported with a separate UOS for each calculus.

- A diagnostic endoscopy is not reported separately. If a diagnostic endoscopy leads to a surgical endoscopy at the same patient encounter, only the surgical endoscopy may be reported.

- When multiple endoscopic procedures are performed at the same patient encounter, the most comprehensive code accurately describing the service(s) performed should be reported. If several procedures not included in a more comprehensive code are performed at the same endoscopic session, multiple HCPCS/CPT codes may be reported with modifier 51. For example, if renal endoscopy is performed through an established nephrostomy with biopsy, fulguration of a lesion, and foreign body (calculus) removal, the following codes would be reported: 50557 and 50561–51, not codes 50551, 50555, 50557, and 50561. This policy

AUDITOR'S ALERT

When an endoscopic procedure is performed as an integral part of an open procedure (such as a scout endoscopy), only the open procedure is reportable.

applies to all endoscopic procedures, not only those of the genitourinary system.

- For urethral therapeutic drug delivery via cystourethroscopy, see 0499T.

Coding Traps

- The insertion and removal of a temporary ureteral catheter during diagnostic or therapeutic cystourethroscopy is an integral part of 52320–52356 and should not be reported.

- Cystourethroscopy and transurethral procedures include fluoroscopy when performed. CPT codes describing fluoroscopy or fluoroscopic guidance (e.g., 76000, 77002) should not be reported separately with a cystourethroscopy or transurethral procedure code.

Endoscopic Procedures via Urethra: Prostate and Vesical Neck (52400–52700)

This subsection includes codes for reporting a transurethral resection of the prostate (TURP). Correct code assignment depends on whether the resection requires one or more operative sessions.

Procedure Differentiation

The code used for a complete TURP procedure (including vasectomy, meatotomy, cystourethroscopy, urethral calibration and/or dilation, and internal urethrotomy) and two-stage resection are all reported with 52601.

It is important to code the different stages of transurethral partial resection of the prostate correctly:

- First stage should be reported as 52601

- Second stage should be reported as 52601 with modifier 58 appended

- Regrowth or residual of prostate obstructive tissue should be reported with 52630

Contracture of the bladder neck outlet usually occurs from scarring after a transurethral resection of the prostate. Transurethral resection of the bladder neck obstruction is reported using 52640.

Laser coagulation, vaporization or enucleation of the prostate is reported using 52647–52649. Documentation must indicate that a laser was used to coagulate (52647), vaporize (52648), or enucleate (52649) the prostate through an endoscope or resectoscope inserted through the urethra. Documentation may also indicate that the physician performed a vasectomy, meatotomy, cystourethroscopy, urethral calibration/dilation, transurethral resection, or internal urethrotomy or a combination of these services.

Code 52647 may also be referred to as visual laser ablation of the prostate (VLAP) and utilizes a transurethral approach with a rigid cystoscope, YAG continuous wave laser, and dilation of the urethra. A laser is inserted through a cystoscope, and the physician directs the laser onto the prostate, without allowing the laser to touch the prostate tissue. In this procedure, the effects of the laser procedure cannot be visualized during the operative session. The prostate will shrink and slough tissue over a period of weeks. This is typically performed for patients who have benign hypertrophy of the prostate (BHP).

Transurethral vapor resection of the prostate (TUVRP), also known as electrovaporization of the prostate, is reported with 52648. Documentation

DEFINITIONS

enucleate. Removal of a growth or organ cleanly so as to extract it in one piece.

AUDITOR'S ALERT

Code 52647 describes noncontact laser coagulation of the prostate. Code 52648 describes contact laser vaporization. Both of these procedures may require the physician to make a small incision. It should also be noted that if a small amount of contact laser vaporization is performed during laser coagulation, code 52648 should not be reported.

must indicate that a laser is inserted through a cystoscope, and the physician allowed the laser to touch the prostate where it immediately began to destroy the hypertrophied tissue. Unlike the noncontact laser coagulation procedure, the effects of the procedure can be visualized during the operative session.

For other approaches for resection of the prostate, see 55801–55845. In addition, transurethral surgery can be performed on the urethra and bladder, as well as ureter and pelvis. Identify the primary site before selecting a code.

Medical Necessity

Most payers consider laser prostatectomy medically necessary for the treatment of bladder neck obstruction secondary to benign prostatic hyperplasia (BPH).

Most often these procedures will be covered for the following indications:

- American Urology Association (AUA) symptom score greater than nine
- Duration of BPH three months or longer
- Urodynamics and Post-void Residual Volume examinations used as appropriate (e.g., patients with suspected neurologic disease or those who have failed prostate surgery)

Key Documentation Terms

Documentation should indicate the surgical procedure that was performed. Terms such as coagulate, enucleate, vaporize, meatotomy, cystourethroscopy, resection, urethral calibration/dilation, or internal urethrotomy provide the guidance needed to ensure correct code assignment.

In addition to the documentation supporting the procedure reported, it is important that the medical record indicate the diagnosis, the duration of the condition, AUA symptoms index, and the urodynamics studies and/or postvoid residual volume results if performed.

Coding Tip
- For open excisional procedures on the prostate gland, see 55801–55845.

Coding Trap
- Endoscopic procedures include all minor related functions performed at the same encounter. For example, transurethral resection of the prostate includes:
    - meatotomy
    - ureteral calibration and/or dilation
    - urethroscopy
    - cystoscopy

These services are not usually reported separately. However, if significant additional time and effort is documented, modifier 22 may be appended. A cover letter and operative report should accompany the claim in these instances.

Procedures Performed on the Male Genital System

The male genital system contains codes for reporting procedures on the penis, testis, epididymis, tunica vaginalis, scrotum, vas deferens, spermatic cord, seminal vesicles, and prostate.

Biopsy and Resection: Testis (54500–54535)

Procedure Differentiation

Correct code selection is dependent upon the nature of the procedure being performed. For example, when coding a biopsy, determine the type (needle, incisional, or excisional) of biopsy performed. Orchiectomy code selection is dependent upon the complexity of the procedure.

As indicated above, orchiectomy code selection is dependent upon the complexity of the procedure. Documentation supporting code 54520 must indicate that an incision was made in one side of the scrotum and removed the testis after the spermatic cord was opened and the individual bundles making up the cord were cross-clamped, cut, and secured with nonabsorbable suture material. Alternatively, this code is also supported when documentation indicates that an incision in the groin was made and the testis is pulled up through the incision after cutting and tying the cord in a fashion similar to the scrotal approach.

Documentation supporting code 54522 must state that a partial excision of one testis or both testes was performed. A longitudinal incision midline in the scrotum is made to expose the testis. The tunica vaginalis is incised, and the testicular vessels and vas deferens are identified, clamped separately, and divided. The cords are ligated at a level slightly above the area of infection, abscess, neoplasm, or trauma and the spermatic cord is isolated for manipulation of the testicle. The testis is delivered to the wound and dissected below the ligated cords.

Documentation indicating that a radical orchiectomy (54530) was performed must indicate the removal en bloc the contents of half of the scrotum. A deep incision is made in the inguinal area from the pubic bone up toward the lateral pelvic bone and the spermatic cord is dissected free and cross-clamped. The testis and all its associated structures are pushed up from the scrotum into the incision and removed. Packing is then placed in the empty scrotum. When the spermatic cord is opened and the individual bundles making up the cord are cross-clamped, cut, and secured with nonabsorbable suture material, care is taken to avoid important nerves and vessels in the area. Code 54535 is supported when documentation states that a midline incision is made from the upper to the lower abdomen and the abdominal cavity is entered. The back wall of the abdomen is exposed and the lymph nodes are checked for spread of tumor. Some may be removed and/or biopsied and the abdominal wound is closed in multiple layers by suturing.

Key Documentation Terms

Documentation should indicate the surgical procedure that was performed. Terms such as biopsy, excision, simple, partial, radical, or with abdominal exploration provide the guidance needed to ensure correct code assignment. Above all else, the documentation should support the medical necessity of the procedure.

Coding Tips

- A vasotomy for vasogram performed in addition to the incisional biopsy of the testis is reported as follows: 55300, 54505–51, and 74440 for the supervision and interpretation (S&I) of the vasogram.

- For repair of strangulated organs or structures, such as testis and truncus vaginalis, code the repair of the organ in addition to the repair of the hernia.

Coding Traps

- For laparoscopic orchiectomy, see 54690.

- Code 54660 for the insertion of a testicular prosthesis when performed during the same operative session should be reported with modifier 59 appended when appropriate.

Open Testicular Procedures (54600–54680)

Procedure Differentiation

Orchiopexy, suspension and fixation of testis, is reported with 54640–54650, according to inguinal or abdominal approach. Insertion of a testicular prosthesis is reported with 54660. Repair of a wound or an injury to the testes is reported with 54670. When the scrotum is damaged or destroyed, the testes may be transplanted to the thigh (54680).

Torsion of the testes is a twisting, turning, or rotation of the testicle upon itself, so as to compromise or cut off the blood supply. Torsion of testis that is surgically reduced is reported with 54600 for one or both testes repaired in the same session. If the contralateral testis is fixated at another operative session, code 54620 should be reported.

Orchiopexy is the surgical fixation of an undescended testicle into the scrotum.

In 54640, an incision is made in the scrotum or the inguinal area from the pubic bone to the upper lateral pelvic area in the skin crease made by the thigh and the lower abdomen. The physician searches for a testis that failed to descend into the scrotum during development. The tissues are separated by dissection to find the testis in the inguinal canal area. The spermatic cord is mobilized to allow positioning of the testis in the scrotum. In the scrotum, a small pouch is created for the testis where the testis is sutured in place to prevent retraction back into the inguinal canal. The incision is closed in layers by suturing.

When 54650 is performed, documentation must state that an incision was made in the inguinal area from the pubic bone to the upper lateral pelvic area or in the skin fold made by the thigh and the lower abdomen. The physician searches the abdominal cavity for a testis that failed to descend into the scrotum during development. The tissues are separated by dissection and the incision is extended into the abdominal cavity to find the testis in the abdominal area. The tissues are separated by dissection to find the testis in the area. At this point several surgical options are available. The one chosen depends on the mobility of the testis and how far it can be brought down through the inguinal canal and into the scrotum. The procedure may take two stages approximately six to 12 months apart. Eventually, the spermatic cord is mobilized sufficiently to allow positioning of the testis in the scrotum. In the scrotum a small pouch is created for the testis where the testis is sutured in place to prevent retraction back into the inguinal canal or into the abdominal cavity.

 DEFINITIONS

inguinal. Within the groin region.

orchiopexy. Surgical fixation of an undescended testicle within the scrotum.

Key Documentation Terms

Documentation should indicate the surgical procedure that was performed. Terms such as torsion, fixation, abdominal approach, inguinal approach, insertion, suture, or transplantation provide the guidance needed to ensure correct code assignment. Above all else, the documentation should support the medical necessity of the procedure.

Coding Tips

- If documentation states that a strangulated testis due to an inguinal hernia is excised and the hernia is surgically repaired, report 54520 and 49507.

- Orchiopexy procedures are unilateral procedures. If performed bilaterally, some payers require that the service be reported twice with modifier 50 appended to the second code while others require identification of the service only once with modifier 50 appended. Check with individual payers. Modifier 50 identifies a procedure performed identically on the opposite side of the body (mirror image).

- When documentation indicates a laparoscopic approach at the time of an orchiopexy, see 54692.

- For exploration of undescended testis only, see 54550–54560.

Coding Traps

- Codes 54620 and 54660 are separate procedures by definition and are usually a component of a more complex service and is not identified separately. When performed alone or with other unrelated procedures/services it may be reported. If performed alone, list the code; if performed with other procedures/services, list the code and append modifier 59.

- Some payers may consider code 54660 a cosmetic procedure and therefore the procedure may be noncovered. Check with payer guidelines for their specific policies.

Procedures Performed on the Tunica Vaginalis (55000–55060)

Procedure Differentiation

The tunica vaginalis is the serous membrane that partially covers the testes formed by an outpocketing of the peritoneum when the testes descend.

The procedures in this section include aspiration, excision, and repair of a hydrocele. Pay close attention to the type of procedure performed and whether it was performed unilaterally or bilaterally as it is important in ensuring correct code selection.

When documentation indicates that a needle was inserted into a hydrocele of the tunica vaginalis and fluid was aspirated (including injection of medications), code 55000 is supported. However, when documentation states that an incision is made and the hydrocele is dissected free while care is taken to keep the hydrocele intact, code 55040 is appropriate when performed unilateral, or 55041 when performed bilaterally.

Documentation supporting 55060 must indicate that the physician treated a hydrocele by removing the abnormal fluid filled sac in the scrotum or in the inguinal canal. After injecting an area with local anesthetic and using aseptic techniques, the physician makes an incision in the scrotum or in the inguinal area. Care is taken to keep the hydrocele intact while it is dissected free of its attachments to the testis and other structures. The sac is opened high along its front surface and the testis is pushed up through the sac and out through the incision. This inverts the hydrocele sac, which is tacked by suturing to the spermatic cord structures behind the testis. The testis is returned to the scrotum and is anchored to the inside of the scrotum with three sutures to prevent later torsion or twisting of the testis. A rubber drain may be left in the scrotum and the incision closed in layers by suturing.

Key Documentation Terms
Documentation should indicate the surgical procedure and support the medical necessity of the procedure performed. Terms such as aspiration, drainage, excision, or repair provide the guidance needed to ensure correct code assignment.

Coding Tips
- When documentation indicates that the hydrocele of the spermatic cord is excised see 55500.

- Careful attention to the type of hydrocele is necessary for correct ICD-10-CM code assignment. There are many types of hydroceles, including female, infected, newborn (congenital), and encysted.

Coding Trap
- The puncture aspiration of a hydrocele (e.g., code 55000) is included in services involving the tunica vaginalis and proximate anatomy (e.g., scrotum, vas deferens) and in inguinal hernia repairs and should not be reported separately.

Procedures of the Male Genital Duct (55200–55400)
The vas deferens is a duct that arises in the tail of the epididymis and stores and carries sperm from the epididymis toward the urethra. The vas deferens is part of the spermatic cord.

Procedure Differentiation
Incision, including cannulization, unilateral or bilateral, is reported with 55200. A vasectomy performed either unilateral or bilateral, is reported with 55250. Report 55300 for a vasotomy for vasograms, seminal vesiculograms, or epididymograms, unilateral or bilateral. Repair or suture of the vas deferens is reported with 55400.

Documentation for 55200 must indicate that the physician entered the vas deferens (the tube that carries spermatozoa from the testis) for purposes of obtaining a sample of semen or testing the patency of the tubes. Under local anesthesia, an incision is made in the upper outer scrotum overlying the spermatic cord. The tissues are dissected to expose the vas deferens. The tube is entered by puncturing with a small needle and fluid samples removed or solution injected to check for blockages. An alternate method involves the tube being cut open with a scalpel. A blunt needle is placed in the tube under direct vision and fluid samples removed or the tube checked for patency. If an incision is made in the tube, the tube must be repaired using microsurgical techniques before the scrotal incisions are closed in layers by suturing.

Documentation supporting 55250 must indicate that the physician grasped the upper scrotum near the inguinal area and held the spermatic cord between the thumb and the index finger. The skin overlying the immobilized cord is injected with a local anesthetic and an incision is made through the scrotal wall to expose the tubular structures. Another incision is made to expose the vas deferens

DEFINITIONS

cannula. Tube inserted into a blood vessel, duct, or body cavity to facilitate passage.

hydrocele. Serous fluid that collects in the tunica vaginalis, the spermatic cord, or the canal of Nuck. Hydroceles may be congenital, due to a defect in the tunica vaginalis, or secondary, due to fluid accumulation, injury, infection, or radiotherapy.

scrotum. Skin pouch that holds the testes and supporting reproductive structures.

(spermatic tube) and the tissues dissected to free it from the adjacent vessels and supporting tissues. The isolated vas deferens is cut in two places and the intervening section of tube is removed. The cut ends of the vas deferens are cauterized and tied with suture material. The incisions are closed in layers by suturing. The procedure is usually repeated on the opposite side.

Documentation indicating that a vasotomy (55300) was performed must state that the physician entered the vas deferens (the tube that carries spermatozoa from the testis) for purposes of testing the patency of the spermatozoa collecting system. An incision is made in the upper outer scrotum overlying the spermatic cord and the tissues dissected to expose the vas deferens.

Documentation for 55400 must indicate that a blockage in the vas deferens was surgically treated. Dye injection studies and semen sampling is often done during the operation to determine the site of the blockage and to accurately choose the segment of tube for excision. The vas deferens is transected in two places, one on each side of the blocked area, and the abnormal segment removed. The created cut ends are sutured together in one or two layers with care to align accurately the lumens of the tubes. The testis and associated structures are returned to the scrotum. A rubber drain is often placed in the scrotum and the incisions closed by suturing.

Key Documentation Terms
Documentation should indicate the surgical procedure that was performed. Terms such as blockage or patency provide the guidance needed to ensure correct code assignment. Above all else, the documentation should support the medical necessity of the procedure.

Coding Tip
- Code 55400 is unilateral. When performed bilaterally, append modifier 50 to the procedure code.

Coding Traps
- Postoperative semen evaluations are an integral part of code 55250.
- Codes 55200 and 55250 are separate procedures by definition and are usually a component of a more complex service and are not identified separately. When performed alone or with other unrelated procedures/services they may be reported. If performed alone, list the code; if performed with other procedures/services, list the code and append modifier 59.

Resection: Spermatic Cord (55500–55540)
This subsection includes excision of a lesion, hydrocele (a confined collection of fluid in the tunica vaginalis of the testicle or spermatic cord), or varicocele (an abnormal dilation of the veins of the spermatic cord in the scrotum).

Procedure Differentiation
Excision of a hydrocele of the spermatic cord, unilateral, is reported with 55500. If performed bilaterally, report 55500 with modifier 50. Excision of a lesion of the spermatic cord is reported with 55520. Excision of a varicocele or ligation of spermatic veins is reported with 55530–55540, according to approach or concurrent hernia repair.

DEFINITIONS

varicocele. Abnormal dilation of the veins of the spermatic cord in the scrotum, most commonly seen on the left side, that prevents proper blood flow, which leads to swelling and widening of the veins, essentially creating varicose veins. Varicoceles are slow to develop, typically seen in males between the ages of 15 and 25 and are very often a cause of male infertility.

Key Documentation Terms

Terms such as excision, hernia repair, hydrocele, lesion, or varicocele provide the guidance needed to ensure correct code assignment.

Coding Tip

- Laparoscopic ligation of spermatic veins is reported with 55550.

Coding Traps

- When a lipoma of the spermatic cord is excised during an inguinal hernia repair, do not assign 55520 to indicate the excision. The excision is performed commonly as an integral part of an inguinal hernia repair and is not reported separately.

- Codes 55500–55540 are separate procedures by definition and are usually a component of a more complex service and are not identified separately. When performed alone or with other unrelated procedures or services they may be reported. If performed alone, list the code; if performed with other procedures or services, list the code and append modifier 59.

Procedures Performed on the Prostate (55700–55866)

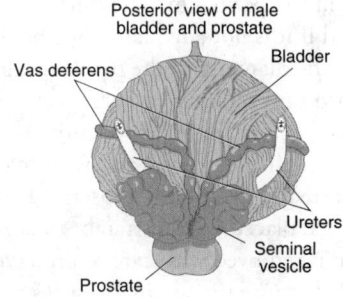

Procedure Differentiation

To select a code for biopsy of the prostate, check the operative notes to determine whether the procedure was performed by needle or punch (55700), incision (55705), or with stereotactic guidance (55706).

For simple incision and drainage of an abscess, report 55720; when complicated, report 55725. Transurethral drainage is reported with 52700.

When documentation indicates that a biopsy needle was passed into the suspect area of the prostate through the skin of the perineum, report 55700. However, when documentation states that the prostate was approached by an incision through the skin of the perineum or through the rectum, report 55705. Documentation for 55706 must indicate that the physician used stereotactic template-guided saturation sampling biopsies to map prostate cancer in high-risk patients. Transrectal ultrasound is used to visualize the prostate. Zones or reference planes of the prostate are determined, and a brachytherapy grid is placed against the perineum and rectum. Using the transperineal route under ultrasonic guidance, multiple biopsies are taken of the prostate. Typically, from 20 to 40 biopsies are taken using the grid as a guide, beginning at the highest point in the prostate and moving right to left in a row, down row by row until the grid is complete. In deeper planes, both a proximal and distal biopsy may be obtained. Each biopsy sample is marked for its coordinates, and all are mapped in 3D to determine the extent and exact position of malignant cells.

Documentation supporting drainage of a prostate abscess must indicate that the physician performed a simple prostatotomy (cutting or puncturing the prostate) through one of two usual approaches. An aspirating needle is passed into the abscessed area of the prostate by puncturing through skin of the perineum (the area between the base of the scrotum and the anus), or by advancing the needle into the rectum by guidance with the index finger and puncturing through the rectal mucosa. The needle is inserted into the abscess in the prostate guided by an index finger or by ultrasound and the contents of the abscess removed by aspiration. The needle is withdrawn and the puncture site bandaged. Report 55720 for simple drainage or 55725 if the procedure is complicated by excessive bleeding, infection, or other problem.

Prostatectomy (55801–55866)

Excision of the prostate, other than by transurethral methods, is reported with 55801–55845. Before assigning a code, determine the approach (perineal or retropubic), extent (radical or subtotal), method (one or two stages), and whether lymphadenectomy was performed.

Documentation for a subtotal perineal prostatectomy (55801) must indicate that the physician performed a prostatectomy (removal of the prostate gland) through an incision made in the perineum. The caliber (internal diameter) of the urethra is measured and if it is not adequate, the opening of the urethra is enlarged (meatotomy) and the diameter of the penile urethra is enlarged with an instrument (internal urethrotomy). A curved instrument (Lowery Tractor) is advanced up the urethra to the prostate to help identify the structures and aid in the dissection. Through the perineal incision and with manipulation of the tractor, the tissues are dissected to expose the prostate. The curved tractor instrument in the urethra is replaced with a straight tractor. A portion of the prostate or the entire gland is removed with care to preserve the seminal vesicles. The operation is "subtotal" because the seminal vesicles remain intact. The bladder outlet is revised and the vas deferens is ligated and may be partially removed (vasectomy). Bleeding is controlled by ligation or cautery. A Foley catheter is placed in the bladder. A rubber drain may be placed in the site of the operative wound and brought out through a separate stab wound. The dissected tissues and the skin incision are closed in layers by suturing.

Documentation indicating that a perineal radical prostatectomy (55810) was performed must first indicate that an incision was made in the skin between the base of the scrotum and the anus and the entire gland was removed along with the seminal vesicles and the vas deferens. In 55812, documentation must state that the local lymph nodes were also removed for analysis. In 55815, a pelvic lymphadenectomy through a separate lower abdominal incision is documented. A midline abdominal incision is made from the upper to the lower abdomen and the back wall of the abdomen is exposed. All lymph nodes along the back wall of the pelvic and abdominal cavities are removed. The abdominal wound is closed in multiple layers by suturing.

Code selection of a subtotal prostatectomy is dependent upon the approach taken. Documentation for a suprapubic subtotal prostatectomy (55821) must indicate that an incision was made in the lower abdomen just above the pubic area and the physician approached the prostate above the pubic bone. However, the documentation for a retropubic subtotal prostatectomy (55831) must indicate that an incision was made in the lower abdomen and the physician approached the prostate by going behind the pubic bone subtotal prostatectomy.

In 55840, the physician performs a radical prostatectomy through an incision made in the lower abdomen just above the pubic area. The gland with the capsule intact and the seminal vesicles and the portions of the vas deferens in the area are removed by freeing the prostate by blunt dissection and by transecting the urethra and by cutting through the bladder outlet. In 55842, the physician performs a radical prostatectomy and a pelvic lymph node biopsy through a midline abdominal incision (this may be done in two stages within seven to 10 days). A midline incision is made from the upper to the lower abdomen and the abdominal cavity is entered. The back wall of the abdomen is exposed and the lymph nodes are checked for spread of tumor. Some may be removed and/or biopsied. Documentation for a bilateral pelvic lymphadenectomy (55845) must indicate that the external iliac, hypogastric, and obturator nodes were removed.

Key Documentation Terms
Documentation should indicate the surgical procedure that was performed. Terms such as biopsy, lymphadenectomy, perineal, retropubic, radical, subtotal, or nerve sparing provide the guidance needed to ensure correct code assignment. Above all else, the documentation should support the medical necessity of the procedure.

Coding Tips
- Use 52000 in conjunction with 55700 or 55705 to indicate a cystoscopy with prostate biopsy. Modifier 59 should be appended to code 52000 due to the fact that it is a separate procedure and modifier 51 for multiple procedures.

- For transurethral methods of prostate excision, see codes in the urinary section (52601–52640).

- Other procedures used to treat benign hypertrophy of the prostate (BHP) include:
  - transurethral resection of the prostate (TURP) (52601–52640)
  - transurethral microwave thermotherapy (TUMT) (53850)
  - transurethral radiofrequency thermotherapy (TUNA) (53852)
  - transurethral radiofrequency generated water vapor thermotherapy (53854)
  - insertion of a temporary prostatic urethral stent (53855)
  - transurethral ultrasound-guided laser-induced prostatectomy (VLAP) coagulation (52647)
  - laser vaporization of the prostate (TUVRP) (52648)
  - laser enucleation of the prostate with morcellation (52649)
  - laparoscopic prostatectomy, radical retropubic (55866)

- For transurethral ablation malignant prostate tissue using high-energy water vapor thermotherapy, see Category III code 0582T. This code includes intraoperative imaging and needle guidance.

Coding Trap
- Transurethral drainage of a prostatic abscess (52700) is included in male transurethral prostatic procedures and should not be reported separately.

Procedures Performed on the Female Genital System

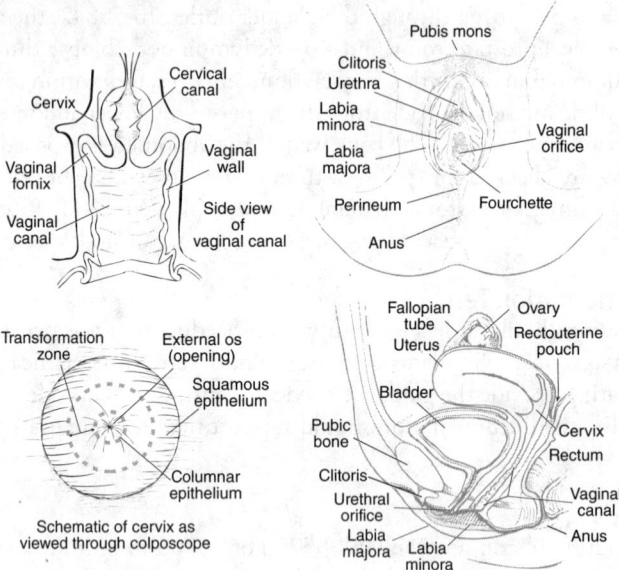

This section of codes (56405–58999) includes the procedures performed on the female genital tract including the perineum, vulva, vagina, cervix, uterus, ovaries, and oviducts.

The following is a discussion of some of the more difficult areas in this section that an auditor may want to consider in a review.

Surgical Procedures of the Vulva, Perineum, and Introitus (56405–56821)

These codes report the incision, incision and drainage, destruction, excision, or repair of conditions that affect the following parts of the female:

- **Vulva.** The vulva is the area on the female external genitalia that includes the labia majora and minora, mons pubis, clitoris, bulb of the vestibule, vaginal vestibule and orifice, and the greater and lesser vestibular glands.

- **Perineum.** The perineum pertains to the pelvic floor area between the thighs: the diamond-shaped area bordered by the pubic symphysis in front, the ischial tuberosities on the sides, and the coccyx in back.

- **Introitus.** The entrance into the vagina.

Incisional Procedures (56405–56442)

Codes in this section are used to report the incision into the vulva, perineum, or introitus for the purposes of draining an abscess, the freeing of adhesions, or incising the hymen.

Procedure Differentiation

Codes within this heading are selected based upon the anatomical site of the procedure. Code 56405 should be reported when documentation indicates that the physician made an incision into the abscess at its softest point and drained the purulent contents. The cavity of the abscess is flushed and often packed with medicated gauze to facilitate drainage.

DEFINITIONS

abscess. Circumscribed collection of pus resulting from bacteria, frequently associated with swelling and other signs of inflammation.

Bartholin's gland. Mucous-producing gland found in the vestibular bulbs on either side of the vaginal orifice and connected to the mucosal membrane at the opening by a duct.

cyst. Elevated encapsulated mass containing fluid, semisolid, or solid material with a membranous lining.

furuncle. Inflamed, painful cyst or nodule on the skin caused by bacteria, often Staphylococcus, entering the hair follicle.

marsupialization. Creation of a pouch in surgical treatment of a cyst in which one wall is resected and the remaining cut edges are sutured to adjacent tissue creating an open pouch of the previously enclosed cyst.

perineal. Pertaining to the pelvic floor area between the thighs; the diamond-shaped area bordered by the pubic symphysis in front, the ischial tuberosities on the sides, and the coccyx in back.

Skene's gland. Paraurethral ducts that drain a group of the female urethral glands into the vestibule.

If the documentation indicates that incision and drainage of a cutaneous or subcutaneous cyst, furuncle, or abscess was performed, report 10060 and 10061. For drainage of a Skene's gland abscess or cyst, see 53060.

However, if documentation specifies that the abscess is of the Bartholin's gland, a mucous-producing gland in the vestibular bulbs on either side of the vaginal orifice, also known as the greater vestibular gland, report 56420. Code 56440 marsupialization of Bartholin's gland cyst, is reported when the documentation indicates that the cyst was everted and approximated to the vaginal mucosa creating a pouch. Marsupialization is performed to prevent recurrent cysts and infections.

Key Documentation Terms
The documentation should be carefully examined to determine the nature of the condition in which the incision and drainage was performed.

Documentation should indicate the surgical procedure that was performed. Terms such as incision and drainage, marsupialization, lysis, vulva, perineal, or Bartholin's gland provide the guidance needed to ensure correct code assignment. Above all else, the documentation should support the medical necessity of the procedure.

Coding Tips
- If a specimen is transported to an outside laboratory, report 99000 for conveyance.

- Report the incision and drainage of a subcutaneous abscess/cyst/furuncle using the appropriate code from the integumentary system (10060, 10061).

- If culture and sensitivity is performed on the contents of the abscess, the appropriate laboratory code should be reported separately.

- When documentation indicates that the Bartholin's gland is removed, or that the Bartholin's gland cyst is removed in total, report 56740.

- Procedures on the Bartholin's gland are unilateral. If performed bilaterally, append modifier 50 to the procedural code.

Destruction of Vulvar Lesions, Any Method (56501–56515)
Destruction of lesions of the vulva is reported with a code from range 56501–56515.

Procedure Differentiation
Appropriate code assignment is dependent upon the extent of the destruction (simple or extensive). Code 56501 should be used to report single, simple lesion destruction, or 56515 to report multiple or complicated destruction of extensive vulvar lesions. These codes are reported regardless of the method used to destroy the lesion (e.g., laser, electrosurgery, freezing, or chemical).

Medical Necessity
As stated in National Coverage Decision 140.5, "The determination of coverage for a procedure performed using a laser is made on the basis that the use of lasers to alter, revise, or destroy tissue is a surgical procedure. Therefore, coverage of laser procedures is restricted to practitioners with training in the surgical management of the disease or condition being treated." The coverage decision also indicates that Medicare contractors have discretion to determine when a laser is reasonable and necessary and therefore covered in the event that there is

 DEFINITIONS

chemosurgery. Application of chemical agents to destroy tissue, originally referring to the in situ chemical fixation of premalignant or malignant lesions to facilitate surgical excision.

electrosurgery. Use of electric currents to generate heat in performing surgery.

laser surgery. Use of concentrated, sharply defined light beams to cut, cauterize, coagulate, seal, or vaporize tissue. The color and wavelength of the laser light is produced by its active medium, such as argon, CO_2, potassium titanyl phosphate (KTP), Krypton, and Nd:YAG, which determines the type of tissues it can best treat.

no specific national coverage policy or Food and Drug Administration approved marketing decision.

Key Documentation Terms
Both the anatomical location and the methodology used for the destruction of the lesion should be well documented. Additionally, look for terms such as numerous, proliferated, or extensive to determine the level of destruction performed.

Genital lesions are often present in multiple anatomical sites. Each site should be reported. The table below helps identify other codes that may be appropriate.

Destruction of Genital Lesions

Anatomical Site	Code
Vulva and perineum	56501–56515
Vagina	57061–57065
Anal	46900–46917, 46924
Rectum	45190

Coding Tips
- For removal or destruction by electric current (fulguration) of Skene's glands, see 53270.
- For destruction of vaginal lesions, see 57061–57065.
- For lysis of labial adhesions, see 56441.

Coding Traps
- Because there is a code that can be reported for the extensive destruction of lesions, modifier 22 should not be reported with 56501.
- When lesions are removed from multiple sites, the multiple procedure payment reduction is applicable.

Biopsy and Resection: Vulva (56605–56740)
The physician performs a biopsy of a lesion (56605–56606) or removes part or all of the vulva to treat premalignant or malignant lesions (56620–56640). This heading also includes codes used to report the revision or partial removal of the hymenal ring (56700) and the removal of a Bartholin's gland or cyst (56740).

Procedure Differentiation
When documentation indicates that the physician excised a piece of tissue from the vulva or perineum, report 56605. When more than one biopsy is performed, report 56606 in addition to code 56605.

A simple complete vulvectomy includes removal of all of the labia majora, labia minora, and clitoris, while a simple, partial vulvectomy (56620) may include removal of part or all of the labia majora and labia minora on one side and the clitoris. The physician examines the lower genital tract and the perianal skin through a colposcope. A wide semi-elliptical incision that contains the diseased area is made. In 56625, two wide elliptical incisions encompassing the vulvar area are made. One elliptical incision extends from well above the clitoris around both labia majora to a point just in front of the anus. The second elliptical incision starts at a point between the clitoris and the opening of the urethra and is carried around both sides of the opening of the vagina. The underlying subcutaneous fatty tissue is removed along with the large portion of excised skin. Vessels are clamped and tied off with sutures or are electrocoagulated to control

AUDITOR'S ALERT

Modifier 22 should not be appended to codes for laser destruction. Therefore, modifier 22 should not be appended to code 56501 as 56515 describes the more extensive service.

AUDITOR'S ALERT

Biopsy of the vulva (56605-56606) is a separate procedure by definition and is usually a component of a more complex service and is not identified separately. When performed alone or with other unrelated procedures or services it may be reported. If performed alone, list the code; if performed with other procedures or services, list the code and append modifier 59.

bleeding. The considerable defect is usually closed in layers using separately reportable plastic techniques.

A partial radical vulvectomy (56630) includes partial or complete removal of a large, deep segment of skin from the following structures: abdomen and groin, labia majora, labia minora, clitoris, mons veneris, and terminal portions of the urethra, vagina, and other vulvar organs. The clitoris may or may not be included in the partial vulvectomy. Through incisions in the lower abdomen, thighs, and vulvar area, the physician removes skin, subcutaneous fatty tissue, and deeper tissue. Also included in the en bloc removal of tissue are portions of the saphenous veins and ligaments and the target lesion. The resulting large and disfiguring defect is usually closed using separately reported plastic surgical techniques, which may include pedicle flaps or free skin grafts. The physician also removes superficial and deep inguinal lymph nodes and adjacent femoral lymph nodes on one side in 56631 and on both sides in 56632.

A complete radical vulvectomy (56633) includes the removal of a large, deep segment of skin and tissue from the following structures: abdomen and groin, labia majora, labia minora, clitoris, mons veneris, and terminal portions of the urethra, vagina, and other vulvar organs. Deep tissue from more than 80 percent of the vulva is excised. Through incisions in the lower abdomen, thighs, and vulvar area, the physician removes skin, subcutaneous fatty tissue, and deeper tissues. Also included in the en bloc removal of tissue are portions of the saphenous veins and ligaments and the target lesion. In 56634, documentation must indicate that the physician also removed the inguinal and femoral lymph nodes on one side; if removed on both sides, report 56637.

A complete radical vulvectomy (56640) includes the removal of a large, deep segment of skin and tissue from the following structures: lower abdomen and groin, labia majora, labia minora, clitoris, mons veneris, and terminal portions of the urethra, vagina, and other vulvar organs. Through incisions in the lower abdomen, thighs, and vulvar area, the physician removes skin, subcutaneous fatty tissue, and deeper tissue. The physician also removes the inguinal and femoral lymph nodes on both sides, as well as the iliac and pelvic lymph nodes in the pelvic cavity, which is entered through an abdominal incision. Also included in the en bloc removal of tissue are portions of the saphenous veins and ligaments and the target lesion. The resulting large and disfiguring defect is usually closed in layers using separately reported plastic surgical techniques, which may include pedicle or free skin grafts.

Medical Necessity
The following conditions may warrant the removal of vulvar tissue (vulvectomy or partial vulvectomy) (this list is not all inclusive):

- Diagnosis or treatment of benign, premalignant, or malignant lesions
- In association with surgery that was performed to treat underlying medical conditions that may include but are not limited to:
    - congenital anomalies
    - cystocele, enterocele, or rectocele
    - fused labia
    - imperforate hymen
- Reconstruction following surgery (e.g., pelvic exenteration)
- Removal of areas involved with persistent infection and/or scarring that has not responded to conventional medical management

AUDITOR'S ALERT

Some lesions of the genitourinary tract occur at mucocutaneous borders. The most appropriate code from either the Female Genital System or Integumentary section of the CPT book that best describes the procedure should be reported. Separate codes from the both sections may be reported if separate procedures are performed on completely separate lesions (i.e., skin and genitourinary tract). Modifier 59 should be reported to indicate that the procedures are on separate lesions.

Vulvar or vaginal surgery performed to change the appearance or reduce the size of the labia, clitoral hood, introitus, hymen, or vagina would be considered cosmetic and therefore is not a covered service for most third-party payers.

The ICD-10-CM coding system classifies malignancies of the labia majora, labia minora, and clitoris individually. Report the individual subcategory code for each area affected when more than one area is involved.

Key Documentation Terms
When coding vulvectomies, the documentation must clearly indicate the anatomical structures removed in order to determine the extent of the procedure. The following table can assist in determining the type of vulvectomy performed.

Skin and superficial tissue	Simple
Skin and deep tissue	Radical
<80 percent of vulvar area	Partial
>80 percent of vulvar area	Complete

Coding Tips
- As an add-on code, 56606 is not subject to multiple procedure rules. No reimbursement reduction or modifier 51 is applied. Add-on codes describe additional intraservice work associated with the primary procedure. They are performed by the same provider on the same date of service as the primary service/procedure, and must never be reported as a stand-alone code. The following table provides additional information for these codes as found in the Medicare Physician Fee Schedule Database.

Parent Code	Add-On	GLOB DAYS	MULT PROC	BILAT SURG	ASST SURG	CO-SURG	TEAM SURG
56605		000	2	0	1	2	0
	56606	ZZZ	0	0	1	2	0

- Skin grafts required for procedures in this section should be reported separately with 15004–15005, 15120–15121, and 15240–15241, when appropriate.
- Vulvectomy (56620–56640), the removal of the vulva, is classified by the extent of the tissue that is removed, if a lymphadenectomy is performed, and if the lymphadenectomy was unilateral or bilateral.

Coding Trap
- Vulvectomy procedures have a 90-day global period. Only those services provided within that time frame that are unrelated to the vulvectomy may be reported separately.

Repairs/Reconstruction External Female Genitalia (56800–56810)
This subsection contains codes that are used to report the repair of vulva, perineum, and introitus including the clitoris.

Procedure Differentiation
When documentation states that excision of scar tissue and strengthening the supporting tissues using tissue flaps and suturing techniques was performed (plastic repair of introitus), report 56800. Treatment of intersex state with clitoroplasty is reported with 56805.

DEFINITIONS

subcutaneous. Below the skin.

vulva. Area on the female external genitalia that includes the labia majora and minora, mons pubis, clitoris, bulb of the vestibule, vaginal vestibule and orifice, and the greater and lesser vestibular glands.

Code 56810 is reported when documentation states that the physician made an incision from the lower vaginal opening to a point just in front of the anus. The underlying weakened tissues are dissected and repaired and tightened by suturing. This restores strength to the pelvic floor, closes tissue defects, and improves function of the perineal muscles. The physician may also document this service as a perineorrhaphy.

Coding Tip

- Code 56810 is a separate procedure by definition and is usually a component of a more complex service and is not identified separately. When performed alone or with other unrelated procedures or services it may be reported. If performed alone, list the code; if performed with other procedures or services, list the code and append modifier 59.

Procedures Performed on the Vagina (57000–57426)

Incisional Procedures: Vagina (57000–57023)

Procedure Differentiation

Colpotomy (57000–57010) is an incision in the wall of the vagina, usually to access a recess between the rectum and uterus formed by a fold in the peritoneum (cul-de-sac). Through a speculum inserted in the vagina, the physician grasps the posterior lip of the cervix with a toothed instrument called a tenaculum. The cervix is lifted up exposing the posterior vaginal pouch. An incision is made through the back wall of the vagina into the posterior pelvic cavity. Through this opening, the pelvic cavity can be explored using instruments. After exploration, the physician closes the incision with absorbable sutures. When performed for exploratory purposes, code 57000 is assigned; for drainage of an abscess, report 57010.

Colpocentesis (57020) is the aspiration of fluid in the peritoneum through the wall of the vagina. Documentation must indicate that a speculum was inserted in the vagina, the posterior lip of the cervix was grasped with a toothed instrument called a tenaculum, and the cervix was lifted, exposing the posterior vaginal pouch and deep back wall of the vagina. A long needle attached to a syringe is inserted through the exposed vaginal wall and the posterior pelvic cavity is entered. Fluid is aspirated through the needle into the syringe.

Codes 57022–57023 are reported to indicate the incision and drainage of a vaginal hematoma. Codes are differentiated by the reason for the hematoma (e.g., obstetrical vs. nonobstetrical).

Coding Tips

- A colposcopy is considered an integral part of a colpotomy. When a colpotomy is performed during the same operative session as a colposcopy, report only the colpotomy as it has a higher relative value.

- A colpocentesis (57020) is a separate procedure by definition and is usually a component of a more complex service and is not identified separately. When performed alone or with other unrelated procedures or services it may be reported. If performed alone, list the code; if performed with other procedures or services, list the code and append modifier 59.

Coding Trap

- Pelvic examination under anesthesia is an integral part of these procedures and should not be reported separately.

AUDITOR'S ALERT

When the medical record documentation indicates that a repair was performed due to nonobstetrical wounds, the appropriate repair code from the integumentary section should be reported.

DEFINITIONS

colpocentesis. Aspiration of fluid from the retrouterine cul-de-sac by puncture of the vaginal vault near the midline between the uterosacral ligaments.

colpotomy. Incision into the vaginal wall for diagnostic or therapeutic purposes.

Destruction of Vaginal Lesions, Any Method (57061–57065)

Codes within this subsection are used to report the destruction by any method of lesions of the vaginal mucosa.

Procedure Differentiation

Destruction of lesions of the vagina is reported with 57061 or 57065. Code assignment is dependent upon the extent of the destruction (e.g., simple [57601] or extensive [57065]). Extensive is reported if the lesions are numerous, large, or difficult. These codes are reported regardless of the method used to destroy the lesion (e.g., laser, electrosurgery, freezing, or chemical).

Coding Tip

- When documentation indicates that anal warts are destroyed during the same operative session, report the appropriate code from range 46900–46917 or 46924.

Coding Trap

- Colposcopy is considered an integral part of this procedure and should not be reported separately.

Excisional Procedures: Vagina (57100–57135)

These codes report the removal of a piece of vaginal tissue (biopsy) or the partial or total removal of the vaginal wall.

Procedure Differentiation

Codes 57100–57111 are differentiated by the amount of tissue removed. For example, when small pieces of tissue are removed (biopsy), 57100–57105 are reported. When part or the entire vaginal wall is removed, 57106–57111 are reported.

When performing a Le Fort procedure (57120), also referred to as a colpoclesis, documentation must indicate that the procedure involved everting the vagina. Two large flaps of vaginal wall removed from opposite sides of the prolapsed vagina are sutured to one another and inverted back inside the body. The former vaginal opening is sutured closed obliterating the vagina and preventing uterine prolapse.

Code 57130 is reported when the vaginal septum is excised. The septum is an anomaly that separates the vagina into two portions. It can be longitudinal, creating two vaginal canals, or transverse, blocking the vagina and preventing menstrual flow. For a small, thin septum, the procedure is often done by injecting a local anesthetic in the tissues around the septum and making an incision through the narrowest portion of the septum. The divided tissue is tied off with suture material and the tissue is excised. For a thicker and more extensive septum, the procedure may be done under general anesthesia. The tissue is excised and the resulting vaginal lining defects are closed. The vagina is packed with medicated gauze or a support device. Report 57135 when documentation states that a vaginal lesion is excised with a scalpel or scissors.

Key Documentation Terms

Documentation must indicate the size and anatomical location of the tissues removed (i.e., paravaginal tissue, lymph node sampling, etc.). When biopsies are performed, the size of the sample, as well as any repair necessary, should also be documented.

Coding Tip

- Code 57120 is rarely used. For vaginectomy other than Le Fort procedure, see 57106–57109 and 57110–57111 with appropriate code selection dependent upon the structures removed.

Coding Trap

- Note that 57100 is a separate procedure and therefore should not be reported when performed at the time of a related, more complex procedure.

Irrigation/Insertion/Introduction Vaginal Medication or Supply (57150–57180)

Codes within this subsection are used to report the introduction of a treatment device into the vagina. Correct code selection is dependent upon the type of device inserted.

Procedure Differentiation

When documentation indicates that the physician inserted a pessary, report 57160. Payer guidelines regarding the removal of a pessary differ. Most payers consider the removal to be included in the insertion. When removed by a physician other than the physician who inserted the device, some payers may allow 58999 Unlisted procedure, female genital system (non-obstetrical), to be reported. A report describing the service should be attached. Other payers may bundle the removal into the evaluation and management code. Check with the specific payer for coverage guidelines.

Clinical brachytherapy performed by means of a uterine tandem or vaginal ovoids is reported with 57155; by means of a vaginal radiation afterloading apparatus, report 57156.

Coding Tips

- The supply of the pessary is not included in the code description and may be reported separately using the appropriate HCPCS Level II code.

- When radioelement sources or ribbons are inserted, a code from range 77761–77763 or 77770–77772 should be reported separately.

- When reporting 57170, the diaphragm or cervical cap may be reported separately using the appropriate HCPCS Level II code when it is provided by the physician.

Vaginal Repair and Reconstruction (57200–57335)

This subsection includes codes for vaginal and paravaginal repairs. Paravaginal wall defects are common and usually have associated cystocele formation, ureterovaginal prolapse, and stress urinary incontinence due to the disruption of the fibromuscular connective tissue that firmly supports the vaginal sulcus to the pelvic wall.

Procedure Differentiation

Codes 57200 and 57210 report the repair of the vagina and/or perineum (nonobstetrical). Documentation must indicate that after accessing the extent of the vaginal laceration or wound, the wound was closed using absorbable sutures. A local anesthetic or general anesthesia may be used, depending on the extent of the wound, age of the patient, patient's general condition, etc. Report 57200 when only the vagina is repaired. In 57210, after the speculum is removed, the perineal laceration is closed in layers with sutures.

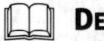

DEFINITIONS

pessary. Device placed in the vagina to support and reposition a prolapsing or retropositioned uterus, rectum, or vagina.

DEFINITIONS

colporrhaphy. Plastic repair or reconstruction of the vagina by suturing the vaginal wall and surrounding fibrous tissue.

cystocele. Herniation of the bladder into the vagina.

enterocele. Intestinal herniation into the vaginal wall.

incontinence. Inability to control urination or defecation.

placation. Surgical technique involving folding, tucking, or pleating to reduce the size of a hollow structure or organ.

prolapse. Falling, sliding, or sinking of an organ from its normal location in the body.

urethrocele. Urethral herniation into the vaginal wall.

SPECIAL ALERT

The use of a prosthesis such as a synthetic implant and mesh to strengthen the vaginal defect area may be reported separately using add-on code 57267. This code is reported once for each site (i.e., anterior, posterior) and is listed in addition to the code for the repair. Note that this is an add-on code and, as such, modifier 51 should not be appended.

Code 57220 is used to report the repair of the urethral sphincter and documentation must indicate that the approach was from the vagina and that sutures were placed on each side of the urethra.

Urethrocele, Cystocele, and Enterocele Repairs

CPT contains a number of codes that are used to report the repair of a urethrocele, cystocele, or enterocele. Correct code selection is dependent upon the type of herniation repaired and the approach.

A urethrocele (57230) is reported when the documentation indicates that the prolapsed urethral tissue is excised from the meatus in a circular manner and the cut edges of the urethral mucosa and vaginal mucosa are then sutured.

A colporrhaphy (57240–57265) is the plastic repair or reconstruction of the vagina by suturing the vaginal wall and surrounding fibrous tissue and may be performed either on the front of the vagina (anterior), back of the vagina (posterior), or both and is frequently performed because of prolapse. The code descriptions should be read thoroughly as colporrhaphies commonly include repair of rectoceles, cystoceles, and enteroceles.

An anterior colporrhaphy (57240) is performed to correct a cystocele, which is a herniation of the bladder, its support tissues, and against the anterior vaginal wall causing it to bulge downward. The physician may also repair a urethrocele, which is a prolapse of the urethra. The repair involves an incision from the apex of the vagina to within 1 cm of the urethral meatus. Plication sutures are placed along the urethral course from the meatus to the bladder neck. A suture is placed through the pubourethral ligament to the posterior symphysis pubis on each side of the urethra. The sutures are tied (ligated), and the posterior urethra is pulled upward to a retropubic position. Cystourethroscopy is included when performed with this procedure.

Code 57250 is used to report a posterior colporrhaphy or the herniation of the rectum into the vagina. A posterior midline incision that includes the perineum and posterior vaginal wall is made. To strengthen the area, the rectovaginal fascia is plicated by folding and tacking, and it is closed with layered sutures. The physician may also perform a perineorrhaphy, the plastic repair of the perineum, which should not be reported separately. Excess fascia in the posterior vaginal wall is excised.

Codes 57260 and 57265 are reported when the physician performs an anterior AND posterior repair. Code 57265 is reported when there is an enterocele or intestinal herniation into the vaginal wall. These codes also include the repair of the enterocele and/or perineum and cystourethroscopy, when performed.

This procedure differs from 57268 and 57270, which is only the repair of the enterocele, in that the vagina is not "lifted" or "tightened" and that only the herniation is repaired.

Codes 57268–57270 describe the repair of an enterocele, which is a herniation of the bowel contents of the rectouterine pouch that protrudes into the septum of tissue between the bladder and vagina or between the vagina and rectum. Through the vaginal approach in 57268, the physician incises and ligates the enterocele sac and approximates the uterosacral ligaments and endopelvic fascia anterior to the rectum. In 57270, the approach is made through an incision in the lower abdominal wall. A vaginal hysterectomy, anterior (cystocele) and posterior (rectocele) colporrhaphy, and perineorrhaphy may also be performed to augment the support.

In some instances, mesh is placed to add strength and stability. When this occurs, add-on code 57267 is reported in addition to the appropriate repair code.

Medical Necessity

Colporrhaphy is generally covered for the herniations described above, which are often accompanied by urinary incontinence. However, a diagnosis of urinary incontinence without indication of cystocele, urethrocele, or urethral hypermobility may not support the medical necessity of the service.

Key Documentation Terms

When documentation indicates the incision was made into the anterior vagina or states that an incision was carried to the apex of the vagina, an anterior repair was performed. The documentation for a posterior repair must state that the incision was made in the posterior vagina or that a posterior midline incision was made. When documentation states both, then a combined anteroposterior (AP) approach was used.

Coding Tip

- As an "add-on" code, 57267 is not subject to multiple procedure rules. No reimbursement reduction or modifier 51 is applied. The following table provides additional information for these codes as found in the Medicare Physician Fee Schedule Database.

Parent Code	Add-On	GLOB DAYS	MULT PROC	BILAT SURG	ASST SURG	CO-SURG	TEAM SURG
45560		090	2	0	2	1	0
57240		090	2	0	2	1	0
57250		090	2	0	2	1	0
57260		090	2	0	2	1	0
57265		090	2	0	2	1	0
	57267	ZZZ	0	0	2	1	0
57285		090	2	0	2	2	0

- Report 57250 only when a colporrhaphy and rectocele are repaired. Report the repair of a rectocele only using 45560.

- Code 57240 includes any repair of a urethrocele the physician may perform together with the cystocele repair and cystourethroscopy, when performed.

- When a plastic repair of a urethrocele is performed, code 57230 should be reported.

Coding Trap

- When documentation indicates that via abdominal incisions the bladder was suspended using sutures, a Marshall-Marchetti-Krantz (MMK) or Burch urethral suspension may have been performed, see 51840 and 51841.

Colpopexy (57280–57283)

A colpopexy is the suturing a prolapsed vagina to its surrounding structures for vaginal fixation. This can be done by an abdominal approach (57280), extra-peritoneal approach (57282), or intra-peritoneal approach (57283).

Procedure Differentiation

Documentation must indicate that the apex of the vagina was firmly sutured to the bridge. This stabilizes the vaginal vault and prevents prolapse of the vagina. When documentation indicates that an incision was made into the abdominal cavity, report 57280.

Code 57282 is reported when documentation indicates that the approach was extraperitoneal. The documentation must also state that a sacrospinous ligament fixation was performed using an anterior transvaginal approach and an iliococcygeus fascial suspension was performed by extraperitoneal transvaginal approach.

When documentation indicates that a colpopexy was performed by transvaginal, intraperitoneal approach, report 57283. In this procedure, uterosacral ligament suspension is performed. Levator myorrhaphy uses the levator musculature to repair the vaginal vault prolapse. The levator musculature is brought together and a high levator shelf created. The shelf is created by tagging and tying together the levator muscles at a site slightly above the junction of the levator and rectum. The vaginal vault is anchored to the shelf.

Key Documentation Terms

Anatomical terms such as iliococcygeus fascia, sacrospinous ligaments, myorrhaphy, abdominal, extra-peritoneal, or intra-peritoneal provide the guidance needed to ensure correct code assignment.

Coding Tips

- For laparoscopic repair of stress incontinence only, see 51990 and 51992.
- The repair of a paravaginal defect is reported with 57284 for an open approach and 57285 for a vaginal approach.

Billing and Payment Issues

These procedures are considered inherently bilateral and modifier 50 would not be used.

Endoscopic Vaginal Procedures (57420–57426)

Surgical procedures performed on the vagina endoscopically or laparoscopically are found in this subsection.

Procedure Differentiation

Codes 57420–57421 describe the visualization of the vagina and/or cervix using a colposcope. If the entire vagina, including the cervix (if present), was visualized, report 57420. Documentation must state that the vagina was inspected through the colposcope, to look for discharge, inflammation, ulceration, or any lesions. The cervix is exposed, cleansed, and gently examined for any lesions or ulceration. Acetic acid may be applied to help make any lesions and the columnar villi more visible. When documentation further states that a biopsy was taken of the area in question under direct vision, report 57421.

Documentation supporting 57423 must indicate that through a laparoscope the physician repaired a paravaginal defect in which there was a loss of the lateral vaginal attachment to the pelvic sidewalls. The physician inserts the nondominate hand into the vagina, lifts the anterior vaginal and pubocervical

AUDITOR'S ALERT

Additional codes may be assigned with modifier 51 for vaginal neck suspension, repair of cystocele, colopexy, repair of vaginal prolapse, and Pereyra procedure.

AUDITOR'S ALERT

These codes represent examination of the vagina as well as the cervix. For colposcopic examination of the cervix with or without surgical intervention, see 57452-57461.

fascia to the normal position, and places four to six sutures along the defect from the ischial spine toward the urethra. This may be performed bilaterally when the defect is bilateral in nature. During the procedure, a herniation of the bladder into the lateral wall may also be repaired.

Code 57425 reports a laparoscopy colpopexy. The documentation must indicate that the peritoneum is incised over the vaginal apex. The vaginal vault is elevated into its normal position and the cul-de-sac is obliterated. If necessary, a suture is placed through the base of the right uterosacral ligament and through the apex of the vagina, securing it posteriorly to the top of the rectovaginal fascia and anteriorly to the pubocervical fascia (to a dermal or mesh graft, if placed) and secured. Four total sutures are used to elevate the vagina, this being done twice through each ligament and the vaginal apex on each side.

When documentation indicates that the physician completely or partially excised the vaginal graft revising or removing eroding mesh, report 57426.

Key Documentation Terms
Documentation should indicate the surgical procedure that was performed. Terms such as apex, biopsy, herniation, paravaginal, retrovaginal fascia, and uterosacral ligament provide the guidance needed to ensure correct code assignment. Above all else, the documentation should support the medical necessity of the procedure.

Coding Tips
- If documentation indicates that the ectocervix and endocervix are examined, see 57452–57461. Code selection is determined by diagnostic service or the surgical procedure performed. Note that these codes may also use a loop electrode.

- For colposcopy performed on the vulva, see 56820–56821.

- When documentation indicates that an endometrial biopsy was performed with colposcopy, see 58110.

- When documentation indicates that a prosthetic vaginal graft (mesh) was removed via a vaginal approach, see 57295; through an abdominal approach, see 57296.

- Report code 57465 when computer-aided mapping of the cervix uteri is used while performing a colposcopy.

Procedures Performed on the Cervix Uteri (57452–57800)

Endoscopic Cervical Procedures (57452–57461)
Colposcopy of the cervix, including portions of the adjacent vagina, is reported with 57452–57461. Code selection is determined by the diagnostic service or surgical procedure performed. Note that these codes may also use a loop electrode.

Procedure Differentiation
When documentation indicates only visualization of the cervix (including portions of the upper/adjacent vagina), report 57452.

When the documentation indicates that the physician swabbed the vaginal walls and cervix with vinegar, iodine, or another type of solution to remove mucus and highlight abnormal cells by turning them white, making them more easily identifiable for biopsy, and removed tissue with a biopsy punch or forceps and endocervical curettage was also performed, report 57454. When the tissue was

DEFINITIONS

laparoscopy. Direct visualization of the peritoneal cavity, including outer fallopian tubes, uterus, ovaries and other structures utilizing a laparoscope, a thin, flexible fiberoptic tube. Laparoscopy can be performed for diagnostic purposes alone or included as part of other surgical procedures accomplished by this approach.

removed from the cervix using a biopsy punch or forceps, report 57455; when documentation indicates that endocervical curettage alone was performed, report 57456.

For the LEEP procedure (57460), the cervix, including the upper/adjacent portion of the vagina, are viewed through a colposcope, a binocular microscope used for direct visualization of the vagina, ectocervix, and endocervix. The physician inserts a speculum into the vagina to fully expose the cervix. The physician swabs the vaginal walls and cervix with vinegar or another type of solution (acetic acid) to remove mucus and highlight abnormal cells by turning them white, making them more easily identifiable for possible biopsy. Sometimes a Schiller test, iodine solution used to coat the cervix, is performed. The solution may cause a slight tingling or burning sensation. Local anesthesia may be used to numb the area. A biopsy specimen of cervical tissue is removed by the loop electrode excision procedure. LEEP uses a thin wire loop carrying an electrical cutting current that acts as a cutting instrument to remove abnormal cells. Due to the electrical current, a grounding pad is attached to the patient's leg during the procedure.

Conization or total excision of the cervix is reported with code 57461. In this procedure the cervix, including the upper/adjacent portion of the vagina, are viewed through a colposcope, a binocular microscope used for direct visualization of the vagina, ectocervix, and endocervix. The physician swabs the vaginal walls and cervix with vinegar or another type of solution (acetic acid) to remove mucus and highlight abnormal cells by turning them white, making them more easily identifiable for possible biopsy. Sometimes a Schiller test, iodine solution used to coat the cervix, is performed. The solution may cause a slight tingling or burning sensation. Local anesthesia may be used to numb the area. LEEP uses a thin wire loop carrying an electrical cutting current that acts as a cutting instrument to remove abnormal cells and, due to the electrical current, a grounding pad is attached to the patient's leg during the procedure. Using the loop, the lesion and transformation zone (the boundary of the excision to assure complete removal of the dysplasia) is removed as one specimen. If the lesion is large and another pass is required, two equal specimens are removed and labeled for the axis of orientation. The same procedure is done again with a smaller loop if an endocervical excision is necessary.

Medical Necessity

Cervical colposcopy is usually considered medically necessary when:

- The patient is at high risk for conditions such as human papilloma virus (HPV)
- There is a lesion or other problem such as genital warts present on or around the cervix and vagina
- There is a previous abnormal Pap test
- There is a previously abnormal colposcope

Coding Tips

- Local anesthesia is included in these procedures. However, these procedures may be performed under general anesthesia, depending on the age and/or condition of the patient.
- For a colposcopy performed on the vulva, see 56820–56821.

Coding Traps

- Visualization of the vulva perineum is reported with an E/M code.

DEFINITIONS

cervical intraepithelial neoplasia. Classification system used to report abnormalities in the epithelial cells of the cervix uteri: **CIN I:** Cervical intraepithelial neoplasia I; low-grade abnormality; mild dysplasia. **CIN II:** Cervical intraepithelial neoplasia II; high-grade abnormality; moderate dysplasia. **CIN III:** Cervical intraepithelial neoplasia III; carcinoma in situ; severe dysplasia.

colposcopy. Procedure in which the physician views the cervix and vagina through a colposcope, which is a binocular microscope used for direct visualization of the vagina, ectocervix, and endocervix.

conization. Excision of a cone-shaped piece of tissue.

curettage. Removal of tissue by scraping.

human papilloma virus. Virus of several different species transmitted by direct or indirect contact and causing plantar and genital warts on skin and mucous membranes. HPV is most commonly associated with increased risk for cervical dysplasia and cancer in women.

- These codes are used only when the procedure is performed with colposcopic visualization. When performed with direct visualization, see 57520–57522.

Cervical Procedures: Multiple Techniques (57500–57558)

This subsection classifies biopsy, curettage, and cautery of the cervix uteri using direct visualization instead of colposcopy.

Procedure Differentiation

When documentation indicates that the physician, under direct visualization, obtains biopsies of the cervix, report 57500.

Cautery of the cervix (57510–57513) is performed for a number of reasons. Documentation must indicate that a speculum was inserted into the vagina to view the cervix. The code choice for cauterization is determined by the equipment/method of cautery used.

Report 57520 when a cold knife or laser is used to perform conization of the cervix. Code 57522 is used to report open loop electrode excision (LEEP) of the cervix (e.g., conization of the cervix without the use of an endoscope).

Coding Tips

- It should be noted that 57500 (biopsy of cervix) is a separate procedure by definition and is usually a component of a more complex service and is not identified separately. When performed alone or with other unrelated procedures or services it may be reported. If performed alone, list the code; if performed with other procedures or services, list the code and append modifier 59.

- Code 57520 includes multiple procedures, including conization of the cervix, with or without fulguration, with or without dilation and curettage, with or without repair. They should not be reported separately.

- Control of bleeding, by any method, is not reported separately.

DEFINITIONS

corpus uteri. Main body of the uterus, which is located above the isthmus and below the openings of the fallopian tubes.

D&C. Dilation and curettage.

Procedures Performed on the Corpus Uteri (58100–58579)

The corpus uteri is the main body of the uterus. The uterus is shaped like an inverted pear, with the body of the uterus forming the wide, superior region and the cervix of the uterus forming the narrow, inferior region. Several distinct regions make up the body of the uterus. The domed, higher region is known as the fundus. At the sides of the fundus, the fallopian (uterine) tubes connect with the uterus and expand into the central fluid-filled uterine cavity. Where the fallopian tubes join the body, the uterus narrows until it joins with the cervix.

The corpus uteri is divided into three separate tissue layers, which can affect code assignment:

- Endometrium (inner layer): Lining of the uterus, that thickens in preparation for fertilization. A fertilized ovum embeds into the thickened endometrium. When no fertilization takes place, the endometrial lining sheds during the process of menstruation.

- Myometrium (middle layer): Muscular middle layer of the uterine wall responsible for contractions associated with childbirth.

- Perimetrium (outer layer): Thin outer layer of tissue made of epithelial cells.

Biopsy and Resection: Corpus Uteri (58100–58294)

Procedure Differentiation

Procedures in this section are differentiated by the amount of tissue removed. For example, if a small sample of tissue is removed (a biopsy), 58100 is reported. Removal of a myoma is reported with the appropriate code from range 58140–58146. Removal of the corpus uteri (hysterectomy) is reported with codes from range 58150–58294.

When a biopsy is obtained from the uterus, the documentation may state that an endometrial sampling was performed. Code 58100 describes an endometrial biopsy with or without endocervical sampling. Add-on code 58110 is used to report an endometrial biopsy performed concurrently with a colposcopy.

When documentation states that after dilating the cervix, the physician placed a curette in the endocervical canal, passed it into the uterus, and then the entire endometrial lining of the uterus was thoroughly scraped on all sides to obtain tissue for diagnosis or to remove unhealthy tissue, a D&C has been performed. Dilation and curettage, nonobstetrical, may be reported with 58120. This code includes a biopsy, single or multiple, whether being performed with a curette or another method. When performed because of postpartum hemorrhage, report 59160.

Key Documentation Terms

Documentation should indicate the surgical procedure that was performed. Terms such as biopsy, endometrial, or nonobstetrical provide the guidance needed to ensure correct code assignment. Above all else, the documentation should support the medical necessity of the procedure.

Coding Trap

- As an "add-on" code, 58110 is not subject to multiple procedure rules. No reimbursement reduction or modifier 51 is applied. The following table provides additional information for these codes as found in the Medicare Physician Fee Schedule Database.

Parent Code	Add-On	GLOB DAYS	MULT PROC	BILAT SURG	ASST SURG	CO-SURG	TEAM SURG
57420		000	2	0	1	0	0
57421		000	2	0	1	0	0
57452		000	2	0	1	0	0
57454		000	3	0	1	0	0
57455		000	3	0	1	0	0
57456		000	3	0	1	0	0
57460		000	3	0	1	0	0
57461		000	3	0	1	0	0
	58110	ZZZ	0	0	0	0	0

Myomectomy (58140–58146)

A myomectomy is the removal of a uterine fibroid. Correct code selection is dependent upon the number of fibroids removed or the weight of the lesions, as well as the approach.

Procedure Differentiation

Myomectomy codes are differentiated by the number of myomas removed, legion weight, and the approach.

When the documentation indicates that the physician removed one to four fibroid tumors from the wall of the uterus (intramural myomas) with a total weight of 250 gm or less and/or removed surface myomas by an abdominal approach, code 58140 is supported. A transverse incision is made in the abdomen, the anterior sheath of the rectus abdominis muscle is dissected, and muscles are retracted. A scalpel, electrocautery, and/or laser may be used to remove small surface myomas. The physician incises the uterus through the myometrium to expose the myoma, which is grasped with a clamp and dissected free from the surrounding myometrium with sharp and blunt dissection. The pedicle is isolated, clamped, and ligated and the myoma is dissected down to the pedicular blood supply. Other myomas are identified by palpating the uterine wall through the defect created by the already excised myoma. Adjacent myomas are reached and removed by tunneling further through the initial incision to avoid additional uterine trauma.

Code 58145 must contain documentation that indicates a vaginal approach. This approach is used for pedunculated myomas protruding through the cervix and prolapsed myomas. The cervix is dilated with laminaria to facilitate exposure and a tonsil snare or other appropriate device is passed through to reach the myoma. Prolapsed myomas are usually attached to the cervical or endometrial cavity by a stalk. The tumor is removed by ligating or twisting the stalk or a tonsil snare is employed to encircle the tumor, cut it from its stalk, and remove it.

Documentation for 58146 must indicate that a transverse incision is made in the abdomen (a midline incision is made for large myomas). Five or more intramural myomas or any number of intramural myomas whose totaled weight is over 250 grams must be indicated for the code to be supported.

Key Documentation Terms

Terms such as total number of myomas, weight, intramural, prolapsed, abdominal or vaginal approach provide the guidance needed to ensure correct code assignment. Above all else, the documentation should support the medical necessity of the procedure.

Coding Trap

- These codes are often misused when fibroid tumors are excised through laparoscopy or hysteroscopy. For the laparoscopic removal of intramural myomas, see 58545–58546. If removal of leiomyomata is performed through a hysteroscope, see 58561.

 DEFINITIONS

intramural uterine leiomyoma. Benign, smooth muscle tumor within the wall of the uterus.

Abdominal and Vaginal Hysterectomies (58150–58294)

A hysterectomy is the removal of the uterus. It may or may not include the removal of the tubes or ovaries. If only the ovaries are removed, then an oophorectomy is performed. When only the tubes are removed, then a salpingectomy is performed.

Procedure Differentiation

The appropriate selection of a hysterectomy code is dependent upon a number of factors including the approach and the complexity of the procedure.

Abdominal Hysterectomy

When the documentation indicates that the physician made an incision into the abdomen, an abdominal hysterectomy was performed. The incision is usually horizontal within the pelvic hairline but may be midline.

Code 58150 is used to report the removal of the uterus and cervix with or without the removal of the tubes and ovaries. This differs from supracervical abdominal hysterectomy (58180) where the uterus is cut free from the cervix leaving the cervix attached to the vagina. When a pelvic lymphadenectomy and para-aortic lymph nodes are sampled in additional to the removal of the uterus, a radical abdominal hysterectomy (58210) is performed. Pelvic exenteration (58240) includes the removal of the bladder and ureteral transplantations and/or an abdominal perineal resection of the rectum and colon and creation of a colostomy.

Documentation should support the description of the procedure as identified below.

> **58150:** Through a horizontal incision just within the pubic hairline, the physician removes the uterus including the cervix and may elect to remove one or both of the ovaries and one or both of the fallopian tubes (salpingo-oophorectomy). The supporting pedicles containing the tubes, ligaments, and arteries are clamped and cut free. The uterus and cervix are removed along with a narrow rim or cuff of vaginal lining. The vaginal defect may be left open for drainage. The abdominal incision is closed by suturing.

> **58152:** This procedure also includes a colpo-urethrocystopexy. The documentation must state that the uterus and cervix were removed. One or both of the ovaries and one or both of the fallopian tubes (salpingo-oophorectomy) may also be removed. The bladder neck is suspended by placing sutures through the tissue surrounding the urethra and into the back of the symphysis pubis, which is the midline junction of the pubic bones in the front (Marshall- Marchetti-Krantz) or sutures are placed in the fascia on either side of the bladder and through the Cooper's ligaments above. The sutures are tied, which elevates the vesical neck (the junction of the bladder and urethra), in the direction of the Cooper's ligament (Burch procedure). The sutures are pulled tight so that the tissues are tacked to the symphysis pubis and the urethra is moved forward. The abdominal incision is closed by suturing.

> **58180:** Through a horizontal incision just within the pubic hairline, the physician removes the uterus above the cervix and may elect to remove one or both of the ovaries and one or both of the fallopian tubes (salpingo-oophorectomy). The supporting pedicles containing the tubes, ligaments, and arteries are clamped and cut free. The uterus is cut free

AUDITOR'S ALERT

Per the *CPT Assistant,* July 2019, there are no CPT codes or unique modifiers for surgical procedures performed using robot-assistance. Physicians are advised to use a CPT code that accurately describes the surgical procedure via a laparoscopic approach. If there is not an existing laparoscopic CPT code describing the procedure performed, an unlisted laparoscopic code in the appropriate CPT subsection should be reported.

DEFINITIONS

Marshall-Marchetti-Krantz. Surgical procedure to correct urinary stress incontinence in which the bladder is suspended by placing several sutures through the tissue surrounding the urethra and into the vaginal wall. The sutures are pulled tight so that the tissues are tacked up to the symphysis pubis and the urethra is moved forward.

from the cervix leaving the cervix still attached to the vagina. The abdominal incision is closed by suturing.

58200: Through a horizontal incision just within the pubic hairline, the physician removes the uterus, including the cervix and part of the vagina. The supporting pedicles containing the tubes, ligaments, and arteries are clamped and cut free and the uterus, cervix, and part of the vagina are removed. A biopsy is taken of the para-aortic and pelvic lymph nodes. The physician may elect to remove one or both of the ovaries and one or both of the fallopian tubes (salpingo-oophorectomy). The abdominal incision is closed by suturing.

58210: Through a horizontal incision just within the pubic hairline, the physician removes the uterus, including the cervix and the pelvic lymph nodes on both sides, and takes a biopsy of the para-aortic lymph nodes. The supporting pedicles containing the tubes, ligaments, and arteries are clamped and cut free and the uterus, cervix, all or part of the vagina, and all pelvic lymph nodes are removed. The physician may elect to remove one or both of the ovaries and one or both of the fallopian tubes (salpingo-oophorectomy). The abdominal incision is closed by suturing.

58240: Through a horizontal incision just within the pubic hairline, the physician removes all of the organs and adjacent structures of the pelvis, including the cervix, uterus, and all or part of the vagina. The supporting pedicles containing the tubes, ligaments, and arteries are clamped and cut free and the uterus, cervix, and all or part of the vagina are removed. The physician may remove one or both of the ovaries and one or both of the fallopian tubes (salpingo-oophorectomy). The physician removes the bladder and diverts urine flow by transplanting the ureters to the skin or colon. The rectum and part of the colon may be removed and an artificial abdominal opening in the skin surface created for waste (colostomy). The abdominal incision is closed by suturing.

Key Documentation Terms

In order to assign the most appropriate code, the medical record documentation must be reviewed to determine the procedure that was performed (e.g., total, subtotal, or radical hysterectomy). In addition, terms such as with or without removal of tubes or ovaries, pelvic or para-aortic lymph node sampling, or lymphadenectomy provide the guidance needed to ensure correct code assignment.

Coding Tips

- When the findings of a D&C result in the decision to perform a hysterectomy, both procedures are reported. Report the D&C with 58120 and the hysterectomy with 58150, appending modifier 58 to indicate a staged procedure.

- Pelvic examination under anesthesia (57410) should not be reported separately.

- When documentation states an urethrocystopexy without a hysterectomy (Marshall-Marchetti-Krantz procedure) was performed, code 51840 or 51841 should be reported.

- When a vaginal hysterectomy is performed with additional dissection to repair a rectocele, the vaginal hysterectomy code and 57250 (posterior colporrhaphy for repair of rectocele including perineorrhaphy if performed) may be reported together with modifier 51 on the lesser procedure.

- When a vaginal hysterectomy is performed with additional dissection to repair a cystocele, the vaginal hysterectomy code and 57240 (anterior colporrhaphy for repair of cystocele including repair of urethrocele if performed) may be reported together with modifier 51 on the lesser procedure.

Coding Trap

- When using 58150 Total abdominal hysterectomy (corpus and cervix), with or without removal of tube, with or without removal of ovaries, do not code the salpingectomy (58700), the salpingectomy-oophorectomy (58720), or oophorectomy (58940) separately.

Vaginal Hysterectomies

These codes are further differentiated by the weight of the uterus, whether or not the tubes and ovaries are removed, and if other repairs are performed during the same operative session.

Documentation should support the description of the procedure as identified below.

58260: The physician performs a vaginal hysterectomy for a uterus 250 gm or less. An incision is made around the cervix through the full thickness of the vaginal membrane. The cut vaginal edge is pulled toward the lower cervix and vaginal dissection is continued with countertraction. The posterior peritoneum is opened to admit a finger examination of the pelvis. The uterosacral ligaments are clamped and possibly shortened, cut from the uterus, and secured to the vagina. The vesicovaginal space is entered. The connective tissue fusing the bladder and vagina is dissected and the bladder is separated from the cervix. The bladder pillars are clamped, cut, and ligated near their cervical attachments, as well as the cardinal ligament tissue on each side of the cervix and the left and right uterine vessels. The physician clamps, cuts, and ligates the upper cardinal and lower broad ligament complex. Traction applied to the cervix moves the uterus down until the fundus is low in the pelvis. Hemostats are applied to the angle of the uterus on each side and the uterus is removed. The peritoneum is closed with purse-string sutures that incorporate the proximal part of the uterosacral ligaments.

58262-58263: The physician performs a vaginal hysterectomy for a uterus 250 gm or less and removes the tubes and/or ovaries. An incision is made around the cervix through the full thickness of the vaginal membrane. The cut vaginal edge is pulled toward the lower cervix and vaginal dissection is continued with countertraction. The posterior peritoneum is opened to admit a finger examination of the pelvis. The uterosacral ligaments are clamped and possibly shortened, cut from the uterus, and secured to the vagina. The vesicovaginal space is entered. The connective tissue fusing the bladder and vagina is dissected and the bladder is separated from the cervix. The bladder pillars are clamped, cut, and ligated near their cervical attachments, as well as the cardinal ligament tissue on each side of the cervix and the left and right uterine vessels. The physician clamps, cuts, and ligates the upper cardinal and lower broad ligament complex. Traction applied to the cervix moves the uterus down until the fundus is low in the pelvis. Hemostats are applied to the angle of the uterus on each side and the uterus is removed. After the uterus is exteriorized, care is taken to ensure ligation of the ovarian vessels. The ovary is excised under direct vision. For removal of both tubes and ovaries, the round ligament on one side at a time is clamped and divided. A tunnel is made through the layers of the uterine broad ligament that enclose the tube and the tube and ovary are clamped together. The structure is pulled forward, the two sheets of the broad ligament are each cut, and the broad ligament is opened completely. The whole specimen is separated from its attaching ligament, which is clamped, and the tube and ovary on that side are removed. Report 58263 if an enterocele is repaired in addition to removing the tube and/or ovary. An enterocele is a hernia of the intestine protruding against the vaginal wall. The hernia sac is bluntly and sharply dissected from the surrounding connective tissue, excised and ligated, and the surrounding tissues are strengthened and sutured. The peritoneal and vaginal wall incisions of the hysterectomy procedure are closed.

58267: The physician performs a vaginal hysterectomy, for a uterus 250 gm or less with colpourethrocystopexy, with or without endoscopic control. An incision is made around the cervix through the full thickness of the vaginal membrane. The cut vaginal edge is pulled toward the lower cervix and vaginal dissection is continued with countertraction. The posterior peritoneum is opened to admit a finger examination of the pelvis. The uterosacral ligaments are clamped and possibly shortened, cut from the uterus, and secured to the vagina. The vesicovaginal space is entered. The connective tissue fusing the bladder and vagina is dissected and the bladder is separated from the cervix. The bladder pillars are clamped, cut, and ligated near their cervical attachments, as well as the cardinal ligament tissue on each side of the cervix and the left and right uterine vessels. The physician clamps, cuts, and ligates the upper cardinal and lower broad ligament complex. Traction applied to the cervix moves the uterus down until the fundus is low in the pelvis. Hemostats are applied to the angle of the uterus on each side and the uterus is removed. Colpourethrocystopexy is done in cases of urinary incontinence to elevate the lower part of the bladder that connects to the urethra (bladder neck) and the urethra to a new position higher in the pelvis so the muscles of the pelvic floor can help control urination. After the uterus has been exteriorized and the bladder and urethra separated from surrounding structures, the physician lifts the vagina upward, suspends the bladder neck and urethra by placing sutures through the fibromuscular wall of the vagina lateral to the tissue surrounding the urethra, and sutures the tissue to the symphysis pubis—the midline junction of the pubic bones at the front. An endoscope may be placed to ensure no sutures pass through the lining of the bladder and to evaluate ureteral patency. The sutures are pulled tight to tack the structures to the pubic bone and provide support.

58270: The physician performs a vaginal hysterectomy for a uterus 250 gm or less, with repair of an enterocele. An incision is made around the cervix through the full thickness of the vaginal membrane. The cut vaginal edge is pulled toward the lower cervix and vaginal dissection is continued with countertraction. The posterior peritoneum is opened to admit a finger examination of the pelvis. The uterosacral ligaments are clamped and possibly shortened, cut from the uterus, and secured to the vagina. The vesicovaginal space is entered. The connective tissue fusing the bladder and vagina is dissected and the bladder is separated from the cervix. The bladder pillars are clamped, cut, and ligated near their cervical attachments, as well as the cardinal ligament tissue on each side of the cervix and the left and right uterine vessels. The anterior peritoneum is opened under direct vision to avoid damaging the bladder and admit finger exploration. The physician clamps, cuts, and ligates the upper cardinal and lower broad ligament complex now that the peritoneum is open both anterior and posterior to the uterine fundus. Hemostats are applied to the angle of the uterus on each side and the uterus is removed, usually posteriorly. The physician also repairs an enterocele, a herniation of intestine that protrudes against the vaginal wall, discovered during finger exploration. The hernia sac is bluntly and sharply dissected from the surrounding connective tissue, excised and ligated, and the surrounding tissues are strengthened and sutured. The peritoneum is closed with purse-string sutures that incorporate the proximal part of the uterosacral ligaments.

58275–58280: The physician performs a vaginal hysterectomy with total or partial vaginectomy in 58275–58280 and with enterocele repair in 58280. An incision is made around the cervix through the full thickness of the vaginal membrane. The cut vaginal edge is pulled toward the lower cervix and vaginal dissection is continued with countertraction. The posterior peritoneum is opened to admit a finger examination of the pelvis. The uterosacral ligaments are clamped and possibly shortened, cut from the uterus, and secured to the vagina. The vesicovaginal space is entered. The connective tissue fusing the bladder and vagina is dissected and the bladder is separated from the cervix. The bladder pillars are clamped, cut, and ligated near their cervical attachments, as well as the cardinal ligament tissue on each side of the cervix and the left and right uterine vessels. The anterior peritoneum is opened under direct vision to avoid damaging the bladder and admit finger exploration. The physician clamps, cuts, and ligates the upper cardinal and lower broad ligament complex now that the peritoneum is open both anterior and posterior to the uterine fundus. Traction applied to the cervix moves the uterus down until the fundus is low in the pelvis. Hemostats are applied to the angle of the uterus on each side and the uterus is removed, usually posteriorly. The vagina is everted out through its opening and totally or partially removed in sections by blunt and sharp dissection. Any remaining vaginal tissue and the supporting tissues are inverted back into the resulting defect and are sutured in place with total vaginectomy obliterating the space. Report 58280 if the physician also repairs an enterocele, a herniation of intestine protruding through the vaginal wall. The hernia sac is bluntly and sharply dissected from the surrounding connective tissue, excised and ligated, and the surrounding tissues are strengthened and sutured. The peritoneum is closed with purse-string sutures that incorporate the proximal part of the uterosacral ligaments.

58285: The physician performs a radical vaginal hysterectomy. This includes the uterus, its surrounding tissues, and the pelvic lymph nodes. An incision is made around the cervix through the full thickness of the vaginal membrane. The cut vaginal edge is pulled toward the lower cervix and vaginal dissection is continued with countertraction. The posterior peritoneum is opened to admit a finger examination of the pelvis. The uterosacral ligaments are clamped and possibly shortened, cut from the uterus, and secured to the vagina. The vesicovaginal space is entered. The connective tissue fusing the bladder and vagina is dissected and the bladder is separated from the cervix. The bladder pillars are clamped, cut, and ligated near their cervical attachments, as well as the cardinal ligament

 DEFINITIONS

vaginectomy. Surgical excision of all or a portion of the vagina.

tissue on each side of the cervix and the left and right uterine vessels. The anterior peritoneum is opened under direct vision to avoid damaging the bladder and admit finger exploration. The physician clamps, cuts, and ligates the upper cardinal and lower broad ligament complex now that the peritoneum is open both anterior and posterior to the uterine fundus. Traction applied to the cervix moves the uterus down until the fundus is low in the pelvis. Hemostats are applied to the angle of the uterus on each side and the uterus is removed, usually posteriorly. The physician also removes the surrounding tissues, including part or all of the vagina and the pelvic lymph nodes. Any incisions are closed by suturing.

58290: The physician performs a vaginal hysterectomy, for a uterus greater than 250 gm. An incision is made around the cervix through the full thickness of the vaginal membrane. The cut vaginal edge is pulled toward the lower cervix and vaginal dissection is continued with countertraction. The posterior peritoneum is opened to admit a finger examination of the pelvis. The uterosacral ligaments are clamped and possibly shortened, cut from the uterus, and secured to the vagina. The vesicovaginal space is entered. The connective tissue fusing the bladder and vagina is dissected and the bladder is separated from the cervix. The bladder pillars are clamped, cut, and ligated near their cervical attachments, as well as the cardinal ligament tissue on each side of the cervix and the left and right uterine vessels. The anterior peritoneum is opened under direct vision to avoid damaging the bladder and admit finger exploration. The physician clamps, cuts, and ligates the upper cardinal and lower broad ligament complex now that the peritoneum is open both anterior and posterior to the uterine fundus. Traction applied to the cervix moves the uterus down until the fundus is low in the pelvis. Hemostats are applied to the angle of the uterus on each side and the uterus is removed, usually posteriorly. When the uterus is too large to permit delivery through the anterior or posterior peritoneal opening, the myometrium may be incised circumferentially parallel to the uterine cavity axis and removed or the uterus can be dissected and removed one half at a time. The peritoneum is closed with purse-string sutures that incorporate the proximal part of the uterosacral ligaments. Colporrhaphy may be performed before the vaginal wall is closed by running or interrupted sutures placed side to side longitudinally.

58291–58292: The physician performs a vaginal hysterectomy, for a uterus greater than 250 gm and removes the tubes and/or ovaries. An incision is made around the cervix through the full thickness of the vaginal membrane. The cut vaginal edge is pulled toward the lower cervix and vaginal dissection is continued with countertraction. The posterior peritoneum is opened to admit a finger examination of the pelvis. The uterosacral ligaments are clamped and possibly shortened, cut from the uterus, and secured to the vagina. The vesicovaginal space is entered. The connective tissue fusing the bladder and vagina is dissected and the bladder is separated from the cervix. The bladder pillars are clamped, cut, and ligated near their cervical attachments, as well as the cardinal ligament tissue on each side of the cervix and the left and right uterine vessels. The anterior peritoneum is opened under direct vision to avoid damaging the bladder and admit finger exploration. The physician clamps, cuts, and ligates the upper cardinal and lower broad ligament complex now that the peritoneum is open both anterior and posterior to the uterine fundus. Traction applied to the cervix moves the uterus down until the fundus is low in the pelvis. Hemostats are applied to the angle of the uterus on each side and the uterus is removed, usually posteriorly. After the uterus is exteriorized, care is taken to ensure ligation of the ovarian vessels. The ovary is excised under direct vision. For removal of both tubes and ovaries, the round ligament on one side at a time is clamped and divided. A tunnel is made through the layers of the uterine broad ligament that enclose the tube and the tube and ovary are clamped together. The structure is pulled forward, the two sheets of the broad ligament are each cut, and the broad ligament is opened completely. The whole specimen is separated from its attaching ligament, which is clamped, and the tube and ovary on that side are removed. Report 58292 if an enterocele is repaired in addition to removing the tube and/or ovary. An enterocele is a hernia of the intestine protruding against the vaginal wall. The hernia sac is bluntly and sharply dissected from the surrounding connective tissue, excised and ligated, and the surrounding tissues are strengthened and sutured. The peritoneal and vaginal wall incisions of the hysterectomy procedure are closed.

58294: The physician performs a vaginal hysterectomy, for a uterus greater than 250 gm, with repair of an enterocele. An incision is made around the cervix through the full thickness of the vaginal membrane. The cut vaginal edge is pulled toward the lower cervix and vaginal dissection is continued with countertraction. The posterior peritoneum is opened to admit a finger examination of the pelvis. The uterosacral ligaments are clamped and possibly shortened, cut from the uterus, and secured to the vagina. The vesicovaginal space is entered. The connective tissue fusing the bladder and vagina is dissected and the bladder is separated from the cervix. The bladder pillars are clamped, cut, and ligated near their cervical attachments, as well as the cardinal ligament tissue on each side of the cervix and the left and right uterine vessels. The anterior peritoneum is opened under direct vision. The physician clamps, cuts, and ligates the upper cardinal and lower broad ligament complex now that the peritoneum is open both anterior and posterior to the uterine fundus. Traction applied to the cervix moves the uterus down until the fundus is low in the pelvis. Hemostats are applied to the angle of the uterus on each side and the uterus is removed, usually posteriorly. The physician also repairs an enterocele, a herniation of intestine that protrudes against the vaginal wall, discovered during finger exploration. The hernia sac is bluntly and sharply dissected from the surrounding connective tissue, excised and ligated, and the surrounding tissues are strengthened and sutured. The peritoneum is closed with purse-string sutures that incorporate the proximal part of the uterosacral ligaments.

Key Documentation Terms

To appropriately report vaginal hysterectomy codes (58260–58294), the size of the uterus must be determined. If the surgeon does not indicate the size in the operative report, the coder may refer to the pathology report to see whether the uterus was weighed. Other common procedures performed at the same time must be reviewed for final code selection. Terms such as total, subtotal, radical, with or without removal of tubes or ovaries, enterocele, or vaginectomy provide the guidance needed to ensure correct code assignment.

Laparoscopic Hysterectomies (58541–58544 and 58548–58554)

These codes describe procedures performed via a laparoscope or hysteroscope. Documentation should support the description of the procedure as identified below.

58541–58542: The physician performs a laparoscopic hysterectomy, removing a uterus with a total weight of 250 gm or less while preserving the cervix. The patient is placed in the dorsal lithotomy position. After the insertion of a speculum in the vagina, the physician grasps the cervix with an instrument to manipulate the uterus during the surgery. A trocar is inserted periumbilically and the abdomen is insufflated with gas. Additional trocars are placed in the right and left lower quadrants. The uterus is dissected free from the bladder and surrounding tissue and its body is separated from the cervix. Coagulation is achieved with the aid of electrocautery instruments. Alternatively, some vessels may be ligated. The uterus is morcellized and removed using endoscopic tools. In 58542, one or both ovaries and/or one or both fallopian tubes are removed in similar fashion. Once the excisions are complete, the abdominal cavity is deflated and instruments and trocars removed. The fascia and skin are closed with sutures.

58543–58544: The physician performs a laparoscopic hysterectomy, removing a uterus with a total weight of more than 250 gm while preserving the cervix. The patient is placed in the dorsal lithotomy position. After the insertion of a speculum in the vagina, the physician grasps the cervix with an instrument to manipulate the uterus during the surgery. A trocar is inserted periumbilically and the abdomen is insufflated with gas. Additional trocars are placed in the right and left lower quadrants. The uterus is dissected free from the bladder and surrounding tissue and its body is separated from the cervix. Coagulation is achieved with the aid of electrocautery instruments. Alternatively, some vessels may be ligated. The uterus is morcellized and removed using endoscopic tools. In 58544, one or both ovaries and/or one or both fallopian tubes are removed in similar fashion. Once the excisions are complete, the abdominal cavity is deflated and instruments and trocars removed. The fascia and skin are closed with sutures.

58548: The physician performs a laparoscopic hysterectomy, bilateral total pelvic lymphadenectomy, and para-aortic lymph node sampling, and may remove all or portions of the fallopian tubes and ovaries. The patient is placed in the dorsal lithotomy position. After the insertion of a speculum in the vagina, the physician grasps the cervix with an instrument to manipulate the uterus during the surgery. A trocar is inserted periumbilically and the abdomen is insufflated with gas. Additional trocars are placed in the right and left lower quadrants. The uterus is dissected free from the bladder and surrounding tissue and its body with the cervix is dissected from the vagina. Alternately, the vagina may also be excised. Coagulation is achieved with the aid of electrocautery instruments. Some vessels may be ligated. The uterus is morcellized and removed using endoscopic tools. One or both ovaries and/or one or both fallopian tubes are removed in similar fashion. The physician removes the pelvic lymph nodes on both sides and takes samples or biopsies of the para-aortic lymph nodes. Once the excisions are complete, the abdominal cavity is deflated and instruments and trocars removed. The fascia and skin of the abdomen and vagina are closed with sutures.

58550–58552: The physician performs surgical laparoscopy with vaginal hysterectomy for a uterus with a total weight of 250 gm or less. The laparoscope is used to perform the initial operative portion of the hysterectomy. The patient is placed in the dorsal lithotomy position for the endoscopic portion. For the vaginal portion, the patient is positioned in stirrups. A trocar is inserted periumbilically and the abdomen is insufflated with gas. Additional trocars are placed in the right and left lower quadrants. An intra-abdominal and pelvic survey is done and any adhesions are lysed. The round ligaments are ligated and incised. Starting on the left round ligament, the vesicouterine peritoneal fold is incised and the peritoneal vessels are dissected and desiccated. The physician continues the incision across the lower uterine segment to the round ligament on the other side and dissects the bladder off the uterus and cervix. Staples are inserted through one port on the side to be stapled or a bipolar coagulation unit is inserted for electrocautery. At this point, if tubes and/or ovaries are to be removed, the infundibulopelvic ligament is now ligated lateral to the ovary. If not, the ligation is done medial to the ovary. Staple-ligation or electrodesiccation of the uterine vasculature is accomplished on both sides, followed by that of the cardinal ligaments. An anterior colpotomy incision is made to enter the vagina and the vaginal portion of the procedure is begun. The vaginal hysterectomy proceeds through a posterior cul-de-sac incision. The uterus is removed, the vagina is closed, and hemostasis is confirmed before the trocars are removed and the skin incisions are closed. Report 58550 for removal of uterus or 58552 if uterus, tubes, and/or ovaries are removed.

58553–58554: The physician performs surgical laparoscopy with vaginal hysterectomy for a uterus with a total weight of more than 250 gm. The laparoscope is used to perform the initial operative portion of the hysterectomy. The patient is placed in the dorsal lithotomy position for the endoscopic portion. For the vaginal portion, the patient is positioned in stirrups. A trocar is inserted periumbilically and the abdomen is insufflated with gas. Additional trocars are placed in the right and left lower quadrants. An intra-abdominal and pelvic survey is done, and any adhesions are lysed. The round ligaments are ligated and incised. Starting on the left round ligament, the vesicouterine peritoneal fold is incised, and the peritoneal vessels are dissected and desiccated. The physician continues the incision across the lower uterine segment to the round ligament on the other side and dissects the bladder off the uterus and cervix. Staples are inserted through one port on the side to be stapled or a bipolar coagulation unit is inserted for electrocautery. At this point, if tubes and/or ovaries are to be removed, the infundibulopelvic ligament is now ligated lateral to the ovary. If not, the ligation is done medial to the ovary. Staple-ligation or electrodesiccation of the uterine vasculature is accomplished on both sides, followed by ligation or electrodesiccation of the cardinal ligaments. An anterior colpotomy incision is made to enter the vagina, and the vaginal portion of the procedure is begun. The remaining supporting structures attached to the cervix and uterus are detached, and the hysterectomy proceeds through a posterior cul-de-sac incision. The uterus is removed, the vaginal incision is closed, and hemostasis is confirmed before the trocars are removed and the skin incisions are closed. Report 58553 for removal of uterus or 58554 if uterus, tubes, and/or ovaries are removed.

Medical Necessity

No matter which approach is used, most third-party payers have medical necessity guidelines for hysterectomy services. In most instances hysterectomies are covered for:

- Abnormal uterine bleeding

- recurrent, lasting longer than 7 days and repetitive at less than 21 days
- unresponsive to medical management
- Chronic pelvic pain
  - impairs ability to complete daily activities
  - nongynecologic sources of pain have been ruled out
  - persistent for more then six months
  - unresponsive to medical management
- Endometrial hyperplasia
- Endometriosis that does not respond to more conservative treatments
- Malignancies
- Pelvic inflammatory diseases unresponsive to medical management
- Postpartal bleeding
- Recurrent, high-grade squamous intraepithelial neoplasia following conservative treatment
- Symptomatic pelvic relaxation such as uterine prolapse that has not responded to more conservative treatments
- Uterine leiomyomata that are of:
  - a significant size
  - are symptomatic, for example:
    - anemia due to chronic bleeding
    - bowel dysfunction
    - chronic pain including pelvic, back and/or rectal
    - failure to respond to other less invasive techniques
    - recurrent and profuse bleeding
    - urinary symptoms found to be due to uterine fibroid

Payer policies vary so it is recommended that payer policies for hysterectomy procedures be included in the practice's compliance policy.

Key Documentation Terms
Terms such as supracervical, weight of uterus, with or without removal of tubes or ovaries, or radical provide the guidance needed to ensure correct code assignment. Above all else, the documentation should support the medical necessity of the procedure.

Coding Tip
- A diagnostic laparoscopy is not reported separately.

Billing and Payment Issues
It is also important to note that some payers may require that a hysterectomy procedure be precertified unless performed in an emergency situation.

Laparoscopic/Hysteroscopic vs. Open Techniques
Many codes for laparoscopic/hysteroscopic procedures performed on the female genital system are available. These codes are listed in separate subsections by anatomic structure. Remember, when a surgical laparoscopy is performed it always includes a diagnostic laparoscopy.

Procedure Differentiation
The following reference has been created to help identify the appropriate code for laparoscopic procedures. Carefully review the index and surgery section

 DEFINITIONS

endometriosis. Aberrant uterine mucosal tissue appearing in areas of the pelvic cavity outside of its normal location, lining the uterus, and inflaming surrounding tissues often resulting in infertility and spontaneous abortion.

hyperplasia. Abnormal proliferation in the number of normal cells in regular tissue arrangement.

uterine fibroid tumor. Benign tumor consisting of smooth muscle in the uterus classified according to the site of the growth: intramural or interstitial tumors are found in the wall of the uterus; subserous fibromas are found beneath the serous membrane lining the uterus; and submucosal fibromas are found beneath the inner lining of the uterus. Although often asymptomatic, these fibroid tumors can cause reproductive problems, pain and pressure, and abnormal menstruation.

 AUDITOR'S ALERT

The diagnostic hysteroscopy is considered an integral part of a therapeutic hysteroscopy and should not be coded separately when done during the same surgical encounter.

before assigning codes. Final code assignment should be made based upon documentation in the medical record and review of the CPT tabular listing and guidelines.

Procedure	Open Code	Laparoscopic/ Endoscopic Code
Ablation, uterine fibroids w/ultrasound guidance	58356	58674
Endometrial ablation (any method)	49203–49205	58563
Fimbrioplasty	58760	58672
Fulguration of oviducts (with or without transection)	N/A	58670
Fulguration or excision of lesions of the ovary, pelvic viscera, or peritoneal surface by any method	49203–49205 (intra-abdominal, retroperitoneal) 56501, 56515 (vulva), 57061, 57065 (vagina), 57500 (cervix)	58662
Hysteroscopy, diagnostic	N/A	58555
Hysteroscopy, with sampling of endometrium or polypectomy, with or without D&C	N/A	58558
Hysteroscopy, with lysis of intrauterine adhesions	N/A	58559
Hysteroscopy, with division or resection of intrauterine septum	N/A	58560
Hysteroscopy, with occlusion of fallopian tube(s) by permanent implant placement	N/A	58565
Lysis of adhesions	58740 (oviduct)	58660
Occlusion of fallopian tube(s) by device (e.g., band, clip, or Falope ring) vaginal or suprapubic approach	58615	58671
Removal of adnexal structures (partial or total oophorectomy and salpingectomy)	58700, 58720, 58940, 58943	58661
Removal of impacted foreign body	49402 (peritoneal cavity), 57415 (vagina)	58562
Removal of leiomyomata (single or multiple)	58140–58146	58545–58546, 58561
Salpingostomy (salpingoneostomy)	58770	58673
Vaginal hysterectomy with or without removal of tube(s), with or without removal of ovary(s)	58260, 58262, 58263	58550, 58552, 58553, 58554
Total hysterectomy with or without removal of tube(s), with or without removal of ovary(s)	58150	58570, 58571, 58572, 58573
Total hysterectomy, with debulking, with omentectomy, with or without removal of tube(s), with or without removal of ovary(s), unilateral or bilateral	58951-58952	58575

Procedures Performed on the Ovary (58800–58960)

Biopsy and Resection: Ovary (58900–58960)

This subsection includes codes for procedures such as biopsy of the ovary, wedge resection of ovary, and excision of ovary.

Procedure differentiation

These procedures are differentiated by the amount of tissue removed and the other procedures that are performed during the surgical encounter.

The descriptions below indicate the type of information that is needed to support code assignment for that particular procedure code.

58900: The physician takes a tissue sample from one or both ovaries for diagnosis. This procedure may be done through the vagina or abdominally through a small incision just above the pubic hairline.

58920: Through a small abdominal incision just above the pubic hairline, the physician takes a pie-shaped section or half of one or both of the ovaries to reduce the size and repairs each ovary with sutures.

58925: Through a small abdominal incision just above the pubic hairline, the physician removes a cyst or cysts on one or both of the ovaries.

58940: Through a small abdominal incision just above the top of the pubic hairline, the physician removes part or all of one or both of the ovaries.

58943: Through an abdominal incision extending from the top of the pubic hairline to the rib cage, the physician removes part or all of one or both ovaries depending on the extent of the malignancy. The physician takes a sampling of the lymph nodes surrounding the lower aorta within the pelvis and flushes the peritoneum, which is the lining of the abdominal cavity, with saline. The saline solution is suctioned from the peritoneum for separately reportable examination. Multiple tissue samples are excised. The physician also examines and takes tissue samples of the diaphragm. The physician may elect to remove one or both fallopian tubes and the omentum. The abdominal incision is closed with layered sutures.

58950: The physician performs the initial resection of an ovarian, tubal, or primary peritoneal malignancy. Through a full abdominal incision, the physician removes both tubes, both ovaries, and the omentum, which is a membrane of lymph nodes, blood vessels, and fat that forms a protective layer extending from the stomach to the transverse colon. The abdominal incision is closed with layered sutures.

58951: Through a full abdominal incision extending from just above the pubic hairline to the rib cage, the physician treats an ovarian, tubal, or peritoneal malignancy by taking out both tubes, both ovaries, and the omentum. The physician also removes the uterus, the pelvic lymph nodes, and a portion of the lymph nodes surrounding the lower aorta. The abdominal incision is closed with layered sutures. This code is to be used only for the initial surgical resection of the malignancy.

58952: Through a full abdominal incision extending from just above the pubic hairline to the rib cage, the physician treats an ovarian, tubal, or peritoneal malignancy by excising both tubes, both ovaries, and the omentum, which is a membrane containing fat, lymph, and blood vessels that acts as a protective layer extending from the stomach to the transverse colon. The physician also reduces the size of a tumor that has grown large enough to cause discomfort or problems. Due to the size and location, it may not be possible to remove the tumor. The abdominal incision is

DEFINITIONS

omentum. Fold of peritoneal tissue suspended between the stomach and neighboring visceral organs of the abdominal cavity.

closed with layered sutures. This code is to be used only for the initial surgical resection of the malignancy.

58953–58954: Through a full abdominal incision extending from just above the pubic hairline to the rib cage, the physician treats an ovarian malignancy. The physician makes a full abdominal incision and carries dissection down to the abdominal cavity. The physician excises the fallopian tubes, both ovaries, the uterus, and the omentum, which is a membrane containing lymph, blood vessels, and fat in a protective layer that extends from the stomach to the transverse colon. The physician removes or reduces metastatic ovarian cancer implants from the abdominal cavity. The abdominal incision is closed with layered sutures. In 58954 the physician also excises pelvic lymph nodes and partially removes para-aortic lymph nodes.

58956: The physician performs a bilateral salpingo-oophorectomy with total omentectomy and total abdominal hysterectomy to treat a malignancy. A full abdominal incision is made extending from just above the pubic hairline to the rib cage. Dissection is carried down to the abdominal cavity. The physician excises the fallopian tubes, ovaries, the uterus, and the omentum. The supporting pedicles containing the tubes, ligaments, and arteries are clamped and cut free. The uterus and cervix are removed along with a narrow rim or cuff of the vaginal lining. The vaginal defect is often left open for drainage. Attention is directed to the omentum, a membrane of lymph, blood vessels, and fat that forms a protective layer that extends from the stomach to the transverse colon. The omentum is mobilized from the stomach and colon, divided from its blood supply, and removed. The physician inspects the abdominal cavity and removes any metastatic lesions. The abdominal incision is closed with layered sutures. This is a bilateral procedure. If salpingo-oophorectomy is performed only on one side, append modifier 52.

58957–58958: These codes report tumor debulking in recurrent ovarian, uterine, tubal, or peritoneal malignancies. Through a full abdominal incision extending from just above the pubic hairline to the rib cage, the physician explores the abdomen, pelvis, and viscera. In addition to debulking recurrent malignancy, the physician releases intestinal adhesions or excises all or portions of the omentum, ovaries, or fallopian tubes. The physician may remove all visible tumors or only reduce their size, depending on the nature of the malignancy and the structures involved. The abdominal incision is closed with layered sutures. Report 58958 when pelvic and para-aortic lymph nodes are also removed.

58960: This procedure is the second operation to check for a recurrence of the ovarian malignancy. Through a full abdominal incision extending from just above the pubic hairline to the rib cage, the physician may elect to remove the omentum, a membrane of lymph, blood vessels, and fat that forms a protective layer that extends from the stomach to the transverse colon. The physician may flush the lining of the abdominal cavity (peritoneum) and remove the liquid to check for cancerous cells. A tissue sample of the abdominal and pelvic peritoneum may be taken. The physician also may examine and take tissue samples of the diaphragm. The pelvic lymph nodes are removed and a portion of the lymph nodes that surrounds the lower aorta within the pelvis is removed. The abdominal incision is closed with layered sutures.

Key Documentation Terms

Documentation should indicate the surgical procedure that was performed. Terms such as biopsy, resection, cystectomy, lymphadenectomy, omentectomy, radical dissection, partial, or total provide the guidance needed to ensure correct code assignment. Above all else, the documentation should support the medical necessity of the procedure.

Coding Tips

- Code 58900 is a separate procedure by definition is usually a component of a more complex service and is not identified separately. When performed alone or with other unrelated procedures/services it may be reported. If performed alone, list the code; if performed with other procedures/ services, list the code and append modifier 59.

- The documentation or pathology report for 58950–58952 should verify a total removal of both tubes, ovaries, and the omentum due to malignancy. These are bilateral codes and are reported once even if the procedure is performed on both sides.

Billing and Payment Issues

These codes reflect unilateral or bilateral procedures and are therefore modifier 50 exempt.

Pregnancy, Delivery, and the Puerperium

This section includes all codes related to pregnancy, delivery, abortion, diagnostic procedures such as amniocentesis and fetal nonstress testing, and postpartum care.

Surgical Treatment of Ectopic Pregnancy or Hydatidiform Mole (59100–59160)

These codes are used to report surgical treatment of an ectopic pregnancy or hydatidiform mole. Assign the code that describes both main and minor procedures performed.

Procedure Differentiation

When determining what the appropriate codes are to report services performed for the treatment of abnormal products of conception, the medical record must be reviewed to determine:

- The type of pregnancy (e.g., tubal, ovarian, abdominal, interstitial)
- The treatment performed (e.g., salpingectomy, oophorectomy, hysterectomy)
- Approach (e.g., abdominal, vaginal, laparoscopic)

A hysterotomy is an incision through the abdominal wall and into the uterus. Code 59100 is assigned when documentation not only indicates that this was the service performed, but also when the reason for the procedure was related to an abnormal pregnancy, such as a hydatidiform mole or embryo.

Ectopic pregnancies may be treated by a number of methods depending on the site of the pregnancy. Documentation that states that a tubal or ovarian pregnancy requires the removal of the tube or ovary is reported using 59120. If the documentation does not state that a salpingectomy was performed, 59121 should be reported.

 DEFINITIONS

ectopic pregnancy. Fertilized ovum that implants and develops outside the uterus. The ovum may implant itself in different sites, such as the fallopian tube, the ovary, the abdomen, or the cervix.

hydatidiform mole. Trophoblastic neoplasm that mimics pregnancy by proliferating from a pathologic ovum and resulting only in a mass of cysts resembling grapes, 80 percent of which are benign, but require surgical removal. Hydatidiform moles can be complete, in which there is no fetal tissue, or partial, in which fetal tissue is frequently present.

interstitial. Within the small spaces or gaps occurring in tissue or organs.

The removal of an embryo or fetus implanted directly in the abdomen (primary) or implanted after escaping from the tube through a rupture or through the fimbriated end (secondary) is reported using 59130. Documentation supporting this service must state that after making an abdominal incision, the physician surgically removed the fetus from the abdomen. The membranes are also removed and the cord is ligated near the placenta. The placenta is usually not removed unless attached to the fallopian tube, ovary, or uterine broad ligament. Abdominal lavage may also be documented.

In 59135, documentation must state that a fertilized ovum that implanted in the portion of the tube that transverses the uterine wall was treated by removing the uterus and cervix. Through an incision extending from just above the pubic hairline to the rib cage, the physician clamps and cuts free the supporting pedicles containing the tubes, ligaments, and arteries. The physician removes the uterus and cervix and may elect to remove the tubes and/or ovaries. Abdominal or pelvic lavage may also be indicated.

When the fertilized ovum implants into the tube where it transverses the uterine wall and a portion of the uterus is removed and then the uterus is reconstructed, code 59136 is appropriate.

When documentation indicates that an embryo at less than 12 weeks gestation has implanted in the cervix, the physician usually removes the embryo through the vagina and 59140 is reported. Curettage of the endocervix and endometrium may stop heavy bleeding. Sutures and gauze packing may also be necessary.

When documentation indicates that an ectopic pregnancy was treated via a laparoscope, see 59150 or 59151 as appropriate. Correct code assignment is dependent upon whether or not the documentation indicates that the tube and/or ovary are removed.

Key Documentation Terms
Documentation should indicate the surgical procedure that was performed. Terms such as abdominal, tubal, ovarian, interstitial, salpingectomy, oophorectomy, hysterectomy, hysterotomy, and the approach (e.g., abdominal, vaginal, laparoscopic) provide the guidance needed to ensure correct code assignment. Above all else, the documentation should support the medical necessity of the procedure.

Coding Tip
- In the event that a tubal ligation is performed during the same operative session as a hysterotomy, code 59100 would be reported in conjunction with add-on code 58611. Code 58611 should only be used for a tubal ligation completed during a cesarean section or during intra-abdominal surgery. For transection, occlusion, or ligation of the fallopian tube(s) at the time of non-obstetrical procedures, see 58600–58615 and 58670–58671.

Coding Traps
- Complications such as control of hemorrhage resulting from the ectopic pregnancy are not included and are reported separately.

- Hysterotomy for abortion or for hydatidiform molar pregnancy (59100) is rarely performed. Suction curettage has replaced hysterotomy as the method of choice in the treatment of hydatidiform mole. For treatment of hydatidiform mole by suction curettage, see 59870.

Obstetrical Care (59400–59622)

Obstetrical care includes antepartum care, delivery, and postpartum care. The global obstetrical package is very similar to the global surgery package in that it combines a set of services and procedures that are included in a single code. The global surgery package includes:

- Antepartum care
- Delivery
- Postpartum care

Coding Tips
- Services that are not part of the normal obstetrical care may be reported separately. A diagnosis code indicating the medical necessity of the service must be reported.
- Visits that are medically necessary above and beyond those in the global obstetrical package should be reported using the appropriate level of evaluation and management code.

Antepartum care (59425–59426)
Antepartum care (59425–59426) is defined as follows:

- History
- Physical examinations
- Recording of weight, blood pressures, fetal heart tones
- Routine chemical urinalysis
- Visits:
  - monthly up to 28 weeks gestation
  - biweekly visits to 36 weeks gestation
  - weekly visits until delivery

Procedure Differentiation
These codes should be reported when documentation indicates that the physician or other qualified health care professional provides all or part of the antepartum care but does not perform the delivery due to termination of the pregnancy or referral to another physician for delivery. When patients are seen for prenatal care over and above the visits described in the global obstetrical package because of complications, these services and procedures should be reported separately. To indicate the encounter with the provider, the appropriate level of E/M service code should be used. Any laboratory, radiologic, and other procedures or services should also be identified, using the appropriate CPT code.

Coding Tips
- For antepartum care provided for one to three visits only, do not report codes from range 59425–59426. Assign the appropriate E/M service code for each visit.
- Codes 59409–59410, 59425–59426, 59430, 59514–59515, 59612–59614, and 59620–59622 can be reported individually only if the patient relocates, the pregnancy was terminated, or complications or other circumstance necessitated the referral of the patient to another provider.
- Antepartum services that are separately billable include amniocentesis, cordocentesis, chorionic villus sampling, fetal contraction stress test, fetal nonstress test, and fetal scalp monitoring.

- Intrauterine fetal surgical procedures, including amnioinfusion, umbilical occlusion, fluid drainage, and shunt placement, are reported with 59070–59076. These services also include ultrasonic guidance in the description.

- All other fetal invasive procedures using ultrasonic guidance are reported with 59897.

- Amniocentesis (59000) may be performed as early as 12 weeks, although it is usually performed between 16 to 18 weeks of gestation. Amnioinfusion (59070) is used to treat problems associated with decreased intra-amniotic volume.

- Code 59050 includes supervision and interpretation of fetal monitoring during labor. Report 59051 for interpretation only.

- Antepartum care includes urinalysis and is not reported separately.

Delivery Services

Delivery services are defined as including:

- Admission to the hospital or birthing center

- Admission history and physical

- Management of uncomplicated labor

- Vaginal (with or without episiotomy, with or without forceps) or cesarean delivery

- Any postdelivery management as discharge services

Postpartum Care

Postpartum care consist of office or other outpatient services that are provided following the delivery whether or not the delivery was vaginal or cesarean.

Vaginal Delivery

Codes within this section allow the provider to report routine obstetrical care, including all antepartum, delivery, and postpartum care or a portion of the global surgery package. Codes from this section should not be used to report the vaginal delivery when the patient has had a previous cesarean delivery (vaginal birth after cesarean or VBAC). In those instances a code from the 59610–59622 range is used. Correct code assignment depends on the services rendered.

Procedure Differentiation

Vaginal deliveries are reported with 59400–59410 and 59610–59614. Appropriate code selection is dependent upon whether or not the patient has had a previous cesarean delivery.

Codes 59400–59410 are used to report a vaginal delivery when there is no history of a previous cesarean section. Code selection is dependent upon if the entire global obstetrical package was provided (59400), if only the delivery was provided (59409), or if delivery and postpartum care is provided (59410).

When the patient has had a previous cesarean section and the patient successfully delivers a subsequent infant vaginally, the appropriate code from range 59610–59614 is assigned. Again, code selection is dependent upon if all or only a portion of the global obstetrical package is provided.

 DEFINITIONS

classical cesarean section. Delivery of the fetus by an incision made in the upper part of the uterus, or corpus uteri, via an abdominal peritoneal approach. This type of delivery is performed when a vaginal delivery is not possible or advisable.

VBAC. Vaginal birth after cesarean section. Because of the uterine incision made for cesarean section, the mother has a higher risk for complications when delivering a subsequent infant vaginally.

Key Documentation Terms

It is crucial that the medical record is examined and the components of the global obstetrical package provided are identified. Also any previous cesarean sections must be documented as this affects code selection.

In ICD-10-CM, most codes require the assignment of a final character to indicate the pregnancy trimester at the time of the encounter. The final character indicates the gestational age of the fetus; for example, to report pre-existing type 2 diabetes mellitus affecting the care of the patient in the first trimester, report code O24.111; however, the same condition in the second trimester is reported with O24.112, and in the third trimester with O24.113. For other conditions it may be necessary to report the fetus affected. When coding for premature infants, the exact gestational age of the fetus must be reported in addition to the weight in grams.

Coding Tips

- An episiotomy is included in these procedures and should not be billed separately.

- For repair of an episiotomy by a provider other than the attending, see 59300.

Cesarean Delivery

Procedure Differentiation

Cesarean deliveries are reported using the appropriate code from range 59510–59515 or 59618–59622.

Codes within this range are used to report all or a portion of the global obstetrical package when the delivery is by cesarean section. As with the vaginal delivery codes, correct code selection depends on what portions of the global obstetrical package are provided and whether the patient who has had a previous cesarean delivery unsuccessfully attempted a vaginal delivery.

Report 59510 for a normal cesarean delivery, including antepartum and postpartum care; 59514 for cesarean delivery only; 59515 for cesarean delivery, including postpartum care. These codes are used to report an unscheduled initial or scheduled cesarean delivery.

Also within this section is code 59525, which is used to report a subtotal or total hysterectomy that is performed at the same surgical encounter as the cesarean delivery. Note that this is an add-on code and is listed in addition to the cesarean delivery code.

Delivery after previous cesarean is reported with codes 59618–59622. As mentioned above, there are times when a patient has had a previous cesarean birth and presents with the expectation of delivering vaginally (VBAC). Because previous cesarean delivery can complicate the vaginal delivery and the patient may require a cesarean delivery, separate codes have been developed to report these services.

Codes 59610–59614 are used to report a vaginal delivery after previous cesarean delivery. Correct code selection depends on how much of the global obstetrical package was provided.

For those patients who have had a previous cesarean delivery and are expecting to deliver vaginally but require a cesarean delivery, a code from the

59618–59622 range is reported. Again, correct code assignment depends on the level of care provided.

Key Documentation Terms

It is crucial that the medical record is examined and the components of the global obstetrical package provided are identified. Also any previous cesarean sections must be documented as this affects code selection.

Multiple pregnancies are often delivered by cesarean; each baby is identified in ICD-10-CM. A seventh-character will be required in categories that designate maternal care for a fetal anomaly, damage, or other problem is required in order to indicate the affected fetus.

Coding Tips

*   To report elective cesarean deliveries, see 59510, 59514, or 59515.

Cesarean Section Crosswalk

Procedure	First Delivery	Subsequent w/o mention of previous C-Section	Following trial vaginal delivery	Subsequent, elective
Cesarean delivery including ante- and postpartum care	59510	59510	59618	59510
Cesarean delivery only	59514	59514	59620	59514
Cesarean delivery w/postpartum care	59515	59515	59622	59515

Billing and Payment Issues

Some payers do not reimburse additionally for multiple gestations; however, many will. In the case of delivery of multiple gestation, the appropriate global code for the first delivery is assigned and the second delivery is reported using the appropriate delivery only code. For example, if a patient who has received routine obstetrical care from the provider delivers twins vaginally, twin A delivery is reported using 59400 and twin B delivery is reported using 59409. Modifier 59 should be appended to the subsequent codes.

Payers may or may not reduce the second delivery code depending upon their policy.

Abortion: Spontaneous/Elective (59812–59857)

Codes 59812–59841 are reported for surgical services related to an abortion.

Procedure Differentiation

Codes within this subsection are selected based on the type of abortion and the trimester.

Determine code assignment for the surgical treatment of abortion based upon the following factors:

*   Trimester of pregnancy

*   Incomplete spontaneous or missed abortion

*   Induced abortion

*   Treatment of septic abortion

Often referred to as a miscarriage, the surgical treatment of a spontaneous abortion is reported with 59812. Unless the documentation indicates some type of surgical procedure, usually a dilation and curettage, this code should not be used.

Codes 59820 and 59821 are selected based on the gestational age of the fetus. After inserting a dilator into the endocervix and up through the cervical canal to enlarge the opening, a cannula is placed in the endocervical canal, passing into the uterus. A suction machine is then activated and the uterine contents are evacuated by rotation of the cannula. After suction curettage, a sharp curette may be used to gently scrape the uterus to ensure that it is empty.

Surgical treatment of a septic abortion (59830) must be supported by documentation that indicates that prompt evacuation of the uterus and vigorous medical treatment of the patient was provided. A septic abortion is one complicated by generalized fever and infection. There is also inflammation and infection of the endometrium and in the cellular tissue around the uterus. The physician treats the infection with intravenous antibiotics and blood transfusions as necessary. To evacuate the uterus, the physician inserts a speculum into the vagina to view the cervix. Suction curettage and a sharp curette are used to gently scrape the uterus to ensure that it is empty.

An induced abortion is the legal termination of the pregnancy by dilation and curettage, dilation and evacuation, or intra-amniotic injections.

Code 59840 is used to report the termination by dilation and curettage. The physician inserts a speculum into the vagina to view the cervix. A tenaculum is used to grasp the cervix, pull it down, and exert traction. A dilator is inserted into the endocervix and through the cervical canal to enlarge the opening. The physician places a curette in the endocervical canal and passes it into the uterus. The uterine contents are removed by rotating the curette and gently scraping the uterus until all the products of conception are removed.

Code 59841 describes the termination by dilation and evacuation (D&E). Because D&E requires wider cervical dilation than curettage, the physician may dilate the cervix with a laminaria several hours to several days before the procedure. At the time of the procedure, the physician inserts a speculum into the vagina to view the cervix. A tenaculum is used to grasp the cervix, pull it down, and exert traction. The physician places a cannula in the dilated endocervical canal and passes it into the uterus. The suction machine is activated, and the uterine contents are evacuated by rotation of the cannula. For pregnancies through 16 weeks, the cannula usually evacuates the pregnancy. For later pregnancies, the cannula is used to drain amniotic fluid and to draw tissue into the lower uterus for extraction by forceps. In either case, a sharp curette may be used to gently scrape the uterus to ensure that it is empty.

When a pregnancy is terminated by inducing labor with amniocentesis and intra-amniotic injections, the appropriate code from the 59850–59852. Code 59850 describes a method that is usually used after the first trimester (13 weeks or more). The physician inserts an amniocentesis needle into the abdomen to obtain a free flow of clear amniotic fluid. A hypertonic solution is then administered by gravity drip. The hypertonic solution results in fetal death and labor usually results. Code 59851 is used when this method fails to expel all products of conception, and a dilation and curettage and/or evacuation is used to remove the remaining tissue. Code 59852 is used when this method fails to expel all products of conception and a hysterotomy, through an incision in the

DEFINITIONS

abortion. Premature expulsion or extraction of the products of conception.

failed attempted abortion. Induced medical abortion that does not eliminate the pregnancy.

illegally induced abortion. Intentional termination of pregnancy that is performed outside the legal boundaries of state law or performed by someone or within a facility failing to meet qualification requirements.

legally induced abortion. Elective or therapeutic termination of pregnancy performed within legal parameters by a licensed physician or other qualified medical professionals.

missed abortion. Retention of a dead fetus within the uterus in cases where fetal demise occurred before 20 weeks gestation. Abortion in this context refers to retained products of conception from the death of a normal fetus that does not result in spontaneous or induced abortion, or missed delivery. Indications are cessation of growth, hardening of the uterus, or a reduction in its size. Fetal electrocardiography or ultrasonography is used to confirm this diagnosis.

selective abortion. Selective reduction, most often using potassium chloride injections, performed to eliminate one or more fetuses of a multiple pregnancy in an attempt to increase the viability of the remaining fetuses. Fetuses are usually eliminated in this procedure until only a twin or triplet pregnancy remains.

DEFINITIONS

spontaneous abortion. Early expulsion of the products of conception from the uterus that occurs naturally, without chemical intervention or instrumentation, before completion of 22 weeks of gestation. Spontaneous abortion may be complete, in which all of the products of conception are expelled, or incomplete, in which parts of the placental material or fetus are retained. Symptoms may include lower abdominal cramping and vaginal bleeding. In cases of incomplete spontaneous abortion, surgical intervention in the form of curettage is required in order to remove the remaining tissue. Medical intervention is generally not required with complete spontaneous abortion.

threatened abortion. Signs and symptoms of a potential miscarriage that occur in early pregnancy, defined by ICD-10-CM as before 20 weeks of completed gestation. Primary symptoms include vaginal bleeding with or without uterine cramping, and a closed cervical os.

abdominal wall and uterus, is used to remove the remaining tissue. Following removal, the incision is closed with sutures.

Termination can also be by means of vaginal suppositories, which induce labor. Before using the suppositories, a laminaria, which is an applicator made of kelp or synthetic material, may be inserted in the cervix to soften and expand the cervical canal. Once the cervix is ready, the physician inserts the vaginal suppositories and labor usually results. The fetus and placenta are delivered through the vagina (59855). Code 59856 is used when this method fails to expel all products of conception and a dilation and curettage and/or evacuation is used to remove the remaining tissue. Code 59857 is used when this method fails to expel all products of conception and a hysterotomy, through an incision in the abdominal wall and uterus, is used to remove the remaining tissue.

Medical Necessity

Some payer contracts may only provide coverage for the treatment of spontaneous abortions.

Legally induced abortions are not covered Medicare procedures except when:

- A woman suffers from a physical disorder, physical injury, or physical illness, including a life-endangering physical condition caused by or arising from the pregnancy itself that would, as certified by a physician, place the patient at the risk of death.

- The pregnancy is the result of an act of rape or incest

Key Documentation Terms

Documentation should indicate the surgical procedure that was performed. Terms such as incomplete, missed, induced, intra-amniotic injection, suppositories, or dilation and curettage provide the guidance needed to ensure correct code assignment. Above all else, the documentation should support the medical necessity of the procedure.

Coding Tips

- When complete spontaneous abortions are treated medically, use the appropriate E/M codes from range 99202–99233.

- A blighted ovum is considered a fertilized egg and treatment is reported using the appropriate code from range 59812–59830.

- Antepartum care associated with a pregnancy that terminates in an abortion is coded in one of the following ways:

  - antepartum care only: four to six visits, see 59425

  - antepartum care only: seven or more visits, see 59426

  - office visit reported for each visit up to four visits, see 99202–99215

- Verify that the procedure code reported is supported by the ICD-10-CM code reported. For example, the surgical treatment of a spontaneous abortion is not supported by the diagnosis of a missed abortion.

Procedures Performed on the Nervous System

Craniectomy/Craniotomy/Decompression Brain by Surgical Approach/Specific Area of Brain (61304–61576)

When auditing craniotomy and craniectomy procedures it is important to know that codes are determined based upon the reason for the surgery (abscess, tumor, etc.), the surgical approach (subtemporal, suboccipital, transcranial), the site of the opening, and the extent of the opening as defined by the subsequent definitive procedure. A craniotomy involves removal of part of the skull (bone flap) to access the brain. When a larger area of the skull is removed, it is usually retained and then refitted. In craniectomy, the skull flap is not replaced.

Surgical procedures involving the skull base are categorized according to approach, definitive procedure, and repair and reconstruction (reported separately).

A burr hole is often necessary for a craniotomy or craniectomy to access intracranial contents, to alleviate pressure, or to place an intracranial pressure monitoring device. When this service is integral to the performance of other services, CPT codes describing these services are not reported separately if performed at the surgical encounter. A burr hole may be reported separately with another cranial procedure only if performed at a separate site unrelated to the other cranial procedure or at a separate surgical encounter on the same date of service.

Procedure Differentiation

Codes 61304 and 61305 report exploration only. Code 61304 reports supratentorial, 61305 reports infratentorial. If followed by a therapeutic procedure during the same surgical session, report only the therapeutic procedure.

Evacuation of a hematoma is reported with 61312–61315 depending on the location of the hematoma.

If a cranial bone graft is placed onto a part of the skull for repair following craniectomy, craniotomy, or other intracranial surgery, report add-on code 61316.

Codes 61320 and 61321 describe drainage of an abscess via a craniectomy or a craniotomy. Code selection is dependent upon supratentorial or infratentorial.

Codes 61322 and 61323 report decompression procedures performed for treatment of intracranial hypertension, with or without a lobectomy.

Procedures of the orbit are reported with 61330–61333.

Other decompression procedures are reported with 61340–61345, depending on approach. Code 61340 is generally performed for benign intracranial hypertension (pseudotumor cerebri) or slit ventricle syndrome. Code 61343 is for Arnold-Chiari malformation. Code 61345 reports other cranial decompressions. Exploration or decompression of the cranial nerves is reported with 61458–61460.

DEFINITIONS

evacuation. Removal or purging of waste material.

extradural. Located outside of the dura mater.

hematoma. Tumor-like collection of blood in some part of the body caused by a break in a blood vessel wall, usually as a result of trauma.

infratentorial. Located below or beneath the tentorium of the cerebellum, which is the dura mater supporting the occipital lobes and covering the cerebellum.

subdural. Potential space between the dura matter and arachnoid membrane around the brain.

supratentorial. Located above the tentorium. The tentorium is the covering of dura mater in the brain supporting the occipital lobes and covering the cerebellum.

DEFINITIONS

Arnold-Chiari syndrome.
Congenital malformation of the brain in which the cerebellum protrudes through the foramen magnum into the spinal canal. There are three types of official Chiari malformation, classified by the severity of herniation. Type II is referred to as the syndrome. This malformation is seen with hydrocephalus, mental defects, and always with a lumbosacral myelomeningocele.

corpus callosum. Mass of thick fibers in the white matter of the brain that connects the right and left hemisphere.

electrocorticography. Electrodes are placed onto specific areas of the brain to record the brain's electrical activity while the cortex is irrigated to localize areas of seizure activity in patients with intractable epileptic seizures who are surgical candidates for excising the epileptic focus or a lobectomy.

innervation. Nerve distribution to a body part.

meningioma. Slow growing, benign vascular tumor originating in the meninges of the brain or spinal cord.

Decompression or compression of the gasserian ganglion is reported with 61450. The gasserian ganglion supplies sensory innervation to the face via the trigeminal nerve.

Excision of brain abscess, cyst, meningiomas, or tumors are reported with 61500–61516 and 61518–61530. Pituitary tumors are reported with 61546–61548; cranial bone tumors 61563–61564. Foreign body removal is reported with 61570–61571.

Add-on code 61517 is reported when a chemotherapeutic agent is implanted into a brain cavity at the time a craniectomy or craniotomy is done to excise the brain tumor. It is reported in conjunction with 61510 or 61518.

Codes 61531–61533 report subdural implantation of electrodes, for long-term seizure monitoring. In 61531, the physician uses a burr or trephine holes to reach the subdural layer. Linear strip electrodes are implanted in each hole. Subdural electrodes are placed just below the dura and do not penetrate the cerebral tissue. In 61533, a bone flap is elevated to implant a subdural electrode array along the cerebral hemispheres. In 61534 and 61536, the epileptogenic focus (the seizure center) is excised. Code 61535 is reported for removal of epidural or subdural electrode array.

Craniotomies with elevation of bone flaps including lobectomies are reported with 61537–61540, temporal lobe lobectomy with or without electrocorticography (61537–61538); other than temporal lobe lobectomy with or without electrocorticography, partial or total (61539–61540).

In 61541, the corpus callosum is transected. This procedure may be staged, with the anterior two-thirds of the corpus callosum being sectioned on the first procedure. If the anterior section is not satisfactory, the posterior third will be sectioned in a second procedure. To report a staged procedure, one that is planned prospectively at the time of the original procedure and performed during the postoperative period of the first procedure, append modifier 58 to the staged or related procedure.

Code 61543 reports a partial or subtotal (functional) hemispherectomy. Report 61543 when the procedure is described as subtotal hemispherectomy with hemispherotomy or when it is described as a cerebral hemicorticectomy. It is performed for a variety of seizure disorders.

Code 61544 reports the excision or coagulation of choroid plexus. In this procedure the physician excises or destroys the choroid plexus. The choroid plexus produces spinal fluid. This procedure is generally performed for removal of tumors and hydrocephalus.

Excision of craniopharyngioma is reported with 61545. This is an excision of a benign tumor located at the base of the skull in the area of the pituitary gland. Although it is benign, it can cause symptoms by exerting localized pressure on the brain or blocking the flow of spinal fluid with resulting hydrocephalus. This type of tumor represents 2 to 3 percent of all primary brain tumors, and 5 to 13 percent of brain tumors in children.

Codes 61550–61559 report procedures for craniectomies and craniotomies for craniosynostosis. Craniosynostosis is a premature closure of the sutures of the skull. In the procedures described by 61550–61552, the physician incises and retracts the scalp over the fused suture line and cuts the bones to reshape the skull into an anatomically correct position. The recreated suture line is left open,

© 2020 Optum360, LLC

and the scalp is reanastomosed and sutured in layers. Report 61550 for a single suture; 61552 for multiple sutures. In 61556, the frontal or parietal bones are raised; in 61557, bifrontal bone flaps are raised; in 61558–61559 multiple suture lines are involved. In these procedures, the bones are reshaped. In 61558, no bone grafts are used to reshape the skull. In 61559, a bone flap is created from the harvested bones to enlarge and reshape the skull. Code 61559 includes obtaining bone grafts; therefore, any bone graft harvest is not reported separately.

Codes 61566–61567 describe a craniotomy performed to treat seizures. Code 61566 is specific to selective amygdalohippocampectomy (AH), which is done to treat intractable mesial temporal lobe epilepsy. This surgical procedure (61566) describes AH in which excision is limited to the anterior hippocampus, amygdala, and parahippocampal gyrus and preserves the fusiform gyrus and the lateral temporal lobe. In 61567, multiple subpial transections are done to reach the areas in the cortex where a focal point of the seizures is identified, as in the frontal, central, or temporal region, and cut the horizontal fibers responsible for the seizure while preserving the vertical fibers responsible for motor and speech. This procedure is done for chronic, intractable, complex partial seizures.

Codes 61575–61576 are reported for biopsy, decompression, or excision of a lesion of the skull base, brain stem, or upper spinal cord. In 61575, the physician accesses the affected area through the patient's mouth. In 61576, the physician performs a tracheostomy and cuts through the mandible and tongue to reach an extensive defect. The physician places a gag retractor in the patient's mouth and makes a posterior pharyngeal wall incision. The mucosa is retracted to the deep muscle layers, which are dissected to reach the skull base or superior spinal cord. The bone is removed to expose the area of interest. A lesion may be biopsied or excised. Decompression is accomplished by removing bone from around the structure. If incised, the dura is closed and the posterior pharyngeal wall is reapproximated and sutured in layers. Arthrodesis is reported separately when used with this procedure, see 22548.

Medical Necessity

The following conditions may warrant this procedure (this list is not all inclusive):

- Benign neoplasms
- Brain abscess
- Brain injury
- Cerebellar tremor
- Foreign body
- Implanting deep brain stimulators for the treatment of Parkinson's disease, epilepsy
- Malignant neoplasms
- Meningioma
- Seizure control

Key Documentation Terms

Documentation should indicate the surgical procedure that was performed. Terms such as anatomical location (e.g., extradural, subdural, or infratentorial), compression/decompression, excision, hematoma, bone flap, lobectomy, or seizure control provide the guidance needed to ensure correct code assignment. Above all else, the documentation should support the medical necessity of the procedure.

DEFINITIONS

Parkinson's disease. Neurologic condition progressive in nature caused by a decrease in dopamine. Symptoms include tremors, rigidity, slow movement, and weakened balance.

tremor. Involuntary trembling movement of a part or parts of the body due to alternate contractions of opposing muscles.

Coding Tips

- If in the course of a craniotomy/craniectomy a ventricular catheter, pressure recording device, or other intracerebral monitoring device is placed through the same skull hole, code 61107 Twist drill hole(s) for subdural, intracerebral, or ventricular puncture; for implanting ventricular catheter…, should not be reported separately.

- Code 61107 may be reported separately with an NCCI-associated modifier when placed through a different hole in the skull.

- A craniotomy is performed through a skull defect resulting from reflection of a skull flap. Replacing the skull flap during the same procedure is an integral component of a craniotomy procedure and should not be reported separately utilizing the cranioplasty codes 62140 and 62141. A cranioplasty may be reported separately with a craniotomy procedure if the cranioplasty is performed to replace a skull bone flap removed during a procedure at a prior patient encounter or if the cranioplasty is performed to repair a skull defect larger than that created by the bone flap.

- As "add-on" codes, 61316 and 61517 are not subject to multiple procedure rules. No reimbursement reduction or modifier 51 is applied. The following table provides additional information for these codes as found in the Medicare Physician Fee Schedule Database.

Parent Code	Add-On	GLOB DAYS	MULT PROC	BILAT SURG	ASST SURG	CO-SURG	TEAM SURG
61304		090	2	0	2	1	0
61312		090	2	0	2	1	0
61313		090	2	0	2	1	0
	61316	ZZZ	0	0	1	0	0
61322		090	2	0	2	1	0
61323		090	2	0	2	1	0
61340		090	2	1	2	1	0
61510		090	2	0	2	1	0
	61517	ZZZ	0	0	1	0	0
61518		090	2	0	2	1	0
61570		090	2	0	2	1	0
61571		090	2	0	2	1	0
61680		090	2	0	2	1	0
61682		090	2	0	2	1	0
61684		090	2	0	2	1	0
61686		090	2	0	2	1	0
61690		090	2	0	2	1	0
61692		090	2	0	2	1	0
61697		090	2	0	2	1	0
61698		090	2	0	2	1	0
61700		090	2	0	2	1	0
61702		090	2	0	2	1	0
61703		090	2	0	2	1	0
61705		090	2	0	2	1	0

- For orbital decompression using a lateral wall approach (Kroenlein type), see 67445.

Posterior Midline Approach: Laminectomy/Laminotomy/Laminoplasty/Decompression (62380, 63001–63051)

Laminotomy and laminectomy are performed to remove the lamina from the vertebral body and gain access to the spinal cord, disc, and nerves. The key procedure is not the access or laminal procedures, but the treatment of the nerves and intervertebral discs. If the lamina is removed for an arthrodesis without neural procedures it is considered part of the arthrodesis and is not reported separately.

Procedure Differentiation

Codes in this section are determined by level (e.g., cervical, thoracic, lumbar, each additional) and the extent of the procedure performed. The number of segments involved varies according to the levels of disc or nerve impingement.

Exploration and decompression of the spinal cord without discectomy is reported with 63001–63011 if one to two vertebral segments are accessed and 63015–63017 if more than two vertebral segments are accessed. A Gill type procedure is reported with 63012 and includes removal of abnormal facets with decompression of the cauda equina and is performed only on the lumbar spine.

Decompression of nerve roots, including excision of a herniated disc if performed, is reported with 63020–63035 for each interspace accessed with a combination of laminotomy, hemilaminectomy, facetectomy, or foraminotomy and 63040–63044 if a re-exploration. For endoscopic decompression of spinal cord and nerve roots including laminotomy, partial facetectomy, foraminotomy, discectomy, and/or excision of herniated intervertebral disc, see 62380.

Decompression of the spinal cord, cauda equina, and nerve roots accessed by a combination of laminectomy, facetectomy, and foraminotomy is reported with 63045–63048. These codes specifically include unilateral or bilateral services and are reported per vertebral segment.

Cervical laminoplasty is reported with 63050 and includes two or more vertebral segments. Report 63051 if the posterior bony portions are reconstructed.

Medical Necessity

The following conditions may warrant this procedure (this list is not all inclusive):

- Cauda equina syndrome
- Congenital spondylolisthesis
- Disc degeneration
- Herniated disc
- Injury/fracture to the vertebrae
- Spinal stenosis
- Spondylosis

Key Documentation Terms

Documentation should indicate the surgical procedure that was performed. Terms such as vertebrae level (e.g., cervical, thoracic, lumbar), facetectomy, foraminotomy, laminotomy or laminectomy provide the guidance needed to ensure correct code assignment. Above all else, the documentation should support the medical necessity of the procedure.

 DEFINITIONS

discectomy. Surgical excision of an intervertebral disk.

facetectomy. Surgical excision of a vertebral articular facet, performed with laminectomy or laminotomy.

hemilaminectomy. Excision of a portion of the vertebral lamina.

interspace. Space between two similar objects.

laminoplasty. Creation of a gutter in the vertebral lamina, with one side acting like a hinge, and the other opening like a door to decompress a pinched spinal cord. The hinge is held in place with small bone struts and a bone graft may be fitted into the open door position with miniplates, wires, or suture.

laminotomy. Surgical incision to divide the lamina, forming the posterior arch of a vertebra, to take pressure off nerve roots, sometimes caused by the rupture of a herniated vertebral disk.

Coding Tips

- Cervical laminoplasty procedures (63050–63051) should not be performed during the same operative session as other procedures on the same vertebral segment (cervical). See the CPT book for complete guidelines.

- Arthrodesis (22590–22614) is reported separately when performed with 63001–63048.

- Codes 63020–63044 are considered unilateral. Report codes 63020, 63030, 63040, and 63042 with modifier 50 if performed bilaterally. For codes 63035, 63043, and 63044 report the procedure code twice if performed bilaterally; do not report with modifier 50.

- The use of an operating microscope (69990) may be reported separately.

- As "add-on" codes, 63035, 63043, 63044, and 63048, are not subject to multiple procedure rules. No reimbursement reduction or modifier 51 is applied. The following table provides additional information for these codes as found in the Medicare Physician Fee Schedule Database.

Parent Code	Add-On	GLOB DAYS	MULT PROC	BILAT SURG	ASST SURG	CO-SURG	TEAM SURG
63020		090	2	1	2	2	0
63030		090	2	1	2	2	0
	63035	ZZZ	0	1	2	2	0
63040		090	2	1	2	2	0
63042		090	2	1	2	2	0
	63043	ZZZ	0	1	2	2	0
	63044	ZZZ	0	1	2	2	0
63045		090	2	2	2	2	0
63046		090	2	2	2	2	0
63047		090	2	2	2	2	0
	63048	ZZZ	0	0	2	2	0

YIELD **DENIAL ALERT**

Manipulation of the spine is integral to spinal procedures. Code 22505 Manipulation of the spine requiring anesthesia, any region, will be denied when reported with a spinal procedure.

Procedures Performed on the Eye and Ocular Adnexa

Anterior Sclera Procedures: By Indication/Specific Area of Eye (66130–66250)

This subsection includes procedures of the anterior sclera, a dense fibrous tissue that forms the "white" of the eye. The sclera helps to maintain the shape of the eyeball and is where the extrinsic muscles of the eye are attached. It is covered with the vascular episclera, the Tenon capsule (fascial bulbi), and the conjunctiva. The sclera comprises five-sixths of the eye surface, with the remaining one-sixth covered by the cornea, which bridges the anterior scleral foramen, one of the two large openings in the sclera. Procedures in this part of the eye are performed primarily for glaucoma, using a variety of techniques including aqueous shunt procedures.

Procedure Differentiation

Removal of a sclera lesion by cutting through the conjunctiva is reported with 66130.

Codes 66150–66172 describe fistulization of the sclera. Each code listed below includes an additional procedure or a different technique to achieve the fistulization.

- Code 66150 reports procedures using a trephine to remove a circular portion of the sclera and iris.

- Code 66155 describes thermocauterization where a portion of the sclera and iris are destroyed by burning with a hot probe.

- Code 66160 reports a sclerectomy using a punch or scleral scissors and includes an iridectomy. Various methods of sclerectomy include Lindner's, Lagrange, Knapp's, Holth's, and Herbert's operations.

- Code 66170 is reported for a trabeculectomy performed in the absence of previous surgery.

- Code 66172 reports a trabeculectomy performed on a patient who has scarring from previous ocular surgery or trauma. This code is to be used only when a trabeculectomy is performed on an eye that has conjunctival scarring from previous ocular surgery or injury. Examples include history of cataract surgery, history of strabismus surgery, history of failed trabeculectomy ab externo, history of penetrating trauma to the eyeball, or conjunctival lacerations. This procedure includes the injection of antifibriotic agents, such a 5-Fluorouracil (5-FU). The technique of injecting 5-FU is recognized as effective in reducing the number of failed procedures caused by the formation of scar tissue and fistula closure.

Aqueous outflow canal transluminal dilation is reported with codes 66174–66175. Report 66175 if a polypropylene suture is placed within the canal to improve aqueous outflow and preserve canal patency. This procedure is usually performed for open-angle glaucoma.

Procedures that pertain to aqueous shunt to extraocular reservoirs are reported with 66179–66185. Shunt procedures are performed in the anterior segment of the eye to reduce and control intraocular pressure (IOP). An aqueous shunt creates an alternate path for aqueous humor to leave the anterior chamber of the

DEFINITIONS

shunt. Surgically created passage between blood vessels or other natural passages, such as an arteriovenous anastomosis, to divert or bypass blood flow from the normal channel.

trabeculectomy. Surgical incision between the anterior portion of the eye and the canal of Schlemm to drain the aqueous humor.

eye and thus lower IOP. In 66179, the physician places an ocular speculum in the patient's eye, makes an incision in the conjunctiva, places tubing into the anterior portion of the eye at the juncture of the sclera and cornea (the limbus), and sutures tubing to the sclera. This improves the aqueous flow in the anterior chamber. The tube implant connects to an equatorial reservoir plate (a bleb) sutured into place behind the pars plana between the extraocular muscles. The physician stretches conjunctival tissue over the shunt and reservoir and sutures it into place. The physician closes the incision with sutures and may restore the intraocular pressure with an injection of water or saline. A topical antibiotic or pressure patch may be applied. Report 66180 when a graft is performed.

Code 66183 describes a procedure in which the physician treats a refractory, primary, open-angle glaucoma by draining aqueous humor from the anterior chamber directly into the Schlemm's canal by shunting or stenting, lowering intraocular pressure (IOP) without the formation of a filtering bleb using an external approach. The physician inserts an implant via a superficial scleral flap through the trabeculum and into the anterior chamber. IOP is reduced by diverting the excess aqueous fluid from the anterior chamber to a subconjunctival bleb rather than to an extraocular reservoir.

When the documentation states that the physician revises a previously placed aqueous shunt to extraocular equatorial plate reservoir, report 66184. The physician places an ocular speculum in the patient's eye and opens the previous incision in the conjunctiva. The tubing from the anterior chamber to the reservoir is revised or replaced. The physician stretches conjunctival tissue over the shunt and reservoir and sutures it into place. The physician may restore the intraocular pressure with an injection of water or saline, and a topical antibiotic or pressure patch may be applied. Report 66184 for revision without graft and 66185 for revision with graft.

Repair of the sclera is reported with 66225 and revision of an operative wound with 66250.

Medical Necessity
The following conditions may warrant these procedures (this list is not all inclusive):

- Essential or progressive iris atrophy
- Glaucoma
- Plateau iris syndrome

Key Documentation Terms
Documentation should indicate the surgical procedure that was performed. Terms such as excision, fistulization, revision, or repair provide the guidance needed to ensure correct code assignment. Above all else, the documentation should support the medical necessity of the procedure.

Coding Tips
- These procedures are generally performed with a subconjunctival injection, retrobulbar injection, or a topical anesthetic rather than general anesthesia.
- Codes 66180 and 66185 should not be reported with scleral reinforcement with graft procedures (67255).
- The use of an operating microscope (69990) is not reported separately.

DEFINITIONS

iridectomy. Surgical removal of part of the iris.

Plateau iris syndrome. Primary angle-closure glaucoma in the absence of classic pupillary block, identifiable by an angle-closure attack. Occurs in the presence of a patent iridectomy caused by an abnormality of the peripheral iris.

Iris, Ciliary Body Procedures: Destruction/Iridectomy/Iridotomy/Repair (66500–66770)

The iris, which lies in front of the lens and ciliary body, separates the anterior chamber from the posterior chamber. The posterior portion of the iris rests on the front of the lens. It contains the pupil, which controls the amount of light that enters the eye.

The ciliary body is a ring of tissue, about 6 mm wide, that is primarily responsible for the production of aqueous humor, accommodation, and maintenance of the lens zonules. Many of the procedures performed on the iris and ciliary are for the treatment of glaucoma.

Procedure Differentiation

Incision into the iris, iridotomy, is reported with 66500 for stab incision; 66505 is reported for transfixion for iris bombe. Iris bombe is a condition where the iris balloons forward blocking aqueous outflow channels. In this procedure, the surgeon pierces the iris in two places.

Excision of the iris (iridectomy) codes (66600–66635) are selected according to the extent of the procedure and concomitant procedures. Codes 66625–66635 are separate procedures by definition and are usually a component of a more complex service and are not identified separately. When performed alone or with other unrelated procedures/services they may be reported. If performed alone, list the code; if performed with other procedures/services, list the code and append modifier 59.

Code 66600 describes the excision of a full-thickness piece of the iris, which is usually accomplished with an argon laser.

In 66605, excision of a piece of the ciliary body (cyclectomy) is performed, the burn is deeper, and goes through the iris into the ciliary body.

Code 66625 is reported for a peripheral iridectomy. In the procedure, a piece of the iris is removed, providing a direct passageway for aqueous. This causes the intraocular pressure to fall as aqueous from behind the iris can flow forward and drain from the eye. This procedure is also called basal, buttonhole, or stenopeic iridectomy and is performed for glaucoma.

In 66630, a sector iridectomy is performed. An incision is made at the juncture of the cornea and sclera (the limbus). The physician removes a wedge piece from the iris leaving what is often referred to as a keyhole pupil.

Code 66635 describes an optical iridectomy. In this procedure an incision is made at the juncture of the cornea and sclera (the limbus). The physician trims the inner ring of iris as a means of widening an abnormally small pupil and improving vision. This is usually performed for pupillary abnormalities (e.g., Argyll Robertson pupil or miosis).

Repair of the iris is reported with 66680 or 66682. Report 66680 for tears at the base of the iris, separating it from the ciliary body; code 66682 for sutures of the iris or ciliary body. These procedures are also performed due to degenerative changes.

 DENIAL ALERT

Repair of laceration codes 65270–65286 will be denied when reported separately for closure of a surgical incision of the conjunctiva, cornea, or sclera.

 DEFINITIONS

Argyll Robertson pupil. Absence of light reflex in the pupil, with no change in the pupil's focus functions.

miosis. Sustained abnormal contraction of the pupil less than 2 mm that is not caused by miotics.

Medical Necessity
The following conditions may warrant these excision and repair procedures (unless noted by the individual code above):

- Atrophy
- Benign neoplasms
- Cysts
- Glaucoma
- Malignant neoplasms
- Plateau iris syndrome

Destruction of a ciliary body is reported with 66700–66740 based upon the method of destruction used.

In 66700, heat probe or diathermy is used to burn holes in the ciliary body.

If a cyclophotocoagulation (laser) is used as a means of destruction, 66710 should be reported for transscleral and 66711 if performed endoscopically. Code 66711 is performed without simultaneous removal of the crystalline lens. If endoscopic cyclophotocoagulation is performed during the same encounter as removal of an extracapsular cataract with the insertion of an intraocular lens, 66987 or 66988 should be reported.

In 66720, a freezing probe (cryotherapy) is used for destruction.

Code 66740 describes cyclodialysis, which is a procedure used to separate the ciliary body from the sclera (a result of trauma or glaucoma surgery).

Laser iridotomy or iridectomy is reported with 66761 per session, and a treatment series using photocoagulation is reported with 66762.

Destruction of a lesion or cyst is reported with 66770.

The following conditions may warrant destruction procedures (unless noted by the individual code above):

- Aniridia
- Atrophy
- Blind hypertensive eye
- Glaucoma
- Hyphema
- Iridodialysis
- Plateau iris syndrome

Key Documentation Terms
Documentation should indicate the surgical procedure that was performed. Terms such as destruction, excision, incision, or repair provide the guidance needed to ensure correct code assignment. Above all else, the documentation should support the medical necessity of the procedure.

 DEFINITIONS

aniridia. Congenital anomaly in which there is incomplete formation or absence of the iris, resulting in loss of vision. Aniridia is typically bilateral and other health or developmental problems may be present.

atrophy. Reduction in size or activity in an anatomic structure, due to wasting away from disease or other factors.

hyphema. Pooled blood in the anterior segment of the eye.

Coding Tips

- These procedures are generally performed with a subconjunctival or retrobulbar injection rather than general anesthesia.

- The use of an operating microscope (69990) is not reported separately.

- When endoscopic cyclophotocoagulation is performed in the same operative session as an extracapsular cataract removal with intraocular lens insertion, see 66987 and 66988.

- When an extracapsular cataract removal is performed with a simultaneous endoscopic cyclophotocoagulation, see 66988.

Lens and Cataract Procedures (66820–66988)

The lens of the eye is the transparent, biconvex structure that is located behind the iris and pupil and anterior to a shallow depression in the face of the vitreous, the lenticular fossa.

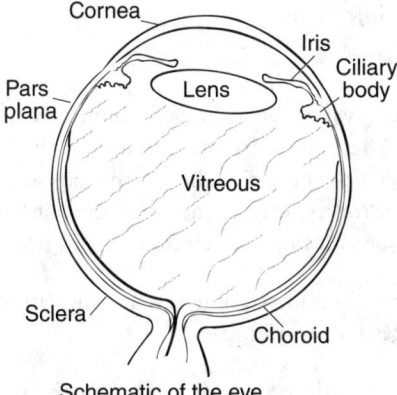

Schematic of the eye

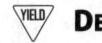

DENIAL ALERT

An iridectomy performed in order to complete a cataract extraction will be denied by most payers. The iridectomy is considered an integral part of the cataract procedure.

A cataract is a condition that involves the partial or total opacity of the crystalline lens or lens capsule. They are most commonly due to degenerative changes associated with the aging process; although they may occur in infants, children, or young adults.

Procedure Differentiation

Code selection for this section is based on the type of procedure performed. This section is further divided with subheadings for incision and removal.

The incision subheading includes codes for discission by stab incision or laser and a code for repositioning of an intraocular prosthesis.

Codes 66820–66821 report discission of the secondary membrane of the lens. The patient initially had extracapsular cataract surgery in which the posterior shell of the lens was not removed from the eye. But the capsule and/or the membrane adjacent to it (the anterior hyaloid) has since become opaque and must be opened in this new surgery. Code 66821 reports a stab incision technique and 66822 uses a laser.

Code 66825 describes a procedure in which the physician makes an incision to access the artificial lens and then adjusts the artificial lens so that the attachments (haptics) of the implant are secured. The incision may be closed with sutures, and the intraocular pressure is restored with an injection of water or saline.

The removal subheading includes various codes for removal of cataract or lens material.

The following procedures are included in the code for the extraction of a lens (66830–66988). Do not reporting the following separately:

- Lateral canthotomy
- Iridectomy
- Iridotomy
- Anterior capsulotomy
- Posterior capsulotomy
- Use of viscoelastic agents (liquid inside connective tissue that helps maintain the shape of the anterior chamber during surgery)
- Enzymatic zonulysis (enzymes injected to break up fibrosis or adhesions of the anterior chambers)
- Pharmacological agents
- Subconjunctival injections
- Subtenon injections

Code 66830 reports removal of the secondary membrane of the lens. Documentation should describe a patient who initially had extracapsular cataract surgery, in which the posterior shell of the lens was not removed from the eye. The capsule and/or the membrane adjacent to it (the anterior hyaloid) has since become opaque and must be removed in this new surgery.

Codes 66840–66940 report removal of lens material, with code selection being dependent upon approach or technique.

In 66840, the lens is removed by aspiration. This procedure is reserved for only the softest of cataracts, such as infantile cataracts, and largely has been replaced by automated irrigation and aspiration techniques.

In 66850, the lens is removed by phacofragmentation. A needle that vibrates 40,000 times per second (phacofragmentation) or sound waves (phacoemulsification, ultrasound) are used to break up the lens. The physician uses irrigation and suction to remove the once hard nucleus, now liquefied by mechanical or sound vibrations.

Code 66852 reports lens removal using a pars plana approach. This approach is used to remove a cataract obstructing the view of the retina during retinal surgery, or to remove a piece of natural lens retained following cataract surgery. The physician makes an incision in the conjunctiva, sclera, and choroid of the pars plana. The physician approaches the lens capsule from behind. If a retained portion of the lens is removed, a portion of the clear gel in the back of the eye may be removed as well (vitrectomy).

Code 66920 reports intracapsular removal of the lens. Intracapsular cataract extraction (ICCE) is when the lens and capsule are removed intact. Report 66930 if removal is for a dislocated lens.

Extracapsular cataract extraction (ECCE) is when the anterior shell and the nucleus of the lens capsule are both removed, leaving the posterior shell of the lens capsule in place. This is reported with 66940 if methods other than described in 66840–66852 are used.

The minimal vitreous loss during cataract surgery does not warrant separate reporting as a vitrectomy no more than an iridectomy performed to accomplish

 DEFINITIONS

canthotomy. Horizontal incision at the canthus (junction of upper and lower eyelids) to divide the outer canthus and enlarge lid margin separation.

iridotomy. Surgical incision into the iris.

vitrectomy. Surgical removal of all or part of the vitreous body.

vitreous. Clear gel filling the posterior segment of the eye and functioning as a refractive component in vision and as a method of maintaining pressure in the posterior segment.

© 2020 Optum360, LLC

the cataract procedure does. However, there are situations when an iridectomy, trabeculectomy, or an anterior vitrectomy may be medically indicated and performed in conjunction with cataract removal and reported separately. For instance, an iridectomy performed to control glaucoma at the same time as a cataract extraction may be reported separately using a different diagnosis (e.g., glaucoma). Performing any of these services due only to an anticipated rise in intraocular pressure postoperatively is not reported separately.

Intraocular lens procedures are reported with range 66982–66988. These codes describe cataract removals replaced with intraocular lens (IOL) prostheses. The procedures are further differentiated by extracapsular and intracapsular extraction. An extracapsular extraction includes the removal of the lens material with the posterior capsule left intact. Intracapsular extraction (ICCE) is removal of the entire lens including the capsule.

Code 66982 reports an extracapsular cataract removal with insertion of intraocular lens prosthesis, without endoscopic cyclophotocoagulation, that is complex. Per the *CPT Assistant* March 2016, indications that justify reporting a complex cataract surgery (66982) include:

- The presence of a miotic pupil that will not dilate sufficiently to allow operative access to the lens, which requires the insertion of one of the following:
  - four iris retractors through four additional incisions
  - a Beehler expansion device
  - a sector iridectomy with subsequent suture repair of an iris sphincter
  - sphincterotomies created with scissors
- The presence of a disease state that produces lens support structures that are abnormally weak or absent, which requires the need to support the lens implant with permanent intraocular sutures, or, alternately, a capsular tension ring may be necessary to allow placement of an intraocular lens
- Pediatric cataract surgery

The documentation for code 66982 should indicate the physician makes a small horizontal incision where the cornea and sclera meet and, upon entering the eye through the incision, gently opens the front of the capsule and removes the hard center, or nucleus, of the lens. Using a microscope, the ophthalmologist suctions out the soft lens cortex, leaving the capsule in place. The area is irrigated and aspirated and an intraocular lens (IOL) (plastic disc that replaces the natural lens) is inserted. The ophthalmologist sutures the incision and instills antibiotic ointment and applies an eye patch. A metal shield is secured over the eye with tape. Standard phacoemulsification may be performed if the lens capsule is intact and sufficient zonular support remains. In capsulorrhexis, the ophthalmologist shatters the cataract nucleus with an ultrasonic oscillating probe. After fragmentation, the phaco probe is inserted into the eye and the cataract is suctioned out through an irrigation-aspiration probe. An IOL is inserted once all of the material is removed. Suture fixation is chosen if both capsular and zonular supports are insufficient and the angle is minimally damaged. In 66987, endoscopic cyclophotocoagulation (ECP) is also performed on the ciliary body and may be accomplished by different methods. In one method, with the pupil dilated, a limbal incision is made and any posterior synechiae are lysed. Viscoelastic material is injected under the iris to partially fill and expand the ciliary sulcus. The ECP probe is inserted under the iris. The probe allows simultaneous visualization with the photocoagulation.

Approximately half the circumference of the ciliary body is treated through the first limbal incision. Another incision is made 180 degrees from the first and the other half of the ciliary body circumference is treated. The viscoelastic material is removed by irrigation and aspiration and the wounds are closed.

Codes 66983–66984 describe the typical lens removal (not complex): with insertion of a lens; intracapsular 66983 and extracapsular, without endoscopic cyclophotocoagulation, 66984. When this procedure is performed with endoscopic cyclophotocoagulation, 66988 should be reported.

Code 66985 reports insertion of an IOL performed during a subsequent surgery.

Other services and supplies may be reported separately during the IOL insertion (66985), if applicable. If a determination of intraocular lens power is required at the time of insertion, code 76519 can be reported separately. When reporting an IOL insertion, the IOL itself is not included. If the surgeon provides the IOL, code 99070 should be used to report the supply of the lens. If performed in a surgery center, it would not be appropriate for the surgeon to bill for the supply.

Code 66986 is reported when an IOL is replaced.

When an ophthalmic endoscope (66990) is used with 66985 or 66986, it may be reported separately.

Medical Necessity

The following conditions may warrant cataract procedures (this list is not all inclusive):

- Cataract
- Dislocated lens
- Ectopic lens
- Glaucoma
- Injury/trauma
- Marfan syndrome
- Pseudoexfoliation syndrome
- Uveitis

Key Documentation Terms

Documentation should indicate the surgical procedure that was performed. Terms such as cyclophotocoagulation, discission, removal, reposition, extracapsular, intracapsular, or intraocular provide the guidance needed to ensure correct code assignment. It must be clearly documented that the patient has impairment of visual function due to cataracts. A decreased ability to carry out activities of daily living, including (but not limited to) reading, watching television, driving, or meeting occupational or vocational expectations, should be documented if applicable. Due to the fact that payer guidelines vary greatly on documentation requirements, it is wise to consult the payer prior to performing the procedure. When reporting 66982 and 66987, the details that contribute to the complexity of the procedure must be documented to receive appropriate reimbursement.

DEFINITIONS

ectopic. Organ or other structure that is aberrant or out of place.

glaucoma. Rise in intraocular pressure, restricting blood flow and decreasing vision.

Marfan syndrome. Disorder that affects the connective tissue of multiple systems, including disproportionally long or abnormal bone structure and eye and cardiovascular complications.

pseudoexfoliation of lens. Deposits of unknown composition and origin appearing on lens surfaces of the eye.

uveitis. Inflammaton of the middle eye layer including the iris and ciliary body.

Coding Tips

- An anterior capsulotomy, iridectomy, iridotomy, lateral canthotomy, posterior capsulotomy, the use of viscoelastic agents, enzymatic zonulysis, and other pharmacologic agents, as well as subconjunctival or sub-tenon injections, are integral to the extraction of a lens.

- The use of an operating microscope (69990) is not reported separately, except with 66985-66986.

- Do not code the injection of Healon or other medications used in conjunction with cataract surgery. Code 66030 Injection of medication into the anterior chamber, is often used inappropriately. The injection is considered an integral part of the cataract procedure and should not be reported separately.

- If a medically necessary iridectomy, vitrectomy, or trabeculectomy is performed with a cataract extraction under a separate diagnosis, modifier 59 should be appended to the service and the medical documentation needs to clearly state the need for the service.

- All of the cataract removal procedures are mutually exclusive of each other when performed on the same eye.

- These procedures are generally performed with a local anesthetic or a retrobulbar injection rather than general anesthesia.

- When an extracapsular cataract removal and IOL insertion are performed with a simultaneous endoscopic cyclophotocoagulation, report 66988.

- When a complex extracapsular cataract removal is performed with a simultaneous endoscopic cyclophotocoagulation, report 66987.

Strabismus and Other Procedures of Extraocular Muscles (67311–67340)

Strabismus is a disorder of the eyes in which the eyes are not able to focus together on an object because of eye muscle imbalance. There are many different types of strabismus, including concomitant, convergent, divergent, vertical, and nonconcomitant. There are also many techniques for correcting the disorder, with code selection based on the specific procedure performed on one or more of the horizontal (lateral and medial rectus muscles), vertical (superior and inferior rectus muscles), or inferior and superior oblique muscles.

CPT codes for strabismus surgery refer to each eye individually. If the same operation is performed in both eyes, the muscle code for the first eye should be reported twice. If horizontal and vertical surgery is performed in the same eye, all of the appropriate codes should be reported. See the table below for classification of the eye muscles.

Horizontal	Vertical
Lateral rectus	Inferior oblique
Medial rectus	Inferior rectus
	Superior oblique
	Superior rectus

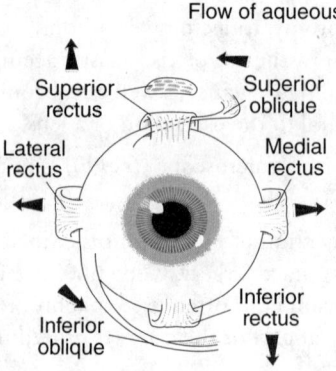

Flow of aqueous

Muscles and actions (right eye)

Procedure Differentiation

In 67311 a speculum is placed in the patient's eye (no previous surgery). The physician makes incisions in the conjunctiva at the juncture of the sclera and cornea (the limbus) or in the cul-de-sac (Parks incision). Radial relaxing incisions in the conjunctiva are made and the muscle (either medial or lateral rectus) is isolated with a muscle hook. The muscle is strengthened by resection (removal of a measured segment) or weakened by recession (retroplacement of the muscle attachment). The muscles are secured with sutures. The operative wound is closed with sutures. In 67311, one horizontal muscle is treated; in 67312, two horizontal muscles in the same are treated. When 67311 is billed twice, it cannot be documented that both procedures have been performed on the same side, since the description clearly states one horizontal muscle. Code 67311 should be reported for the contralateral eye with modifier 50 appended. The operation is performed for patients whose eyes turn in (esotropia) or turn out (exotropia).

Code 67312 (strabismus surgery, two horizontal muscles) might not be allowed unless the appropriate modifier is reported. It is inappropriate to use this code when one horizontal muscle is operated upon in each eye. The appropriate coding for that situation would be 67311–50 or 67311 and 67311–50 depending on payer guidelines.

Codes 67314–67316 describe procedures on vertical muscles. There are four vertically acting muscles. An operation performed on the inferior oblique, superior rectus, or the inferior rectus is described by these codes. Code 67314 is reported if one vertical muscle is treated and code 67316 would be reported if two or more vertical muscles in the same eye are treated. A procedure performed on the superior oblique muscle is reported with code 67318.

Within this section of codes there are add-on codes (67320, 67331–67340) that are reported to clarify the specific circumstances and additional physical work related to the strabismus surgery being performed.

Transposition performed in addition to strabismus surgery is reported with add-on code 67320. This procedure is performed when a patient has lost function in one of the extraocular muscles. Generally the patient cannot turn the eye to the outside or inward.

Code 67331 indicates that a patient has had previous eye surgery or injury not involving the extraocular muscles.

Code 67332 reports the patient has scarring of extraocular muscles or restrictive myopathy.

Code 67334 reports the use of posterior fixation sutures.

Code 67335 is used to indicate the placement of adjustable sutures.

Code 67340 is used to report the exploration and repair (if performed) of detached extraocular muscles, usually as a complication of surgery.

Code 67343 reports the release of extensive scar tissue from an extraocular muscle. This code may be reported with other strabismus surgical procedures (67311–67340) when they are used to report a procedure performed on other than the affected muscle. This separate procedure by definition is usually a component of a more complex service and is not identified separately. When performed alone or with other unrelated procedures/services it may be reported. If performed alone, list the code; if performed with other procedures/services, list the code and append modifier 59.

Medical Necessity
The following conditions may warrant this procedure (this list is not all inclusive):

- Diplopia
- Esotropia
- Exotropia
- Strabismus

Key Documentation Terms
Documentation should support the medical necessity of the procedure and a narrative of the procedure performed. The documentation may also include therapies tried to correct the problem and test reports. Terms such as horizontal, vertical, oblique, transposition scarring, or posterior fixation suture provide the guidance needed to ensure correct code assignment.

Coding Tips
- Placement of adjustable sutures (67335) may be reported separately when performed with strabismus surgery (67311–67334).
- These are unilateral procedures. If performed bilaterally, some payers require that the service be reported twice with modifier 50 appended to the second code while others require identification of the service only once with modifier 50 appended. Check with individual payers. Modifier 50 identifies a procedure performed identically on the opposite side of the body (mirror image).
- These procedures include the use of an operating microscope (69990).
- If a wound of the extraocular muscle, tendon, or Tenon's capsule is repaired, code 65290 may be reported.
- As "add-on" codes, 67320, 67331, 67332, 67334, 67335, and 67340 are not subject to multiple procedure rules. No reimbursement reduction or modifier 51 is applied. The following table provides additional information for these codes as found in the Medicare Physician Fee Schedule Database.

DEFINITIONS

diplopia. Double vision.

esotropia. Misalignment of the eye usually evidenced by the eye turning inward.

exotropia. Frequently occurring form of strabismus characterized by permanent or intermittent deviation of the visual axis when one eye turns outward while the other fixes upon an image, affecting one or both eyes.

Parent Code	Add-On	GLOB DAYS	MULT PROC	BILAT SURG	ASST SURG	CO- SURG	TEAM SURG
67311		090	2	1	1	0	0
67312		090	2	1	1	1	0
67314		090	2	1	1	0	0
67316		090	2	1	0	0	0
67318		090	2	1	1	1	0
	67320	ZZZ	0	0	1	0	0
	67331	ZZZ	0	1	1	1	0
	67332	ZZZ	0	1	1	1	0
	67334	ZZZ	0	1	1	1	0
	67335	ZZZ	0	1	1	1	0
	67340	ZZZ	0	0	2	0	0

Procedures Performed on the Auditory System

Myringotomy (69420–69421)

A myringotomy is a surgical procedure in which a small incision is made in the eardrum (tympanic membrane), usually in both ears, to relieve pressure and release pus from an infection. In this procedure, fluid is gently suctioned out of the middle ear. The physician may also document the procedure as myringocentesis, tympanotomy, or paracentesis of the tympanic membrane.

Procedure Differentiation

Code selection is differentiated by whether the procedure was performed with or without general anesthesia.

This procedure is usually done in an ambulatory surgical unit under general anesthesia, although some physicians do it in the office with moderate (conscious) sedation and local anesthesia, especially in older children. Verify that the place of service is correctly reported.

Medical Necessity

The following conditions may warrant this procedure (this list is not all inclusive):

- Acute mastoiditis
- Acute or chronic otitis media (e.g. serous, mucoid, sanguinous)
- Dysfunction of Eustachian tube

Key Documentation Terms

Documentation should support the medical necessity of the procedure and a narrative of the procedure performed. The key terms with or without general anesthesia determines correct code assignment.

Coding Tips

- Code 69420 or 69421 should not be reported when the documentation indicates that a myringotomy with insertion of a ventilating tube was performed, see 69433 and 69436 as appropriate.

DEFINITIONS

conductive hearing loss. Hearing loss due to the inability of sound waves to move from the outer (external ear) to the inner ear.

eustachian tube. Internal channel between the tympanic cavity and the nasopharynx that equalizes internal pressure to the outside pressure and drains mucous production from the middle ear.

mastoiditis. Acute or chronic inflammation and irritation of the air space and air cells in the mastoid section of the temporal bone.

otitis media. Inflammation of the middle ear, often causing pain and temporary hearing loss. Otitis media commonly occurs in children as a result of infection.

paracentesis. Surgical puncture of a body cavity with a specialized needle or hollow tubing to aspirate fluid for diagnostic or therapeutic reasons.

- If a myringotomy or tympanostomy is performed bilaterally, the procedure should be reported with modifier 50.

Tympanoplasty (69631–69646)

This procedure involves repairing or reconstructing the eardrum. It is important to carefully read the code descriptions in this section. The tympanoplasty code description often includes or excludes certain procedures.

Procedure Differentiation

The tympanoplasty may involve one or more of the following procedures:

- Antrotomy, surgical opening into the antrum of the mastoid.

- Atticotomy, cutting an opening in the wall of the "attic"(a cavity of the middle ear that lies above the tympanic cavity and contains the upper portion of the malleus and most of the incus)

- Canaloplasty, the repair of the external ear canal (usually due to trauma, especially basilar skull fracture trauma)

- Mastoidectomy, surgical excision of a portion of the mastoid of the posterior temporal bone often performed in conjunction with other related procedures and not reported separately.

- Ossicular chain reconstruction, the repair of the three small bones in the ear called ossicles-malleus, incus, and stapes; these bones may be replaced with prosthetic bones (this procedure usually is performed for chronic ear infection, trauma, or perforation of the eardrum).

Codes 69631–69633 describe tympanoplasties without mastoidectomy. Code 69631 should be reported for procedures without ossicular chain reconstruction, 69632 includes ossicular chain reconstruction, and 69633 includes ossicular chain reconstruction and prosthesis.

Codes 69635–69537 include an antrotomy or a mastoidotomy in addition to the tympanoplasty. Code 69635 is performed without ossicular chain reconstruction, 69636 includes ossicular chain reconstruction, and 69637 includes ossicular chain reconstruction and prosthesis.

Codes 69641–69646 describe tympanoplasties with a mastoidectomy. Code 69641 is performed without ossicular chain reconstruction and 69642 includes ossicular chain reconstruction. In 69643, the posterior canal is reconstructed with cartilage, bone, or hydroxyapatite (i.e., Wehr's canal wall reconstruction). The procedure does not include ossicular chain reconstruction. Code 69644 includes posterior canal and ossicular chain reconstruction. Codes 69645 and 69646 describe radical or complete procedures. In these procedures, the documentation may indicate that the posterior canal wall is taken down to the level of the facial nerve. In 69645, the ossicles are inspected and all or part of the ossicles may be removed and a piece of Silastic may be placed in the middle ear to develop an air-containing space. In 69646, ossicular chain reconstruction is performed also.

Medical Necessity

The following conditions may warrant these procedures (this list is not all inclusive):

- Acute or chronic otitis media (e.g., sanguinous, suppurative)
- Cholesteatoma

 DEFINITIONS

antrum. Chamber or cavity, typically with a small opening.

ossicular chain. Anatomic structure formed by the three small bones of the middle ear—incus, malleus, and stapes—functioning together to conduct sound vibrations through the ear.

-otomy. Making an incision or opening.

prosthesis. Man-made substitute for a missing body part.

- Chronic mastoiditis
- Hearing loss (e.g., conductive, neural, or sensory)
- Impaired mobility of the ear ossicles
- Perforation of tympanic membrane

Key Documentation Terms
Documentation should indicate the surgical procedure that was performed. Terms such as antrotomy, atticotomy, canaloplasty, mastoidectomy, ossicular chain reconstruction, and radical provide the guidance needed to ensure correct code assignment. Above all else, the documentation should support the medical necessity of the procedure.

Coding Tip
- A myringotomy (69420–69421) is included in a tympanoplasty or tympanostomy procedure and is not reported separately.

Cochlear Implantation (69930)
A cochlear implant is a hearing device used in profoundly deaf individuals, consisting of a battery-operated processor that converts sound waves into an electrical current, an internal and external coil system that transmits the electrical impulses, and an electrode array implanted in the cochlea that stimulates the fibers of the auditory nerve.

CMS determined that cochlear implantation is reasonable and necessary for the treatment of bilateral pre- or postlinguistic, sensorineural, and moderate-to-profound hearing loss in individuals who demonstrate limited benefit from amplification. Limited benefit from amplification is defined by test scores of 40 percent correct or less in the best-aided listening condition on tape recorded tests of open-set sentence cognition.

Medical Necessity
The following conditions may warrant this procedure (this list is not all inclusive):

- Bilateral moderate-to-profound sensorineural hearing impairment with limited benefit from appropriate hearing (or vibrotactile) aids
- The patient's cognitive ability to use auditory clues and a willingness to undergo an extended program of rehabilitation
- Absence of middle ear infection, an accessible cochlear lumen that is structurally suited to implantation, and absence of lesions in the auditory nerve and acoustic areas of the central nervous system
- No contraindications to surgery
- Use of the device in accordance with Food and Drug Administration (FDA)-approved labeling

Key Documentation Terms
Documentation should support the medical necessity of the procedure and a narrative of the procedure performed. The documentation may also include that the patient had limited or no benefit from appropriately fitted hearing aids.

Coding Tip
- For implantation or replacement of an electromagnetic bone conduction hearing device in the temporal bone, see 69710. For other related CPT codes, see 69714–69718.

 DEFINITIONS

cochlea. Bony, spiral-shaped structure forming part of the inner ear labyrinth that leads from the oval window.

Ménière's disease. Distended membranous labyrinth of the middle ear from endolymphatic hydrops, causing ischemia, failure of nerve function, and hearing and balance dysfunction.

© 2020 Optum360, LLC

Chapter 7. **Auditing Radiology Services**

Radiology services have unique components that make coding, billing, and auditing more complex than other services. Some of the unique components include:

- Radiology services consist of two components: the technical and professional component.
- Radiology services may be diagnostic, therapeutic, or interventional.
- Radiology services can be performed in a variety of settings and by more than one provider.

When auditing radiology services, the auditor must determine:

- What service was provided?
- Where was the service performed?
- Who owns the equipment used to perform the service?
- Did the provider perform both the technical and professional components?
- Was more than one procedure performed?
- Are the procedures within the same family and, therefore, should the multiple procedure reduction apply?
- How many providers performed the service, and if more than one, who did what?
- Why was the service performed?
- Was the service for screening purposes?

The CPT® book provides guidelines for radiology codes at the beginning of the radiology section. Notes providing additional instruction may also be found at the beginning of many subsections. Additional instruction is also provided at the code categories or subcategories level, as well as parenthetical notes specific to a code or group of codes.

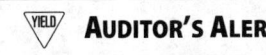

AUDITOR'S ALERT

See Appendix 1 for the audit worksheet for radiology procedures.

Date of Service

When auditing radiology services, the date of service in the medical record should be compared to the date of service on the claim and any discrepancies should be noted.

Medical Necessity

The medical necessity of radiology procedures must be supported by the reason the service was rendered. However, unlike surgical or evaluation and management services, the medical necessity of the service may be established by the provider who orders the service. For example, a patient presents to his or her primary care physician complaining of a cough. The primary care physician orders a chest x-ray from the radiology group located in the same medical building. On the request for the service, the primary care physician should indicate the reason the service is being ordered.

When completing the claim form, ICD-10-CM coding guidelines indicate that the radiologist should identify the reason the service was requested unless another definitive diagnosis was established as a result of the service. In other words, if after interpreting the chest x-ray in the scenario above the radiologist notes that the patient has pneumonia, the diagnosis reported should be pneumonia.

There will be times, however, that the request does not contain a reason for the service. In this instance, the medical record should include documentation that the requesting provider was contacted, and that a reason for the service was provided. Additionally, there may be times when the radiology practice may contact the referring provider to obtain additional information regarding the patient's condition to further substantiate the medical necessity of the service. This, too, should be well documented.

Medical record documentation must also necessitate the need for certain screening services. When a service such as a screening mammography is performed, it is imperative that the claim indicates the appropriate Z code to identify the screening nature of the service. Failure to do so can result in claim denial, inappropriate payment, or inappropriate costs to the patient.

Procedure Coding

As mentioned earlier, radiology procedure coding can be more difficult due to the complexity of the services and the number of variances that can occur.

Modifiers

The modifiers discussed below may be appended to codes from the radiology section of the CPT book.

22	Increased procedural services
26	Professional component
32	Mandated services
33	Preventive service
50	Bilateral procedure
51	Multiple procedures
52	Reduced services
53	Discontinued procedure
58	Staged or related procedure or service by the same physician or other qualified health care professional during the postoperative period
59	Distinct procedural service
76	Repeat procedure or service by the same physician or other qualified health care professional
77	Repeat procedure by another physician or other qualified health care professional
99	Multiple modifiers

GG Performance and payment of a screening mammogram and diagnostic mammogram on the same patient, same day.

GH Diagnostic mammogram converted from screening mammogram on same day

LC Left circumflex coronary artery

LD Left anterior descending coronary artery

LT Left side

RC Right coronary artery

RT Right side

TC Technical component

See chapter 3 for a detailed explanation of these modifiers.

Components of Radiology Services
Radiology procedures generally consist of two components: the professional component (PC) and the technical component (TC).

Professional Component
The professional component (PC) is defined by Medicare and most other third-party payers as the portion of the radiology procedure that represents the physician's (or other practitioner's) work in providing the service, including interpretation and report of the procedure.

The PC portion of radiology services should be reported when it is furnished by a provider to a patient in any setting as long as the above definition has been met and documented in the medical record (such as a formal written radiology report). When services are furnished to hospital patients, most payer guidelines require that the PC portion of the procedure be billed only when "the services meet the conditions for fee schedule payment and are identifiable, direct, and discrete diagnostic or therapeutic services to an individual patient, such as an interpretation of diagnostic procedures and the PC of therapeutic procedures."

When submitting claims for only the PC portion of a service, the appropriate procedure code with CPT modifier 26 should be assigned.

Technical Component
The technical component (TC) of a radiology procedure represents the equipment, supplies, technical personnel, and costs necessary for the performance of the procedure. It does not include the physician's (or other practitioner's) work in providing the service, including interpretation and report of the procedure.

When reporting only the technical component of the service, modifier TC should be appended to the procedure code.

Supervision and Interpretation
Many radiology CPT codes indicate supervision and interpretation (S&I) services, which occur only when the procedure is performed by the radiologist and the provider as a team. In this situation, a combination of codes is used: one code reporting the nonradiologic portion (usually, but not always from the surgical section of CPT) and another code from the 70000 series to report the radiological supervision and interpretation of the image.

For example, an ankle arthrography is performed. The orthopedist injects the contrast material and the radiologist supervises the imaging and interprets the films. The orthopedist reports the injection procedure using CPT code 27648 Injection procedure for ankle arthrography. The radiologist reports the S&I using 73615 Radiologic examination, ankle, arthrography, radiologic supervision and interpretation. The appropriate modifier indicating the technical or professional components would also be appended, if appropriate.

Number of Views

Correct procedure code assignment may also be affected by the number of images taken. For example, when reporting imaging of the mandible, code 70100 is reported if less than four views are obtained, 70110 if four or more views are taken.

Contrast Material

Some radiologic services require the use of contrast materials to enhance imaging. These may include:

- Intra-articular
- Intrathecally
- Intravascularly

Note: Oral or rectal administration of contrast does not meet the criteria to report a "with contrast" procedure code.

Medicare and most other payers will not pay separately for high osmolar contrast materials (HOCM), as the cost of this type of contrast is included in the reimbursement rate for the service unless there is documentation supporting medical necessity.

However, additional payment is often made for low osmolar contrast materials (LOCM). These should be reported using the appropriate HCPCS Level II codes. Payment is made to the provider who incurs the expense of the contrast. For example, no additional payment will be made to a provider when only the professional component of the service is provided as the facility where the service was performed incurs the expense.

Correct Coding Policies for Radiology Services

Physicians should report the HCPCS/CPT code that describes the procedure performed to the greatest specificity possible. A HCPCS/CPT code should be reported only if all services described by the code are performed. A physician should not report multiple HCPCS/CPT codes if a single HCPCS/CPT code exists that describes the services. This type of unbundling is incorrect coding.

HCPCS/CPT codes include all services usually performed as part of the procedure as a standard of medical/surgical practice. A physician should not separately report these services simply because HCPCS/CPT codes exist for them.

Non-interventional Diagnostic Imaging

Non-invasive/interventional diagnostic imaging includes but is not limited to standard radiographs, single or multiple views, contrast studies, computed/computerized tomography and magnetic resonance imaging. There are various combinations of codes to address the number and type of radiographic views. For a given radiographic series, the procedure code that most

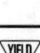

AUDITOR'S ALERT

The following should be reported on the claim when billing for LOCM:

- Report intrathecal injections separately using the appropriate CPT code.

accurately describes what was performed should be reported. Because the number of views necessary to obtain medically useful information may vary, a complete review of CPT coding options for a given radiographic session is important to assure accurate coding with the most comprehensive code describing the services performed rather than billing multiple codes to describe the service.

If imaging studies (e.g., radiographs, computerized tomography, magnetic resonance imaging) are repeated during the course of a radiological encounter due to substandard quality or need for additional views, only one unit of service for the appropriate code may be reported. If the radiologist elects to obtain additional views after reviewing initial films in order to render an interpretation, the Medicare policy on the ordering of diagnostic tests must be followed. The code describing the total service should be reported, even if the patient was released from the radiology suite and had to return for additional services. The CPT descriptors for many of these services refer to a "minimum" number of views. If more than the minimum number specified is necessary and no other more specific code is available, only that service should be reported. However, if additional films are necessary due to a change in the patient's condition, separate reporting may be appropriate.

CPT code descriptors that specify a minimum number of views include additional views if there is no more comprehensive code specifically including the additional views. For example, if three views of the shoulder are obtained, code 73030 Radiologic examination, shoulder; complete, minimum of two views, with one unit of service should be reported rather than code 73020 Radiologic examination, shoulder; one view, plus code 73030.

When a comparative imaging study is performed to assess potential complications or completeness of a procedure (e.g., postreduction, postintubation, post-catheter placement, etc.), the professional component of the CPT code for the postprocedure imaging study is not separately payable and should not be reported. The technical component of the CPT code for the postprocedure imaging study may be reported.

Some studies may be performed without contrast, with contrast, or both with and without contrast. There are separate codes to describe all of these combinations of contrast usage. When studies require contrast, the number of radiographs obtained varies between patients. All radiographs necessary to complete a study are included in the CPT code description.

Fluoroscopy is inherent in many radiological supervision and interpretation procedures. Unless specifically noted, fluoroscopy necessary to complete a radiologic procedure and obtain the necessary permanent radiographic record is included in the radiologic procedure and should not be reported individually.

Preliminary "scout" radiographs prior to contrast administration or delayed imaging radiographs are not reported individually.

A complete retroperitoneal ultrasound study (76770) includes the following:

- Complete assessment of kidneys and bladder if history indicates urinary pathology
- Real time scans of:
  - abdominal aorta
  - common iliac artery origins

- inferior vena cava
- kidneys

A limited retroperitoneal ultrasound (76775) plus limited pelvic ultrasound (76857) should not be reported in lieu of the complete retroperitoneal ultrasound (76770).

Code 76380 Computed tomography, limited or localized follow-up study, should not be reported with other computed tomography (CT), computed tomography angiography (CTA), or computed tomography guidance codes for the same patient encounter.

When a central venous catheter is inserted, a chest radiologic examination is usually performed to confirm the position of the catheter and absence of pneumothorax. Similarly when an emergency endotracheal intubation procedure (31500), chest tube insertion procedure (e.g., codes 32550, 32551, 32554, 32555), or insertion of a central flow directed catheter procedure (e.g., Swan Ganz) (93503) is performed, a chest radiologic examination is usually performed to confirm the location and proper positioning of the tube or catheter. The chest radiologic examination is integral to the procedures, and a chest radiologic examination (e.g., codes 71045, 71046) should not be reported separately.

Code 77075 includes radiologic examination of all bones. Codes for radiologic examination of other bones should not be reported in addition to code 77075. However, if a separate and distinct radiologic examination with additional films of a specific area of the skeleton is performed to evaluate a different problem, the appropriate code for the additional radiologic examination may be reported with an NCCI-associated modifier.

Code 77073 includes radiologic examination of the lower extremities. Codes for radiologic examination of lower extremity structures should not be reported in addition to code 77073 for examination of the radiologic films for the bone length studies. However, if a separate and distinct radiologic examination with additional films of a specific area of a lower extremity is performed to evaluate a different problem, the appropriate code for the additional radiologic examination may be reported with an NCCI-associated modifier.

Code 75635 describes computed tomographic angiography of the abdominal aorta and bilateral iliofemoral lower extremity runoff. This code includes the services described by codes 73706 (Computed tomographic angiography, lower extremity, with contrast material(s), including noncontrast images, if performed, and image postprocessing) and 74175 (Computed tomographic angiography, abdomen, with contrast material(s), including noncontrast images, if performed, and image postprocessing). Codes 73706 and 74175 should not be reported with code 75635 for the same patient encounter. Code 73706 in addition to code 74175 should not be reported in place of code 75635.

Ultrasound examination of a transplanted kidney and retroperitoneal structures at the same patient encounter may be reported with code 76770 (Ultrasound, retroperitoneal, complete). It should not be reported with code 76776 (Ultrasound, transplanted kidney) and code 76775 (Ultrasound, retroperitoneal, limited).

Computed tomography (CT) of the spine with intrathecal contrast should not be reported with myelography (e.g., codes 72240–72270) unless both studies are medically reasonable and necessary. Radiography after injection of intrathecal contrast to perform a CT of the spine to confirm the location of the contrast is not reported separately as myelography.

Code 77063 is an add-on code describing screening digital tomosynthesis for mammography. Since this procedure requires performance of a screening mammography producing direct digital images, code 77063 may be reported; however, it should not be reported with 77067, which describes screening mammography using radiography.

Screening and diagnostic mammography are normally not performed on the same date of service. However, when the two procedures are performed on the same date of service, Medicare requires that the diagnostic mammography code be reported with modifier GG and the screening mammography code be reported with modifier 59 or XU.

Codes 72081–72084 describe radiologic examination of the entire spine, the codes differing based on the number of views. The other codes in code range 72020–72120 describe radiologic examination of specific regions of the spine differing based on the region of the spine and the number of views. If a physician performs a procedure described by codes 72081–72084 and at the same patient encounter performs a procedure described by one or more other codes in the code range 72020–72120, the physician should sum the total number of views and report the appropriate code in the code range 72081–72084. The physician should not report a code from the code range 72081–72084 in addition to one from code range 72020–72120 for services performed at the same patient encounter.

Since the foot includes the toes and calcaneus bone, code 73630 (radiologic examination, foot; complete, minimum of 3 views) includes radiologic examination of the toes and calcaneus. A physician should not report code 73650 (radiologic examination; calcaneus, minimum of 2 views) or 73660 (radiologic examination; toe[s], minimum of 2 views) with code 73630 for the same foot on the same date of service.

Interventional/Invasive Diagnostic Imaging

If a radiologic procedure requires that contrast be administered orally (e.g., upper GI series) or rectally (e.g., barium enema), the administration is integral to the radiologic procedure, and the administration service is not separately reportable. If a radiologic procedure requires that contrast material be administered parenterally (e.g., IVP, CT, MRI), the vascular access (e.g., codes 36000, 36406, 36410) and contrast administration (e.g., codes 96360–96376) are integral to the procedure and are not reported separately.

Many services utilizing contrast are composed of a procedural component (codes outside the 70000 section) and a radiologic supervision and interpretation component (code in the 70000 section). If a single provider performs both components of the service, the provider may report both codes. However, if different providers perform the different components, each provider reports the code corresponding to that component.

Many interventional procedures require contrast injections for localization and/or guidance. Unless there are CPT instructions directing the physician to report specific codes for the localization or guidance, the localization or guidance is integral to the interventional procedure and is not reported separately.

Diagnostic angiography (arteriogram/venogram) performed on the same date of service by the same provider as a percutaneous intravascular interventional procedure should be reported with modifier 59 or XU. If a diagnostic angiogram (fluoroscopic or computed tomographic) was performed prior to the date of the percutaneous intravascular interventional procedure, a second diagnostic angiogram cannot be reported on the date of the percutaneous intravascular interventional procedure unless it is medically reasonable and necessary to repeat the study to further define the anatomy and pathology. Report the second angiogram with modifier 59 or XU. If it is medically reasonable and necessary to repeat only a portion of the diagnostic angiogram, append modifier 52 in addition to modifier 59 or XU to the angiogram CPT code. If the prior diagnostic angiogram (fluoroscopic or computed tomographic) was complete, the provider should not report a second angiogram for the dye injections necessary to perform the percutaneous intravascular interventional procedure.

The individual CPT codes in the 70000 section identify which injection or administration code, if any, is appropriate for a given procedure. In the absence of a parenthetical CPT note, the injection or administration service is integral to the procedure and is not reported individually. If an intravenous line is inserted (e.g., code 36000) for access in the event of a problem with the procedure or for administration of contrast, it is integral to the procedure and is not separately reportable. Code 36005 describes the injection procedure for contrast venography of an extremity and includes the introduction of a needle or an intracatheter (e.g., code 36000). Code 36005 should not be reported for injections for arteriography or venography of sites other than an extremity.

For lymphangiography procedures, injection of dye into subcutaneous tissue is integral to the procedure. Code 96372 Therapeutic, prophylactic, or diagnostic injection; subcutaneous or intramuscular, should not be reported separately for this injection of dye.

When urologic radiologic procedures require insertion of a urethral catheter (e.g., code 51701–51703), this insertion is integral to the procedure and is not reported separately.

Fluoroscopy reported with code 76000 is integral to many procedures including, but not limited, to most spinal, endoscopic, and injection procedures and should not be reported individually. For some of these procedures, there are separate fluoroscopic guidance codes that may be reported separately.

Computed tomography (CT) and computed tomographic angiography (CTA) procedures for the same anatomic location may be reported together in limited circumstances. If a single technical study is performed that is utilized to generate images for separate CT and CTA reports, only one procedure, the CT or CTA, for the anatomic region may be reported. Both a CT and CTA may be reported for the same anatomic region if they are performed at separate patient encounters or if two separate and distinct technical studies, one for the CT and one for the CTA, are performed at the same patient encounter. The medical necessity for the latter situation is uncommon.

Similarly, magnetic resonance imaging (MRI) and magnetic resonance angiography (MRA) procedures for the same anatomic location may be reported together in limited circumstances. If a single technical study is performed that is utilized to generate images for separate MRI and MRA reports, only one procedure, the MRI or MRA, for the anatomic region may be reported. Both an MRI and MRA may be reported for the same anatomic region if they are

© 2020 Optum360, LLC

performed at separate patient encounters or if two separate and distinct technical studies, one for the MRI and one for the MRA, are performed at the same patient encounter. The medical necessity for the latter situation is uncommon.

Computed tomography of the heart (75571–75573) and computed tomographic angiography of the heart (75574) include electrocardiographic monitoring if performed. Codes 93000–93010 and 93040–93042 should not be reported individually with codes 75571–75574 for the ECG monitoring integral to these procedures.

If a breast biopsy, needle localization wire, metallic localization clip, or other breast procedure is performed with mammographic or stereotactic guidance (e.g., 19281–19282), the physician should not separately report a post-procedure mammography code (e.g., 77065, 77066, 77067) for the same patient encounter. The radiologic guidance codes include all imaging by the defined modality required to perform the procedure.

3D rendering of an imaging modality (e.g., codes 76376, 76377) should not be reported for mapping the sites of multiple biopsies or other needle placements under radiologic guidance. For example, a provider performing multiple prostate biopsies under ultrasound guidance (e.g., code 76942) should not report 76376 or 76377 for developing a map of the locations of the biopsies.

Nuclear Medicine

The general policies described above apply to nuclear medicine, as well as standard diagnostic imaging.

The injection of a radiopharmaceutical is an integral component of a nuclear medicine procedure. Codes for vascular access (e.g., code 36000) and injection of the radiopharmaceutical (e.g., codes 96360–96376) are not reported separately.

Single photon emission computed tomography (SPECT) studies represent an enhanced methodology over standard planar nuclear imaging. Several nuclear medicine CPT codes describe combinations of planar, single photon emission computed tomography (SPECT), flow imaging, or SPECT with CT imaging for evaluation of a specific anatomic area. Unless specified by a single code that combines two or more imaging modalities, no additional information is procured by obtaining both planar and SPECT studies for a limited anatomic area.

Myocardial perfusion imaging (78451–78454) is not reportable with cardiac blood pool imaging by gated equilibrium (78472–78473) because the two types of tests use different radiopharmaceuticals.

Codes 76376 and 76377 (3D rendering) are not reported individually for nuclear medicine procedures (78012–78999). However, code 76376 or 76377 may be separately reported with modifier 59 or XS on the same date of service as a nuclear medicine procedure if the 3D rendering procedure is performed in association with a third procedure (other than nuclear medicine) for which 3D rendering is appropriately reported.

Codes 78451–78452 include calculation of the heart-lung ratio if obtained. Code 78580 should not be reported for calculation of the heart-lung ratio during the processing of a SPECT myocardial perfusion procedure.

Positron emission tomography (PET) imaging requires use of a radiopharmaceutical diagnostic imaging agent. HCPCS Level II codes A9555 and A9526 may only be reported with PET scan codes 78491 and 78492. HCPCS Level II code A9552 may only be reported with PET scan codes 78459, 78608, and 78811–78816.

Positron emission tomography (PET) procedures include a finger stick blood glucose level. Code 82948 (glucose; blood, reagent strip) or 82962 (glucose, blood by glucose monitoring devices) should not be reported individually for the measurement of the finger stick blood glucose included in a PET procedure.

HCPCS Level II code A9512 describes a radiopharmaceutical utilized for nuclear medicine studies. Technetium Tc-99m pertechnetate is also a component of other Technetium Tc-99m radiopharmaceuticals with separate AXXXX codes. Code A9512 should not be reported with other AXXXX radiopharmaceuticals containing Technetium Tc-99m for a single nuclear medicine study. However, if two separate nuclear medicine studies are performed on the same date of service, one with the radiopharmaceutical described by HCPCS Level II code A9512 and one with another AXXXX radiopharmaceutical labeled with Technetium Tc-99m, both codes may be reported utilizing an NCCI-associated modifier. HCPCS Level II codes A9500, A9540, and A9541 describe radiopharmaceuticals labeled with Technetium Tc-99m that may be utilized for separate nuclear medicine studies on the same date of service as a nuclear medicine study utilizing the radiopharmaceutical described by HCPCS Level II code A9512.

Generally diagnostic nuclear medicine procedures are performed on different dates of service than therapeutic nuclear medicine procedures. However, if a diagnostic nuclear medicine procedure is performed on an organ and the decision to proceed with a therapeutic nuclear medicine procedure on the same organ on the same date of service is based on results of the diagnostic nuclear medicine procedure, both procedures may be reported on the same date of service utilizing an NCCI-associated modifier. A physician should not report a radiopharmaceutical therapy administration code for the radionuclide administration that is integral to diagnostic nuclear imaging procedures.

A three phase bone and/or joint imaging study (78315) includes initial vascular flow imaging. Code 78445 (non-cardiac vascular flow imaging) should not be reported individually for the vascular flow imaging integral to 78315.

Non-cardiac vascular flow imaging (78445), when performed, is integral to a nuclear medicine procedure. Code 78445 should not be reported with any other nuclear medicine procedure code.

Supervision and handling of radionuclides is integral to nuclear medicine procedures (e.g., codes 78012-79999). Physicians should not separately report code 77790 (supervision, handling, and loading of radiation source) for this service.

Radiation Oncology

Except for an initial visit evaluation and management (E/M) service at which the decision to perform radiation therapy is made, E/M services are not separately reportable with radiation oncology services with the following exceptions as noted below. Effective January 1, 2010, CMS eliminated payment for consultation E/M codes 99241–99255. The initial visit E/M for radiation oncology services may be reported with office/outpatient E/M codes

99202–99215, initial hospital care E/M codes 99221–99223, subsequent hospital care E/M codes 99231–99233, or observation/inpatient hospital care with same day admission and discharge E/M codes 99234–99236.

E/M services in addition to an initial visit E/M service may be reported with codes 77770–77772. E/M services reported with these brachytherapy codes must be significant, separate, and distinct from radiation treatment management services.

E/M services (i.e., 99211–99213) in addition to an initial visit E/M service may be reported with code 77401 Radiation treatment delivery, superficial and/or ortho voltage, per day, with modifier 25 for the purpose of reporting physician services for certain aspects of radiation therapy planning.

Continuing medical physics consultation (77336) is reported "per week of therapy." It may be reported after every five radiation treatments. (It may also be reported if the total number of radiation treatments in a course of radiation therapy is less than five.) Since radiation planning procedures (77261–77334) are generally performed before radiation treatment commences, the NCCI contains edits preventing payment of 77336 in conjunction with 77261–77295, 77301–77321, and 77332–77334. Because radiation planning procedures may occasionally be repeated during a course of radiation treatment, the edits allow modifiers 59 or -X{EPSU} to be appended to code 77336 when the radiation planning procedure and continuing medical physics consultation are reported on the same date of service.

The *Internet-Only Manuals* (IOM), *Medicare Claims Processing Manual,* Pub. 100-04, Chapter 13, Section 70.2 (Services Bundled Into Treatment Management Codes) defines services that may not be reported separately with radiation oncology procedures. Based on these requirements, the NCCI contains edits bundling the following codes into all radiation therapy services:

- Tattooing (11920–11921)
- Treatment of burns (16000–16030)
- Venipuncture or introduction of catheter (36000, 36410, 36425)
- Urinary bladder catheterization (51701–51703)
- Intravenous infusion (96360–96368)
- Psychotherapy (90832–90840 and 90846–90847)
- Pharmacologic management (90863)
- Medical nutrition therapy (97802–97804)
- Moderate conscious sedation (99151–99153)
- Evaluation and management (99202–99215, 99217–99239, 99281–99498)

Brachytherapy (77750–77790) includes radiation treatment management (77427 and 77431) and continuing medical physics consultation (77336). Codes 77427, 77431, and 77336 should not in general be reported separately with brachytherapy services. However, if a patient receives external beam radiation treatment and brachytherapy treatment during the same time period, radiation treatment management and continuing medical physics consultation may be reported for the external beam radiation treatments. Additionally, if a patient has multi-step brachytherapy, it may be appropriate to report separately continuing medical physics consultation with the brachytherapy.

Stereotactic radiosurgery (SRS) treatment delivery (77371–77373) includes stereotactic guidance for placement of the radiation therapy fields for treatment delivery. Codes 77014 and 77387 should not be reported additionally for guidance for placement of the radiation therapy field for SRS treatment delivery.

The procedure described by CPT code 77778 requires that a radiation source be applied interstitially. Reporting a code requires that all essential components of the procedure are performed. These codes should not be reported by a radiation oncologist for intraoperative work with another physician who surgically places catheters interstitially unless the radiation oncologist also applies the radiation source at the same patient encounter. The intraoperative work of the radiation oncologist may be reportable with a non-brachytherapy code. If the radiation source application occurs postoperatively in a different room, the radiation oncologist may report 77770–77772 for the radiation source application.

Partial breast high dose rate brachytherapy may be performed two times a day. The first therapeutic radiology simulation for the course of therapy may be complex and reported as code 77290. However, subsequent simulations during the course of therapy should be reported with 77280.

Intensity modulated treatment (IMRT) delivery (e.g., codes 77385, 77386) is not normally reported with treatment device design and construction codes 77332–77334. The latter codes are generally reported for treatment device(s) design and construction for external beam radiation therapy. IMRT planning (77301) includes many treatment device(s) required for IMRT. Multi-leaf collimator (MLC) device(s) (77338) may be reported separately once per IMRT plan. However, patients receiving IMRT occasionally require an additional treatment device at a later date due to decreased tumor volume or patient weight. This device may be reported with codes 77332–77334.

Calculations described by 77300, if performed, are integral to some clinical brachytherapy procedures (e.g., 77767–77772, 77778). Code 77300 should not be reported with these clinical brachytherapy procedure codes.

Intensity modulated radiotherapy (IMRT) plan (77301) includes therapeutic radiology simulation-aided field settings. Simulation field settings for IMRT should not be reported separately with codes 77280–77290. Although procedure to procedure edits based on this principle exist in NCCI for procedures performed on the same date of service, these edits should not be circumvented by performing the two procedures described by a code pair edit on different dates of service.

Codes 77280–77290 (simulation-aided field settings) should not be reported for verification of the treatment field during a course of intensity modulated radiotherapy (IMRT) treatment.

Medically Unlikely Edits (MUE)

Providers/suppliers should be cautious about reporting services on multiple lines of a claim utilizing modifiers to bypass MUEs. MUEs were set so that such occurrences should be uncommon. If a provider/supplier does this frequently for any HCPCS/CPT code, the provider/supplier may be coding units of service incorrectly. The provider/supplier should consider contacting his/her national health care organization or the national medical/surgical society whose members commonly perform the procedure to clarify the correct reporting of units of service. A national health care organization, provider/supplier, or other interested third party may request a reconsideration of the MUE value of a

HCPCS/CPT code by submitting a written request to: NCCIPTPMUE@cms.hhs. The request should include a rationale for reconsideration, as well as a suggested remedy.

Codes 76942, 77002, 77003, 77012, and 77021 describe radiologic guidance for needle placement by different modalities. CMS payment policy allows one unit of service for any of these codes at a single patient encounter regardless of the number of needle placements performed. The unit of service for these codes is the patient encounter, not number of lesions, number of aspirations, number of biopsies, number of injections, or number of localizations.

The MUE values for J0153 Injection, adenosine, 1 mg (not to be used to report any adenosine phosphate compounds) and J1245 Injection, dipyridamole, per 10 mg, were set for single pharmacologic stress tests. For the unusual patient who requires two different types of pharmacologic stress tests (e.g., myocardial perfusion and echocardiography) on the same date of service, the amount of drug used for each stress test should be reported on separate lines of a claim with modifier 59 or XU appended to the code on one of the claim lines.

The code descriptor for code 77417 states: "Therapeutic radiology port image(s)." The MUE value for this code is one (1) since it includes all port films.

General Policy Statements
Any abdominal radiology procedure that has a radiological supervision and interpretation code (e.g., code 75625 for abdominal aortogram) includes abdominal x-rays (e.g., codes 74018–74022) as part of the total service.

Guidance for placement of radiation fields by computerized tomography or by ultrasound (77014 or 77387) for the same anatomical area are mutually exclusive of one another.

Evaluation of an anatomic region and guidance for a needle placement procedure in that anatomic region by the same radiologic modality at the same or different patient encounter(s) on the same date of service are not reported separately. For example, a physician should not report a diagnostic ultrasound code and code 76942 (ultrasonic guidance for needle placement...) when performed in the same anatomic region on the same date of service. Physicians should not avoid these edits by requiring patients to have the procedures performed on different dates of service if historically the evaluation of the anatomic region and guidance for needle biopsy procedures were performed on the same date of service.

Code 77790 is not reported separately with any of the remote afterloading brachytherapy codes (e.g., 77767–77772) since these procedures include the supervision, handling, and loading of the radioelement.

Bone studies such as 77072–77076 require a series of radiographs. Separate reporting of a bone study and individual radiographs obtained in the course of the bone study is inappropriate.

Radiological supervision and interpretation codes include all radiological services necessary to complete the service. Codes for fluoroscopy/fluoroscopic guidance (e.g., 76000, 77002, 77003) or ultrasound/ultrasound guidance (e.g., 76942, 76998) should not be reported separately.

Radiological guidance procedures include all radiological services necessary to complete the procedure. Codes for fluoroscopy (e.g., 76000, 76001) should not be reported separately with a fluoroscopic guidance procedure. Codes for ultrasound (e.g., 76998) should not be reported separately with an ultrasound guidance procedure. A limited or localized follow-up computed tomography study (76380) should not be reported separately with a computed tomography guidance procedure.

Abdominal ultrasound examinations (76700–76775) and abdominal duplex examinations (93975, 93976) are generally performed for different clinical scenarios although there are some instances where both types of procedures are medically reasonable and necessary. In the latter case, the abdominal ultrasound procedure code should be reported with an NCCI-associated modifier.

Tumor imaging by positron emission tomography (PET) may be reported with 78811–78816. If a concurrent computed tomography (CT) scan is performed for attenuation correction and anatomical localization, 78814–78816 should be reported rather than 78811–78813. A CT scan for localization should not be reported separately with 78811–78816. However, a medically reasonable and necessary diagnostic CT scan may be reported separately with an NCCI-associated modifier.

Axial bone density studies may be reported with 77078 or 77080. Peripheral site bone density studies may be reported with 77081, 76977, or G0130. Although it may be medically reasonable and necessary to report both axial and peripheral bone density studies on the same date of service, NCCI edits prevent the reporting of multiple codes for the axial bone density study or multiple codes for the peripheral site bone density study on the same date of service.

When existing vascular access lines or selectively placed catheters are used to procure arterial or venous samples, reporting sample collection separately is inappropriate. Codes 36500 and 75893 may be reported for venous blood sampling through a catheter placed for the sole purpose of venous blood sampling with or without venography. Code 75893 includes concomitant venography. If a catheter is placed for a purpose other than venous blood sampling with or without venography (75893), it is a misuse of 36500 or 75893 to report them in addition to codes for the other venous procedures. Codes 36500 and 75893 should not be reported for blood sampling during an arterial procedure.

Codes 70540–70543 are utilized to report magnetic resonance imaging of the orbit, face, and/or neck. Only one code may be reported for an imaging session regardless of whether one, two, or three areas are evaluated in the imaging session.

An MRI study of the brain (70551–70553) and MRI study of the orbit (70540–70543) are reported separately only if they are both medically reasonable and necessary and are performed as distinct studies. An MRI of the orbit is not reported separately with an MRI of the brain if an incidental abnormality of the orbit is identified during an MRI of the brain since only one MRI study is performed.

If the code descriptor of a HCPCS/CPT code includes the phrase "separate procedure," the procedure is subject to NCCI edits based on this designation. CMS does not allow separate reporting of a procedure designated as a "separate procedure" when it is performed at the same patient encounter as another procedure in an anatomically related area through the same skin incision, orifice, or surgical approach.

© 2020 Optum360, LLC

Code 36005 (injection procedure for extremity venography (including introduction of needle or intracatheter)) should not be utilized to report venous catheterization unless it is for the purpose of an injection procedure for extremity venography. Some physicians have misused this code to report any type of venous catheterization.

Most NCCI edits for codes describing procedures that may be performed on bilateral organs or structures (e.g., arms, eyes, kidneys, lungs) allow use of NCCI-associated modifiers (modifier indicator of "1") because the two codes of the code pair edit may be reported if the two procedures are performed on contralateral organs or structures. Most of these code pairs should not be reported with NCCI-associated modifiers when the corresponding procedures are performed on the ipsilateral organ or structure unless there is a specific coding rationale to bypass the edit. The existence of the NCCI edit indicates that the two codes generally should not be reported together unless the two corresponding procedures are performed at two separate patient encounters or two separate anatomic sites. However, if the corresponding procedures are performed at the same patient encounter and in contiguous structures, NCCI-associated modifiers should generally not be utilized.

Physicians should not report radiologic supervision and interpretation codes, radiologic guidance codes, or other radiology codes where the radiologic procedure is integral to another procedure being performed at the same patient encounter. Procedure to procedure edits that bundle these radiologic codes into the relevant procedure codes have modifier indicators of "1" allowing use of NCCI-associated modifiers to bypass them. An NCCI-associated modifier may be used to bypass such an edit only if the radiologic procedure is performed for a purpose unrelated to the procedure to which it is integral. For example, fluoroscopy is integral to a cardiac catheterization procedure and should not be reported separately with a cardiac catheterization. However, if on the same date of service the physician performs another procedure in addition to the cardiac catheterization, the additional procedure requires fluoroscopy, and fluoroscopy is not integral to the additional procedure, the fluoroscopy procedure may be reported separately with an NCCI-associated modifier.

Auditing Supplies

In most instances, the only additional supply that is reported with radiology claims is the low osmolar contrast material. This is reported using the appropriate HCPCS Level II code. Correct code assignment is dependent upon the specific contrast used and the amount. The provider should only bill for LOCM the cost of the contrast incurred. The following table lists the contrast agents.

 AUDITOR'S ALERT

See Appendix 1 for the audit worksheet for radiology procedures.

Contrast Material

Code	Description
A4641	Radiopharmaceutical, diagnostic, not otherwise classified
A4642	Indium In-111 satumomab pendetide, diagnostic, per study dose, up to 6 millicuries
A9500	Technetium Tc-99m sestamibi, diagnostic, per study dose
A9501	Technetium Tc-99m teboroxime, diagnostic, per study dose
A9502	Technetium Tc-99m tetrofosmin, diagnostic, per study dose
A9503	Technetium Tc-99m medronate, diagnostic, per study dose, up to 30 millicuries
A9504	Technetium Tc-99m apcitide, diagnostic, per study dose, up to 20 millicuries
A9505	Thallium Tl-201 thallous chloride, diagnostic, per millicurie
A9507	Indium In-111 capromab pendetide, diagnostic, per study dose, up to 10 millicuries
A9508	Iodine I-131 iobenguane sulfate, diagnostic, per 0.5 millicurie
A9509	Iodine I-123 sodium iodide, diagnostic, per millicurie
A9510	Technetium Tc-99m disofenin, diagnostic, per study dose, up to 15 millicuries
A9512	Technetium Tc-99m pertechnetate, diagnostic, per millicurie
A9513	Lutetium Lu 177, dotatate, therapeutic, 1 mCi
A9515	Choline C-11, diagnostic, per study dose up to 20 millicuries
A9516	Iodine I-123 sodium iodide, diagnostic, per 100 microcuries, up to 999 microcuries
A9517	Iodine I-131 sodium iodide capsule(s), therapeutic, per millicurie
A9520	Technetium tc-99m, tilmanocept, diagnostic, up to 0.5 millicuries
A9521	Technetium Tc-99m exametazime, diagnostic, per study dose, up to 25 millicuries
A9524	Iodine I-131 iodinated serum albumin, diagnostic, per 5 microcuries
A9526	Nitrogen N-13 ammonia, diagnostic, per study dose, up to 40 millicuries
A9528	Iodine I-131 sodium iodide capsule(s), diagnostic, per millicurie
A9529	Iodine I-131 sodium iodide solution, diagnostic, per millicurie
A9530	Iodine I-131 sodium iodide solution, therapeutic, per mCi
A9531	Iodine I-131 sodium iodide, diagnostic, per microcurie (up to 100 microcuries)
A9532	Iodine I-125 serum albumin, diagnostic, per 5 microcuries
A9536	Technetium Tc-99m depreotide, diagnostic, per study dose, up to 35 millicuries
A9537	Technetium Tc-99m mebrofenin, diagnostic, per study dose, up to 15 millicuries
A9538	Technetium Tc-99m pyrophosphate, diagnostic, per study dose, up to 25 millicuries
A9539	Technetium Tc-99m pentetate, diagnostic, per study dose, up to 25 millicuries
A9540	Technetium Tc-99m macroaggregated albumin, diagnostic, per study dose, up to 10 millicuries
A9541	Technetium Tc-99m sulfur colloid, diagnostic, per study dose, up to 20 millicuries
A9542	Indium In-111 ibritumomab tiuxetan, diagnostic, per study dose, up to 5 millicuries
A9543	Yttrium Y-90 ibritumomab tiuxetan, therapeutic, per treatment dose, up to 40 mCi
A9546	Cobalt Co-57/58, cyanocobalamin, diagnostic, per study dose, up to 1 microcurie
A9547	Indium In-111 oxyquinoline, diagnostic, per 0.5 millicurie
A9548	Indium In-111 pentetate, diagnostic, per 0.5 millicurie

Code	Description
A9550	Technetium Tc-99m sodium gluceptate, diagnostic, per study dose, up to 25 millicurie
A9551	Technetium Tc-99m succimer, diagnostic, per study dose, up to 10 millicuries
A9552	Fluorodeoxyglucose F-18 FDG, diagnostic, per study dose, up to 45 millicuries
A9553	Chromium Cr-51 sodium chromate, diagnostic, per study dose, up to 250 microcuries
A9554	Iodine I-125 sodium iothalamate, diagnostic, per study dose, up to 10 microcuries
A9555	Rubidium Rb-82, diagnostic, per study dose, up to 60 millicuries
A9556	Gallium Ga-67 citrate, diagnostic, per millicurie
A9557	Technetium Tc-99m bicisate, diagnostic, per study dose, up to 25 millicuries
A9558	Xenon Xe-133 gas, diagnostic, per 10 millicuries
A9559	Cobalt Co-57 cyanocobalamin, oral, diagnostic, per study dose, up to 1 microcurie
A9560	Technetium Tc-99m labeled red blood cells, diagnostic, per study dose, up to 30 millicuries
A9561	Technetium Tc-99m oxidronate, diagnostic, per study dose, up to 30 millicuries
A9562	Technetium Tc-99m mertiatide, diagnostic, per study dose, up to 15 millicuries
A9563	Sodium phosphate P-32, therapeutic, per mCi
A9564	Chromic phosphate P-32 suspension, therapeutic, per mCi
A9566	Technetium Tc-99m fanolesomab, diagnostic, per study dose, up to 25 millicuries
A9567	Technetium Tc-99m pentetate, diagnostic, aerosol, per study dose, up to 75 millicuries
A9568	Technetium Tc-99m arcitumomab, diagnostic, per study dose, up to 45 millicuries
A9569	Technetium Tc-99m exametazime labeled autologous white blood cells, diagnostic, per study dose
A9570	Indium In-111 labeled autologous white blood cells, diagnostic, per study dose
A9571	Indium In-111 labeled autologous platelets, diagnostic, per study dose
A9572	Indium In-111 pentetreotide, diagnostic, per study dose, up to 6 millicuries
A9575	Injection, gadoterate meglumine, 0.1 ml
A9576	Injection, gadoteridol, (ProHance multipack), per ml
A9577	Injection, gadobenate dimeglumine (MultiHance), per ml
A9578	Injection, gadobenate dimeglumine (MultiHance multipack), per ml
A9579	Injection, gadolinium-based magnetic resonance contrast agent, not otherwise specified (NOS), per ml
A9580	Sodium fluoride F-18, diagnostic, per study dose, up to 30 millicuries
A9581	Injection, gadoxetate disodium, 1 ml
A9582	Iodine I-123 iobenguane, diagnostic, per study dose, up to 15 millicuries
A9583	Injection, gadofosveset trisodium, 1 ml
A9584	Iodine I-123 ioflupane, diagnostic, per study dose, up to 5 millicuries
A9585	Injection, gadobutrol, 0.1 ml
A9586	Florbetapir F18, diagnostic, per study dose, up to 10 millicuries
A9587	Gallium ga-68, dotatate, diagnostic, 0.1 millicurie
A9588	Fluciclovine f-18, diagnostic, 1 millicurie
A9589	Instillation, hexaminolevulinate hydrochloride, 100 mg
A9590	Iodine I-131, iobenguane, 1 mCi

Code	Description
A9597	Positron emission tomography radiopharmaceutical, diagnostic, for tumor identification, not otherwise classified
A9598	Positron emission tomography radiopharmaceutical, diagnostic, for non-tumor identification, not otherwise classified
A9600	Strontium Sr-89 chloride, therapeutic, per mCi
A9604	Samarium Sm-153 lexidronam, therapeutic, per treatment dose, up to 150 mCi
A9606	Radium RA-223 dichloride, therapeutic, per mcCi
A9698	Non-radioactive contrast imaging material, not otherwise classified, per study
A9699	Radiopharmaceutical, therapeutic, not otherwise classified
A9700	Supply of injectable contrast material for use in echocardiography, per study
Q9951	Low osmolar contrast material, 400 or greater mg/ml iodine concentration, per ml
Q9953	Injection, iron-based magnetic resonance contrast agent, per ml
Q9954	Oral magnetic resonance contrast agent, per 100 ml
Q9955	Injection, perflexane lipid microspheres, per ml
Q9956	Injection, octafluoropropane microspheres, per ml
Q9957	Injection, perflutren lipid microspheres, per ml
Q9958	High osmolar contrast material, up to 149 mg/ml iodine concentration, per ml
Q9959	High osmolar contrast material, 150–199 mg/ml iodine concentration, per ml
Q9960	High osmolar contrast material, 200–249 mg/ml iodine concentration, per ml
Q9961	High osmolar contrast material, 250–299 mg/ml iodine concentration, per ml
Q9962	High osmolar contrast material, 300–349 mg/ml iodine concentration, per ml
Q9963	High osmolar contrast material, 350–399 mg/ml iodine concentration, per ml
Q9964	High osmolar contrast material, 400 or greater mg/ml iodine concentration, per ml
Q9965	Low osmolar contrast material, 100-199 mg/ml iodine concentration, per ml
Q9966	Low osmolar contrast material, 200-299 mg/ml iodine concentration, per ml
Q9967	Low osmolar contrast material, 300-399 mg/ml iodine concentration, per ml

Radiological Procedures

Procedures in the radiology section generally establish a diagnosis or follow the progression or remission of a disease process. However, also included in this section are procedures that are therapeutic in nature. These therapeutic procedures are often referred to as interventional or invasive radiology services. Codes in this section of the CPT book report the radiological supervision and interpretation of these interventional and invasive procedures.

The codes in this section of the CPT book are separated by radiologic modality:

- Diagnostic radiology (diagnostic imaging)
- Diagnostic ultrasound
- Radiologic guidance
- Breast, mammography
- Bone/joint studies
- Radiation oncology
- Nuclear medicine

© 2020 Optum360, LLC

When auditing radiology services, the guidelines found in the CPT book should be reviewed carefully. Guidelines found at the beginning of certain radiology sections clarify the use of codes within that section. Code categories, subcategories, and parenthetical phrases also may be presented. The guidelines are arranged similar to other sections of the CPT book and are unique to the individual code, category, subcategory, or range of codes.

Other procedures frequently performed by radiologists may be found outside the radiology section, such as noninvasive vascular diagnostic studies found in the medicine section. Services involving the invasive or interventional component of interventional radiology services are found in the surgery section. These include percutaneous biopsies, injection procedures, and transcatheter procedures.

Procedures performed with contrast material often do not specify the type of contrast; however, other codes are more specific.

Many radiologic procedures may also be reported with a surgical component based on the nature of the radiologic portion of the procedure. Many of the surgical procedures have parenthetical notes that follow the surgical procedure indicating that the radiologic portion may be reported separately when done in conjunction with the procedure. Radiology procedure codes may also be billed with visit type services, and modifier 25 should be appended to the visit codes.

Diagnostic Radiology/Imaging Procedures: By Specific Area (70010–76499)

Radiological x-rays, computed tomography (CT) scans, magnetic resonance imaging (MRI), computed tomographic angiography (CTA), magnetic resonance angiography (MRA), and therapeutic radiological procedures with supervision and interpretation are included in this section. The subdivisions of this section are grouped by anatomic site.

Codes for the supervision and radiological interpretation for selective and nonselective catheterization are included in this section.

The type of radiological exam must first be determined. The term "radiologic examination" in this section usually refers to "flat plate" or the most common type of x-ray exam. These use a cassette with the x-ray film or digital receiver under or behind the area to be viewed. X-rays are then used to provide images of the bones and internal organs obtained by sending small amounts of radiation through the body, leaving a shadow-like image of internal structures. This type of imaging exam usually involves multiple views, or x-rays taken from different angles.

In addition, codes are selected based upon the number of views taken. The example below illustrates how the number of views affects code assignment.

73120	Radiologic examination, hand; 2 views
73130	Radiologic examination, hand; minimum of 3 views

For a standard two-view exam, report 73120. If only one view is taken, report 73120 with modifier 52. Code 73130 is used when three or more views are taken. A unit of one is indicated in the units column, not the number of views obtained. Documentation must include the number of views take if that is a component of the code.

Computed tomography or CT exams are computer regeneration of x-ray images taken of a plane from multiple sources or angles. CT may be performed without contrast agent, with a contrast agent, or without contrast followed by administration of contrast and additional contrasted sequences. Codes should be selected based upon anatomic site and use of contrast agent.

Magnetic resonance imaging or MRI is a radiation-free, noninvasive technique that produces high quality, multiple plane images of the inside of the body by using the natural magnetic properties of the hydrogen atoms within the body that emit radiofrequency signals when exposed to radio waves in a strong magnetic field.

Magnetic resonance angiography (MRA) is performed in a similar manner but allows visualization of the vessels. MRA procedures differ from other forms of MRI in that the provider is able to perform a physiologic evaluation of cardiac function. Often more than one code is required: one for the imaging (determine if stress imaging was performed when selecting this code) and a second code to report velocity flow mapping. When pharmacologic stress is also performed by the same provider, report the appropriate stress testing code from 93015–93018. Velocity flow mapping (75565) is an add-on code that may be reported in addition to 75557, 75559, 75561, or 75563.

Other radiologic procedures include angiography or discography, a radiographic imaging of the arteries or spinal canal. Imaging may be performed to study the vasculature of any given organ, body system, or area of circulation such as the brain, heart, chest, kidneys, limbs, gastrointestinal tract, aorta, and pulmonary circulation to visualize the formation and the function of the blood vessels to detect problems such as a blockage or stricture. A catheter is inserted through an accessible blood vessel or spine, a radiopaque contrast material is injected, and x-rays are taken.

DEFINITIONS

discography. Radiographic imaging of an intervertebral disk, done after the injection of a contrast agent.

radiopaque dye. Medium injected into the body that is impenetrable by x-rays.

stricture. Narrowing of an anatomical structure.

Diagnostic Ultrasound Procedures: By Specific Area (76506–76999)

Ultrasonography refers to a radiographic recording by rapidly oscillating crystals that produce the sound waves used in the ultrasound beam. A transducer, which must be in close contact with the skin, transmits the sound waves and receives the echo. A gel substance placed on the skin improves the transmission of sound. Ultrasound is sound with a frequency over 20,000 Hz, which is about the upper limit of human hearing, although inaudible.

Ultrasound procedures may be found in other sections of the CPT book. For example, echocardiography procedures are in the medicine section under "Cardiovascular Services." Color mapping in conjunction with fetal echocardiography (76825–76826) is reported with 93325 in the medicine section. Duplex scans and Doppler studies of the vascular system are found in the medicine section under the heading "Noninvasive Vascular Diagnostic Studies," codes 93880–93990.

Diagnostic ultrasound codes are arranged by anatomic site. Code selection is also based upon the type of ultrasonic procedure.

Head and neck ultrasounds include evaluation of the eyes and soft tissue of the head and neck. Intracranial ultrasound is reported with 93886–93893. Ultrasound of the chest does not include intravascular ultrasound; this is reported with 92978.

Ultrasound of the pelvis is subdivided into obstetrical and nonobstetrical procedures. Obstetrical (76801–76828) include evaluation of the fetus. Nonobstetrical pelvic ultrasound is reported with 76830–76857, male genitalia with 76870–76873, and extremities with 76881–76886.

For code 76881, the documentation requirements are very specific. A complete extremity joint evaluation requires **all** of the following components:

- Joint space
- Peri-articular soft tissue structure surrounding the joint
  - muscles
  - tendons
  - other soft structures
- Any identifiable abnormalities
- Permanent recorded images
- Written report
  - must contain a description of each of the required elements or a reason why the element could not be visualized, such as surgical absence

In the event that a complete evaluation cannot be performed, code 76882 may be reported. A limited extremity joint evaluation requires the following components:

- Evaluation of one of the following:
  - joint space
  - muscle
  - tendon
  - other soft structures that surround the joint
- Permanent recorded images
- Written report
  - must contain a description of each element evaluated

Ultrasonic guidance is reported with 76932–76965. These codes are specific to the use of ultrasound and not other methods of imaging used as guidance. Code selection is determined based upon the type of procedure performed.

Other ultrasound procedures include breast (76641–76642), gastrointestinal (76975), bone density (76977), using microbubbles as an intravascular contrast agent (76978-76979), elastography for tumor detection (76981-76983), and intraoperative guidance (76998).

Radiologic Guidance: By Technique/Specific Area (77001–77022)

This section includes the codes used for radiologic guidance. Codes are determined by the procedure being performed.

There are many methods used for guidance including, but not limited to:

- Computed tomography guidance
- Fluoroscopic guidance
- Magnetic resonance guidance

Codes for ultrasound guidance are found in the diagnostic ultrasound section (76932–76965).

It is crucial to read the instructional notes within this subsection, as many procedures are considered an integral part of other procedures in the radiology section.

Radiography: Breast (77046–77067)

The codes for mammography services are combined under the subsection of breast mammography. Mammography services include screening, diagnostic, magnetic imaging, and other breast procedures.

Report modifier GG if both a screening and diagnostic mammogram are performed on the same date. Report modifier GH if the screening mammogram is converted to a diagnostic mammogram.

Additional Evaluations of Bones and Joints (77071–77086)

Bone joint studies include stress and bone age and length studies, osseous survey, joint survey, bone mineral density studies, absorptiometry, and magnetic resonance imagery of bone marrow blood supply.

Radiation Oncology Procedures: By Technique/Specific Area (77261–77799)

Radiation oncology is a therapeutic modality as opposed to a diagnostic service. Radiation therapy is used as a treatment method for patients who have malignant neoplasms. Treatment modes include:

- Brachytherapy
- Teletherapy

Procedure codes within this section include:

- Initial consultation

- Clinical treatment planning
- Clinical treatment management procedures
- Dosimetry
- Follow-up care during treatment and for three months after the completion of treatment
- Medical radiation physics
- Respiratory motion management simulation
- Simulation
- Special services
- Treatment devices

Any special or rarely performed services that require using an unlisted procedure code must be accompanied by a special report.

Radiosurgery is a term that describes the use of high-energy beams of radiation that are precisely directed at the selected target cells. There are six types of radiation currently used in radiosurgery: electromagnetical waves (gamma and photon x-rays), subatomic particles (electrons, protons, and neutrons), and carbon ions. Some radiosurgery is performed using gamma rays or a gamma knife. Others are performed using a linear accelerator (Linac), proton beam therapy, image guided radiation therapy (IGRT), or intensity modulated radiation techniques (IMRT). Neutron therapy is still experimental and is not routinely used. Radiosurgery can be performed in one session or fractionated (divided into multiple sessions).

Important definitions in radiation oncology include:

- Simulation (the process of targeting abnormal/normal anatomy, acquiring images and data so that a radiation plan may be developed for the patient)
  - simple
    - single treatment area
  - intermediate
    - two separate treatment areas
  - complex
    - three or more treatment areas or any area using the following:
    - brachytherapy simulation
    - complex blocking
    - custom shield blocks
    - hyperthermia probe verification
    - particle
    - rotation or arc therapy
    - any use of contrast material

Note: A treatment area is an adjacent anatomic location that is also being treated (e.g., primary tumor organ, the resection bed, and lymph nodes). If the treatment areas are not adjacent (e.g., tibia, and lumbar spine), each area is considered a separate treatment area.

Hyperthermia is used in addition to radiation therapy or chemotherapy. It may be induced in the following ways:

- Low-energy radiofrequency conduction
- Microwave
- Probes
- Ultrasound

Clinical brachytherapy requires the use of natural or man-made radioelements applied to the treatment areas.

- Simple: one to four sources/ribbons
- Intermediate: five to 10 sources/ribbons
- Complex: greater than 10 sources/ribbons

Note: Some of the procedures in this section represent professional or technical services only, and other codes in this section are a combination of professional and technical services. Read the codes carefully and use modifier 26 to identify professional services if the technical portion is reported by another entity.

Coverage Information

The Centers for Medicare and Medicaid Services, as well as many other third-party payers, bundle the following services into the radiation therapy; therefore, they are not paid separately:

11920-11921	Tattooing
16000-16030	Treatment of burns
36000, 36410, 36425	Venipuncture or Introduction of catheter
51701-51703	Urinary bladder catheterization
90832-90840	Psychotherapy
90846-90847	Psychotherapy
90863	Pharmacologic management
96360-96368	Intravenous infusion
97802-97804	Medical nutrition therapy
99151-99153	Moderate conscious sedation
99202-99215	Evaluation and Management
99217-99239	Evaluation and Management
99281-99498	Evaluation and Management

Nuclear Radiology Procedures (78012–78999)

Nuclear medicine involves radioactive elements for diagnostic imaging or radiopharmaceutical imaging. A radioactive element, such as uranium, spontaneously emits energetic particles by the disintegration of the nuclei.

Nuclear medicine is different from other radiology services. In nuclear medicine, the radioelement is ingested, placed, or infused. The images obtained are based upon the emission of the radioelement. These services can be helpful in diagnosing specific illnesses such as cancer as the diseased cells attract the radioelement. An example of this is tumor imaging. Note that oral and intravenous administration of contrast media is included in the procedure codes. When intra-arterial, intra-cavitary, intrathecal, intra-articular, and other nonoral or IV administration of contrast media is performed, it may be reported separately.

The nuclear medicine codes do not include the radionuclides used in the performance of the service. Code these materials separately using HCPCS Level II codes.

Diagnostic procedures are grouped by the system examined and further delineated by anatomic site and type of procedure or examination performed. Therapeutics describes specific procedures and methods of contrast administration.

Interventional Procedures

The development of cross-sectional imaging techniques, such as ultrasound, CT, MRI, and digital processing of fluoroscopy forced a shift in the use of angiographic studies from purely diagnostic to include therapeutic applications. Thus the name interventional radiology is now used to describe the specialty. The techniques include percutaneous biopsy (obtaining tissue specimens from inside the body without surgery), percutaneous drainage (removing fluid and bypassing obstructions), intravascular therapy (delivery of vasoactive drugs, clot-dissolving drugs, and chemotherapy), angioplasty (intraluminal dilatation of vascular narrowing), and embolization (injection of substances that stop bleeding).

Documentation

Documentation of interventional procedures is different from other radiology services. The dictated operative report is the best and most appropriate document to support procedure charges as images are usually destroyed after five or seven years.

In 2014, the American College of Radiology (ACR) revised the standards of communication for diagnostic radiology's written interpretations. The following is a summary of a policy statement by the ACR in an attempt to promote optimal patient care and enhance effective documentation supporting appropriate coding methods of all diagnostic and therapeutic interventional radiology procedures performed by physicians.

For example, a dictated operative report should be organized as follows:

- The facility or location where the procedure was performed
- Patient name
- Name(s) of ordering physician(s) or other health care provider(s)
- Date of the procedure (and time if relevant)
- Preoperative diagnosis
- Postoperative diagnosis (conclusion or impression)
- Precise name or title of procedures performed (specific selective catheter placement)

The body of a procedure report should contain descriptions of:

- Actual process and events of how procedures were approached and performed

- Utilized materials, drugs, contrast, guidewires and catheters
- Precise anatomic terminology and names of vessels observed or studied
- Identifiable limiting factors
- Other pertinent clinical issues, such as patient condition, complications, etc.
- Comparisons with previous studies where applicable

Summary of findings (conclusion, impression or diagnosis) should contain:

- A precise diagnosis if possible
- Recommendations for follow-up or additional diagnostic or therapeutic procedures

Patient demographic and other pertinent information should be contained in the procedure report format such as patient name, facility name, patient account number, patient date of birth, referring physician name, date and time procedure dictated, date and time report was transcribed, as well as name of physician performing procedure.

Transcribed report revisions or edits should be performed per individual facility health information and medical staff guidelines.

Special Report

Services that are unusual or rarely performed may require a special report in order to be reimbursed by the payer.

This report should include the following:

- Adequate description of the service
- Complexity of symptoms
- Concurrent problems
- Diagnostic and therapeutic procedures
- Follow-up care
- Nature, extent, medical appropriateness of the service
- Pertinent physical findings
- Time, effort, equipment necessary to provide the service

Chapter 8. **Auditing Pathology and Laboratory Procedures**

The pathology and laboratory CPT® codes (80047–89398 and 0001U–0241U) are used for those services provided by a reference, hospital, or physician laboratory. **Note:** A draw station is not a laboratory. It is a place where a specimen is collected but no laboratory testing is performed on the specimen.

Laboratory and Pathology Coding and Billing Considerations

A laboratory is defined as any facility that performs laboratory testing on specimens derived from humans for the purpose of providing information for the diagnosis, prevention, and treatment of disease or impairment, or assessment of health. A diagnostic laboratory test is considered a laboratory service for billing purposes, regardless of where it is performed.

Some factors that can influence billing and payment of laboratory services include:

- Clinical Laboratory Improvement Amendment (CLIA) status
- Point of service
- Billing authority
- Code selection
- Modifier assignment
- Units of service
- Qualifying circumstances

 AUDITOR'S ALERT

See Appendix 1 for the audit worksheet for laboratory procedures.

Clinical Laboratory Improvement Amendments Status

CMS regulates all laboratory testing (except research) performed on humans in the U.S. through the Clinical Laboratory Improvement Amendments (CLIA). The objective of the CLIA program is to ensure quality laboratory testing. All clinical laboratories must enroll in CLIA and they must be certified to test in order to receive Medicare or Medicaid payments. The type of certification is dependent upon the complexity of the test being performed. There are three basic levels of CLIA tests: waived, moderate, and high-complexity. Each level of complexity has a set of personnel requirements, as well as proficiency standards that must be met in order for that entity to be certified. This information can be found on the Center for Disease Control website at http://www.cdc.gov/CLIA/default.aspx. CLIA certified laboratories are able to bill for laboratory procedures that fall within their certification level. The CLIA number must be entered on the claim as a condition for payment. Medicare contractors deny claims for diagnostic clinical laboratory tests performed if the laboratory CLIA certificate is expired or the laboratory performs a testing outside the scope of their certificate.

CODING AXIOM

Modifier QW must be appended to the procedure code when billing for CLIA waived tests, unless otherwise indicated by the payer.

There are five types of certification that a laboratory can receive:

- **Certificate of Waiver:** Permits the laboratory or physician practice to perform only waived tests. Waived tests have been deemed simple and accurate and have little risk of error. Examples of waived tests include fecal occult blood tests and some types of urinalysis. A list of CLIA waived tests can be found at https://www.cms.gov/Regulations-and-Guidance/ Legislation/CLIA/downloads/waivetbl.pdf.

- **Certificate for Provider-Performed Microscopy (PPMP):** PPMP is a subset of the moderate complexity testing methodology. This certificate is required when a physician, dentist, or other mid-level provider (e.g., nurse midwife, nurse practitioner, physician assistant) performs only certain microscopy procedures, such as urine microscopic examination or KOH smear examinations. The physician, mid-level practitioner (under supervision if required by the state), or dentist must personally perform the procedure on specimens obtained during the visit. A laboratory or practice that has this type of waiver may also perform waived tests. While routine on-site surveys are not required for the PPMP Certificate, any PPMP certified entity is subject to the same moderate complexity requirements and can be surveyed by CMS as part of a routine survey for nonwaived tests or when a complaint is reported. A complete list of tests considered to be PPMP can be found at https://www.cms.gov/Regulations-and-Guidance/Legislation/CLIA/ Downloads/ppmplist.pdf.

- **Certificate of Registration (COR):** A Certificate of Registration is issued to laboratories that apply for but have not yet received a Certificate of Compliance or a Certificate of Accreditation. A COR enables the laboratory to perform tests that are considered to be moderate or high complexity until such a time that the laboratory has demonstrated through a CMS survey or a CMS approved accrediting organization that all requirements are met.

- **Certificate of Compliance (COC):** A COC is issued by CMS to laboratories that are in compliance with CLIA requirements after an on-site survey. The surveyor observes the laboratory's past and current practices, interviews employees, and reviews relevant documentation.

- **Certificate of Accreditation (COA):** A laboratory may also choose to become accredited by a CMS accrediting organization. This allows the laboratory to perform moderate and/or high complexity tests. The accrediting organization inspects the laboratory every two years to determine that the CLIA requirements are being met.

Note: Some laboratory procedures are excluded from the CLIA regulations and do not require CLIA certification. Examples of these types of procedures are included in the following table.

Code	Description
80502	Clinical pathology consultation; comprehensive, for a complex diagnostic problem, with review of patient's history and medical records
81050	Volume measurement for timed collection, each
82075	Alcohol (ethanol); breath
83013	Helicobacter pylori; breath test analysis for urease activity, non-radioactive isotope (eg, c-13)
83014	Helicobacter pylori; drug administration

 © 2020 Optum360, LLC

Code	Description
86077	Blood bank physician services; difficult cross match and/or evaluation of irregular antibody(s), interpretation and written report
86078	Blood bank physician services; investigation of transfusion reaction including suspicion of transmissible disease, interpretation and written report
86079	Blood bank physician services; authorization for deviation from standard blood banking procedures (eg, use of outdated blood, transfusion of Rh incompatible units), with written report
86485	Skin test; candida
86486	Skin test; unlisted antigen, each
86490	Skin test; coccidioidomycosis
86510	Skin test; histoplasmosis
86580	Skin test; tuberculosis, intradermal

A complete list of excluded laboratory tests may be found at https://www.cms.gov/Regulations-and-Guidance/Legislation/CLIA/Downloads/cpt4exc.pdf.

Billing Authority

There are numerous, complicated laws that dictate who can bill for laboratory services and how much can be charged. There are antimarkup provisions in some states, self-referral prohibitions, Stark, Shell Lab, and other federal regulations that must be considered. Health care providers and laboratories are urged to determine billing authority prior to submitting any claim for laboratory services. Proposed contractual agreements between laboratories and other providers should be reviewed by a health care attorney to ensure compliance with existing laws.

The prices that laboratories charge physicians for laboratory services should be at or above fair market value for nonfederal health care program tests. Pricing below fair market value to induce physicians to refer their federal health care program business may put the laboratory at risk for antikickback enforcement.

Code Selection

With few exceptions, outpatient laboratory services must be reported with HCPCS Level II and CPT codes. Codes reported should be selected by an individual technically familiar with laboratory testing methodologies and specimen sources, as these factors can influence code selection.

The pathology and laboratory codes are used to indicate laboratory services performed by a physician or by a technologist under the responsible supervision of a physician.

The HCPCS Level II code book also contains a section titled "Pathology and Laboratory Services." This section is divided into the following subsections:

- Chemistry and Toxicology Tests (P2028–P2038)
- Pathology Screening Tests (P3000–P3001)
- Microbiology Tests (P7001)
- Miscellaneous (P9010–P9615)

Other sections of the HCPCS Level II coding system may contain codes for laboratory services. For example, the Q code section (temporary codes) includes Q0113 Pinworm examinations and Q0114 Fern test. The S code section (temporary national codes [non-Medicare]) contains many codes for genetic testing.

Claims submitted for laboratory services must also include ICD-10-CM codes. ICD-10-CM codes explain the reason for the service. If a particular procedure code is identified on a national or local coverage policy and that policy requires a specific diagnosis to support the medical necessity of that service, then that diagnosis must be submitted in order to receive payment. However, it is important to remember that the selection of ICD-10-CM codes must be based on information provided by the provider that is substantiated in the medical record and relevant to the testing episode. It is inappropriate to select an ICD-10-CM code based on coverage decisions. Some key items to remember when selecting ICD-10-CM codes are:

- Diagnostic information from earlier dates of service (other than standing orders) should not be reported on laboratory claims.

- Diagnostic information that has triggered reimbursement in the past should not be used to simply receive coverage and/or reimbursement. Diagnostic information should be what is documented in the medical record for that date of service.

- Computer programs that automatically insert diagnosis codes without receipt of diagnostic information from the ordering provider or other authorized individual should not be reported.

Modifier Assignment

There are a number of factors that may require the assignment of a modifier to the laboratory code in order to identify the specific procedure or portion of the procedure that was performed. For example, the majority of codes represent a technical component only, but certain codes represent a global service—a combination of professional and technical components. When only a portion of these global services is provided, it is imperative that modifier TC (technical component) or 26 (professional component) be appended to the procedure code. This applies mostly to laboratory services that are paid under the Medicare physician fee schedule. More information about fee schedules is provided below.

The most common modifiers used when reporting laboratory services include:

26	Professional component
32	Mandated services
59	Distinct procedural service
90	Reference (outside) laboratory
91	Repeat clinical diagnostic laboratory test
92	Alternative laboratory platform testing

© 2020 Optum360, LLC

CS   Cost-sharing waived for specified COVID-19 testing-related services that result in an order for, or administration of, a COVID-19 test and/or used for cost-sharing waived preventive services furnished via telehealth in Rural Health Clinics and Federally Qualified Health Centers during the COVID-19 public health emergency

GA   Waiver of liability statement issued, as required by payer policy, individual case

GZ   Item or service expected to be denied as not reasonable and necessary

QW   CLIA waived test

TC   Technical Component

For more information regarding the appropriate use of modifiers, see chapter 3.

Billing Guidelines

When billing Medicare for laboratory services, there are a number of requirements that must be followed. Many of these requirements are specific to laboratory services and differ from those for medical or surgical procedures.

Medicare uses several different methods to reimburse for laboratory services, including:

- Medicare Physician Fee Schedule (MPFS)
- 101 percent of reasonable cost (critical access hospitals)
- Laboratory Fee Schedule
- Outpatient Prospective Payment System
- Reasonable charge

Most commonly, laboratory services are paid using the Clinical Laboratory Fee Schedule. The Medicare Physician Fee Schedule may be used to pay for services such as routine venipuncture (36410) or physician interpretation. Medicare pays in full for covered laboratory. Neither the Medicare annual deductible nor the 20 percent coinsurance is applicable to laboratory services.

The Social Security Act (SSA) § 1834A, as required by the Protecting Access to Medicare Act (PAMA) of 2014, required changes to the methodology to develop the Clinical Laboratory Fee Schedule (CLFS). The Centers for Medicare and Medicaid Services (CMS) implemented this new methodology on January 1, 2018. Under this method rates for laboratory services are based on weighted median private payer rates. Payment rates under the private payer rate-based CLFS are generally updated every three years. The payment amounts established are not subject to any geographic adjustments.

Additionally, SSA § 1834A and CMS regulations at 42 Code of Federal Regulations (CFR) § 414.507(d) limit the amounts the CLFS rates for most CDLTs can be reduced as compared to the payment rates for the preceding year. For the first three years after implementation (calendar year [CY] 2018 through CY 2020), the reduction could not be more than 10 percent per year and for the next three years (CYs 2021 through 2023), the reduction cannot be more than 15 percent per year.

Under the final rule, laboratories, including physician office laboratories, were required to report private payer rates and volume data if they:

- Had more than $12,500 in Medicare revenues from laboratory services on the CLFS, not including revenue from Medicare Advantage payments under Medicare Part C.

- Received more than 50 percent of their Medicare revenues from laboratory and physician services during a data collection period

The new process that CMS implemented contains the following elements:

- **Data Collection Period.** The data collection period is the six months from January 1 through June 30 during which applicable information is collected.

- **Six-Month Review and Validation Period.** A six-month review and validation period follows the data collection period and precedes the data reporting period (the period where applicable information must be submitted to CMS). During the six-month review and validation period, laboratories should assess whether the applicable laboratory thresholds are met.

- **Data Reporting Period.** The data reporting period is the three-month period, January 1 through March 30, during which a reporting entity reports applicable information to CMS. Applicable information reported during the data reporting period will be used to calculate payment rates effective January 1 of the following year.

Data Collection Period	Six-Month Review & Validation Period	Data Reporting Period	CLFS Rate Years
January 1, 2019 – June 30, 2019	July 1, 2019 – December 31, 2019	January 1, 2021 – March 31, 2021	2022 – 2024
January 1, 2023 – June 30, 2023	July 1, 2023 – December 31, 2023	January 1, 2024 – March 31, 2024	2025 - 2027
Continues for 3 years	Continues for 3 years	Continues for 3 years	New CLFS rate every 3rd year

* Previously January 1, 2020 through March 31, 2020. Reporting entities must report applicable information based on the original data collection period of January 1, 2019 through June 30, 2019. Data reporting for these tests will resume on a three-year cycle, beginning in 2024.

This CLAB contains the following information:

Column 1   Year: Calendar year rates are effective.

Column 2   Code: This column contains all active CPT and HCPCS Level II codes for laboratory services.

Column 3   Modifier: When included, QW denotes a CLIA-waived test (with the exception of codes 81002, 81025, 82270, 82272, 82962, 83026, 84830, 85013, and 85651, which do not require modifier QW to be recognized as a waived test).

Column 4   Effective Date: Date fee schedule rates are effective.

Column 5   Indicator: This indicates if the service is paid at the national level (N) or by the local contactor (L).

    © 2020 Optum360, LLC

Column 6   Rate: The payment rate shown by the dollar amount.

Column 7   Short Description: This is the short description of the service.

Note: Laboratory services are paid by Medicare on an assignment basis. This means that the provider MUST accept assignment for any laboratory service provided to a Medicare patient. When a claim is received that is not assigned, the Medicare contractor will pay that claim as if assignment was accepted. For those providers who do not normally accept assignment, if a claim is received with multiple types of service and one of those services is a laboratory service, the claim will be paid as if assignment was NOT accepted for ALL services EXCEPT the laboratory service.

Medicare requirements prohibit the billing of a laboratory service by an entity other than the performing entity. For physician practices, this means that unless performed by the practice, it cannot be billed. When the physician office performs the laboratory study, the 10-digit CLIA number is identified in item 23 of the CMS 1500 claim form.

Often laboratory tests are not done on the same day as the specimen is obtained. CMS guidelines indicate that a provider should report the date that the specimen was obtained even if the laboratory test is performed on a subsequent date. For example, a patient is seen in the office on February 12 and the physician orders a SGOT and SGPT. Blood is drawn. The laboratory test is performed on February 13. The correct date of service indicated on the claim in February 12 since that is the day that the specimen is obtained.

Automated Tests

Many laboratory tests are performed automatically on multi-channel equipment, allowing multiple testing to be done on a single specimen simultaneously. When three or more tests are reported using the automated testing method, Medicare pays the lower of a disease oriented panel that includes the tests or the cost of the test individually.

The CPT book identifies the individual tests that are included in organ or disease oriented panels (80047–80076 and 80081). For example, the basic metabolic panel (80047) includes the following individual tests:

- Calcium, ionized
- Carbon dioxide
- Chloride
- Creatinine
- Glucose
- Potassium
- Sodium
- Urea Nitrogen (BUN)

Example
The physician orders a glucose, BUN, creatinine, and potassium. The Medicare contractor determines that if billed separately payment would be $24.92. The payment for a basic metabolic panel (code 80047) is $12.42. Because payment is lower for the panel, the Medicare contractor bundles the tests and pays at the panel rate.

☞   **KEY POINT**

Medicare pays laboratory claims in full and on an assignment basis.

Tests that are not usually performed using the automated testing methodology can be billed separately. For example, if in addition to the tests indicated above the physician also orders an A1C (by chromatography) (83036), the Medicare contractor would pay for 80047 and 83036.

Nonpatient Testing

Nonpatient testing is when the hospital performs testing on patients who are not being treated in the facility—the specimen is obtained by personnel other than one employed by the hospital. In these instances, the hospital is acting as a reference laboratory. Claims for nonpatient testing are reported using a bill type of 0141 on the UB-04 claim.

Payment for Review of Laboratory Rest Results by Physician

Reviewing results of laboratory tests, phoning results to patients, filing such results, etc., while considered a Medicare-covered service, are not separately billable. Payment for these services are included in the physician fee schedule payment for the evaluation and management (E/M) service.

Clinical pathology consultation services (80500–80502) include a written report with medical interpretation of the results. More information regarding these codes can be found elsewhere in this chapter.

Billing for Noncovered Tests

Medicare does not allow a provider to bill for services that are denied as not medically necessary unless the provider has had a patient sign a completed Advance Beneficiary Notice (ABN) of noncoverage.

It is very important that the ABN is completed before the patient signs. A common error that physician practices make is to have the patient sign a blank ABN or one that does not indicate the reason a laboratory test is likely to be denied as noncovered.

Medical Necessity

Payers cover laboratory services only when considered reasonable and necessary. Medicare has developed a set of Laboratory National Coverage Determinations (NCD). These NCDs differ from other Medicare NCDs in that ICD-10-CM codes are included. All codes are included on one of three lists: covered codes, noncovered codes, and codes that do not support medical necessity. The laboratory NCDs may be useful in determining when an ABN should be completed and signed by the patient in addition to determining coverage guidelines.

Laboratory-Specific Documentation

Laboratory accrediting agencies, federal law (CLIA and OSHA), and state laws dictate specific documentation requirements for all phases of the analytic process and mandate the retention of:

- Test requisition
- Test records
- Test procedures
- Patient test reports (preliminary and final)

 KEY POINT

The ABN must be completed BEFORE obtaining a patient's signature.

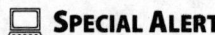 **SPECIAL ALERT**

A revised Advance Beneficiary Notice of Noncoverage (ABN), Form CMS-R-131, has been approved. Use will be mandatory starting 8/31/20. More information can be found at: https://www.cms.gov/Medicare/Med icare-General-Information/BNI/ABN

 FOR MORE INFO

A list of the laboratory national coverage determinations can be found at http://www.cms.gov/ Medicare/Coverage/CoverageGen Info/LabNCDs.html.

- Immunology test reports
- Pathology test reports
- Bone marrow reports
- Histopathology stained slides and blocks
- Cytology slides
- Accession log records
- Quality control activity records
- Blood and blood products quality control records
- Instrument maintenance records
- Personnel records
- Proficiency testing records
- OSHA training, inspection, and exposure records

Documentation must show that all tests were ordered by an authorized individual, correctly performed on the correct patient by qualified personnel, and timely reported to the ordering provider. Test results must be interpretable and accurate. Documentation must also be maintained to substantiate that test systems are operating correctly.

Regulatory agencies have indicated that records do not need to be in hard copy form. Records may be stored in computers, on tapes or disks, compact disks, microfilm, or microfiches as long as they can be retrieved within a reasonable period of time.

Multi-test Laboratory Panels (80047–80076 and 80081)

Organ or disease-oriented panels are used to confirm specific diagnoses. These panels are problem-oriented in scope. There is an instructional note at the beginning of this subsection indicating that additional tests may be performed separately. In addition, each panel contains a list of the tests that must be included in order to report that particular code. This does not mean a provider may not report additional tests. If appropriate, these additional tests may be reported with the panel code. It is also inappropriate to separately report the components of a panel test if the full set of identified tests was performed.

Clinical information derived from results of laboratory data that are mathematically calculated is considered part of the test procedure and not reported separately.

Coding Tips
- Tests that are nonautomated may be billed in addition to organ or disease-oriented panels.

The following table contains some of the most frequently ordered tests and can be a useful tool in determining what tests are contained in which panel and which codes may be billed individually.

 AUDITOR'S ALERT

General health panels performed at the time of a routine physical examination are usually noncovered because they are not considered medically necessary. For Medicare patients, a completed and signed ABN must be obtained or the patient cannot be billed if the panel is denied.

Test	CPT Code	Basic Metabolic (calcium ionized) 80047	Basic Metabolic (calcium total) 80048	Electrolyte 80051	Comprehensive Metabolic 80053	Lipid 80061	Renal Function 80069	Hepatic Function 80076
Albumin	82040				X		X	X
Alkaline Phosphatase	84075				X			X
ALT (SGPT)	84460				X			X
AST (SGOT)	84450				X			X
Total Bilirubin	82247				X			X
Direct Bilirubin	82248							X
Total Calcium	82310		X		X		X	
Ionized Calcium	82330	X						
Chloride	82435	X	X	X	X		X	
Cholesterol	82465					X		
CPK, CK	82550							
CO2	82374	X	X	X	X		X	
Creatinine	82565	X	X		X		X	
GGT	82977							
Glucose	82947	X	X		X		X	
LDH	83615							
HDL	83718					X		
Phosphorus	84100						X	
Potassium	84132	X	X	X	X		X	
Protein	84155				X			X
Sodium	84295	X	X	X	X		X	
Triglycerides	84478					X		
Urea nitrogen	84520	X	X		X		X	
Uric Acid	84550							

Drug Testing Assays (80143–80299 and 80305–80377 and 83992)

Drug testing can be difficult and confusing to report. There are three major subsections: therapeutic drug assays, drug assays, and chemistry. Code assignment depends on why the test is being performed and the type of results obtained. For example, therapeutic drug assays may be used to determine if there is an optimal level of a specific drug in the blood while drug assay is used to determine if the patient is or is not using a particular drug.

It is important to understand some key terms when determining correct code assignment.

Drug assays are divided into two categories:

Presumptive: Commonly assayed first by a presumptive screening method followed by a definitive drug identification method. Presumptive testing may be qualitative, semiquantitative, or quantitative depending on the purpose of the testing. However, presumptive drug testing cannot distinguish between structural isomers (for example, it cannot identify the difference between morphine and hydromorphone).

Definitive (80320–80377 and 83992): These procedures may be quantitative or qualitative and are used to identify possible use or nonuse of a drug. These tests can differentiate between structural isomers. However, they are not usually able to differentiate between stereoisomers.

The specimen for drug assay testing may be any type (i.e., urine, blood, hair, saliva, meconium) unless otherwise specified within the code description. Qualitative testing usually renders results such as positive/negative or present/absent while semiquantitative or quantitative results are usually of a numeric or measured value.

Presumptive Drug Assay

Presumptive drug assays (80305–80307) are usually performed first and, if positive followed by a definitive drug identification method. Presumptive drug assay methodologies include chromatography, direct optical observation, immunoassay, mass spectrometry with or without chromatography immunoassays methods.

Code 80305 should be reported when the documentation states that the results were obtained by direct optical observation, as in the case of viewing urine cups, urine dipsticks, test cards, or cartridges. When documentation states that direct optical observation was used in addition to instrumentation, see 80306. Presumptive tests may be confirmed with a definitive test that designates the drug.

Code 80307 is reported for tests performed utilizing instrument chemistry analyzers, such as immunoassay (e.g., EIA, ELISA, EMIT, FPIA, IA, KIMS, RIA), chromatography (e.g., GC, HPLC), and mass spectrometry with or without chromatography (e.g., DART, DESI, GC-MS, GC-MS/MS, LC-MS, LC-MS/MS, LDTD, MALDI, TOF).

These tests may be requested for all drugs and all drug classes performed. In addition, each code encompasses all sample validations performed and may include, but is not limited to, pH, specific gravity, and nitrite. The specimen type may vary. This code should only be reported once per date of service no matter how many procedures or results are performed.

DEFINITIONS

qualitative. To determine the nature of the component of substance.

quantitative. To determine the amount and nature of the components of a substance.

stereoisomers. Isomeric molecules that have the same molecular formula and sequence of bonded atoms (constitution), but that differ only in the three-dimensional orientations of their atoms in space.

structural isomers. Isomeric molecules share the same molecular formula, but the bond connections or their order differs.

Definitive Drug Testing

As mentioned earlier, definitive drug testing methods may be quantitative or qualitative and are used to identify possible use or nonuse of a drug. These tests can differentiate between structural isomers; however, they usually cannot differentiate between stereoisomers. Examples of the methodologies used for definitive drug testing include but are not limited to gas chromatography with mass spectrometry and liquid chromatography mass spectrography. Immunoassays and enzymatic methods are excluded from definitive drug testing.

The table below indicates the appropriate code for the type of substance being tested. Note that the CPT book contains a table that identifies individual substances included in each type of substance. In some instances, correct code assignment depends on the number of substances.

Substance	CPT Code
Alcohols	80320
Alcohol biomarkers	80321– 80322
Alkaloids	80323
Amphetamines	80324–80326
Anabolic steroids	80327–80328
Analgesics, non-opioid	80329–80331
Antidepressants serotonergic	80332–80334
Antidepressants, tricyclic and other cyclical	80335–80337
Antidepressants, not otherwise classified	80338
Antiepileptics, not otherwise specified	80339–80341
Antipsychotics, not otherwise specified	80342– 80344
Barbiturates	80345
Benzodiazepines	80346–80347
Buprenorphine	80348
Cannabinoids, natural	80349
Cannabinoids, synthetic	80350–80352
Cocaine	80353
Fentanyl	80354
Gabapentin, non-blood	80355
Heroin metabolite	80356
Ketamine and norketamine	80357
Methadone	80358
Methylenedioxyamphetamines (MDA, MDEA, MDMA)	80359
Methylphenidate	80360
Opiates	80361
Opioids and opiate analogs	80362- 80364
Oxycodone	80365
Pregabalin	80366
Propoxyphene	80367
Sedative hypnotics (non-benzodiazepines)	80368
Skeletal muscle relaxants	80369–80370

 © 2020 Optum360, LLC

Substance	CPT Code
Stimulants, synthetic	80371
Tapentadol	80372
Tramadol	80373
Stereoisomer (enantiomer) analysis, single drug class	80374
Drug(s) or substances(s), definitive, qualitative or quantitative, not otherwise specified	80375–80377
Phencyclidine (PCP)	83992

For definitive drug testing billed to Medicare, count the number of drug classes tested, both qualitative and quantitative, any method, and report the corresponding HCPCS Level II code. The description for all of the following HCPCS Level II codes is: Drug test(s), definitive, utilizing (1) drug identification methods able to identify individual drugs and distinguish between structural isomers (but not necessarily stereoisomers), including, but not limited to, GC/MS (any type, single or tandem) and LC/MS (any type, single or tandem and excluding immunoassays (e.g., IA, EIA, ELISA, EMIT, FPIA) and enzymatic methods (e.g., alcohol dehydrogenase)), (2) stable isotope or other universally recognized internal standards in all samples (e.g., to control for matrix effects, interferences and variations in signal strength), and (3) method or drug-specific calibration and matrix-matched quality control material (e.g., to control for instrument variations and mass spectral drift); qualitative or quantitative, all sources, includes specimen validity testing, per day. The only differentiation is the number of classes tested.

Number of Drug Classes	HCPCS Level II Code
1–7 drug classes	G0480
8–14 drug classes	G0481
15–21 classes	G0482
22 or more classes	G0483

Therapeutic Drug Assays (80143–80299)

These services are used to monitor the patient's clinical response to a known medication. For example, a physician may order a therapeutic drug assay to determine the level of theophylline in a patient's blood to determine if the clinically effective level has been obtained. Correct code assignment is determined by the drug being monitored. Note that because of the nature of the test performed, some drugs may require code assignment from the chemistry subsection.

Coding Tips

- For presumptive or definitive drug testing, see the appropriate codes from range 80305–80307or 80320–80377 and 83992.

Stimulation and Suppression Test Panels (80400–80439)

Evocative or suppression testing requires the administration of pharmaceutical agents to determine a patient's response to those agents.

For physician administration of evocative or suppressive agents, codes 96360–96361, 96365–96368, 96372–96374, and 96375 should be used. For supplies and drugs, see 99070 or the appropriate HCPCS Level II supply and drug codes.

 DENIAL ALERT

Definitive drug testing billed to Medicare should be reported with HCPCS Level II codes G0480-G0483, depending on the number of drug classes tested.

 AUDITOR'S ALERT

An NCD applies to code 80162. See Medicare's *National Coverage Determinations Manual*, Pub. 100-03, section 190.24 for more information.

In cases where prolonged infusions (96360–96361) are reported it would be inappropriate to also report prolonged physician care E/M codes.

When billing this section of codes there will be a note under each code description telling the provider how many times a particular analyte must be performed in order to meet the criteria for the service to be reported.

Coding Tips
- The CPT book indicates that aldosterone is tested twice by including "x 2" in the description of 80408.
- For aldosterone suppression evaluation panel (e.g., saline infusion) (80408), this panel must include the following: Aldosterone (82088 x 2) and Renin (84244 x 2).

Consultation by Clinical Pathologist (80500–80502)

Clinical pathology consultation services (80500–80502) include a written report with medical interpretation of the results. Consultative clinical pathology services are eligible for payment by Medicare in accordance with the following requirements. The consultative services must:

- Be requested by the patient's attending physician or other qualified health care professional.
- Relate to a test result that lies outside the clinically significant normal or expected range in view of the condition of the patient.
- Result in a written narrative report included in the patient's medical record.
- Require medical judgment by the consulting pathologist.

Routine conversations a laboratory director has with attending providers about test orders or results are not consultations unless all four requirements are met.

Clinical pathology consultations generally consist of two types. One type involves a review of a patient's history and medical records along with the laboratory test results. Consultations of this nature are considered complex and should be reported with 80502.

Another type is an interpretive consultation, which is a consultation of limited duration requiring medical judgment in interpreting test findings. Interpretive consults provide information directly related to the condition of the patient to the attending provider, which ordinarily cannot be furnished by a nonphysician laboratory specialist. Claims for this service should be reported with 80500.

Note: Clinical pathology consultation services remain a separately payable service for 2020 even though CMS has bundled other consultative services into nonconsultative evaluation and management codes.

Urine Tests (81000–81099)

Urinalysis testing (81000–81099) includes dipstick testing, bacteriuria screening, pregnancy testing, and volume measurement. Code selection is based upon the actual test performed.

Coding Tips
- Codes 81002, 81003, and 81007 may be performed using a CLIA-waived test system. Laboratories with a CLIA-waived certificate must report this code with modifier QW CLIA waived test.

- Do not report 81005 for immunoassay; see 83518.

- For reagent strip using nonimmunoassay methodology, see 81000 (with microscopy) or 81002 (without microscopy).

- To report urine culture, consult code 87086–87088.

Molecular Testing Procedures (81105–81408 and 81479)

Molecular pathology procedures are used to determine if there are variants in genes that may indicate constitutional or somatic disorders by analyzing the nucleic acid.

Codes in this subsection are divided into tier 1 and tier 2. Codes in tier 1 describe more commonly performed procedures than those classified in tier 2.

Code selection is based upon the specific gene(s) being analyzed. Usually, all of the listed variants are included in the procedure, eliminating the need to report multiple codes for the same gene analysis.

These codes include all analytical services that are required to perform the assay, including:

- Amplification

- Cell lysis

- Detection

- Digestion

- Extraction

- Nucleic acid stabilization

Quantitation of extracted DNA is also included in the payment for a molecular pathology procedure. Other HCPCS/CPT codes, such as CPT code 84311 Spectrophotometry, analyte not elsewhere specified, should not be reported for this quantitation.

Scraping a tumor off an unstained slide, if performed, is included in the payment for these procedures. A physician should not report microdissection (codes 88380 or 88381) for this process. The microdissection CPT codes require a pathologist to use laser capture microdissection (88380) or a dissecting microscope (88381) to separate malignant cells from normal cells.

According to Medicare, physician (M.D. or D.O.) interpretation of a molecular pathology procedure (e.g., codes 81105–81408, and 81479) may be reported to Medicare with HCPCS Level II code G0452 when medically reasonable and necessary. It should not be reported with code 88291 (cytogenetics and molecular cytogenetics, interpretation and report). Check with payers to see what their policy is to report these services.

Codes under the heading "Genomic Sequencing Procedures (GSPs) (81410–81471)" focus on parallel genetic sequencing for genes and mutations associated with a specific set of conditions, as well as whole exome and whole genome sequencing. These include:

- Aortic dysfunction

- Colon cancer

- Fetal aneuploidy

- Hearing loss

- Targeted neoplasm somatic mutations (solid organ and hematolymphoid)
- Whole exome and whole genome
- Whole mitochondrial genome
- X-linked intellectual disability

Providers testing for individual or a small number of targeted genes or mutations in which all of the components of the procedures as described by the codes are not performed report the appropriate tier 1 or tier 2 code instead. If the services are not identified by a tier 1 or tier 2 code, code 81479 Unlisted molecular pathology procedure, should be reported.

Documentation

Documentation regarding the patient's family history of the conditions being tested should be detailed and more specific than what might usually be obtained, including the precise relationship to the patient (i.e., paternal grandfather, maternal aunt, etc.). The patient's past medical history, including pathological findings, should be clearly indicated in the medical record. Any related laboratory examinations that have been performed should be noted. A clear indication of which criteria is met when specified for one of the conditions above should also be noted.

Furthermore, in the case of therapy-directed testing, the documentation must also indicate that the provider anticipates the test result is likely to be of use in the management of the patient's condition.

Coding Tips
- In cases where the interpretation component of the service is the only performed service, append modifier 26 Professional component, to the code.
- A table is included at the beginning of the pathology/lab section that gives detailed information such as the gene name, commonly associated proteins and diseases, and the CPT code.

Multianalyte Assays with Algorithmic Analyses (81490–81599)

These codes represent continued advancements in the highly complex field of molecular testing. Multianalyte assays with algorithmic analyses (MAAA) are typically performed by a single clinical laboratory or manufacturer. These analyses use results obtained from assays of various types, including molecular pathology, fluorescent in situ hybridization, and non-nucleic acid-based assays, to perform proprietary analysis using the results, as well as other patient information, to assess risk. This risk factor is reported typically as a numeric score(s) or as a probability to address specific clinical concerns, such as the likelihood that a tumor will recur in the future or respond to a particular drug treatment regimen, whether or not a patient is experiencing rejection of a heart transplant, the activity of disease in patients with rheumatoid arthritis, and the likelihood that a nodule in the thyroid is benign.

Codes are classified as category 1 codes (81490–81599) or, when a specific procedure has not been assigned a category 1 code, a four-digit alphanumeric administrative code found in appendix O of the CPT book.

Appendix O of the CPT book contains the proprietary name and clinical laboratory or manufacturer of a specific MAAA and crosswalks this to the appropriate CPT code that should be assigned. When a proprietary name is not included in the list, code 81599 should be reported. Appendix O also contains the following list of MAAA codes that have not been assigned a category 1 code. These codes have four numbers followed by the letter M.

The following M codes are identified in appendix O:

- 0002M Liver disease, ten biochemical assays (ALT, A2-macroglobulin, apolipoprotein A-1, total bilirubin, GGT, haptoglobin, AST, glucose, total cholesterol and triglycerides) utilizing serum, prognostic algorithm reported as quantitative scores for fibrosis, steatosis and alcoholic steatohepatitis (ASH)

- 0003M Liver disease, ten biochemical assays (ALT, A2-macroglobulin, apolipoprotein A-1, total bilirubin, GGT, haptoglobin, AST, glucose, total cholesterol and triglycerides) utilizing serum, prognostic algorithm reported as quantitative scores for fibrosis, steatosis and nonalcoholic steatohepatitis (NASH)

- 0004M Scoliosis, DNA analysis of 53 single nucleotide polymorphisms (SNPs), using saliva, prognostic algorithm reported as a risk score

- 0006M Oncology (hepatic), mRNA expression levels of 161 genes, utilizing fresh hepatocellular carcinoma tumor tissue, with alpha-fetoprotein level, algorithm reported as a risk classifier

- 0007M Oncology (gastrointestinal neuroendocrine tumors), real-time PCR expression analysis of 51 genes, utilizing whole peripheral blood, algorithm reported as a nomogram of tumor disease index

- 0011M Oncology, prostate cancer, mRNA expression assay of 12 genes (10 content and 2 housekeeping), RT-PCR test utilizing blood plasma and/or urine, algorithms to predict high-grade prostate cancer risk

- 0012M Oncology (urothelial), mRNA, gene expression profiling by real-time quantitative PCR of five genes (MDK, HOXA13, CDC2 [CDK1], IGFBP5, and CXCR2), utilizing urine, algorithm reported as a risk score for having urothelial carcinoma

- 0013M Oncology (urothelial), mRNA, gene expression profiling by real-time quantitative PCR of five genes (MDK, HOXA13, CDC2 [CDK1], IGFBP5, and CXCR2), utilizing urine, algorithm reported as a risk score for having recurrent urothelial carcinoma

- 0014M Liver disease, analysis of 3 biomarkers (hyaluronic acid [HA], procollagen III amino terminal peptide [PIIINP], tissue inhibitor of metalloproteinase 1 [TIMP-1]), using immunoassays, utilizing serum, prognostic algorithm reported as a risk score and risk of liver fibrosis and liver-related clinical events within 5 years

- 0015M Adrenal cortical tumor, biochemical assay of 25 steroid markers, utilizing 24-hour urine specimen and clinical parameters, prognostic algorithm reported as a clinical risk and integrated clinical steroid risk for adrenal cortical carcinoma, adenoma, or other adrenal malignancy

- 0016M Oncology (bladder), mRNA, microarray gene expression profiling of 209 genes, utilizing formalin-fixed paraffin-embedded tissue, algorithm reported as molecular subtype (luminal, luminal infiltrated, basal, basal claudin-low, neuroendocrine-like)

Because the AMA updates the codes three times a year, before reporting one of the codes above, it is best to determine if a category 1 CPT code has been assigned and if so, check with the payer in question as to which code should be reported. When a category 1 or administrative code is not available, the unlisted MAAA code (81599) is reported.

When reporting an MAAA service it is also appropriate to report additionally those services performed prior to cell lysis such as microdissection (88380–88381). Such services as nucleic acid stabilization, extraction, digestion, application, hybridization and detection, and the cell lysis, however, are included and are not reported separately. It is important to note that when reporting genomic sequencing procedure assays, the most specific code for the primary disorder should be reported, even though genes may be listed in multiple code descriptors.

Chemistry Testing Procedures (82009–84999)

Codes within this subsection are used to report the measurement of a specimen for a specific analyte. Analytes are arranged in alphabetic order. Services are listed alphabetically by the type of analyte. When reporting services performed from the chemistry section, it is important to note the following:

- All examinations are quantitative analysis unless otherwise specified

- Code assignment may vary dependent upon the methodology used

- Mathematically calculated results are an integral part of testing

- Specimen sources can be of any type. However, there are some codes that reference a specific specimen.

  - Example codes 82105 and 82106 are for alpha-fetoprotein (AFP) for serum or amniotic fluid, respectively.

    82105 Alpha-fetoprotein (AFP); serum

    82106 Alpha-fetoprotein (AFP); amniotic fluid

- When multiple specimens from different sources are analyzed, report the appropriate code for *each* individual source.

  - Example: Creatinine analysis of blood and urine is ordered by the physician. Report:

    82565 Creatinine; blood

    82570 Creatinine; other source

    Code 82570 is used to report the urine creatinine since there is no code specific for urine creatinine.

- Codes often indicate the methodology used to perform the analysis. When two different methodologies are used, both codes are reported.

Coding Tips
- Clinical data or calculated values not specifically requested by the ordering provider and derived from the results of other ordered or performed laboratory tests are considered part of the ordered test and are not reported separately. However, if a calculated analysis required values derived from other requested and nonrequested laboratory results, the requested analyte codes, including the codes for those calculated, should be reported individually.

- Analyte testing may be reported separately each time there is a different source or specimen.

✓ QUICK TIP

Blood glucose determination may be done by a various methods (automated testing, colormetric testing such as by dipstick or assay) using whole blood, serum, or plasma. The sample may be obtained by capillary puncture (fingerstick), venipuncture, or arterial sampling. Correct code assignment is dependent upon methodology used.

▽ AUDITOR'S ALERT

Medicare laboratory NCD 190.20 states that medical record documentation must include an evaluation of history and physical preceding the ordering of glucose testing and manifestations of abnormal glucose levels must be present to warrant the testing.

Hematology/Coagulation Testing Procedures (85002–85999)

Included in this section are testing procedures such as blood count, bleeding time, hemograms, clotting factor analysis, coagulation time, prothrombin time, thromboplastin time, and viscosity. Code selection is based upon the actual tests performed and may include differentiation as to manual and automated methods. A number of tests that are commonly performed are listed below.

Prothrombin time (85610): This test may be ordered as prothrombin time, PT, protime, or prothrombin. Used to evaluate the extrinsic coagulation pathway, it is most commonly performed to:

- Evaluate patients taking warfarin
- Evaluate patients with signs or symptoms of abnormal bleeding or thrombosis
- Evaluate patients who have a history of a condition known to be associated with the risk of bleeding or thrombosis
- Evaluate the risk of hemorrhage or thrombosis in patients who are going to have a medical intervention known to be associated with increased risk of bleeding or thrombosis
- Prior to the use of thrombolytic medication

Coding Tips
- A National coverage determination (NCD) exists for this code. This test may be performed using a CLIA-waived test system. When a CLIA waived test system is used, modifier QW should be appended.

Partial thromboplastin time (85730): Also know as activated partial thromboplastin or PTT, this test evaluates the intrinsic coagulation pathway. Common conditions that support the medical necessity of a PTT include:

- Liver disease or failure
- Clinical conditions associated with nephrosis or renal failure
- Certain bleeding disorders

A PTT is not useful for routinely monitoring Warfarin. Most payers allow this test to be repeated when the underlying condition and/or dosing of heparin is changed.

Coding Tips
- A National coverage determination (NCD) exists for this code. This test may be performed using a CLIA-waived test system. When a CLIA waived test system is used, modifier QW should be appended.

Blood Counts: There are a number of CPT codes (85004–85049) that can be used to report CBCs and code selection is dependent upon which components are performed and the methodology used.

Blood counts are used to evaluate and diagnose diseases related to abnormalities of the blood or bone marrow, including conditions such as anemia, leukemia, polycythemia, thrombocytosis, and thrombocytopenia. Many other conditions that secondarily affect the blood or bone marrow, including inflammation and infections, coagulopathies, neoplasms, and exposure to toxic substances, also support the medical necessity of performing a CBC.

Coding Tips
- CBCs are commonly performed at the time of a routine physical examination. Because medical necessity may not be established, this service may be denied as not medically necessary. In those instances, the Medicare patient should not be balance billed unless a completed ABN has been signed. Other third-party payers may allow patient billing without obtaining a waiver. Verify payer billing requirements prior to billing the patient.

Immunology Testing Procedures (86000–86849)

Immunology codes are qualitative or semiqualitative immunoassays performed by multiple-step methods. It is appropriate to code each separate test performed to detect antibodies to organisms. Infectious agent or antibodies detection is reported using 87260–87999. Included in this subsection are codes for the detection of the HIV virus.

Antibody: HIV-1 (86701), HIV-2 (86702), HIV-1 and HIV-2, single result (86703): HIV-1 antibody test (86701) may be ordered as an HIV-1 serological test or HIV-1 antibody. Code 86702 may be ordered as an HIV-2 serological antibody, which is a retrovirus closely related to simian AIDS and found initially in West African nations and Portugal, but with cases also being reported in the United States since 1987. Code 86703 may be ordered as a combined HIV-1 and -2 serological or a combined HIV-1 and -2 antibody, which tests for HIV-1 and HIV-2 with a single result.

Coding Tips
- When HIV-1 antigen is reported with HIV-1 and HIV-2 antibodies as a single result, code 87389 should be reported.
- A National coverage determination (NCD) exists for these codes. Codes 86701 and 86703 represent tests that may be performed using a CLIA-waived test system. Laboratories with a CLIA-waived certificate must report these codes with modifier QW CLIA-waived test. When a CLIA waived test system is used, modifier QW should be appended.
- When codes from range 86701–86703 are performed using a kit or transportable instrument and the single-use requirements are met, modifier 92 should be appended.
- Code 86701 or 86703 is performed initially. Code 86702 is performed when 86701 is negative and clinical suspicion of HIV-2 exists.

Microbiology Testing Procedures (87003–87999)

This section includes direct cultures for bacterial identification, parasite direct smears, tissue examination for fungi, and tissue culture inoculation for virus identification.

Urine culture and sensitivity is one of the frequently reported codes within this section.

Urine Culture and Sensitivity: A bacterial urine culture is performed to establish the etiology of a presumed urinary tract infection. It is common practice to do a urinalysis prior to a urine culture and this may be reported separately. Urine cultures may be reported using a number of codes listed below.

87086   Culture, bacterial, quantitative colony count, urine

87088   Culture, with isolation and presumptive identification of each isolate, urine

These codes report the performance of a urine bacterial culture with a calibrated inoculating device so that a colony count accurately correlates with the number of organisms in the urine. In 87088, isolation and presumptive identification of bacteria recovered from the sample is done by identifying colony morphology, subculturing organisms to selective media, and performing a gram stain or other simple test to identify bacteria to the genus level. There are several automated systems that detect the presence of bacteria using colorimetric, radiometric, or spectrophotometric means. In 87086, quantified colony count numbers within the urine sample are measured.

87184   Susceptibility studies, antimicrobial agent; disk method, per plate (12 or fewer agents)

87186   Susceptibility studies, antimicrobial agent; microdilution or agar dilution (minimum inhibitory concentration [MIC] or breakpoint), each multi-antimicrobial, per plate

Code 87184 is commonly called a Kirby-Bauer or Bauer-Kirby sensitivity test. It is a sensitivity test to determine the susceptibility of a bacterium to an antibiotic. The methodology is disk diffusion and results are reported as sensitive, intermediate, or resistant. As many as 12 antibiotic disks may be used per plate and the procedure is billed per plate not per antibiotic disk. Code 87186 may be referred to as a MIC or a sensitivity test. This test determines the susceptibility of a bacterium to an antibiotic. The methodology is microtiter dilution (several commercial panels use this method). Results are given as a minimum inhibitory concentration (MIC) with an interpretation of sensitive, intermediate, or resistant. The antibiotics on commercial plates are numerous, but predetermined. The procedure is charged by plate not by antibiotic.

Coding Tips
- According to NCD 190.12, codes 87088, 87184, and 87186 may be used multiple times in association with or independent of 87086, as urinary tract infections may be polymicrobial.
- Code 87086 may be used one time per encounter.

AUDITOR'S ALERT

Infectious agents detected by direct fluorescence microscopy or nucleic acid probe are reported with 87260–87300.

Pap Smear Screening (88141–88155, 88164–88167, 88174–88175)

Cytopathology of cervical or vaginal screens is performed using various methods. Code assignment depends on the method of screening, as well as the method of reporting (Bethesda or non-Bethesda system).

When the Bethesda or non-Bethesda systems are utilized, the following codes may be used:

- Code 88142 is reported for manual screening done under physician supervision and 88143 for manual screening followed by manual rescreening, done under physician supervision. These tests may be identified by the name "thin prep."

- Code 88147 is reported for smears screened by an automated system under physician supervision, while 88148 reports automated screening with manual rescreening under physician supervision. These tests may be identified as a cervical smear, Pap smear, or vaginal cytology.

- Code 88150 is used to report manual screening under physician supervision; 88152 is used to report manual screening and computer-assisted rescreening under physician supervision; and 88153 is used to report manual screening and rescreening under physician supervision. These tests may also be identified as a cervical smear, Pap smear, or vaginal cytology.

- Code 88174 should be reported for automated screening done under physician supervision and 88175 when automated screening is followed by manual rescreening or review under physician supervision. These tests may be identified by the brand name ThinPrep.

- Add-on code 88155 should be reported when the method is microscopy examination of a spray or liquid fixated smear. The test may be used to determine the balance of estrogen and progesterone of the vaginal squamous epithelium.

The following codes should be reported when the Bethesda System of evaluating and describing cervical/vaginal cytopathology slides is used.

- Code 88164 describes manual screening under physician supervision; 88165 manual screening and rescreening under physician supervision; 88166 manual screening and computer-assisted rescreening under physician supervision; 88167 manual screening and computer-assisted rescreening using cell selection and review under physician supervision. These tests may be identified as a cervical smear, Pap smear, or vaginal cytology.

Coding Tips
- Code 88141 is used to report physician interpretation of the cytopathology of the smear and is reported in addition to the primary technical service. If the cytopathology interpretation extends to include hormonal evaluation, assign 88155 in addition to the primary technical service. Assign 88141 or 88155, but not both, depending on the level of service performed.

- As an "add-on" code, 88155, is not subject to multiple procedure rules. No reimbursement reduction or modifier 51 is applied. The following table provides additional information for these codes as found in the Medicare Physician Fee Schedule Database.

Parent Code	Add-On	GLOB DAYS	MULT PROC	BILAT SURG	ASST SURG	CO-SURG	TEAM SURG
88142		XXX	9	9	9	9	9
88143		XXX	9	9	9	9	9
88147		XXX	9	9	9	9	9
88148		XXX	9	9	9	9	9
88150		XXX	9	9	9	9	9
88152		XXX	9	9	9	9	9
88153		XXX	9	9	9	9	9
	88155	XXX	9	9	9	9	9
88164		XXX	9	9	9	9	9
88165		XXX	9	9	9	9	9
88166		XXX	9	9	9	9	9
88167		XXX	9	9	9	9	9
88174		XXX	9	9	9	9	9
88175		XXX	9	9	9	9	9

Surgical Pathology (88300–88399)

These services represent the examination of specimens to determine the presence or absence of disease. The examination may be gross only (without the use of a microscope) or gross and microscopic. A specimen is defined as tissue or tissues that are submitted for individual and separate attention and require individual examination as well as pathologic diagnosis. When two or more specimens from the same patient are examined, such as two skin biopsy specimens, each specimen may be reported separately.

There are six levels of service. Refer to the instructional notes within each code.

Code 88300 may be assigned to any specimen the pathologist considers appropriate for diagnosis using gross examination method only. The other codes (88302–88309) include lists of specimens for which the procedure is appropriate. Any unlisted specimen should be assigned the code most closely reflecting the level of service. Please note that codes 88300-88309 do not include the services described in codes 88311–88365 and 88399.

Other Pathology Services (89049–89240)

Codes assigned to this section include cell count for miscellaneous body fluids, nasal smears, intubation aspiration specimen, sweat collection by iontophoresis, and water load test.

Infertility Treatment Services (89250–89398)

This subsection includes procedures to prepare ova and semen, create oocytes, culture and fertilization of the oocytes, storage, and thawing until implanted. These procedures are often performed in a special lab associated with an infertility clinic.

Proprietary Laboratory Analyses (PLA) Codes (0001U–0241U)

CPT includes a Proprietary Laboratory Analyses (PLA) section within Pathology and Laboratory. Codes in this section are available for use by any clinical laboratory or manufacturer that wants their tests specifically identified. A PLA is an alphanumeric CPT code (0001U–0241U) and corresponding descriptor that labs or manufacturers use to identify their particular test with greater specificity. These services are performed by a single "sole source" laboratory or for laboratory services that are cleared or approved by the Food and Drug Administration (FDA) and licensed and/or marketed to multiple providing laboratories. These services are often referred to as Proprietary Laboratory Analyses or PLA services. Correct code selection is dependent upon the service being provided.

PLA code sets are found in the CPT book but are also updated and released quarterly on the AMA CPT public website found at https://www.ama-assn.org/cpt-pla-codes. Users are advised to refer to the on-line file for the most current listing of PLA test codes due to the update frequency.

Chapter 9. **Auditing Medical Services**

The medicine section of the CPT® book contains codes for diagnostic and therapeutic services, such as immunizations, injections, dialysis, specialty specific codes, and special services. Within the medicine section of the CPT book, there are a number of subsections for the type of service being provided (e.g., chemotherapy administration) or for the specialty area providing the service (i.e., cardiovascular). As with other sections of the CPT book, there are general guidelines at the beginning of the section. Most of the subsections have guidelines, which are specific to the codes contained in that subsection. These guidelines contain valuable information regarding the proper use of the codes and should be read carefully.

There are a number of situations that may require the assignment of a modifier to the Medicine codes in order to identify the specific services performed. Each modifier is listed below with its official definition.

22	Increased procedural services
26	Professional component
33	Preventive service
50	Bilateral procedure
51	Multiple procedures
52	Reduced services
53	Discontinued procedure
55	Postoperative management only
56	Preoperative management only
57	Decision for surgery
58	Staged or related procedure or service by the same physician or other qualified health care professional during the postoperative period
59	Distinct procedural service
76	Repeat procedure or service by same physician or other qualified health care professional
77	Repeat procedure by another physician or other qualified health care professional
78	Unplanned return to the operating/procedure room by the same physician or other qualified health care professional following initial procedure for a related procedure during the postoperative period
79	Unrelated procedure or service by the same physician or other qualified health care professional during the postoperative period
95	Synchronous Telemedicine Service Rendered Via a Real-Time Interactive Audio and Video Telecommunications System
96	Habilitative services
97	Rehabilitative services
99	Multiple modifiers

See chapter 3 for a detailed explanation of these modifiers.

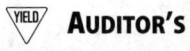 **AUDITOR'S ALERT**

See Appendix 1 for the audit worksheet for medicine section procedures.

DEFINITIONS

Holter monitor. Device worn by the patient for long-term continuous recording of electrocardiographic signals on magnetic tape, replayed at rapid speed, for scanning and selection of significant but brief changes that might otherwise escape notice.

AUDITOR'S ALERT

These codes must be reported in addition to the IV infusion services (96365–96375).

Date of Service

When auditing medical services it is important to pay close attention to the date of service reported. The date of service on the claim must agree with the date of service in the medical record. For those services that may extend beyond a single calendar day, such as holter monitor started at 11:45 a.m. and completed at 11:55 a.m. the next day, the date the procedure was started is usually indicated on the claim.

Immune Globulins Serum or Recombinant Products (90281–90399)

Intravenous immune globulin (IVIg) is a solution of globulins that contains antibodies normally found in adult human blood. (Globulins are proteins that provide disease immunity.) It is defined by Medicare as an approved pooled plasma derivative for the treatment of primary immune deficiency disease.

Medical Necessity
The following conditions may warrant IVIg therapy (this list is not all inclusive):

- Allogeneic bone marrow transplantation
- Chronic B-cell lymphocytic leukemia
- Chronic lymphocytic leukemia
- Chronic inflammatory demyelinating polyneuropathy (CIDP)—Solely Gamunex
- Common variable immunodeficiency (CVID)—A group of approximately 150 primary immunodeficiencies (PID) that have a common set of features, but that have different underlying causes
- Graft versus host disease
- Guillain-Barré syndrome
- Hematopoietic stem cell transplantation in patients older than 20 years of age (Gamimune-N only)
- Immune-mediated thrombocytopenia
- Kawasaki disease (see the Kawasaki Disease Diagnostic Criteria calculator)
- Kidney transplantation with a high antibody recipient or with an ABO incompatible donor
- Pediatric HIV type 1 infection
- Polymyositis/dermatomyositis
- Primary immunodeficiency disorders associated with defects in humoral immunity

Coding Tips
- Medicare regulations state patients must meet at least one of the following criteria:
  - conventional therapy failed (to be defined by the individual contractor)
  - conventional therapy is contraindicated (to be defined by the individual contractor)

- the disease is progressing so quickly that conventional therapy would not effect a response that is fast enough. IVIg may be given concurrently with conventional treatment, and only until the conventional treatment can take effect.

Note: Verify with third-party payers for their specific coverage guidelines.

Administration and Vaccine Products (90460–90756)

Correctly reporting the administration of a vaccine or toxoid is crucial to receive proper reimbursement. This is one area that an error in reporting can be very costly to a practice. The administration code is dependent upon the type of route chosen to deliver the vaccine or toxoid (i.e., percutaneous, intradermal, subcutaneous, intramuscular, intranasal, or oral methods). In addition to the administration code it is also necessary that a code for the vaccine/toxoid product (90476–90756) is reported.

It is important to note that counseling provided to the patient and/or family is included in the administration of a vaccine/toxoid to a patient younger than 18 years of age, codes 90460–90461. CPT guidelines indicate that this must be face-to-face counseling by the physician or qualified health care professional (e.g., nurse practitioner, physician assistant, or certified nurse specialist). When counseling is not provided and documented, codes from range 90471–90474 are used to report the vaccine administration.

When auditing claims for vaccines, it is crucial that the correct number of single or combination vaccines/toxoids administered has been correctly identified when assigning the code. It should be noted that code 90460 is reported for *each* vaccine component administered. For combo vaccines, code 90460 should be reported in conjunction with 90461 for each additional vaccine component. "Component" refers to an antigen in a vaccine that prevents disease(s) caused by one organism. Combination vaccines have multiple vaccine components. Codes 90471–90474 are not reported by component; they are reported once for each single or combination vaccine/toxoid.

Below are a few examples of the appropriate usage of the administration codes.

Example

The intramuscular administration of a measles, mumps, rubella, and varicella vaccine with counseling to a 10-year-old patient would be reported with:

- 90710 Measles, mumps, rubella, and varicella vaccine (MMRV), live, for subcutaneous use
- Code 90460 is billed for the first component (measles).
- Code 90461 is billed with three units for the counseling of additional components: mumps, rubella, and varicella.

Example

The intramuscular administration of human papilloma virus (HPV) vaccine with counseling to a 16-year-old female would be reported with:

AUDITOR'S ALERT

Administration to a patient up to 18 years of age (90460–90461) includes face-to-face physician or other qualified health care professional counseling with the patient and/or family and, therefore, should not be reported separately.

AUDITOR'S ALERT

Modifier 51 should not be appended to vaccine/toxoid codes 90476-90756.

DEFINITIONS

antigen. Substance inducing sensitivity or triggering an immune response and the production of antibodies.

human papilloma virus. Virus of several different species transmitted by direct or indirect contact and causing plantar and genital warts on skin and mucous membranes. HPV is most commonly associated with increased risk for cervical dysplasia and cancer in women.

– 90649 Human Papilloma virus (HPV) vaccine, types 6, 11, 16, 18 (quadrivalent), 3 dose schedule, for intramuscular use

– 90460 Immunization administration through 18 years of age via any route of administration, with counseling by physician or other qualified health care professional; first or only component of each vaccine or toxoid administered

Example

The subcutaneous administration of measles, mumps, and rubella (MMR) and intramuscular injection of diphtheria and tetanus, in a child younger than 7 years old, without counseling, would be assigned codes:

– 90471 Immunization administration (includes percutaneous, intradermal, subcutaneous, intramuscular injections); one vaccine (single or combination vaccine/toxoid)

– 90472 Immunization administration (includes percutaneous, intradermal, subcutaneous, intramuscular injections); each additional vaccine (single or combination vaccine/toxoid)

– 90702 Diphtheria and tetanus toxoids (DT) adsorbed when administered to individuals younger than 7 years, for intramuscular use

– 90707 Measles, mumps and rubella virus vaccine (MMR), live, for subcutaneous use

The appropriate evaluation and management (E/M) service code should be assigned when a significant and separately identifiable service was performed in addition to the administration of the vaccine or toxoid.

Immunizations are usually provided in conjunction with a medical service. This subsection also includes codes for vaccines or immunizations that have been developed by the manufacturer and are awaiting approval from the Federal Drug Administration (FDA). These are identified by the thunderbolt icon [⚡]. The AMA errata released during the year removes the icon when FDA approval is obtained. Due to the fact that these vaccines are awaiting approval from the FDA, it is wise to verify patient coverage before administering the vaccine. This could be a source of denials in a practice.

When assigning influenza codes, the following must be known:

- Vaccine type

  – trivalent vaccines, includes coverage for three (trivalent) strains: two A strains and one B strain (AMA, CPT 2013 Changes, An Insider's View)

  – quadrivalent vaccines, contain three influenza strains (two A strains and one B strain) obtained from the virus lineage that is predicted by the World Health Organization (WHO) and the US Food and Drug Administration (FDA) to be prevalent for the upcoming flu season, plus an additional B strain that is derived from the opposite lineage from the first B strain selected. This fourth strain helps overcome potential mismatches of the first B strain included in the vaccine that has been selected for a given flu season (American Medical Association, CPT 2017 Changes, An Insider's View)

  – pandemic formulation, created for potential use in the event of another pandemic such as H1N1 (swine flu)

- Dosage: 0.25mL or 0.5mL, if applicable
- Whether the vaccine is preservative free or preservative and antibiotic free
- Type of administration/route of administration (intramuscular, intradermal, intranasal, oral, percutaneous, and subcutaneous)
  - immunization administration, patient age through 18 years of age with provider counseling, per vaccine component (90460-90461)
  - immunization administration, without provider counseling, per vaccine (single or a combination vaccine) (intradermal, intramuscular, percutaneous, or subcutaneous) (90471-90472)
  - immunization administration, without provider counseling, per vaccine (single or a combination vaccine) (intranasal or oral) (90473-90474)

Coding Tips

- Identify the number of single or combination vaccines or toxoids administered to determine if the assigned code is correct.
- Immunizations are usually provided in conjunction with a medical service.
- Only one initial code should be reported per visit: 90460, 90471, or 90473.
- As add-on codes, 90461, 90472, and 90474 are not subject to multiple procedure rules. No reimbursement reduction or modifier 51 is applied. Add-on codes describe additional intraservice work associated with the primary procedure. They are performed by the same provider on the same date of service as the primary service/procedure, and must never be reported as a stand-alone code. The following table provides additional information for these codes as found in the Medicare Physician Fee Schedule Database.

Parent Code	Add-On	GLOB DAYS	MULT PROC	BILAT SURG	ASST SURG	CO-SURG	TEAM SURG
90460		XXX	0	0	0	0	0
	90461	ZZZ	0	0	0	0	0
90471		XXX	0	0	0	0	0
	90472	ZZZ	0	0	0	0	0
90473		XXX	0	0	0	0	0
	90474	ZZZ	0	0	0	0	0

Psychiatric Treatment (90785–90899)

Psychotherapy codes are not identified by site of service as are other codes and are based on time spent with the patient and whether an E/M service was performed in conjunction with the psychotherapy. Some highlights of the section are discussed below. Codes 90791–90792 are used to report diagnostic evaluations. A psychiatric diagnostic evaluation is the assessment of the patient's psychosocial history and current mental status, and review and ordering of diagnostic studies, followed by appropriate treatment recommendations. The services described by code 90792 include medical services, such as physical examination and prescription of pharmaceuticals, in addition to the diagnostic evaluation. Interviews and communication with family members or other sources is included in these codes.

Three timed codes are available for psychotherapy:

90832   Psychotherapy, 30 minutes with patient

90834   Psychotherapy, 45 minutes with patient

90837   Psychotherapy, 60 minutes with patient

In addition, add-on codes are available for psychiatric services performed in conjunction with E/M services (99202–99255, 99304–99377, 99341–99350). Many patients see providers for E/M services on the same date of service a psychotherapy service is provided. If the psychotherapy service is separately identifiable, an add-on code may be reported in addition to the E/M service. The time spent fulfilling the criteria for the E/M service is not included in the time reported for the psychotherapy service.

The add-on codes are listed below:

+90833   Psychotherapy, 30 minutes with patient when performed with an evaluation and management service (List separately in addition to the code for primary procedure)

+90836   Psychotherapy, 45 minutes with patient when performed with an evaluation and management service (List separately in addition to the code for primary procedure)

+90838   Psychotherapy, 60 minutes with patient when performed with an evaluation and management service (List separately in addition to the code for primary procedure)

Codes 90832–90838 include the following:

- Face-to-face time with patient. It should be noted that informants may be included in that time, but the patient should be there for the majority of the service.

- Psychotherapy only (90832, 90834, 90837)

- Psychotherapy with separately identifiable medical evaluation and management services includes add-on codes (90833, 90836, 90838)

- Services provided in all settings

- Therapeutic communication to:
  - ameliorate the patient's mental and behavioral symptoms
  - modify behavior
  - support and encourage personality growth and development

- Treatment for:
  - behavior disturbances
  - mental illness

Code	Type of Service	Time
90832	Psychotherapy	16–37 minutes
90833	Psychotherapy & E/M	16–37 minutes
90834	Psychotherapy	38–52 minutes
90836	Psychotherapy & E/M	38–52 minutes
90837	Psychotherapy	53 minutes or greater
90838	Psychotherapy & E/M	53 minutes or greater

When the psychotherapy and E/M service performed last for more than 90 minutes, report prolonged services (99354–99357). If the psychotherapy service performed is less than 16 minutes, it is inappropriate to report these codes.

The psychiatry section also has an add-on code, 90785, for interactive complexity. This code should be reported in addition to diagnostic psychiatric evaluation (90791–90792), psychotherapy (90832, 90834, 90837), group psychotherapy (90853), and psychotherapy when provided at the same visit with an E/M service (90833, 90836, 90838, 99202–99255, 99304–99337, 99341–99350).

Code 90785 includes at least one of the following activities:

- Discussion of a sentinel event demanding third-party involvement (e.g., abuse or neglect reported to a state agency)
- Interference by the behavior or emotional state of caregiver to understand and assist in the plan of treatment
- Management of discordant communication complicating care among participating members (e.g., arguing, reactivity)
- Use of nonverbal communication methods (e.g., toys and other devices or translator) to eliminate communication barriers
- Involved communication with:
  - patients wanting others present during the visit (e.g., family member, translator)
  - patients with third parties responsible for their care (e.g., parents, guardians)
  - third-party involvement (e.g., schools, probation and parole officers, child protective agencies)

Documentation must clearly specify the complexity that indicated the use of this code. Please see the CPT book for additional guidelines.

Codes 90839–90840 describe psychotherapy performed on a patient in crisis. Report these codes when the psychotherapy is urgent for a life-threatening or highly complex psychiatric crisis state in a patient in distress. Code 90839 is used for the first 30 to 74 minutes of intervention and 90840 for each additional 30 minutes. These codes include history of crisis state, mental status examination, psychotherapy, mobilization of resources, and implementation treatment.

For providers not authorized to report E/M service codes, an add-on code 90863 Pharmacologic management, including prescription and review of medication, when performed with psychotherapy services, is available to report. Code 90863 describes the psychiatric services of managing the patient's medications, including the patient's current use of the medicines, a medical review of the benefits and treatment progression, management of side-effects, and review or change of prescription.

The appropriate psychotherapy code without E/M service (90832, 90834, or 90837) should be reported in addition to code 90863. When determining the appropriate psychotherapy code to be reported with this procedure, any time spent providing the medication management should be excluded. For example, if the patient is seen for 45 minutes, and 15 minutes is spent performing medication management, code 90832 Psychotherapy, 30 minutes with patient and/or family, and code 90863 are reported. This code should not be reported with an E/M code as the service is included as part of the E/M code.

Medical record documentation should include the medication prescribed, condition for which the medication is needed, dosage, directions for use, any frequent side-effects, the effect the medication is having on the patient's symptoms or conditions, and any changes or continuation of medications.

Other physicians and other qualified health care professionals who perform psychotherapy and pharmacologic management for a patient are instructed to use the appropriate E/M code (99202–99255, 99281–99285, 99304–99337, 99341–99350) and an add-on code (90833, 90836, or 90838) when the time spent fulfilling the criteria for the E/M service is not included in the time reported for the psychotherapy service.

Coding Tips
- As "add-on" codes, 90785, 90833, 90836, 90838, 90840, and 90863 are not subject to multiple procedure rules. No reimbursement reduction or modifier 51 is applied. Add-on codes describe additional intraservice work associated with the primary procedure. Such services are performed by the same provider on the same date of service as the primary service/procedure and must never be reported as stand-alone codes. Please see the CPT book for the codes that these add-on codes should be reported with.

- Adaptive behavior treatment, 97151–97158, should not be reported in addition to interactive complexity (90785), psychiatric diagnostic evaluations (90791–90792), family psychotherapy (90846–90847), or the interpretation of psychiatric or other medical record documentation (90887).

- It should be noted that many codes in this section have a ★ icon. This indicates that they are telemedicine codes and should be reported with modifier 95 Synchronous Telemedicine Service Rendered Via a Real-Time Interactive Audio and Video Telecommunications System. Please see chapter 3 for more information on this modifier. A complete list of these codes can be found in appendix P in the CPT book.

Diagnostic Gastroenterology Procedures (91010–91299)

These diagnostic procedures are frequently performed with consultations or other E/M services. Evaluation and management services should be reported separately. Even though gastroenterology is a medicine subspecialty, the majority of procedures gastroenterologists perform are endoscopic and are listed in the surgery section.

Procedure Differentiation
Within the gastroenterology section, esophageal motility is one of the more common procedures performed. This study is commonly referred to as esophageal manometry and is reported with code 91010. In this procedure, a sensor is placed in the esophagus via the nose or mouth. The patient is given fluids to drink and the sensor measures the pressure of the contraction waves. This procedure is useful in diagnosing abnormalities of the muscles of the esophagus and/or the gastroesophageal junction, which propel food and water into the stomach.

Esophageal motility is indicated for the diagnosis of esophageal pathology, including achalasia, noncardiac chest pain, aperistalsis, spasm, esophagitis, esophageal ulcer, esophageal congenital webs, diverticula, hiatus hernia, congenital cysts, benign and malignant tumors, hypermobility, hypomobility, scleroderma, and extrinsic lesions. Generally this study is performed in addition to x-rays and endoscopy. This service is usually only covered by payers when it is medically necessary to diagnose a specific condition. When this study is ordered, it is important that the documentation supports the necessity.

Code 91013 is an add-on code to be used in conjunction with 91010 and reports stimulation and/or acid or alkali perfusion, such as a mecholyl provocation test. Code 91020 should be reported for a gastric manometry and 91022 for duodenal manometry.

A Bernstein test or acid perfusion test or study (91030) is performed on the esophagus, not in conjunction with a motility test. The acid perfusion test is done to try and replicate atypical chest pain the patient has been experiencing and aid in diagnosing the pain as noncardiac or due to esophageal reflux/esophagitis. Hydrochloric acid and an alternate saline control solution are infused one after the other via a nasogastric tube, without the patient being aware of the identity of the solution. The symptoms of chest pain are recorded as the patient identifies them.

Codes 91034–91038 are used to report commonly performed esophageal reflux and function tests. Each code has a different element that makes it unique and is briefly described below.

Gastroesophageal reflux testing is reported with 91034. In this test, the physician performs a gastroesophageal reflux test using esophageal pH electrode placement and recording. This procedure evaluates the proper functioning of the lower esophageal sphincter, the strong muscular ring located at the entrance to the stomach. A probe or electrode that measures the pH (acidity) level is inserted through the nose down to the esophagus. The probe records the pH level within the esophagus. The nasal catheter is connected to a small data recorder. The pH recording may be done over the course of a day. This code includes the analysis and interpretation of the recorded results.

Code 91035 is used to report a gastroesophageal reflux test performed via a mucosal attached telemetry pH electrode with recording. A small capsule containing a radiotelemetry pH sensor is inserted endoscopically in the esophagus and temporarily attached to the esophageal wall. The capsule monitors esophageal pH levels over a 48-hour period.

Esophageal function and reflux testing is reported with 91037–91038. These codes are differentiated by time. Code 91037 should be reported for a recording of one hour or less and 91038 for prolonged recording of greater than one hour, up to 24 hours. Time must be documented to report these services appropriately.

Capsule endoscopy, also referred to as gastrointestinal (GI) tract imaging, is reported with 91110. Documentation must indicate that the patient swallowed the endoscopic capsule with a glass of water. Color video images from inside the GI tract are recorded as the natural peristaltic movement passes the capsule smoothly and painlessly through the system. The data is transmitted by sensors, secured to the patient's abdomen, from the capsule to a data recorder, worn like a belt around the patient's waist, while the patient goes about daily ambulatory

DEFINITIONS

achalasia. Failure of the smooth muscles within the gastrointestinal tract to relax at points of junction; most commonly referring to the esophagogastric sphincter's failure to relax when swallowing.

esophagitis. Inflammation of the esophagus.

gastroesophageal reflux. Weakening of the lower esophageal sphincter allowing reflux of the stomach contents into the esophagus. One form is commonly defined as "heartburn."

perfusion. Act of pouring over or through, especially the passage of a fluid through the vessels of a specific organ.

scleroderma. Systemic disease characterized by excess fibrotic collagen build-up, turning the skin thickened and hard.

activities. After eight hours, the patient returns the equipment for processing at the computer workstation. The physician views and interprets the images and prepares a report. Report 91110 when the imaging includes the esophagus through the ileum. Report 91111 when the imaging is of the esophagus only. The difference between codes 91034 and 91035 is how pH is measured: through a nasal catheter or a mucosal attached electrode. Documentation is crucial in these procedures.

Capsule endoscopies are indicted for a patient that has had esophagogastroduodenoscopy (EGD) and colonoscopy. Symptoms generally include small bowel neoplasm or regional enteritis, gastrointestinal blood loss, or anemia due to blood loss, the origin of which is suspected to be in the small intestinal mucosa. Other indications include small intestine neoplasm or regional enteritis. A prior EGD and colonoscopy are not a prerequisite for these indications.

In 91112, gastrointestinal (GI) transit and pressure measurement are performed via wireless capsule. The patient swallows the capsule with a glass of water. Pressure, pH, and temperature are recorded as the natural peristaltic movement passes the capsule smoothly and painlessly through the system. This information is used to calculate regional transit times, including gastric emptying time, small bowel transit time, colonic transit time, combined small/large bowel transit time, whole gut transit time, pressure contraction patterns from the antrum and duodenum, and motility indices. The data is transmitted from the capsule to a data recorder, worn like a belt around the patient's waist or around the neck, for three to seven days, while the patient goes about daily ambulatory activities. The equipment is brought to the provider for processing at the computer workstation. The images are reviewed, interpreted, and a report is prepared. This procedure may be used for assessment of patients with functional or slow transit constipation, suspected gastroparesis, and unexplained diarrhea; conditions that may be due to poor GI motility.

Colonic motility (91117) is measured using various manometric techniques. In one method, a manometric catheter is positioned endoscopically and clipped to the colonic mucosa. A minimum of six hours of continuous recording ensues. Any provocation tests performed are included, as is the interpretation and report.

Rectal sensation, tone, and compliance testing (91120) is performed using graded balloon distention to evaluate anorectal pathology. Tone testing measures relaxation or rigidity in the rectum, compliance tests assess the distensibility of the rectum, and sensation tests assess feelings of fullness and discomfort upon distention. The patient is asked to empty his or her bowels. The patient is then placed in left lateral decubitus position with the head lowered 20 degrees, and the physician inserts a two-lumen catheter containing a cylindrical bag into the rectum. One lumen is used to inflate the bag, and the other is used to measure pressure within the bag. With the distal end of the bag 5 cm from the anal verge, the bag is inflated with air. Inflation is slowly increased and sensation, tone, and compliance monitored. The balloon is deflated when the patient experiences discomfort and urgency lasting more than 30 seconds.

Code 91122 describes the performance of anorectal manometry to help diagnose constipation and/or incontinence due to myotonic dysfunction or suspected cases of Hirschsprung's disease, a congenital absence of ganglion nerve cells in the plexus that innervates the colon and/or rectum to relax the internal anorectal sphincter in response to rectal distension. A manometry probe is

DEFINITIONS

ileum. Lower portion of the small intestine, from the jejunum to the cecum.

mucosa. Moist tissue lining the mouth (buccal mucosa), stomach (gastric mucosa), intestines, and respiratory tract.

neoplasm. New abnormal growth, tumor.

regional enteritis. Chronic inflammation of unknown origin affecting the ileum and/or colon.

advanced into the rectum after a digital exam. The probe is then slowly withdrawn, taking continuous pressure measurements until the high pressure area of the anal sphincters is located. With the patient relaxed, the "basal anal pressure" is recorded, and the highest pressures are recorded as the patient performs a maximum squeeze. The manometry catheter is inserted again with a rectal balloon that is slowly inflated to the patient's first sensation of fullness, and the volume is recorded. The anal sphincter response to the rectal distention is also recorded. Another manometry technique using a 3 balloon apparatus may also be employed in which pressure measurements are taken as the external, middle, and internal rectal balloons are inflated and deflated to note threshold levels and sphincter responses.

In electrogastrography (EGG), electrodes are placed on the skin over the stomach at a specific distance from each other and attached to a recording computer. The electrical activity initiated by the distal two-thirds of the stomach (gastric electrical activity—GEA) is recorded and analyzed by the computer. Report 91132 when diagnostic electrogastrography is performed alone. Report 91133 when diagnostic EGG is performed in conjunction with the administration of a drug in an attempt to manipulate conditions and provoke a measurable abnormality.

A liver elastography (91200) can evaluate liver stiffness and is can help determine the amount of fibrosis and scarring of the liver due to damage. It may also be used to survey any disorder advancement and help evaluate ongoing therapy. During the procedure, a probe is applied to the skin between the ribs focusing on the liver. The shear wave is mechanically generated, causing the probe to discharge pulses that meet the shear wave and bounce back to the probe. This process allows the shear wave to be measured, which leads to values for liver stiffness. This code indicates no imaging; however interpretation and report are required.

Key Documentation Terms

Both the anatomical location and the methodology used in the procedure should be well documented. Terms such as with stimulation, capsule, duodenal, esophagus, ileum, motility, and pH electrode provide the guidance needed to ensure correct code assignment. Above all else, the documentation should support the medical necessity of the procedure.

Coding Tips

- Visualization of the colon is an integral part of code 91110.

- If the ileum is not viewed, append modifier 52 to code 91110.

- As an "add-on" code, 91013 is not subject to multiple procedure rules. No reimbursement reduction or modifier 51 is applied. The following table provides additional information for these codes as found in the Medicare Physician Fee Schedule Database.

Parent Code	Add-On	GLOB DAYS	MULT PROC	BILAT SURG	ASST SURG	CO-SURG	TEAM SURG
91010		000	0	0	0	0	0
	91013	ZZZ	0	0	0	0	0

Coding Traps

- When reporting capsule endoscopy, physician interpretation must be performed to report 91110 and 91111.

- Code 91035 requires attachment of a telemetry pH electrode to the esophageal mucosa. When endoscopy is used for electrode placement guidance, the endoscopy is not reported separately.

Ophthalmology Examinations and Other Services (92002–92499)

Very specific guidelines appear at the beginning of the ophthalmology subsection explaining services included in general ophthalmologic examinations. Special ophthalmologic services, which go beyond the service included under general ophthalmologic services (92002–92014), may be listed in addition to general ophthalmologic services or E/M services.

Procedure Differentiation

There are two levels of ophthalmology services: intermediate and comprehensive. Intermediate ophthalmology services (92002, 92012) include:

- Evaluation of new/existing condition complicated by new diagnostic or management problem

- Integrated services where medical decision making cannot be separated from examination methods

- Problems not related to primary diagnosis

- Biomicroscopy

- External ocular/adnexal examination

- General medical observation

- History

- Mydriasis

- Ophthalmoscopy

- Other diagnostic procedures

- Tonometry

Comprehensive ophthalmology services (92004, 92014) include:

- General evaluation of complete visual system

- Integrated services where medical decision making cannot be separated from examination methods

- Single service that need not be performed at one session

- Basic sensorimotor examination

- Biomicroscopy

- Consultations

- Dilation (cycloplegia)

- External examinations

- General medical observation

- Gross visual fields

- History

© 2020 Optum360, LLC

- Initiation of diagnostic/treatment programs
- Laboratory services
- Mydriasis
- Ophthalmoscopic examinations
- Other diagnostic procedures
- Prescription of medication
- Radiological services
- Tonometry

Ophthalmology services of either level are an integrated service for which medical decision making is not separate from examination techniques and itemization of services is not applicable.

Note: Verify with third-party payers for their specific coverage guidelines.

Key Documentation Terms
Documentation should clearly state the ophthalmology services that were performed.

Special ophthalmology services describe evaluation of a visual system performed to a greater level than considered part of a general service. A physician interpretation and report are an integral part of this service. Special ophthalmology services may be reported in addition to E/M services and general ophthalmological services. Terms such as intermediate and comprehensive provide the guidance needed to ensure correct code assignment.

Coding Tips
- Routine ophthalmoscopy is considered part of the general and special services codes and should not be reported separately.
- Contact lens prescription is not part of the general service. For prescription and fitting of one eye, add modifier 52 to 92310 or 92314.
- Computerized scanning of the eye is reported with 92132–92134. This service includes interpretation and report and is unilateral or bilateral.
- There are multiple indications for which these services can be performed; verify coverage with the payer.
- When fluorescein angiography and indocyanine-green angiography are performed at the same patient encounter, see 92242. If both services are not performed at the same time, see 92235 or 92240.

Coding Trap
- Codes 92002–92015 should not be reported with visual screening services (99173–99174 or 99177).

DEFINITIONS

keratometry. Taking measurements relating to the curvature of the cornea.

Schirmer test. Test for moisture in the eye, using a sterile paper strip between the lower lid and globe and measuring how much moisture is wicked into the strip within five minutes. If local anesthesia is applied, it is called a basic Schirmer test.

slit lamp biomicroscope. Microscope with fine, intense light used to visualize structures at the front of the eye.

Diagnostic Otorhinolaryngologic Services (92502–92700)

The procedures in this section include examinations and diagnostic services of speech, language, voice, communication, and/or auditory function. Services that are included in an E/M service should not be reported separately, such as:

- Anterior rhinoscopy
- Otoscopy
- Removal of cerumen (non-impacted)
- Tuning fork testing

Procedure Differentiation

Codes 92502 and 92504 describe otolaryngologic examinations. Occasionally, a child or an adult is uncooperative and an otolaryngologic examination cannot be performed until the patient is placed under general anesthesia. At other times, as in the case of a trauma victim, the patient is already anesthetized. In this case, it is appropriate to report 92502. In 92504 the physician uses an operating binocular microscope to examine the ear and occasionally the nose for direct, detailed visualization.

Codes 92507 and 92508 are reported for treatment of disorders in auditory processing, speech, language, voice, and communication. These activities may include oral strength and control exercises, sound production drills, and receptive language therapy. In group sessions, the therapist may present situations that patients may encounter in daily living and the group analyzes and discusses how to solve each situation (e.g., how would you invite a friend to coffee?). These codes are differentiated by whether the treatment was performed for an individual or in a group setting.

An endoscopic nasopharyngoscopy (92511) is also found in this section. In this procedure the physician introduces the flexible fiberoptic endoscope through the nose and advances it into the pharynx to determine whether there are any fixed blockages such as a deviated septum, nasal polyps, or enlarged adenoids and tonsils. The physician may position the tip of the endoscope at the level of the hard palate and instruct the patient to perform simple maneuvers that demonstrate airway activity under conditions that promote or prevent collapse. The test may be performed to identify anatomic factors contributing to sleep disorder and to determine the stability of the upper airway and treatments.

In codes 92521–92524, the physician takes a history of the patient, including speech and language development, hearing loss, and physical and mental development. A physical examination is performed. Speech and language evaluations are performed. Assessment of deficits and a plan for the patient are made. These plans may involve speech therapy, hearing aids, etc. In auditory processing disorders, the patient (usually children) cannot process the information heard due to lack of integration between the ears and the brain, even though hearing may be normal. Central auditory processing disorder (CAPD) is often confused with or functions as an underlying factor to a number of learning disabilities. In code 92521, speech fluency, including stuttering and cluttering, are evaluated. Code 92522 is reported when evaluation of phonics and speech/sound production is performed. Report code 92523 when language comprehension is addressed in addition to the evaluation described in code 92522. Code 92524 is reported for evaluation of voice and resonance.

Coding Tips

- Note that 92511, a separate procedure by definition, is usually a component of a more complex service and is not identified separately. When the service it describes is performed alone or with other unrelated procedures/services, the code may be reported. If performed alone, list the code; if performed with other procedures/services, list the code and append modifier 59.

- When reporting a single laryngeal function study (92520), append modifier 52 to code 92520.

- To report a nasopharyngoscopy with dilation of the eustachian tube, see code 69705 for unilateral; code 69706 for bilateral.

Vestibular Balance Testing (92531–92549)

Vestibular function testing is often an area of confusion. Services may be performed with or without recordings and are dependent upon the type of testing performed. Often testing is performed due to nystagmus.

Procedure Differentiation

Codes 92531–92534 are reported for services performed without recordings.

In 92531, the patient's eyes are observed for spontaneous nystagmus as the patient is asked to look straight ahead, 30 degrees to 45 degrees to the right, and 30 degrees to 45 degrees to the left. No electrodes are used and no recording made. The documentation should state spontaneous nystagmus and without a recording. Code 92541 should be reported when a recording is obtained.

In 92532, a positional nystagmus test measures whether the eyes can maintain a static position when the head is in different position. The test may be performed to help document and quantify a patient's complaint of dizziness in certain positions. In addition it may also be performed to determine if there is an abnormality in the central or peripheral nervous system. The documentation should state positional nystagmus and without a recording. Code 92542 should be reported when a recording is obtained.

Code 92533 is used to report caloric vestibular testing without recording. In this test, each ear is separately irrigated with cold water and then warm water to create nystagmus in the patient. The physician or audiologist observes the patient to detect any difference between the reaction of the right side and the left side. Report 92537 or 92538 if a recording is obtained. When reporting 92533 or 92537, the service should be reported four times. In other words, if only one ear is irrigated, or only one water temperature was used, then the equivalent number of codes should be reported. For example, one irrigation should be reported as 92533 or 92537 x 1, two irrigations 92533 or 92537 x 2, three irrigations 92533 or 92537 x 3. Code 92538 describes monothermal irrigation, which is one irrigation in each ear for a total of two irrigations.

It is important that the provider's documentation clearly identifies the number of irrigations performed.

In 92534, a rotating drum made of alternating light and dark vertical stripes is placed in front of the patient and the patient is instructed to stare at the drum without focusing on any one stripe. The eyes are observed for nystagmus while the drum is rotated in one direction. The direction of the drum is then reversed. No electrodes are used. Report 92544 when a recording is obtained.

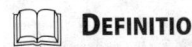

DEFINITIONS

nystagmus. Rapid, rhythmic, involuntary movements of the eyeball in vertical, horizontal, rotational, or mixed directions that can be congenital, acquired, physiological, neurological, or due to ocular disease.

Note: The CPT description for 92544 states bidirectional, foveal, or peripheral stimulation. Documentation should include at least one of these terms.

In 92540, electronystagmography (ENG) electrodes are placed and the patient is asked to look straight ahead, 30 degrees to 45 degrees to the right, and 30 degrees to 45 degrees to the left. Recordings are made to detect spontaneous nystagmus. In the positional nystagmus test, an ENG recording is made of the rapid eye movements occurring with the patient's head placed in a minimum of four positions (e.g., supine with head extended dorsally, left, right, and sitting). This is often done using infrared video recording systems. An optokinetic nystagmus test is usually done with a rotating drum of alternating light and dark vertical stripes. The drum is placed in front of the patient and the patient is instructed to stare at the drum without focusing on any one stripe. The drum is rotated in one direction and reversed and rotated in the opposite direction. ENG electrodes are used to record nystagmus. In an oscillating tracking test, the patient is asked to follow a swinging object such as a ball on a string. ENG electrodes are in place and a recording is made of the eye tracking the motion. The recording is analyzed for smoothness.

The documentation should state that each aspect of the test was performed and that a recording was made. If all the aspects of this test are not performed another code may be more appropriate.

In 92545, documentation will state that ENG electrodes were in place and the patient was asked to follow a swinging object such as a ball on a string. A recording is made of the eye tracking the motion. The recording is analyzed for smoothness.

Code 92546 would be reported when documentation states that the patient is placed in a rotary chair with the head positioned at a 30 degree angle and the eyes closed. Electronystagmography (ENG) electrodes are placed on the face near the eyes, and the chair is rotated via computer control for 30 to 40 minutes while normal eye movement and involuntary rapid eye movements are recorded. The recording is evaluated to determine whether there is an abnormal labyrinthine response on either side.

Code 92547 is an add-on code to be used when the documentation states ENG electrodes are placed to measure vertical and rotary nystagmus.

Code 92548 reports computerized dynamic posturography sensory organization test (CDP-SOT). This test evaluates a patient's ability to utilize information from the sensory systems (vestibular, visual, and proprioceptive) to achieve and maintain balance and postural control. The patient is placed in the posturography system. The system is made up of a force plate that controls foot support and a visual surround reference that can be controlled. Force transducers measure the vertical and horizontal force output of the patient's feet. The patient's center-of-force is used as an estimate of body sway during testing. The patient is placed in a harness during the test for support and to prevent falls while standing on the plate within the system. Tests performed within the system assess the patient's ability to remain balanced during varying conditions that represent situations similar to those encountered in daily living. The walls of the system as well as the force plate move, and testing occurs with eyes open and/or closed. The testing typically takes about 20 minutes and is provided by a qualified technician with results interpreted by a physical therapist to determine a therapy program specific to the patient's needs. Report 92548 for evaluation of six components, including eyes open, eyes closed, visual sway, platform sway, eyes closed platform sway, and platform and visual sway. Report 92549 if the above testing includes a motor control test (MCT) and adaptation test (ADT). The MCT assesses the patient's automatic motor reflex responses and their effectiveness in balance restoration following sudden forward and backward movements of the support surface. The test is useful in identifying impaired motor function and evaluating performance changes following treatment. In one version of an upright motor control test evaluating knee extension and flexion, the patient stands with knees flexed, then lifts the foot of the extremity that is least affected, transferring full weight onto the extremity that is more affected. The patient then attempts to extend the more affected knee. To test extension, the patient stands with knees straight and then lifts the knee of the lower extremity that is more affected toward the chest as rapidly and as high as possible; this is performed three times. These tests are useful in measuring voluntary movement and muscle control in chronic stroke victims. Motor ADT evaluates the performance in repeated movements to determine changes in neuromuscular responses and motor function.

Codes 92517–92519 report vestibular evoked myogenic potential testing (VEMP). This test is useful in diagnosing superior canal dehiscence syndrome (SCDS), a little-known cause of vertigo and auditory symptoms. Caused by an abnormal opening or dehiscence in the bony roof of the superior semicircular canal in the temporal bone, SCDS may present with excessive sound sensitivity, tinnitus, or dizziness brought on by changes in pressure or sound. This vestibular function test is performed by stimulating one ear repeatedly with pulse or click sounds. Surface EMG responses are then measured over selected muscles, averaging the reaction of the muscle's electrical activity related to each pulse or sound click. In cervical VEMP (cVEMP) (92517), the sound stimulus that is applied to one ear elicits a response within the sternocleidomastoid muscles on the same side (ipsilateral) that can be recorded with surface electrodes and then averaged. In ocular VEMP (oVEMP) (92518), this sound stimulus elicits a response that is greatest when recorded from the opposite (contralateral) inferior oblique muscle by a surface electrode and averaged. Report 92519 if both cVEMP and oVEMP are performed. These codes include interpretation and report.

Medical Necessity
The following conditions may warrant the reporting of 92540–92547 (this list is not all inclusive):

- Dizziness
- Labyrinthine dysfunction
- Ménière's disease
- Vertigo

Key Documentation Terms
In 92537–92547, a recording must be obtained at the time the service is rendered. These recordings must be maintained in the patient's medical record. In 92517–92519 an interpretation and report must be documented. The procedure report by itself is not enough to show that the services being reported are medically reasonable and necessary.

Coding Tip
- Code 92542 requires four or more positions to be performed in order to report one unit.

Coding Traps

- Codes 92531 and 92532 should not be reported in conjunction with E/M services or other outpatient services.

- Codes 92540–92542 or 92544–92545 should not be reported together.

- When performing a vestibular function test that includes a recording (92537–92549) it should not be reported with electro-oculography with interpretation and report (92270) or with another vestibular function test in the same section. It is important to read the section guidelines thoroughly.

- As add-on code, 92547 is not subject to multiple procedure rules. No reimbursement reduction or modifier 51 is applied. Add-on codes describe additional intraservice work associated with the primary procedure. They are performed by the same provider on the same date of service as the primary service/procedure, and must never be reported as a stand-alone code. The following table provides additional information for these codes as found in the Medicare Physician Fee Schedule Database.

Parent Code	Add-On	GLOB DAYS	MULT PROC	BILAT SURG	ASST SURG	CO-SURG	TEAM SURG
92540		XXX	0	0	0	0	0
92541		XXX	0	0	0	0	0
92542		XXX	0	0	0	0	0
92544		XXX	0	0	0	0	0
92545		XXX	0	0	0	0	0
92546		XXX	0	0	0	0	0
	92547	ZZZ	0	0	0	0	0

Cardiography and Cardiovascular Monitoring (93000–93278)

Codes in this section are distinct from other sections of the CPT book as the codes are separated into the professional component only (interpretation and report), the technical component only (tracing), physician supervision only, or the total procedure. For example, cardiovascular stress testing has a code for each of the three components and a code for the total procedure, including:

93015   Cardiovascular stress test using maximal or submaximal treadmill or bicycle exercise, continuous electrocardiographic monitoring, and/or pharmacological stress; with supervision, with interpretation and report

93016   supervision only, without interpretation and report

93017   tracing only, without interpretation and report

93018   interpretation and report only

Procedure Differentiation

If the total procedure is performed and reported by a single entity, only 93015 is reported. If the tracing is taken at a facility that does not employ the provider, 93017 is reported by the facility. The provider who supervises the testing reports 93016 and the provider who performs the official interpretation and report uses 93018.

Note: Not every procedure in this section includes provider supervision. Code selection includes those from the following table.

Codes	Cardiography Procedure
93000–93010	12 lead EKG
93015–93018	Cardiovascular stress test
93024	Ergonovine provocation
93025	Microvolt T-wave alternans assessment
93040–93042	1–3 lead rhythm EKG
93050	Arterial pressure waveform analysis
93224–93227	External EKG monitor, up to 48 hours
93228–93229	Cardiovascular telemetry, external, mobile, > 24 hours
93241–93244	External EKG monitor, more than 48 hours, up to 7 days
93245–93248	External EKG monitor, more than 7 days, up to 15 days
93268–93272	Auto activated, rhythm derived EKG event recording, up to 30 days
93278	Signal averaged electrocardiography (SAECG)

The following is a discussion of the most frequently billed codes in this section.

In EKG codes 93000–93010, 12 electrodes are placed on a patient's chest to record the electrical activity of the heart. A physician interprets the findings. Code 93000 reports the combined technical and professional components of an EKG. Code 93005 reports the technical component only. Code 93010 reports the professional component only.

Medical Necessity

The following circumstances may warrant an EKG (93000–93010) (this list is not all inclusive):

- Coronary artery disease (CAD) and/or heart muscle disease that presents with symptoms such as increasing shortness of breath (SOB), palpitations, angina, etc.

- Evaluation of a patient on a cardiac medication for a cardiac arrhythmia or other cardiac condition that affects the electrical conduction system of the heart (e.g., inotropics such as digoxin; antiarrhythmics such as Tambocor, Procainamide, or Quinidine; and antianginals such as Cardizem, Isordil, Corgard, Procardia, Inderal, and Verapamil). The EKG is necessary to evaluate the effect of the cardiac medication on the patient's cardiac rhythm and/or conduction system.

- Evaluation of a patient with a pacemaker with or without clinical findings (history or physical examination) that suggest possible pacemaker malfunction.

- Evaluation of a patient's response to a newly established therapy for angina, palpitations, arrhythmias, SOB, or other cardiopulmonary disease process.

- Evaluation of a patient's status postcoronary artery revascularization by coronary artery bypass grafting (CABG), percutaneous transluminal coronary angiography (PTCA), thrombolytic therapy (e.g., TPA, Streptokinase, Urokinase), and/or stent placement.

- Evaluation of a patient's response to the administration of an agent known to result in cardiac or EKG abnormalities (for patients with suspected, or

DEFINITIONS

acidosis. Reduction of alkaline in the blood and tissues caused by an increase in acid and decrease in bicarbonate.

alkalosis. Increased alkaline balance in the blood and tissues.

arrhythmia. Irregular heartbeat.

EKG. Electrocardiogram. Graphic recording of the changes in electrical voltage and polarity caused by the heart muscle's electrical excitation. The tracing follows atrial and ventricular activity over time, captured through electrodes placed on the skin.

hyperthyroidism. Condition caused by the production of excessive quantities of thyroid hormones resulting in fibrillations, nervousness, weight loss, heat intolerance, excessive sweating, and weakness. This may stem from a goiter, malfunctioning thyroid gland, or the ingestion of a high dose of thyroid hormones in medication form or from iodine as a dietary supplement or contrast medium.

hypothyroidism. Underproduction of thyroid hormone.

infarction. Area of necrosis in tissue, due to ischemia from lack of circulation, usually from a thrombus or an embolus.

ischemia. Deficiency in blood supply causing tissues to be deprived of oxygen, resulting from trauma, mechanical or functional constriction of blood vessels, or a physical obstruction.

at increased risk of developing, cardiovascular disease or dysfunction). Examples of these agents are antineoplastic drugs, lithium, tranquilizers, anticonvulsants, and antidepressant agents.

- Initial diagnostic workup for a patient that presents with complaints of symptoms such as chest pain, palpitations, dyspnea, dizziness, syncope, etc. that may suggest a cardiac origin.

- Patients presenting with symptoms of a myocardial infarction (MI).

- Significant cardiac arrhythmia or conduction disorder in which an EKG is necessary as part of the evaluation and management of the patient. These disorders may include, but are not limited to, the following:

  - complete heart block
  - second-degree AV block
  - left bundle branch block
  - right bundle branch block
  - paroxysmal VT
  - atrial fib/flutter
  - ventricular fib/flutter
  - cardiac arrest
  - frequent PVCs
  - frequent PACs
  - wandering atrial pacemaker
  - any other unspecified cardiac arrhythmia

- Symptomatology that may indicate a cardiac origin, especially in patients who have a history of an MI, CABG surgery, or PTCA or patients who are being treated medically after a positive stress test or cardiac catheterization.

- Preoperative evaluation of the patient when:

  - the patient is undergoing cardiac surgery such as CABGs, automatic implantable cardiac defibrillator, or pacemaker
  - the patient has a medical condition associated with a significant risk of serious cardiac arrhythmia and/or myocardial ischemia such as diabetes, history of myocardial infarction (MI), angina pectoris, aneurysm of heart wall, chronic ischemic heart disease, pericarditis, valvular disease, or cardiomyopathy to name a few

- When performed as a baseline evaluation prior to the initiation of an agent known to result in cardiac or EKG abnormalities. An example of such an agent is verapamil.

When a cardiovascular stress test (93015–93018) is performed, a continuous recording of electrical activity of the heart is acquired while the patient is exercising on a treadmill or bicycle and/or given medicines. The stress on the heart during the test is monitored. Code 93015 reports the test, provider supervision, and provider interpretation of the report; 93016 reports the provider's supervision of the test; 93017 reports tracing only; and 93018 reports the provider's interpretation and report.

The following conditions may warrant stress tests (this list is not all inclusive):

- A patient who has signs or symptoms consistent with CAD:

  - angina pectoris or anginal equivalent symptoms
  - cardiac rhythm disturbances

- heart failure
- significant atherosclerotic vascular disease elsewhere in the body (e.g., carotid obstructive disease, peripheral vascular disease involving the lower extremities, or abdominal aortic aneurysm
- syncope
- A patient who has a metabolic disorder known to cause CAD:
  - atherogenic hypercholesterolemia
  - diabetes mellitus
  - syndrome X
- A patient who has an abnormal ECG consistent with CAD
  - needs an evaluation for progression of CAD with the potential for a change in treatment:
  - following coronary artery bypass graft (CABG) surgery
  - following medical treatment to reverse or stabilize CAD
  - following a myocardial infarction (MI) procedure
  - following a percutaneous transluminal coronary angioplasty (PTCA), atherectomy, intracoronary thrombolysis, or other coronary revascularization
  - for a history of a coronary artery ischemic event without symptoms (i.e., a prior "silent MI")
- Needs an evaluation as part of a preoperative assessment when intermediate- or high-risk for CAD is present and surgery is likely to induce significant cardiac stress

In ECG codes 93040-93042, one to three electrodes are placed on the patient's chest to record electrical activity of the heart. The physician interprets the report. Code 93040 reports the combined technical and professional components of an ECG; 93041 reports the technical component only; and 93042 reports the professional component only.

The following conditions may warrant an ECG (93040-93042) (this list is not all inclusive):

- Acid-base disorders
- Arteriovascular disease, including coronary, central, and peripheral disease
- Cardiac hypertrophy
- Cardiac rhythm disturbances
- Chest pain or angina pectoris
- Conduction abnormalities
- Drug cardiotoxicity
- Electrolyte imbalance
- Endocrine abnormalities
- Heart failure
- Hypertension
- Myocardial ischemia or infarction
- Neurological disorders affecting the heart
- Palpitations
- Paroxysmal weakness

 DEFINITIONS

angina. Chest pain that occurs secondary to the inadequate delivery of oxygen to the heart muscle and may be described as a heavy or squeezing pain in the midsternal area of the chest.

revascularization. Restoration of blood flow and oxygen supply to a body part. This may apply to an extremity, the heart, or penis.

syncope. Light-headedness or fainting caused by insufficient blood supply to the brain.

- Pericarditis
- Pulmonary disorders
- Sudden lightheadedness
- Structural cardiac conditions
- Syncope
- Temperature disorders

A preoperative EKG may be reasonable and necessary under one of the following conditions:

- In the presence of preexisting heart disease such as angina, congestive heart failure, coronary artery disease, dysrhythmias, or prior myocardial infarction
- In the presence of known comorbid conditions that may affect the heart, such as chronic pulmonary disease, diabetes, peripheral vascular disease, or renal impairment
- When the pending surgical procedure requires a general or regional anesthetic

Arterial blood pressure pulse wave analysis is reported with code 93050. This procedure measures the blood pressure at the heart rather than in the arm as with traditional blood pressure cuffs, as well as provides information regarding the interaction of the heart and blood vessels. The brachial blood pressure is obtained to calibrate the radial pressure waveform. The pressure sensor wand (tonometer) is placed on the wrist where the strongest pulse is present. The pressure waveforms are transmitted and displayed on a data collection screen on a computer. After there is at least 10 seconds of data displayed, the data is captured. The data reflects average central aortic waveform, pressure measurements, and central parameters, as well as reference ranges. The augmentation index can be acquired by direct measurement or acquired pressure waveforms. This index is a percentage of pressure from systolic rise over pressure waves. The nonlinear mathematical transformation can be utilized to differentiate between active and rest blood pressure coinciding with the systolic and diastolic process. This code includes the digitization of the data, as well as the use of nonlinear mathematical transformation to determine pressure, augmentation index, and the provider interpretation and report.

Key Documentation Terms

Documentation for these services must contain the patient's history of recent, past, ongoing, or suspected cardiac disease or symptoms. When an EKG is being performed for chest pain, the documentation must demonstrate that the ordering clinician has a legitimate concern that the chest pain etiology or other symptoms are cardiac in origin. The documentation must establish the medical necessity for the service being performed.

Coding Tips

- When only the interpretation and report are performed for code 93278, append modifier 26.
- Codes 93228 and 93229 should only be reported once per 30 day period.
- For 93224–93227, if the monitoring is less than 12 hours append modifier 52.
- Cardiovascular stress tests include insertion of a needle and/or a catheter, infusion/injection (pharmacologic stress tests), and ECG strips (e.g., CPT

codes 36000, 36410, 96360–96376, 93000–93010, 93040–93042).
These services should not be reported separately.

Coding Traps
- Do not report external mobile telemetry with external EKG recording

Monitoring of Cardiovascular Devices (93260–93264, 93279–93298)

These services include evaluation, programming, and monitoring of pacemakers, implantable defibrillators (ICD), and implantable, insertable, and wearable cardiac device systems.

- Implantable defibrillator
  - Transvenous implantable defibrillator (ICD)
    - single, dual, or multiple leads
    - provides antitachycardia pacing or chronic pacing
  - Subcutaneous implantable defibrillator (SICD)
    - single electrode
    - treats ventricular tachyarrhythmias
- Pacemaker
  - single chamber (pacing in the ventricle) or dual chambers (pacing in the atrium and ventricle)
  - May be permanent, temporary, or leadless
    - a permanent pacemaker is used to maintain cardiac stability.
    - a temporary pacemaker is used to treat transient bradycardias that may be due to an acute myocardial infarction or drug toxicity.
    - leadless cardiac pacemakers systems that are implanted into the cardiac chamber
- Implantable cardiovascular physiologic monitor
  - Assists in the management of cardiac conditions that are non-rhythm related (i.e., heart failure)
  - Collects longitudinal physiologic cardiovascular data elements
- Subcutaneous cardiac rhythm monitor
  - A device that continuously and automatically monitors the heart's electrical activity when sensing the patient's rapid, irregular, or slow heartrate or can also be prompted by the patient in the course of experiencing symptoms
  - Capable of recording heartrates and rhythms for over one year
  - The device may work independently or as component of a pacemaker or implantable defibrillator system

Procedure Differentiation
Programming services (93260, 93279–93285) include an in-person evaluation of the patient and the device and iterative changes to the programming. At the end of the service, the device parameters may remain unchanged, but the patient and device must have been fully evaluated, including interrogation services and interim changes.

Programming services are reported when performed, and although they include interrogation services, they are separate from the interrogation. Programming, when performed, may be reported during the 30 or 90 day interrogation time period.

Remote monitoring of a wireless pulmonary artery pressure sensor is reported with 93264. This code is reported once for up to 30 days and weekly downloads. A pulmonary pressure monitoring system—a device comprised of a battery-free sensor such as the CardioMEMS™—permits ongoing monitoring and measurement of a patient's heart rate as well as systolic, diastolic, and mean pressures in a patient diagnosed with non-rhythm-related cardiac conditions (i.e., heart failure). Pulmonary arterial pressure (PAP) readings transmitted from an internally implanted sensor to a wireless electronic unit are subsequently transmitted to an internet-based file server or monitored by a surveillance technician with results sent to an online portal that can be accessed by the patient's treating health care provider. Through accurate monitoring of patients diagnosed with heart failure (HF) for exacerbations, it is possible to minimize the need for additional hospitalizations and the associated complications and allow for early pharmacological intervention.

Patients with a previously implanted pacemaker or defibrillator systems may require adjustment of the device to patient-specific settings prior to a surgery, test, or procedure. This is reported with codes 93286–93287. The device system data is interrogated to evaluate the battery, leads, and sensors, as well as the stored patient and system measurements. If necessary, the device is programmed to settings appropriate for the surgery, test, or procedure. A postprocedure evaluation and programming may also be performed, with adjustments as required. Report 93286 for evaluation of a single-, dual-, or multiple-lead implantable pacemaker system or leadless pacemaker system. Report 93287 for evaluation of a single-, dual-, or multiple-lead implantable defibrillator system. Both codes include physician or other qualified health care professional analysis, review, and report. If both evaluation services (pre and post) are performed by one physician, 93286 or 93287 may be reported twice. If two physicians perform the service, each may report 93286 or 93287 one time as appropriate.

Patients with a previously implanted device, such as a cardiac pacemaker, subcutaneous and transvenous implantable defibrillators, implantable cardiovascular physiologic monitor (ICM), or subcutaneous cardiac rhythm monitor system require periodic interrogation device evaluations. This diagnostic procedure includes a face-to-face assessment of all device functions. Components that must be evaluated in order to assign 93288 include the battery, lead(s), capture and sensing function, heart rhythm, and programmed parameters of a single-, dual-, or multiple-lead pacemaker system. Code 93289 requires evaluation of the battery, lead(s), capture and sensing function, heart rhythm derived elements, presence or absence of therapy for ventricular tachyarrhythmias, and programmed parameters of a single-, dual-, or multiple-lead transvenous implantable defibrillator system. Code 93290 requires analysis of at least one recorded physiologic cardiovascular data element obtained from internal or external sensors and evaluation of programmed parameters of an ICM. Code 93291 requires evaluation of heart rate and rhythm during recorded episodes (from both patient-initiated and device algorithm detected events), as well as evaluation of programmed parameters of a subcutaneous cardiac rhythm monitor system. Code 93292 reports an interrogation device evaluation of a wearable defibrillation system. Code 93261 reports interrogation device evaluation of an implantable subcutaneous lead defibrillator system. These codes include physician or other qualified health care professional analysis, review, and report. They also include connection, recording, and disconnection, and are assigned per procedure.

Interrogation device evaluations may also be performed remotely and apply to single-, dual-, multiple-lead or leadless devices. Code 93294 reports the remote evaluation of a pacemaker system with interim physician or other qualified health care professional analysis, review, and report. Components that must be evaluated in order to assign this code include the battery, lead(s), capture and sensing function, heart rhythm, and programmed parameters. Code 93295 reports the remote evaluation of an implantable defibrillator system with interim physician or other qualified health care professional analysis, review, and report. Required evaluation components include the battery, lead(s), capture and sensing function, heart rhythm derived elements, presence or absence of therapy for ventricular tachyarrhythmias, and programmed parameters. Code 93296 reports the acquisition of remote data, transmission receipt and technician review, technical support, and result distribution and applies to pacemaker and defibrillator systems. Codes from this range may be reported only once per 90-day period.

Remote interrogation device evaluations may be performed on patients with a previously implanted implantable cardiovascular physiologic monitor (ICM) or subcutaneous cardiac rhythm monitor system using codes 93297–93298. These codes report remote evaluations only and may be reported only once per 30-day period. Code 93297 reports the remote evaluation of an ICM and includes the analysis of at least one recorded physiologic cardiovascular data element obtained from internal or external sensors. Physician or other qualified health care professional analysis, review, and report are also included. Code 93298 reports the remote evaluation of a subcutaneous cardiac rhythm monitor system; it requires the analysis of recorded heart rhythm data and also includes the provider's review and report.

It is important to read the CPT reporting guidelines for interrogation device evaluations as some are every 30 days, where others are 90 days. Interrogation includes download of data, battery voltage, lead impedance, tachycardia detection settings, and rhythm treatment settings. Trained staff may facilitate the remote interrogation. The physician or other qualified health care professional interpretation and review of the interrogation is part of the in-person and remote interrogation. The frequency of the interrogation is dependent upon patient status, device status, and may be performed one or more times. Please refer to CPT guidelines.

Coding Tips
- Code range 93293–93296 should not be reported more than once in a 90 day period. It is inappropriate to report these codes if the monitoring period is less than 30 days.

- Code range 93297–93298 should not be reported more than once in a 30 day period. It is inappropriate to report these codes if the monitoring period is less than 10 days.

- Peri-procedural device evaluation codes (93286–93287) should not be reported with category III codes for permanent cardiac contractility modulation systems (0408T–0415T).

- For an interrogation device evaluation(s) performed remotely for an implantable cardioverter-defibrillator with substernal electrode, report Category III code 0578T or 0579T.

Echocardiography (93303–93355)

Echocardiography records ultrasonic waves reflected from the heart and allows visualization of heart size and shape, myocardial wall thickness, motion, cardiac valve structure, and function. Echocardiography codes represent a global procedure. In echocardiography, ultrasonic waves directed at the heart and great vessels provide a hard copy recording that serves as a diagnostic tool.

Procedure Differentiation

Codes 93303–93308 are used to report a transthoracic echocardiography. Each service contains a unique component.

Code 93303 reports a *complete* evaluation for congenital defects.

Code 93304 reports a *follow-up or a limited* evaluation for congenital defects.

Code 93306 reports real-time with image documentation (2D), includes M-mode recording, when performed, complete, *with* spectral Doppler echocardiography, and with color flow Doppler echocardiography.

Code 93307 reports real-time with image documentation (2D), includes M-mode recording, when performed, complete, *without* spectral or color Doppler echocardiography.

Code 93308 reports real-time with image documentation (2D), includes M-mode recording, when performed, *follow-up or limited study.*

Codes 93350–93351 are also used to report transthoracic echocardiography. In 93350, the test is performed during rest and during a cardiovascular stress test, with interpretation and report. Code 93351 includes all of the elements in 93350, plus continuous electrocardiographic monitoring, with physician or other qualified health care professional supervision.

Medical Necessity

The following conditions may warrant a transthoracic echocardiography (this list is not all inclusive):

- Abnormalities of the great vessels (aorta and pulmonary artery)
- Acute endocarditis
- Acute myocardial infarction and coronary insufficiency
- Arrhythmias and palpitations
- Cardiac transplant and rejection monitoring
- Cardiac tumors and masses
- Congenital heart disease
- Critically ill and trauma patients
- Exposure to cardiotoxic agents (chemotherapeutic and external)
- Hypertensive cardiovascular disease
- Native valvular heart disease
- Pericardial disease
- Prosthetic heart valves (mechanical and bioprostheses)
  - Transthoracic echocardiography (TTE) assessment soon after prosthetic valve implant is important in establishing a baseline

DEFINITIONS

Doppler. Ultrasonography used to augment two-dimensional images by registering velocity. When emitted sound waves reflect back off a moving object, the frequency of the reflected sound waves varies in relation to the speed of the moving object and may be used in many different procedures.

endocarditis. Inflammatory disease of the interior lining of the heart chamber and heart valves, most commonly caused by bacteria.

hypertrophy. Overgrowth or enlargement of normal cells in tissue.

M-mode. One-dimensional procedure with movement of the trace to record amplitude and velocity of moving echo-producing structures.

myocardial infarction. Obstruction of circulation to the heart, resulting in necrosis.

pericardium. Thin and slippery case in which the heart lies that is lined with fluid so that the heart is free to pulse and move as it beats.

stent. Tube to provide support in a body cavity or lumen.

© 2020 Optum360, LLC

structural and hemodynamic profile unique to the individual and the prosthesis. Size, position, underlying ventricular function and concomitant valve pathologies all affect this unique profile. Reassessment following convalescence (three to six months) is appropriate. Thereafter, absent discretely defined clinical events or obvious change in physical examination findings, annual stability assessment is considered medically reasonable and appropriate.

- Pulmonary heart disease
- Suspected cardiac thrombi and embolic sources
- Syncope
- Ventricular function and cardiomyopathies

Codes 93312–93318 and 93355 are used to report transesophageal echocardiography with each service containing a different component.

Codes 93312–93314 describe transesophageal echocardiography with image documentation (2D) (with or without M-mode recordings). Code 93312 includes probe placement, image acquisition, and the interpretation and report. Code 93313 reports placement of a transesophageal probe. Code 93314 reports the image acquisition, and the interpretation and report.

Codes 93315–93317 describe transesophageal echocardiography for congenital cardiac anomalies. Code 93315 includes probe placement, image acquisition, and the interpretation and report. Code 93316 reports placement of a transesophageal probe. Code 93317 reports the image acquisition and the interpretation and report.

Code 93318 reports a transesophageal echocardiography performed for monitoring purposes, which includes probe placement, real time 2-dimensional image acquisition and interpretation leading to ongoing (continuous) assessment of (dynamically changing) cardiac pumping function and to therapeutic measures on an immediate time basis.

Code 93355 reports the guidance during the procedure(s) as well as measurements of the surrounding structures. It includes probe navigation, image acquisition, and the physician's interpretation and report. Diagnostic TEE is included, and contrast administration, Doppler, color flow, and 3D images, when performed, are also included.

The echocardiography section also contains add-on codes 93320, 93321, 93325, 93352, and 93356. They identify other procedures performed in addition to the echocardiography.

Code 93320 reports a Doppler echocardiography, pulsed wave and/or continuous wave with spectral display; complete.

Code 93321 is reported when the study is a follow-up or limited.

Code 93325 reports Doppler echocardiography, with color flow velocity mapping.

Report 93352 when an echocardiographic contrast agent is used during stress echocardiography.

Code 93356 reports myocardial strain imaging, also referred to as echocardiographic strain imaging or deformation (lengthening, shortening, or thickening) imaging, was initially utilized as a feature of Doppler imaging where velocity information is regenerated into strain rate. New technology, known as speckle tracking echocardiography (STE), utilizes image-processing algorithms to track areas of interest. Used in conjunction with two-dimensional or three-dimensional echocardiography for determining the multidirectional components of left ventricular (LV) deformation, these areas contain blocks of 20 to 40 pixels that contain constant patterns referred to as speckles. These markers or fingerprints are helpful in outlining irregularities by comprehensive assessment of regional myocardial function, specifically by discriminating between active and passive myocardial wall movement. Strain rate data assists in early detection of myocardial dysfunction and is beneficial in therapeutic decisions and follow-up of previous cardiac surgery. Code 93356 should be reported in addition to the applicable codes for echocardiography imaging.

The following conditions may warrant transesophageal echocardiography (this list is not all inclusive):

- Aortic pathological conditions (e.g., aortic dissection and aneurysm)
- Aortic ulceration, atherosclerotic plaque, and mural thrombotic material
- Bacterial endocarditis
- Cardiac and pericardiac masses
- Cardiac embolism
- Congenital heart disease
- Critically ill patient
- Endocarditis
- Intraoperative use (e.g., assessment of the adequacy of valvuloplasty or revascularization, determination of proper valve placement, placement of shunts or other devices, assessment of ventricular function, vascular integrity, or detection of intravascular air)
- Native and prosthetic valvular heart disease
- Pericardial disease

Key Documentation Terms

Documentation for an echocardiography must contain the patient's history of recent, past, ongoing, or suspected cardiac disease or symptoms. The patient's medical record must document the medical necessity of services performed for each date of service submitted. When transthoracic and transesophageal studies are performed on the same day, the record must support the medically necessity of each procedure.

Coding Tips

- As add-on codes, 93320, 93321, 93325, 93352, and 93356 are not subject to multiple procedure rules. No reimbursement reduction or modifier 51 is applied. Add-on codes describe additional intraservice work associated with the primary procedure. They are performed by the same provider on the same date of service as the primary service/procedure, and must never be reported as a stand-alone code. The following table provides additional information for these codes as found in the Medicare Physician Fee Schedule Database.

Parent Code	Add-On	GLOB DAYS	MULT PROC	BILAT SURG	ASST SURG	CO-SURG	TEAM SURG
76825		XXX	0	0	0	0	0
76826		XXX	0	0	0	0	0
76827		XXX	0	0	0	0	0
76828		XXX	0	0	0	0	0
93303		XXX	6	0	0	0	0
93304		XXX	6	0	0	0	0
93306		XXX	6	0	0	0	0
93307		XXX	6	0	0	0	0
93308		XXX	6	0	0	0	0
93312		XXX	6	0	0	0	0
93314		XXX	6	0	0	0	0
93315		XXX	0	0	0	0	0
93317		XXX	0	0	0	0	0
	93320	ZZZ	0	0	0	0	0
	93321	ZZZ	0	0	0	0	0
	93325	ZZZ	0	0	0	0	0
93350		XXX	6	0	0	0	0
93351		XXX	6	0	9	9	9
	93352	ZZZ	0	0	0	0	0
	93356	ZZZ	0	0	0	0	0

- Do not report 93350 in conjunction with the global code for cardiac stress testing (93015).

- Do not report 93351 in conjunction with the professional components of complete stress test (93015–93018) or 93350.

- Do not report 93352 more than once for each stress echocardiogram.

- Do not report transesophageal echocardiography procedures 93312–93325 with 93355.

- In the event that an echocardiography procedure detects a congenital abnormality, it is appropriate to report congenital codes 93303-93304 and 93315-93317.

- When a patient who has had a previous childhood cardiac defect repaired presents for an echo for another unrelated acquired cardiac condition, the congenital echo codes should not be reported. However if the echo detects another congenital defect (other than the one previously repaired), the appropriate congenital code should be reported.

- Code 93356 should only be reported once per session.

Heart Catheterization (93451–93572)

Carefully review medicine section codes 93451–93572 and their notes before selecting a code for cardiac catheterization.

Left Heart Catheterization

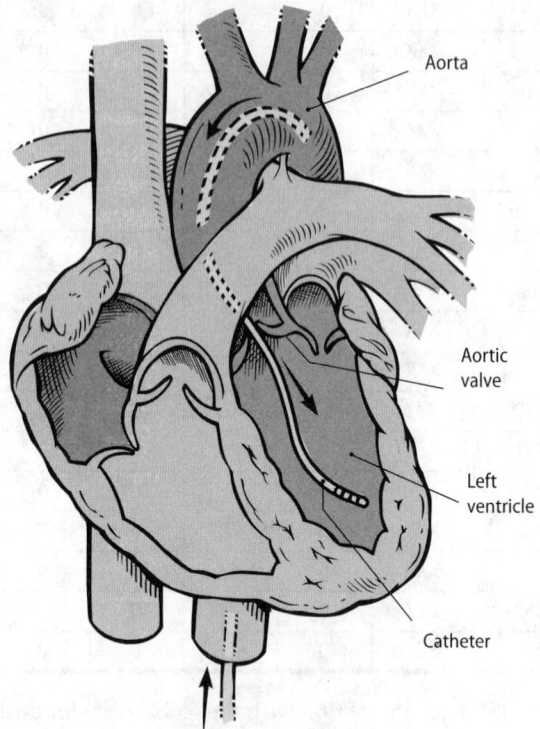

Right Heart Catheterization

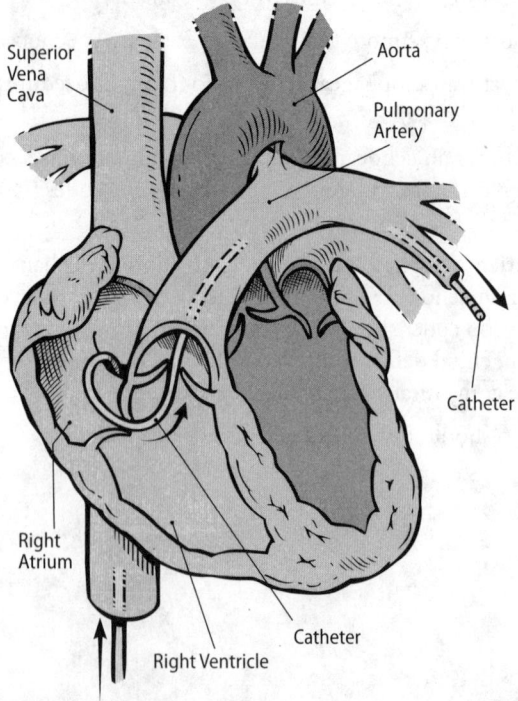

Procedure Differentiation

Codes are built on progressive hierarchies with more intensive services inclusive of lesser intensive services. Supervision and interpretation are included in the codes and are not reported separately as in previous years.

> *Example*
> 93452 Left heart catheterization including intraprocedural injection(s) for left ventriculography, imaging supervision and interpretation, when performed

When reporting codes for cardiac catheterization procedures, the approach is not the determining factor for code selection (e.g., percutaneous, cut-down).

Cardiac catheterization procedure codes include:

- Introduction, positioning, and repositioning of catheter
- Recording of intracardiac and intravascular pressure
- Obtaining blood samples for measurement of blood gases, dye dilution, or other dilution curves
- Cardiac output measurements (Fick or other method)
- Electrode catheter placement
- Final evaluation and report

When auditing these procedures, consider the following:

- What type of cardiac condition exists?
  - congenital cardiac anomalies
  - other cardiac conditions
- What side of the heart is catheterized?
  - left side
  - right and left sides
- Is angiography performed? If yes, on which site?
  - pulmonary
  - right ventricular
  - right atrial
  - left ventricular
  - left atrial
  - selective coronary (injection of radiopaque material may be by hand)
  - aortic root
  - all sites listed above
- Is selective visualization or opacification of bypass graft performed? If yes, on which site?
  - arterial conduits (e.g., internal mammary)
  - aortocoronary venous bypass grafts

Services and procedures that are inclusive of cardiac catheterization include:

- Administration of medications during catheterization
- Anesthesia
- Insertion or use of percutaneous vascular closure devices

 DEFINITIONS

bypass graft. Surgically created alternative blood vessel used to reroute blood flow around an area of obstruction or disease.

DEFINITIONS

congestive heart failure. Condition caused by the heart's inability to adequately pump and circulate blood, resulting in fluid accumulation in the lungs and other tissues.

cor pulmonale. Heart-lung disease appearing in identifiable forms as chronic or acute. The chronic form of this heart-lung disease is marked by dilation and hypertrophy failure of the right ventricle due to a disease that has affected the function of the lungs, excluding congenital or left heart diseases and is also called chronic cardiopulmonary disease. The acute form is an overload of the right ventricle from a rapid onset of pulmonary hypertension, usually arising from a pulmonary embolism.

shunt. Surgically created passage between blood vessels or other natural passages, such as an arteriovenous anastomosis, to divert or bypass blood flow from the normal channel.

tamponade heart. Interference with the venous return of blood to the heart due to an extensive accumulation of blood in the pericardium (pericardial effusion). Tamponade may occur as a complication of dissecting thoracic aneurysm, pericarditis, renal failure, acute myocardial infarction, chest trauma, or a malignancy. Treatment involves the emergent removal of the fluid.

- Prophylactic insertion of temporary transvenous pacemaker
- Repositioning and replacement of catheters

Medical Necessity

The following conditions may warrant right heart catheterization (this list is not all inclusive):

- Congenital heart disease
- Congestive heart failure
- Cor pulmonale
- Endocarditis anticipated to require valvular surgical repair
- Intracardiac shunts (including septal rupture) and extracardiac vascular shunts
- Pulmonary hypertension
- Suspected cardiomyopathy or myocarditis
- Suspected pericardial tamponade or constriction
- Suspected rejection of a transplanted heart
- Valvular heart disease

The following conditions may warrant left heart catheterization (this list is not all inclusive):

- Cardiac trauma
- Congenital heart abnormalities
- Intracardiac shunts
- Pericardial tamponade
- Valvular dysfunction

The following conditions may warrant cardiac angiography (this list is not all inclusive):

- Cardiac trauma
- Congenital heart disease
- Intracardiac shunts
- Suspected ventricular aneurysms
- To assess mitral or tricuspid valve function
- To assess ventricular function or morphology (including tumors and clots)

The tables below may be used to help determine which code is appropriate for the procedures performed.

CPT Coding for Cardiac Catherization Procedures

CPT Code	Procedure Description
93451	Right Heart Cath
93452	Left Heart Cath with or without left ventriculogram
93453	Right and Left Heart Cath with or without left ventriculogram
93454	Coronary Angiograms only
93455	Coronary artery and bypass graft angiograms
93456	Coronary artery angiograms and Right Heart Cath
93457	Coronary artery and bypass graft angiograms and Right Heart Cath
93458	Coronary artery angiograms and Left Heart Cath with or without left ventriculogram
93459	Coronary artery and bypass graft angiograms and Left Heart Cath
93460	Coronary artery angiograms and Right & Left Heart Cath
93461	Coronary artery and bypass angiograms and Right & Left Heart Cath
Add-On Codes:	
93462	Left Heart Cath by transseptal or transapical puncture
93463	Pharmacologic agent administration
93464	Physiologic exercise study
93566	Injection for right ventricular or right atrial angiography
93567	Injection for supravalvular aortography (aortic root)
93568	Injection for pulmonary angiograms
93571	Intravascular Doppler velocity and/or coronary flow reserve measurement, initial vessel
93572	Intravascular Doppler velocity and/or coronary flow reserve measurement, each additional vessel
0523T	Intraprocedural coronary fractional flow reserve (FFR) with 3D functional mapping

CPT Coding for Congenital Cardiac Catherization Procedures

CPT Code	Procedure Description
93530	Right heart cath for congenital cardiac anomalies
93531	Right heart cath & retrograde LHC for congenital cardiac anomalies
93532	RHC and transseptal LHC through intact septum with or without retrograde LHC
93533	RHC and transseptal LHC through existing septal opening with or without retrograde LHC
Add-on Codes	
93563	Injection selective coronary angiograms
93564	Injection for selective opacification coronary bypass
93565	Injection for left ventriculogram or left atrial
93566	Injection for right ventriculogram or right atrial
93567	Injection for supravalvular aorta (aortic root)
93568	Injection for pulmonary angiograms
93571	Intravascular Doppler velocity and/or coronary flow reserve measurement, each additional vessel
93572	Intravascular Doppler velocity and/or coronary flow reserve measurement, each additional vessel

Refer to the table provided to determine the order of the vessels catheterized.

The starting point of the catheterization would be the aorta in this example.

First Order (Aorta)	Second Order (Selective Vessel Order)	Third Order	Beyond Third Order Branches
Innominate	common carotid (right)	internal carotid (right)	ophthalmic (right) posterior communicating (right) middle cerebral (right) cerebral (right, anterior)
		external carotid (right)	superior thyroid (right) ascending pharyngeal (right) facial (right) lingual (right) occipital (right) posterior aurical (right) superficial temporal (right) internal maxillary (right) middle meningeal (right)
	subclavian and axillary (right)	vertebral (right)	basilar
		internal mammary (right)	
		thyrocervical trunk (right)	inferior thyroid (right) suprascapular (right) transverse cervical (right)
		costocervical trunk (right)	highest intercostal (right) deep cervical (right)
		lateral thoracic (right) thoracoacromial (right) humeral circumflex (right)	
		subscapular (right)	circumflex scapular (right)
		brachial (right)	
		brachial, deep (right)	ulnar (right) radial (right) interosseous (right) deep palmar arch (right) superficial palmar arch (right) metacarpals and digitals (right)
Common carotid (left)	internal carotid (left)	ophthalmic (left) posterior communicating (left) middle cerebral (left) anterior cerebral (left)	
	external carotid (left)	superior thyroid (left) ascending pharyngeal (left) facial (left) lingual (left) occipital (left) posterior auricular (left) superficial temporal (left)	
		internal maxillary (left)	middle meningeal (left)

First Order (Aorta)	Second Order (Selective Vessel Order)	Third Order	Beyond Third Order Branches
Subclavian & axillary (left)	vertebral (left) internal mammary (left)		
	thyrocervical trunk (left)	inferior thyroid (left) supracapular (left) transverse cervical (left)	
	costocervical trunk (left)	highest intercostal (left) cervical, deep (left)	
	lateral thoracic (left) thoracoacromial (left) humeral circumflex (left) subscapular (left) brachial, (left)	circumflex scapular (left)	
	deep brachial (left)	radial (left), ulnar (left)	
		interosseous (left)	deep palmar arch (left) superficial palmar arch (left) metacarpals and digitals (left)
Intercostal			
Bronchials			
Esophageal (recurrent)			
Phrenic (inferior)	suprarenal (superior)		
Celiac trunk	gastric (left)	esophageal branch	
	splenic	pancreatic, dorsal pancreatic, great pancreatic, caudal gastroepiploic short gastrics	transverse pancreatic, inferior

	common hepatic	gastroduodenal	posterior superior
			  pancreaticoduodenal
			anterior superior
			  pancreaticoduodenal

		proper hepatic	hepatic (left) hepatic (right) cystic gastroepiploic supraduodenal intermediate hepatic
Middle suprarenal			
Superior mesenteric artery	colic (middle)		

	pancreaticoduodenal (inferior)	posterior inferior
		  pancreaticoduodenal
		anterior inferior
		  pancreaticoduodenal	

	jejunal ileocolic appendicular posterior cecal anterior cecal marginal colic (right)		
Renal	inferior suprarenal		
Testicular/ovarian			
Lumbar			

First Order (Aorta)	Second Order (Selective Vessel Order)	Third Order	Beyond Third Order Branches
Inferior mesenteric artery	colic (left)		
	sigmoid	rectosigmoid superior rectal	
Middle sacral			
Common iliac	internal iliac	iliolumbar lateral sacral superior gluteal umbilical superior vesical obturator inferior vesical rectal, middle inferior rectal inferior pudental inferior gluteal	
	external iliac	inferior epigastric	cremasteric pubic
		circumflex iliac, deep	deep circumflex liliac, ascending
	common femoral	profunda femoris	medial descending perforating branches lateral descending lateral circumflex
		pudendal, deep, external pudendal, superficial, external circumflex femoral, ascending, lateral circumflex femoral, descending, lateral circumflex femoral, transverse, lateral	
		superficial femoral	geniculate popliteal anterior tibial peroneal posterior tibial
Main pulmonary arteries, (right/left)			

© 2020 Optum360, LLC

Teaching Physician Guidelines

Per Medicare guidelines, cardiac catheterization procedures require personal ("at the elbow") supervision of its performance by a physician. When cardiac catheterization is performed in a teaching setting, the teaching physician must be present, in the room, with the resident, for the *entire* procedure. Medicare denies payment for the performance of these services by the resident alone and considers the service not medically necessary.

Key Documentation Terms

Documentation for these procedures should include ICD-10-CM codes that reflect the condition of the patient and indicate the reason(s) for which the service was performed, which in turn establishes the medical necessity for the cardiac catheterization, coronary angiography, and injection procedures. This documentation includes, but is not limited to, relevant medical history, physical examination, and results of pertinent diagnostic tests or procedures.

All services should have a formal procedural and interpretation report. These reports may be requested to support the medical necessity of the service rendered. The record must include documentation of the medical decision making when interventional procedures are not performed during the same session as the diagnostic procedures. The documentation must include the medical necessity for each procedure when multiple catheterizations and angiographic procedures are performed during the same session.

Terms such as catheter placement, heart catheterization, intraprocedural injection, and retrograde provide the guidance needed to ensure correct code assignment.

Coding Tips

- Cardiac catheterizations (93451–93461) include:

  - roadmapping angiography
  - catheter insertion and positioning
  - contrast injection (except as listed below)
  - radiology supervision and interpretation
  - report

  Code also separately identifiable:

  - aortography (93567)
  - noncardiac angiography (see radiology and vascular codes)
  - pulmonary angiography (93568)
  - right ventricular or atrial angiography (93566)

- Cardiac catheterization procedures may require ECG tracings to assess chest pain during the procedure. These ECG tracings are not reported separately. Diagnostic ECGs performed prior to or after the procedure may be reported separately with modifier 59 or XU.

- Report right ventricular or right atrial angiogram (93566) in addition to right heart catheterization when performed.

- Medicare guidelines state selective catheter placement for the left or right pulmonary artery cannot be coded with a right-heart catheter.

- Cardiac catheterizations for congenital anomalies, should be reported with codes 93530–93533.

- For contrast injections performed with cardiac catheterizations for congenital anomalies, see 93563–93568.

- As add-on codes, 93462–93464, 93563–93568, 93571, and 93572 are not subject to multiple procedure rules. No reimbursement reduction or modifier 51 is applied. Add-on codes describe additional intraservice work associated with the primary procedure. They are performed by the same provider on the same date of service as the primary service/procedure, and must never be reported as a stand-alone code. The following table provides additional information for these codes as found in the Medicare Physician Fee Schedule Database.

Parent Code	Add-On	GLOB DAYS	MULT PROC	BILAT SURG	ASST SURG	CO-SURG	TEAM SURG
33477		000	2	0	0	1	1
92920		000	2	0	0	0	0
92924		000	2	0	0	0	0
92928		000	2	0	0	0	0
92933		000	2	0	0	0	0
92937		000	2	0	0	0	0
92941		000	2	0	0	0	0
92943		000	2	0	0	0	0
92975		000	2	0	0	0	0
93451		000	2	0	0	0	0
93452		000	2	0	0	0	0
93453		000	2	0	0	0	0
93454		000	2	0	0	0	0
93455		000	2	0	0	0	0
93456		000	2	0	0	0	0
93457		000	2	0	0	0	0
93458		000	2	0	0	0	0
93459		000	2	0	0	0	0
93460		000	2	0	0	0	0
93461		000	2	0	0	0	0
	93462	ZZZ	0	0	0	0	0
	93463	ZZZ	0	0	0	0	0
	93464	ZZZ	0	0	0	0	0
93530		000	2	0	0	0	0
93531		000	2	0	0	0	0
93532		000	2	0	0	0	0
93533		000	2	0	0	0	0
	93563	ZZZ	0	0	0	0	0
	93564	ZZZ	0	0	0	0	0
	93565	ZZZ	0	0	0	0	0
	93566	ZZZ	0	0	0	0	0
	93567	ZZZ	0	0	0	0	0
	93568	ZZZ	0	0	0	0	0
	93571	ZZZ	0	0	0	0	0
	93572	ZZZ	0	0	0	0	0

Parent Code	Add-On	GLOB DAYS	MULT PROC	BILAT SURG	ASST SURG	CO-SURG	TEAM SURG
93580		000	2	0	0	0	0
93581		000	2	0	0	0	0
93582		000	2	0	0	0	0
93583		000	2	0	0	0	0
93653		000	2	0	0	0	0
93654		000	2	0	0	0	0

- Per Medicare guidelines, diagnostic coronary angiography may not be reported when performed during percutaneous coronary intervention if it has been previously performed within the last six months and resulted in the decision for the beneficiary to undergo the specific interventional procedure.

- Per Medicare guidelines, diagnostic cardiac catheterization with coronary angiography is separately reimbursable when performed prior to an interventional procedure. It may be performed on the same day or on the day before when used as a diagnostic tool to evaluate the need for the intervention, but only once prior to the interventional procedure. In addition, when the diagnostic and interventional procedures are performed on the same day, modifier 51 should be appended to the subsequent procedure. Angiography before, during, or after an interventional procedure to evaluate results or to guide the catheter(s) is considered incidental to the procedure and not reported separately.

- Per Medicare guidelines, each angiography procedure may be reimbursed once regardless of the number of injections of contrast, views, or actual pictures taken.

- Heart catheterization codes 93452–93453 and 93458–93461 should not be reported with category III codes for permanent cardiac contractility modulation systems (0408T–0415T).

Coding Traps
- Do not report 93503 in conjunction with diagnostic cardiac catheterization codes.

- Do not report right heart catheterization when it is a component of another surgical procedure such as in codes 93453, 93456, 93457, 93460, or 93461.

- Do not report left heart catheterization when it is a component of another surgical procedure such as in codes 93453 or 93458–93461.

- Do not report cardiac catheterization injection procedures (93563–93565) with codes 93452–93461.

- Codes 93451–93461 and 93563–93564 should not be reported with diagnostic right heart catheterization procedures intrinsic to the valve repair (33418, 0345T, 0483T–0484T) or annulus reconstruction (0544T–0545T) procedures.

Paravalvular Leak Repair (93590–93592)

A paravalvular leak (PVL) is found in patients that have had valve replacement surgery. Usually when a new valve is placed there are no gaps between the edges of the valve and the surrounding natural heart tissue. Occasionally there may be a gap that was unnoticed or one that develops around the replaced valve—this is known as paravalvular defect. Blood leaks through these defects, known as PVL. Codes 93590–93592 report percutaneous transcatheter closure of a PVL found in the mitral or aortic valve. This procedure can be achieved by antegrade or retrograde approach. There are codes that report the mitral or aortic valve for the initial occlusion and then each additional occlusion.

In these procedures a transesophageal echocardiogram (TEE) for a mitral valve leak or a transthoracic echocardiogram (TTE) for an aortic leak will have been performed within the previous six months—earlier if the patient was symptomatic. Documentation will state that a retrograde transfemoral approach is performed utilizing a catheter and guidewire. Upon crossing the leak, the wire is removed and a stiff wire is inserted along with the device delivery system consisting of a guide catheter or sheath. The wire is removed allowing for advancement and deployment of an occlusion device. In cases where support becomes an issue, a transseptal access and snare may be employed to establish a rail. This entails the snaring of the initial wire within the left atrium or the formation of an apical ventricular rail by left ventricular puncture with the wire crossing the apex. In mitral PVL, if this approach does not achieve the desired result, an antegrade transseptal approach may be used. Upon completion of the procedure for 93590, TEE should indicate fluent leaflets, clear pulmonary veins, and if anterior leak, clear mitral valve. In 93591, the physician must evaluate that the coronary ostia is not covered and leaflets are fluent. For both procedures, the device deployed is dependent upon the defect size. Many closure devices are currently used in these procedures, such as embolization coils, double-umbrella devices, occluders, and plugs approved for other specific defects and may be suitable in most cases. However for PVLs, they are limited by size, shape, specific characteristics, and features of the delivery system. Code 93592 is reported for each additional occlusion device employed.

Key Documentation Terms

Documentation should indicate the surgical procedure that was performed. Terms such as mitral valve, aorta, or documentation of additional occlusion devices provide the guidance needed to ensure correct code assignment. Above all else, the documentation should support the medical necessity of the procedure.

Coding Tips

- When diagnostic heart catheterization is performed in the same operative session and on the same calendar date as a closure of a paravalvular leak (93590–93592), it may be reported with modifier 59 appended.

- Additional diagnostic heart catheterization procedures may be reported separately when they are not an integral component of the PVL repair.

- Codes 93590 and 93591 include angiography, fluoroscopy (76000), and radiological supervision and interpretation when used to assist in the closure of the PVL.

- As an add-on code, 93592 is not subject to multiple procedure rules. No reimbursement reduction or modifier 51 is applied. Add-on codes describe additional intraservice work associated with the primary procedure. It is performed by the same provider on the same date of service as the primary service/procedure, and must never be reported as a stand-alone code.

Parent Code	Add-On	GLOB DAYS	MULT PROC	BILAT SURG	ASST SURG	CO-SURG	TEAM SURG
93590		000	2	0	2	1	0
93591		000	2	0	0	2	1
	93592	ZZZ	0	0	2	1	0

INR Monitoring (93792–93793)

International normalized ratio (INR) monitoring is the management of outpatients receiving warfarin therapy, including monitoring dosage and orders and reviewing and interpreting INR levels. These services are reported with 93792–93793.

Each code has specific guidelines for reporting the service. In 93792, face-to-face, clinician-directed training is started for the patient and/or caregiver for in-home INR monitoring, which includes:

- Proper use and care of the INR monitoring device
- Instructions for obtaining blood samples
- Instructions for reporting INR test results
- Documented determination as to the patient's and/or caregiver's ability to adequately perform testing and reporting

Test materials may be reported with the appropriate HCPCS Level II code or CPT code 99070 in addition to 93792.

Code 93793 is reported for anticoagulant management of warfarin therapy, which includes:

- Review and interpretation of new INR test results that may be done at home, the office, or in a lab
- Patient instructions
- Dosage adjustments, as appropriate

Coding Tips
- When a significant, separately identifiable evaluation and management service is performed on the same day as 93792, modifier 25 is appended to the E/M service. Code 93793 should not be reported on the same day as an E/M service and should only be reported once per date of service, regardless of how many tests were reviewed.

- CPT guidelines state that these services should not be reported with the following codes:
  - telephone services (98966–98968), online digital E/M services (99421–99423, 99441–99443) when they are used to perform home and outpatient INR monitoring
  - care management (99487, 99489, 99490)
  - transitional care services (99495, 99496)

Respiratory Services: Diagnostic and Therapeutic (94002–94799)

These codes are used to report procedures such as ventilator management, spirometry, inhalation services, and ear or pulse oximetry.

Procedure Differentiation

Ventilator management is reported with 94002–94005. Code selection is based upon the site of service, and is reported per day of management.

Code 94005 may be reported by a physician or other qualified health care professional for ventilator management when a patient is also being managed by another physician reporting 99339, 99340, or 99374–99378 within the same 30-day period.

Codes 94010–94799 include all laboratory procedures and interpretation of test results for pulmonary services such as spirometry, bronchospasm evaluation, breathing capacity evaluation, pulse oximetry, circadian respiratory pattern recording, and ventilation assistance and management. Some of these codes are therapeutic services, such as 94011–94012 (spirometric measurements), and 94013 (lung volume measurements), 94610 (surfactant administered by physician or other qualified healthcare professional), 94667–94668 (chest wall manipulation), 94669 (chest wall oscillation, mechanical), and others are diagnostic, such as exercise test for bronchospasm (94617, 96419), pulmonary stress tests (94618), and cardiopulmonary exercise testing (94621). It is important to read the code description carefully as some procedures, such as spirometry (94010), are included in some of the code descriptions.

The most common procedures in this section will be discussed below.

Pulmonary function testing (PFT) measures the capacity of the lungs and the exchange of air. A PFT includes three components:

- Spirometry (94010, 94060, 94070)
- Lung volume determination (94726, 94727, 94728)
- Diffusion capacity (94729)

In 94010, a spirometer in a pulmonary lab is used to measure functions of the lungs, including the amount of air contained in the lungs, the rate of expiration, and the volume of air a patient respires. The physician interprets the results of the spirometry and a graphic record is obtained.

A bronchodilation responsiveness test is performed in 94060, using spirometry completed before and after administering a bronchodilating medicine to the patient. Code 94070 applies to spirometry conducted multiple times to evaluate bronchospasm provocation after exposing the patient to an agent, such as antigen(s), exercise, cold air, or methacholine. This test usually follows performance of 94010 where reduced airflow is indicated.

Medical Necessity

Spirometry may be indicated for one of the following conditions (this list is not all inclusive):

Diagnostic indications:

- To detect the presence or absence of lung dysfunction suggested by history or clinically significant physical signs and symptoms
- Detect the presence or absence of lung dysfunction suggested by other abnormal diagnostic tests (e.g., radiography, arterial blood gas analysis)

Monitoring indications:

- Assess the change in lung function following administration of or a change in therapy
- Assess the change in lung function over time
- Assess the risk for surgical procedures known to affect lung function
- Quantify the severity of known lung disease

Procedure Differentiation

In 94726, the lung volume and possibly the airway resistance are evaluated using a variety of methods. In the oldest method, the patient is enclosed in a pressurized small room, and the volume of air and air resistance are measured as the patient breathes. In a newer method, two belts with sensors are wrapped around the patient at the rib cage and the abdomen to measure the lung volumes, referred to as respiratory inductance plethysmography. In 94727, lung volumes are tested in a pulmonary lab using helium, nitrogen open circuit, or another method to check lung functions to include residual capacity or residual volume, which is the volume of air remaining in the lung after a patient exhales. The physician interprets the results. This code applies to the distribution of inspired gas using multiple breath nitrogen washout curves and including alveolar nitrogen or helium equilibration time. In 94728, airway resistance is tested by oscillometry. In one method, the patient breathes into an apparatus called a pneumotachograph. This device uses soundwaves to detect and analyze airway changes. Code 94728 may be reported in addition to gas dilution techniques. In 94729, diffusing capacity is tested. In this test, the patient takes a deep breath, holds it for 10 seconds, and releases the first half. The second half is collected and analyzed for the amount of carbon dioxide it contains.

Medical Necessity

Lung volume testing may be indicated for one of the following conditions (this list is not all inclusive):

- Assess the effectiveness of a therapy
- Early detection of lung dysfunction
- Evaluation of dyspnea, cough, and other symptoms
- Evaluation of the type and degree of pulmonary dysfunction
- Follow-up and response to therapy
- Pre- and post-op evaluations for Lung Volume Reduction Surgery (LVRS)
- Preoperative evaluation
- Track pulmonary disease progression

 DEFINITIONS

emphysema. Pathological condition in which there is destructive enlargement of the air spaces in the lungs resulting in damage to the alveolar walls, commonly seen in long-term smokers.

hypercapnia. Excess carbon dioxide in the blood.

hypoxemia. Inadequate oxygen in the blood.

sarcoidosis. Clustering of immune cells resulting in granuloma formation. Often affects the lungs and lymphatic system but can occur in other body sites.

Procedure Differentiation

Diffusing capacity is tested in 94729. In this test, the patient takes a deep breath, holds it for 10 seconds, and releases the first half. The second half is collected and analyzed for the amount of carbon dioxide it contains.

Medical Necessity

Diffuse capacity testing may be indicated for one of the following conditions (this list is not all inclusive):

- Assist in the evaluation of some types of cardiovascular disease (e.g., primary pulmonary hypertension, pulmonary edema, acute or recurrent thromboembolism)
- Differentiate between asthma, chronic bronchitis, and emphysema in patient with obstructive patterns
- Evaluate and quantify the disability associated with interstitial lung disease
- Evaluate hemorrhagic disorders
- Evaluate the effects of chemotherapy agents or other drugs known to induce pulmonary dysfunction
- Evaluate the pulmonary involvement in systemic diseases (e.g., rheumatoid arthritis, systemic lupus)
- Evaluation and follow-up of emphysema and cystic fibrosis
- Evaluation and follow-up of parenchymal lung diseases associated with dusts, drug reactions, or sarcoidosis
- Predict arterial desaturation during exercise in chronic obstructive pulmonary disease

Procedure Differentiation

In 94618, a pulmonary exercise stress test is performed to see how much air moves in and out of the lungs during exercise and to determine where breathing problems are occurring, since they may be in the lungs, heart, or circulation. An exercise stress test is done with the patient riding a stationary bike (ergometer) or walking on a treadmill. Heart rate, breathing, and blood pressure are monitored before beginning the exercise.

Code 94621 reports cardiopulmonary exercise testing (CPET). This test uses electrodes placed on the upper body to monitor the heart. Throughout the process, blood samples may be taken to measure oxygen uptake and carbon dioxide waste products in the blood during exercise, as well as other tests including minute ventilation and an electrocardiogram (ECG, EKG). CPET provides assessment of the exercise responses involving the pulmonary, cardiovascular, hematopoietics, neuropsychological, and skeletal muscle systems, which are not adequately reflected through the measurement of individual organ system function.

Medical Necessity

Pulmonary stress tests may be indicated for one of the following conditions (this list is not all inclusive):

- Detection of interstitial lung disease (fibrosis) or exercise-induced bronchospasm, which are only manifested by exercise
- Evaluate a patient's response to a newly established pulmonary treatment regimen

 DEFINITIONS

lupus erythematosus. Inflammatory, autoimmune skin condition in which the body's autoimmune system attacks healthy tissue of the integumentary system.

pulmonary edema. Accumulation of fluid in the air sacs of the lungs, making it difficult to breath.

pulmonary hypertension. Condition that occurs when pressure within the pulmonary artery is elevated and vascular resistance is observed in the lungs.

rheumatoid arthritis. Autoimmune disease causing pain, stiffness, inflammation, and possibly joint destruction.

sarcoidosis. Clustering of immune cells resulting in granuloma formation. Often affects the lungs and lymphatic system but can occur in other body sites.

- Initial diagnostic workup when symptoms (generally dyspnea) are out of proportion to findings on static function (spirometry, lung volume, diffusion capacity)

- To determine whether the patient's exercise intolerance is related to pulmonary disease, cardiac disease, or due to lack of conditioning or poor effort

Procedure Differentiation

Car seat testing airway integrity is reported with 94780 and 94781. A hospital professional trained in car seat/bed safety and positioning, as well as monitoring for apnea, bradycardia, and oxygen saturations, observes an infant, up to 12 months old, for a cardiac or respiratory event. This type of event occurs most often in preterm or low birth weight infants, infants born with hypotonia (e.g., Down syndrome), or infants who undergo congenital cardiac surgery. The newborn is placed in the car seat/bed at a 45-degree angle with the harness clip at chest level. The infant is attached to a monitor that assesses heartrate, respiratory rate, and oxygen saturation. Obstructive apnea monitoring may be performed as well. The infant is constantly observed by clinical staff for 60 to 120 minutes or the amount of time the baby will be in transport home, whichever is longer. This procedure includes the interpretation, recording, and report of the findings. Code 94780 should be reported for the first 60 minutes and 94781 for each additional full 30 minutes. As with other codes reported by time, the start and stop time must be documented.

Key Documentation Terms

Documentation for these procedures in this section should include ICD-10-CM codes that reflect the condition of the patient and indicate the reason(s) for which the service was performed, which in turn establishes medical necessity. Documentation should include, but is not limited to, relevant medical history, physical examination, and results of pertinent diagnostic tests or procedures. All tests require an interpretation with a written report. Computerized reports must have a provider's signature indicating the provider's review and the accuracy.

All providers of pulmonary function tests should have on file a referral (an order, a prescription) with clinical diagnoses and requested tests.

Coding Tips

- If multiple spirometric determinations are necessary to complete the service described by a CPT code, only one unit of service should be reported. For example, code 94070 describes bronchospasm provocation with an administered agent and utilizes multiple spirometric determinations as in code 94010. A single unit of service includes all of the necessary spirometric determinations.

- PFTs are diagnostic, not therapeutic. PFTs are not used to demonstrate breathing exercises.

- As add-on codes, 94645, 94729, and 94781 are not subject to multiple procedure rules. No reimbursement reduction or modifier 51 is applied. Add-on codes describe additional intraservice work associated with the primary procedure. They are performed by the same provider on the same date of service as the primary service/procedure, and must never be reported as a stand-alone code. The following table provides additional information for these codes as found in the Medicare Physician Fee Schedule Database.

 AUDITOR'S ALERT

Codes 94010–94799 include all laboratory procedures and interpretation of test results for pulmonary services, such as spirometry, bronchospasm evaluation, breathing capacity evaluation, pulse oximetry, circadian respiratory pattern recording, and ventilation assistance and management.

Parent Code	Add-On	GLOB DAYS	MULT PROC	BILAT SURG	ASST SURG	CO-SURG	TEAM SURG
94010		XXX	0	0	0	0	0
94060		XXX	0	0	0	0	0
94070		XXX	0	0	0	0	0
94375		XXX	0	0	0	0	0
94644		XXX	0	0	0	0	0
	94645	XXX	0	0	0	0	0
94726		XXX	0	0	0	0	0
94727		XXX	0	0	0	0	0
94728		XXX	0	0	0	0	0
	94729	ZZZ	0	0	0	0	0
94780		XXX	0	0	1	0	0
	94781	ZZZ	0	0	1	0	0

- Code 94610 should be reported only one time per dosing episode.
- Code 94664 should be reported only one time per day.
- Arterial blood gases, may be reported separately with code 36600.
- If more than one inhalation treatment is performed in a day, report 94640 with modifier 76 appended.

Allergy Tests and Immunology (95004–95199)

Allergy and Ingestion Challenge Tests (95004–95079)
Codes in this subsection are used to report percutaneous tests (95004), a combination of percutaneous and intracutaneous (95017–95018), intracutaneous (95024–95028), patch (95044), photo (95052–95056), ophthalmic mucous (95060), nasal mucous (95065), inhalation (95070), and ingestion challenge testing (95076–95079).

Procedure Differentiation
In percutaneous tests (95004), the skin is scratched, punctured, or pricked to introduce specific allergy extracts, drugs, venoms, or other biological agents to determine a patient's allergies. The immediate skin reaction is documented.

A combination of percutaneous and intracutaneous tests use various scratches, punctures, pricks, or intradermal injections to determine a patient's allergies. The immediate skin reaction is documented. This code includes the provider's test interpretation and report. Report 95017 if the allergen being tested is insect venom, and report 95018 if the allergen being tested is drugs or biologicals.

In code 95024, intracutaneous tests are performed, the patient is injected with allergenic extracts for airborne allergens, immediate type reaction, to determine a patient's specific allergies. In 95027 intracutaneous tests, sequential and incremental intracutaneous tests are performed. The number of tests must be specified. These codes includes test interpretation and provider report. Code 95028 is reported when a delayed skin reaction is documented.

In a patch test (95044), a patch containing specific allergenic substances is placed on the patient's arm to determine the patient's specific allergies.

In a photo patch test (95052–95056), a patch is applied as in code 95044 but then the area is exposed to ultraviolet light to determine a patient's specific allergies.

In an ophthalmic mucous test (95060), the allergy extracts are introduced to the patient's eye mucus membranes to determine the patient's specific allergic reactions.

When a nasal mucous test (95065) is performed, allergy extracts are introduced to the patient's mucus membrane in the nose.

In an inhalation test (95070), the patient inhales histamines, methacholamines, or similar medications to determine specific allergies.

In ingestion challenge testing (95076–95079), the patient ingests specific substances such as food or drugs to determine the patient's specific allergies. The reaction is documented. Report 95076 for the first 120 minutes of testing. Report add-on code 95079 for each additional 60 minutes of testing.

Medical Necessity
The following conditions may warrant allergy testing (this list is not all inclusive):

- Allergic gastroenteritis
- Allergic urticaria
- Allergy to medicinal agents
- Anaphylactic shock due to adverse food reaction
- Contact allergic dermatitis
- Contact photosensitization (e.g., photoallergic contact dermatitis)
- Generalized eczema
- Ichthyosis
- Severe dermatographism

Key Documentation Terms
Documentation for these procedures should include ICD-10-CM codes that reflect the condition of the patient and indicate the reason(s) for which the service was performed, which in turn establishes medical necessity. Documentation should include, but is not limited to, relevant medical history, physical examination, and results of pertinent diagnostic tests or procedures. All tests include an interpretation with a written report. The number of tests and substances should also be documented. Terms such as percutaneous, intracutaneous, patch, photo patch, inhalation, incremental, sequential, and ingestion provide the guidance needed to ensure correct code assignment.

Coding Tips
- When allergy is performed using a lab test, report a code from the code range 86000–86999.
- E/M codes reported with allergy testing or allergy immunotherapy are appropriate only if a significant, separately identifiable service is performed. Obtaining informed consent is included in the

 DEFINITIONS

contact dermatitis. Superficial skin inflammation characterized by epidermal edema and irritated vesicles occurring as a reaction to a substance coming in contact with the skin.

eczema. Inflammatory form of dermatitis with red, itchy breakouts of exudative vesicles that leads to crusting and scaling that occurs as a reaction to internal or external agents.

ichthyosis. Congenital condition in which an excessive production of skin cells results in red, dry, scaly skin.

immunotherapy service and should not be reported with an E/M code. If E/M services are reported, modifier 25 should be utilized.

- Drugs administered for intractable/severe allergic reaction (e.g., antihistamines, epinephrine, steroids) may be reported separately with code 96372.

- If percutaneous or intracutaneous (intradermal) single test (95004 or 95024) and "sequential and incremental" tests (95017–95018 or 95027) are performed on the same date of service, both the "sequential and incremental" test and single test codes may be reported if the tests are for different allergens or different dilutions of the same allergen.

- As an add-on code, 95079 is not subject to multiple procedure rules. No reimbursement reduction or modifier 51 is applied. Add-on codes describe additional intraservice work associated with the primary procedure. They are performed by the physician on the same date of service as the primary service/procedure, and must never be reported as stand-alone codes. The following table provides additional information for these codes as found in the Medicare physician fee schedule database.

Parent Code	Add-On	GLOB DAYS	MULT PROC	BILAT SURG	ASST SURG	CO-SURG	TEAM SURG
95076		XXX	0	0	0	0	0
	95079	ZZZ	0	0	0	0	0

Coding Trap
- An evaluation and management service should not be reported separately for the interpretation and report of allergy testing.

Allergy Immunotherapy (95115–95199)
Immunotherapy is the parenteral administration of extracts, such as antigens given in increasing dosages at periodic intervals. The goal is to desensitize the body against the allergen.

Procedure Differentiation
Codes 95115–95117 describe the administration (injection) of the allergenic extract when the extract provision or preparation of the extract is not included. They do not include the provision or preparation of the extract. These services are typically performed by a nurse. In the event that the provider performs an E/M service on the same date of service as an injection, the provider should document the service and report the appropriate level E/M code. In situations when there is not a provider history or exam performed and the nurse must consult with the provider as to whether the patient should receive the injection and whether dosage adjustments are required, CPT code 99211 would be appropriate. When the documentation indicates that one allergy injection is given, report 95115. If two or more injections are given, report 95117 only once.

Codes 95120–95134 report a single or multiple injection(s) of the allergen or venom and include the provision of the substance.

Code 95144 reports the allergist's preparation and supply of an antigen extract for allergen immunotherapy in a single dosage vial. The antigen is to be administered by another provider. Single dose vials contain one dose to be administered in a single injection.

Codes 95145–95170 report the provider's preparation of an antigen for allergen immunotherapy and the provision of the antigen extract itself. They also include the provider's calculations for the concentration and volume to be used in the dosage based upon the patient's previous skin test results and personal history. These codes do not, however, include the administration of the allergen therapy. The number of doses must be specified and the vial(s) (series of vials from a treatment board or one multiple dose vial) from which the dose may be drawn is irrelevant. Report the code based on the type of preparation (e.g., the number of different venoms contained in a single administered injection of the extract). Codes 95145-95149 report stinging insects. Code 95165 reports single or multiple antigens (not stinging insect) and 95170 is for a whole body extract of a biting insect or other arthropod.

Treatment boards are used by many allergists, defined as small amounts of antigens that are drawn from a number of separate bottles containing different antigens. The mixture is injected into the patient. Each time the patient receives an allergenic extract, it is to be reported per dose. For those physicians providing one or more multiple-dose vials for use over a long period of time, the total number of doses provided should be listed in the units box of the CMS-1500 claim form or the electronic equivalent.

> ### Example
> The allergist prepares a multidose vial of antigens (eight doses). Only one injection is given. Code eight doses of the antigen and one injection. When the remaining doses are injected, code only the injection service. For the injection, see 95115 or 95117 and for the extraction, see 95145–95170.

Report the number of hours spent providing desensitization in the units box with code 95180. This procedure is usually done in four to 24 hours.

Medical Necessity
The following conditions may warrant allergen immunotherapy (this list is not all inclusive):

- Allergic conjunctivitis
- Allergic rhinitis due to pollen or animal (cat) (dog) hair and dander
- Anaphylactic reaction
- Asthma
- Atopic conjunctivitis
- Chemical conjunctivitis
- Toxic effect of venom

Key Documentation Terms
Documentation for these procedures should include ICD-10-CM codes that reflect the condition of the patient and indicate the reason(s) for which the service was performed, which in turn establishes medical necessity. The number of injections and substance should be documented. Terms such as supervision of preparation, preparation and provision, and single or multiple antigens provide the guidance needed to ensure correct code assignment.

Coding Tips
- Allergy testing is not performed on the same day as allergy immunotherapy in standard medical practice. These codes should not be reported together for the same date of service.

 AUDITOR'S ALERT

Code 95117 Professional services for allergen immunotherapy not including provision of allergenic extracts; two or more injections, should be reported only once regardless of the number of injections provided.

Additional evaluation and management may be reported if applicable.

 DEFINITIONS

allergic rhinitis. Inflammation of the mucous membranes of the nose due to allergy.

anaphylactic reaction. Type of life threatening, whole body allergic reaction to a substance that has become an allergen. Body tissues in various areas of the body immediately release histamine and other substances that can result in a tightening of the airways making breathing difficult, in addition to other symptoms.

conjunctivitis. Inflammation of the membrane lining the eyelids.

- Allergy testing is an integral component of rapid desensitization kits (code 95180) and is not reported separately.

Hydration, Therapeutic, Prophylactic, and Diagnostic Injections and Infusions (Nonchemotherapy) (96360–96379)

Hydration (96360–96361)

Hydration via intravenous infusion is reported with 96360 and 96361. Hydration services include:

- Direct physician supervision
    - direction of personnel
- Minimal supervision for
    - consent
    - safety oversight
    - supervision of personnel
- Pre-packaged fluid/electrolytes
- Providers report the initial code for the primary reason for the visit regardless of the order in which the infusions or injections are given
- The following if done to facilitate the injection/infusion
    - flush at the end of infusion
    - indwelling IV, subcutaneous catheter/port access
    - local anesthesia
    - start of IV
    - supplies/tubing/syringes
- Treatment plan verification
- Coding hierarchy rules for facility reporting only
    - chemotherapy services are primary to diagnostic, prophylactic, and therapeutic services
    - diagnostic, prophylactic, and therapeutic services are primary to hydration services
    - infusions are primary to pushes
    - pushes are primary to injections

Do not report a second initial service on the same date for accessing a multi-lumen catheter or restarting an IV, or when two IV lines are needed to meet an infusion rate.

Codes are selected based on the amount of time the infusion is running. Drug infusion should not be reported with these codes.

Medical Necessity
The following conditions may warrant hydration (this list is not all inclusive):

- Dehydration
- Diarrhea
- Gastritis

AUDITOR'S ALERT

See Appendix 1 for the audit worksheet for nonchemotherapy injections and infusions.

DEFINITIONS

dehydration. Condition resulting from an excessive loss of water from the body.

volume depletion. Depletion of total body water.

- Hyperemesis
- Persistent vomiting
- Volume depletion

Key Documentation Terms

Documentation for these procedures should include ICD-10-CM codes that reflect the condition of the patient and indicate the reason(s) for which the service was performed.

Documentation should state why the patient required these services to support the medical necessity for hydration therapy. The volume of hydration therapy and the doses of nonchemotherapy drugs administered should also be documented.

These codes are based on time and the start and stop times must be documented. No other service may be billed concurrently with the time represented by these codes.

Terms such as initial or each additional provide the guidance needed to ensure correct code assignment.

Coding Tips

- As an add-on code, 96361 is not subject to multiple procedure rules. No reimbursement reduction or modifier 51 is applied. Add-on codes describe additional intraservice work associated with the primary procedure. They are performed by the same provider on the same date of service as the primary service/procedure, and must never be reported as a stand-alone code. The following table provides additional information for these codes as found in the Medicare Physician Fee Schedule Database.

Parent Code	Add-On	GLOB DAYS	MULT PROC	BILAT SURG	ASST SURG	CO-SURG	TEAM SURG
96360		XXX	0	0	0	0	0
	96361	ZZZ	0	0	0	0	0

- The administration of drugs and fluids other than antineoplastic agents, such as growth factors, antiemetics, saline, or diuretics, may be reported with codes 96360–96379. If the sole purpose of fluid administration (e.g., saline, D5W, etc.) is to maintain patency of an access device, the infusion is neither diagnostic nor therapeutic and should not be reported separately. Similarly, the fluid utilized to administer drugs/substances is incidental hydration and should not be reported separately.

- If therapeutic fluid administration is medically necessary (e.g., correction of dehydration, prevention of nephrotoxicity) before or after transfusion or chemotherapy, it may be reported separately.

- Hydration concurrent with other drug administration services is not reported separately.

Coding Traps

- Do not report hydration infusions of 30 minutes or less.

- Initiation of an IV catheter is included and not reported separately.

- Codes 96360 and 96361 should not be reported if a concurrent service from code range 96365–96549 is performed.

 AUDITOR'S ALERT

Infusions less than 30 minutes are not billable with 96360 and 96361.

diagnostic services. Examination or procedure performed on a patient to obtain information to assess the medical condition of the patient or to identify the nature and cause of a sign or symptom.

prophylactic. Agent or treatment measure intended to prevent or ward off a disease condition.

therapeutic services. Services performed for treatment of a specific diagnosis. These services include performance of the procedure, various incidental elements, and normal, related follow-up care.

Infusions: Diagnostic/Preventive/Therapeutic (96365–96371)

Infusion therapy is described as providing hydration for a diagnostic, prophylactic, or therapeutic purpose. These services include:

- Administration of fluid
- Administration of substances/drugs
- An infusion of 16 minutes or more
- Constant presence of health care professional administering the substance/drug
- Direct physician supervision:
  - consent
  - direction of personnel
  - patient assessment
  - safety oversight
  - supervision of personnel
- The following, if done to facilitate the injection/infusion:
  - flush at the end of infusion
  - indwelling IV, subcutaneous catheter/port access
  - local anesthesia
  - start of IV
  - supplies/tubing/syringes
- Training to assess patient and monitor vital signs
- Training to prepare/dose/dispose
- Treatment plan verification
- Physicians report the initial code for the primary reason for the visit regardless of the order in which the infusions or injections are given

Do not report a second initial service on the same date for accessing a multi-lumen catheter or restarting an IV or when two IV lines are needed to meet an infusion rate.

Codes 96365–96371 are also selected based upon the time the patient receives infusion therapy, what is infused, type of infusion, and whether it is an additional sequential or concurrent infusion. It is important to note that the additional time and sequential therapy are not subject to modifier 51 or fee reduction.

Procedure Differentiation

When reporting intravenous infusion, documentation must indicate that a physician or other qualified health care professional or an assistant under direct physician or other qualified health care professional supervision injects or infuses a therapeutic, prophylactic (preventive), or diagnostic medication other than chemotherapy or other highly complex drugs or biologic agents via intravenous route. Infusions are administered through an intravenous catheter inserted by a needle into a patient's vein or by injection or infusion through an existing indwelling intravascular access catheter or port. Report 96365 for the initial hour and 96366 for each additional hour. Report 96367 for each additional sequential infusion of a different substance or drug, up to one hour, and 96368 for each concurrent infusion of substances other than chemotherapy or other highly complex drugs or biologic agents. Code 96368 should not be reported more than one time per date of service.

When reporting subcutaneous infusion, documentation must indicate that a physician or an assistant under direct physician supervision infuses a therapeutic or prophylactic (preventive) medication other than chemotherapy or other highly complex drug or biologic agent via a subcutaneous route. Infusions are administered through a needle inserted beneath the skin; common infusion sites include the upper arm, shoulder, abdomen, or thigh. Report 96369 for infusions lasting longer than 15 minutes and up to one hour. This code includes pump set-up and the establishment of subcutaneous infusion sites. Report 96370 for each additional hour and 96371 for an additional pump set-up with the establishment of a new subcutaneous infusion site(s). Codes 96369 and 96371 should be reported only once per encounter.

Indications for subcutaneous infusion may include coma, dysphagia, nausea/vomiting, intestinal obstruction, malabsorption, or extreme weakness.

Medical Necessity
There are multiple indications for which these services may be performed. Check with third-party payers to verify coverage.

Key Documentation Terms
Documentation for these procedures should include ICD-10-CM codes that reflect the condition of the patient and indicate the reason(s) for which the service was performed.

Documentation should state why the patient required these services to support the medical necessity for infusion therapy. The volume and doses of nonchemotherapy drugs administered should also be documented.

These codes are based on time and the start and stop times must be documented. No other service may be billed concurrently with the time represented by these codes. Terms such as initial, each additional, concurrent, and sequential provide the guidance needed to ensure correct code assignment.

Coding Tips
As add-on codes, 96366–96368 and 96370–96371 are not subject to multiple procedure rules. No reimbursement reduction or modifier 51 is applied. Add-on codes describe additional intraservice work associated with the primary procedure. They are performed by the same provider on the same date of service as the primary service/procedure, and must never be reported as a stand-alone code. The following table provides additional information for these codes as found in the Medicare Physician Fee Schedule Database.

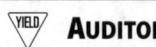 **AUDITOR'S ALERT**

It is important to note that the additional time and sequential therapy are not subject to modifier 51 or fee reduction.

Parent Code	Add-On	GLOB DAYS	MULT PROC	BILAT SURG	ASST SURG	CO-SURG	TEAM SURG
96365		XXX	0	0	0	0	0
	96366	ZZZ	0	0	0	0	0
	96367	ZZZ	0	0	0	0	0
	96368	ZZZ	0	0	0	0	0
96369		XXX	0	0	0	0	0
	96370	ZZZ	0	0	0	0	0
	96371	ZZZ	0	0	0	0	0
96374		XXX	0	0	0	0	0
96409		XXX	0	0	0	0	0
96413		XXX	0	0	0	0	0
96415		ZZZ	0	0	0	0	0
96416		XXX	0	0	0	0	0

- Providers report the initial code for the primary reason for the visit regardless of the order in which the infusions or injections are given. Do not report a second initial service on the same date for accessing a multi-lumen catheter or restarting an IV, or when two IV lines are needed to meet an infusion rate.
- Infusion used to administer drugs is not reported separately.
- Code 96366 or 96370 should be used for infusions that last more than 30 minutes beyond the first hour.
- Code 96369 or 96371 should only be reported once per encounter.
- Code 96368 should not be reported more than one time per date of service.
- Antineoplastic nonhormonal injection therapy, should be reported with code 96401.
- Antineoplastic hormonal injection therapy, should be reported with code 96402.
- Nonantineoplastic hormonal therapy injections, should be reported with code 96372.
- Infusions taking 15 minutes or less, should be reported with code 96372.

Injections: Diagnostic/Preventive/Therapeutic (96372–96375 and 96377)

Injections are reported based upon the route of administration: subcutaneous or intramuscular (96372), intra-arterial (96373), and intravenous push (96374). Intravenous push includes a separate code for subsequent administration of a different drug (96375).

An on-body injector (96377) delivers drug therapy at and for a specified time. Documentation should state that the skin is pierced and a cannula inserted. The cannula is connected to the device which is adhered to the outside of the patient's body, typically the abdomen or arm. The device is filled with the appropriate amount of medication and programmed for dose delivery.

© 2020 Optum360, LLC

Medical Necessity

There are multiple indications for these services to be performed. Verify with third-party payers for coverage.

Key Documentation Terms

Documentation for these procedures should include ICD-10-CM codes that indicate the reason(s) for which the service was performed. Documentation should state the substance and doses of nonchemotherapy drugs administered. Terms such as intramuscular, subcutaneous, intra-arterial, intravenous, on-body, and each additional provide the guidance needed to ensure correct code assignment.

Coding Tip

- As an add-on code, 96375 is not subject to multiple procedure rules. No reimbursement reduction or modifier 51 is applied. Add-on codes describe additional intraservice work associated with the primary procedure. They are performed by the same provider on the same date of service as the primary service/procedure, and must never be reported as a stand-alone code. The following table provides additional information for these codes as found in the Medicare Physician Fee Schedule Database.

Parent Code	Add-On	GLOB DAYS	MULT PROC	BILAT SURG	ASST SURG	CO-SURG	TEAM SURG
96365		XXX	0	0	0	0	0
96374		XXX	0	0	0	0	0
	96375	ZZZ	0	0	0	0	0
96409		XXX	0	0	0	0	0
96413		XXX	0	0	0	0	0

Coding Trap

- Code 96376 may only be reported by facilities.

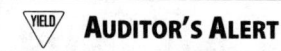 **AUDITOR'S ALERT**

Injections given without direct physician supervision are reported using 99211.

Chemotherapy and Other Complex Drugs, Biologicals (96401–96549)

Chemotherapy codes are reported independent of E/M services provided during the same encounter or on the same day. Most individuals receiving chemotherapy services require an E/M service reported separately at the time of chemotherapy services.

The chemotherapy codes apply to parenteral administration of:

- Antineoplastic agents for noncancer diagnoses
- Monoclonal antibody agents
- Nonradionuclide antineoplastic drugs
- Other biologic response modifiers

Chemotherapy codes include preparation of the chemotherapy agent; however, the supply of chemotherapy agents should be reported with HCPCS Level II J codes or with CPT code 99070. Medicare and most commercial payers require HCPCS Level II codes. Indicate the exact drug and supply for payers and include invoices to answer questions regarding cost.

Administration of other medications provided in conjunction with chemotherapy should be reported separately with codes 96360–96361, 96365, or 96379. These may include:

- Analgesics
- Antibiotics
- Antiemetics
- Narcotics
- Steroids

Chemotherapy codes include:

- Use of local anesthesia
- IV start
- Access to indwelling IV, subcutaneous catheter, or port
- Flush at conclusion of infusion
- Preparation of chemotherapy agent(s)
- Standard tubing, syringes, and supplies

Procedure Differentiation

Documentation for codes 96401 and 96402 must indicate that the physician or supervised assistant prepared and administered nonhormonal anti-neoplastic medication (96401) to combat diseases such as malignant neoplasms or microorganisms. These codes apply to medication injected under the skin (subcutaneous) or into a muscle (intramuscular) often in the arm or leg. Report 96402 for a hormonal anti-neoplastic medication administered to combat diseases, such as malignant neoplasms or microorganisms.

Codes 96405–96406 report intralesional chemotherapy. Report 96405 if medication is injected directly into the lesion or up to seven lesions and 96406 for more than seven lesions.

If documentation indicates that the drug is administered through intravenous (IV) push technique in which the physician or supervised assistant is continuously present to administer the injection and observe the patient or for an infusion of less than 15 minutes, report 96409 for a single or the initial substance or drug given and 96411 for each additional substance or drug given.

When documentation indicates that infusion is through a catheter tubing placed in a vein, report 96413 for a single or the initial substance given for up to one hour of service and report 96415 for each additional hour of service beyond the initial hour. Code 96416 applies to initiating an infusion that will take more than eight hours. Code 96417 applies to initiating a separate additional substance for infusion that is adjunct to the primary chemotherapy infusion service reported by 96413.

Document for code 96420 should describe an intra-arterial push technique, in which the medication is injected in a timed fashion into the nearest port of a catheter already placed in an artery. Placement of the intra-arterial catheter itself is not included. In 96422 and 96423, the drug is administered through an infusion technique, in which the medication is allowed to slowly enter the body through a catheter already in place within an artery. Report 96422 for the first hour of intraarterial infusion and 96423 for each additional hour. In 96425, an infusion is initiated that takes more than eight hours and requires using an implanted pump or a portable pump to infuse the medication very slowly through catheter tubing placed in an artery.

Codes 96440–96450 describe different methods of chemo administration. In 96440, the medication is injected into the lung cavity through a catheter placed into the pleura. In 96446, the medication is injected into the peritoneal cavity through an indwelling port or catheter. In 96450, the medication is injected into the spinal cord through a catheter placed through the space between the lower back bones (lumbar puncture).

Codes 96521–96522 describe services performed on portable or implantable pumps or reservoirs. When a venous access device is used for drug delivery, it is irrigated with an anticoagulant to prevent coagulation at the catheter tip. This service is reported with code 96523.

 DENIAL ALERT

Incorrect units for chemotherapy agents are often responsible for claim downcoding or denial.

When performing a chemotherapy injection (96542), the documentation must indicate the medication that is infused into the central nervous system through a catheter leading from a subcutaneous reservoir of medication in the brain's subarachnoid or intraventricular space.

A concurrent infusion is the administration of multiple infusions at the same time through the same IV line. Sequential infusions are the administration of multiple drugs immediately following another infusion. Sequential and additional hours refer to continued services through the same vascular site. For example, if drug A is administered at the same time as drug B using the same IV line with Y connector, the drug B infusion is concurrent. If drug B was administered through the same IV line, but after the drug A infusion finished, the drug B infusion is sequential. Sequential and additional infusion hours may be more difficult to track particularly when a patient moves between hospital departments.

CMS allows only one initial drug administration service per encounter for each vascular site, regardless of the types of infusion services provided. Additional medications administered through those vascular sites should be reported with the sequential, concurrent, or additional hour codes. Although CPT guidelines differ regarding the initial administration, CMS will continue its current guidelines. If an infusion or injection is of a subsequent or of concurrent nature, report the drug administration code as subsequent or concurrent even if it was the first drug administered. For example, if using the same IV line, an IV push drug is administered first, but the main encounter is for a chemotherapy infusion, the chemotherapy infusion is reported as the initial infusion and the IV push is reported as sequential. When protocol requires two different vascular sites for drug administration or when the route of administration is different, more than one initial drug administration code may be reported.

Official hierarchy has been developed by CMS for facility reporting of drug administration and is followed by most payers for physician administration as well. The following hierarchy applies: chemotherapy services are primary over therapeutic, prophylactic, or diagnostic services, which are primary over hydration services. Infusions are primary to pushes, which are primary to injections.

When timing an infusion for reporting purposes, use the actual time that the infusion was administered and documented. Additional hour add-on codes should be reported only when an infusion runs more than 30 minutes. For example, an infusion that runs 1 hour and 20 minutes is reported only with the initial hour drug administration code. If the infusion was administered over 91 minutes (1 hour and 31 minutes), then the initial hour infusion would be reported as well as one additional hour add-on code. Infusions that are of 15 minutes duration or less should be reported as an intra-arterial or intravenous push injection.

Medical Necessity
There are multiple indications for these services to be performed. Verify with third-party payers for coverage.

Key Documentation Terms
Documentation for these procedures should include ICD-10-CM codes that reflect the condition of the patient and indicate the reason(s) for which the service was performed.

Documentation should state why the patient required these services to support the medical necessity for chemotherapy. The volume and doses of drugs administered should also be documented.

For codes that are based on time, the start and stop times must be documented. No other service may be billed concurrently with the time represented by these codes.

Terms such as initial, each additional, more than eight hours, initial substance, IV push, intralesional, intrathecal, pleura, and peritoneal cavity provide the guidance needed to ensure correct code assignment.

Coding Tips
- Separate codes are reported for each parenteral method of administration utilized when therapy is administered by different techniques.

- Physicians or other qualified health care professional report the initial code for the primary reason for the visit regardless of the order in which the infusions or injections are given. Do not report a second initial service on the same date for accessing a multi-lumen catheter or restarting an IV, or when two IV lines are needed to meet an infusion rate.

- Medicare currently permits separate payment of hydration therapy provided sequentially (but not concurrently) to chemotherapy infusion.

- Administration of anti-anemia drugs and anti-emetic drugs by injection or infusion for cancer patients should be reported using the following codes: 96360–96361, 96365, or 96379, as appropriate.

- As add-on codes, 96411, 96415, 96417, or 96423 are not subject to multiple procedure rules. No reimbursement reduction or modifier 51 is applied. Add-on codes describe additional intraservice work associated with the primary procedure. They are performed by the same provider on the same date of service as the primary service/procedure, and must never be reported as a stand-alone code. The following table provides additional information for these codes as found in the Medicare Physician Fee Schedule Database.

 AUDITOR'S ALERT

Review the documentation to verify the route of administration. Intramuscular injections will note an injection site deep into a muscle in the arm, thigh, or buttock. Subcutaneous injections will be performed just under the skin.

Parent Code	Add-On	GLOB DAYS	MULT PROC	BILAT SURG	ASST SURG	CO-SURG	TEAM SURG
96409		XXX	0	0	0	0	0
	96411	ZZZ	0	0	0	0	0
96413		XXX	0	0	0	0	0
	96415	ZZZ	0	0	0	0	0
	96417	ZZZ	0	0	0	0	0
96422		XXX	0	0	0	0	0
	96423	ZZZ	0	0	0	0	0

- Report 96415 or 96423 when infusion extends more than 30 minutes beyond the first hour.

- Code 96417 should only be reported once per sequential infusion.

- When the medical record documentation clearly identifies that it is medically necessary to separate a substance into two doses (i.e., two injections or infusions in different sites), it is appropriate to code both doses with modifier 59 or the appropriate X [E, S, P, U] modifier. The preparation of chemotherapy agent(s) is included in the service for administration of the agent and is not reported as a separate service.

- To report the intramuscular or subcutaneous administration of antiemetics, narcotics, or analgesics administered, see 96372. The substance used when providing this procedure may be reported with the appropriate HCPCS Level II code. Verify the appropriate dosing requirements and units of service. Experimental or non-Food and Drug Administration (FDA) approved treatment may not be covered by the payer. Check with the specific payer for coverage guidelines or limitations. Examples of hormonal anti-neoplastics include degarelix (SC), infergen (SC), and triptorelin (IM).

- When the encounter is solely for the administration of chemotherapy, immunotherapy, or radiation therapy, assign the appropriate code from category Z51 Encounter for other aftercare and medical care, as the principal or first-listed diagnosis. The specific malignancy code is assigned as a subsequent condition.

Coding Traps

- Time spent for the initial IV or preparation of medications/drugs is not reported separately.

- Fluid used to administer the drug(s) is not reported separately.

- There is no code for concurrent administration of chemotherapeutic drugs. Multiple drugs given at the same session are considered to be sequential, rather than concurrent. The services are reported with 96411 for IV push administration of additional drugs/substances at the same session and 96417 for IV infusion administration of additional drugs/substances at the same session.

Physical/Occupational Therapy and Sports Evaluations (97161–97172)

This section of codes describes physical and occupational therapy and athletic training evaluations. Each of the code sections has specific documentation requirements that should be closely followed.

Procedure Differentiation

Physical therapy evaluations are reported with the following codes:

Code	Medical Decision Making	History- Personal factors or comorbidities	Exam- body structures/ functions, activity limitations, participation	Clinical Presentation	Time Spent Face to Face (avg.)
97161	Low	None	1-2 elements	Stable	20 min
97162	Moderate	1-2	3 or more	Evolving	30 min
97163	High	3 or more	4 or more	Unstable	45 min
97164	Revised plan of care	Review of hx	–	–	20 min

Occupational therapy evaluations are reported with the following codes:

Code	Medical Decision Making	Medical/ Therapy history	Performance Deficits	Time Spent Face to Face (avg.)
97165	Low	Brief	1-3	30 min
97166	Moderate	Expanded	3-5	45 min
97167	High	Extensive	5 or more	60 min
97168	Revised plan of care	Update	Assessment of change	30 min

Athletic training evaluations are reported with the following codes:

Code	Medical Decision Making	History and Activity- Comorbidities	Exam- body structures, physical activity, participation deficiencies	Clinical Presentation	Time Spent Face to Face (avg.)
97169	Low	None	1-2 elements	–	15 min
97170	Moderate	1-2	3 or more	–	30 min
97171	High	3 or more	4 or more	Unstable	45 min
97172	Revised plan of care	Review of hx	–	–	20 min

Coding Tips

- Note the required elements for these codes are different from the codes in the E/M section of the CPT book. For example, in the physical therapy evaluations, the review of body systems includes musculoskeletal, neuromuscular, cardiovascular pulmonary, and integumentary. The review focuses on different details; for instance, the integumentary looks at scar formation, skin texture, color, and integrity. Read each section carefully when auditing these codes.

- These services can be performed at multiple places of service (e.g., patient's home, physical therapist's office, outpatient hospital). The correct place of service should be indicated on the claim form.

- It is appropriate to report the reevaluation if the patient's status should change and the reevaluation is medically reasonable and necessary. It may be necessary to append modifier 59 or XU if performing 97164 or 97168 with other 97000 series codes. Check with payers to determine their specific guidelines.

- A therapeutic procedure may be reported on the same day as an evaluation or reevaluation (97161–97164) when the medical record documentation supports the medical necessity of both services.

Many practices develop excellent policies and procedures for auditing medical records but fail to use the results of the audit. Before an audit can be considered complete, the practice should:

- Compile a complete report of audit findings
- Develop an executive summary
- Calculate potential risks to lost revenue or revenue at risk
- Determine the root cause of the error
- Develop recommendations for a corrective action plan
- Implement an action plan
- Reevaluate the issue

While it seems that these steps can be more difficult to accomplish than the audit itself, by creating templates and using staff input it is not as daunting as it seems.

Developing the Audit Report

An audit report should identify a number of factors:

- Number of records reviewed
- Number of potential errors
- What the errors were
- Financial impact of errors
- Extrapolated impact of errors
- Recommendations
- Corrective action plan
- Potential costs of corrective action
- Implementation time frame
- Reevaluation date

Errors that appear to be isolated do not have to be addressed in the report; however, these errors should be corrected immediately. Patterns of inappropriate coding or billing errors should be specifically addressed in the report.

For example, if upon review a code number was inadvertently transposed on a claim, the claim should be corrected and resubmitted. This does not have to be addressed in the report. However, if during the audit it is noted that 75 percent of claims for colonoscopy with both punch and hot biopsy is performed but only the code for punch biopsy is reported, this should be discussed in detail.

For consistency and to ensure that all factors are addressed, the practice should consider developing an audit report template. The following is an example of the headings that could be used and the type of information that should be included in each.

Type of Audit: _____

Focused (such as a particular provider or specific procedure), Random, Statistically Valid (an SVRS review is an in-depth audit of a provider's utilization, coding, and documentation practices), etc. If there is a specific reason for the review, such as a large number of claim denials or payer inquiries, this should be identified here.

Name of Auditor: _____

Date of Audit: _____

Span of Review: _____

Include this if the review is for a specific time frame (e.g., all level 4 E/M services for the last three months are being reviewed).

Number of Records Reviewed: _____

Number of Errors: _____

If multiple errors are discovered during the review, consider addressing each individually.

Findings: _____
_____
_____
_____

Examples may include such items as incorrect coding, inappropriate use of modifiers, incorrect claim completion, etc.

Financial Impact: _____
_____
_____
_____

When the same error occurs repeatedly, consider including the dollar value found during the audit and extrapolate it. For example, if each error resulted in a $25 loss of reimbursement and the error was found 32 times, the total amount lost would be $800. However, because this procedure is performed an average of 4,200 times per year, the extrapolated revenue lost is $105,000. This helps identify the magnitude of the issue.

Root Cause: _____
_____
_____
_____

Identify the reason for the error. Is it a coding error, a documentation error, or failure to obtain information or precertification?

Recommendations: _____
_____
_____
_____

Include any recommendations that have been created for process improvements. For example, if there is a coding error that occurs repeatedly, the recommendation may be to develop a coding compliance policy and educate staff. If the findings have shown a failure to obtain precertification for a procedure, a recommendation may be to develop a list of procedures that require precertification, post the list, and educate staff.

Cost of Recommendation: _____
_____
_____
_____

Sometimes a recommendation has associated costs, such as software upgrades or additional staffing. These costs should be estimated and included here. These costs should be determined using estimate based methods. For example, the software provider should be contacted for an estimated cost of the upgrade.

Action Plan: _____
_____
_____
_____

A recommendation may require that a task force be developed to review the issue before a final corrective action can be developed. Or, changes in processes may need to be developed with input from appropriate staff members. In these instances, a description of what needs to be completed (such as development of a task force) and how these recommendations will be implemented should be described in detail here.

Implementation Date: _____

Implementation may require weeks or months to complete. If so, provide time span. Include milestones of when specific aspects of the implementation plan will be met.

Reevaluation Date: _____

Depending on the type of error, it may be advisable to reevaluate recommendations and new processes to ensure that the problem has been alleviated. If so, include a date of when this should occur here.

Developing an Executive Summary

Audit findings need to be reported to executive management, such as a practice administrator, chief financial officer, chief executive officer, or the physician. However, most executives want to know two things: the findings and how the errors will be addressed.

High-level management may not be concerned with the details of the individual steps taken to correct an issue; however, they should be kept apprised of the findings, the impact on revenue, and general actions to correct the problem.

Consider including an executive summary at the beginning of each audit report. The information in the executive summary can be pulled directly from the report. By including it with the report, senior management will be able to review the report for specific details if they are interested.

The following should be included in an executive summary:

- **Type of Audit:** Focused (such as a particular provider or specific procedure), Random, Statistically Valid, etc. If there is a specific reason for the review, such as a large number of claim denials or payer inquiries, this should be identified here.

- **Date of Audit:**

- **Span of Review:**

- **Number of Records Reviewed:**

- **Number of Errors:**

- **Findings:** Include only a summary of the findings from the report, such as "E/M codes were assigned a higher level of service than supported by documentation."

- **Financial Impact:** When determining the financial impact, remember to not only include overpayments but also potential underpayments. This is discussed in more detail later in this chapter.

- **Root Cause:** Provide a short synopsis of the reason for the error. For example, for the finding above, the root cause noted could be "Clinician documentation does not provide the level of detail necessary for meeting or exceeding the three key components for a level 4 office or other outpatient evaluation and management service."

- **Recommendations:** Include any recommendations that have been created for process improvements. For example, if there is a coding error the recommendation may be to develop a coding compliance policy and provide staff education. If the findings have shown a failure to obtain precertification for a procedure, a recommendation may be to develop a list of procedures that require precertification, post the list, and educate staff.

- **Cost of Recommendation:** A fact-based estimate of the costs of the recommendations should be included here, including the salary and benefits of additional staff, equipment upgrade, educational materials, etc. If clinician training is recommended, some executives require that the lost revenue from the clinician being unavailable to see patients is also included.

- **Action Plan:** Again, in the situation above, the action plan may be to develop training materials for clinician education or to purchase evaluation and management training.

- **Implementation Date:**

- **Reevaluation Date:**

Calculate Potential Risks to Lost Revenue or Revenue at Risk

As stated above, the amount of risk or loss of revenue should be determined. Not only should the practice determine the specific amount associated with the audit but should also determine an extrapolated—or the possible cumulative amount—that is involved. This is very important because it can stress the impact that the error is having on the financial health of the practice. Also, remember to not only include those services that result in dollars at risk (overcoding) but also those errors that resulted in lost revenue (downcoding). For example, an audit found that 22 out of 100 records (22 percent) were assigned a level 4 visit inappropriately. Of those 22 records, six were undercoded by one level of service, 15 were overcoded by one level, and one encounter was overcoded by two levels. Each level has a $25 payment differential. The extrapolated dollar value would be calculated as follows:

Records undercoded (lost revenue)	6 x $25 = $150
Records overcoded by one level (at risk revenue)	15 x $25 = $375
Records overcoded by two levels (at risk revenue)	1 x $50 = $50
Total Financial Impact	$150 - $-425 = $-275

To extrapolate the dollar amount, many offices use the total number of times a service or procedure was performed the year before. If a level 4 E/M service was billed 32,000 times in the previous year, the following figures could be determined based on the audit:

Records undercoded (lost revenue)	1,920 x $25 = $48,000
Records overcoded by one level (at risk revenue)	4,800 x $25 = $120,000
Records overcoded by two levels (at risk revenue)	320 x $50 = $16,000
Total Financial Impact	$48,000 - $-136,000 = $-88,000

Determine the Root Cause of the Error

Determining the root cause of an error can be as simple as noting a transposed code number to as complex as trying to differentiate between two similar procedures. Careful attention should be given to the documentation, as well as official coding guidelines and guidance from third-party payers. Determining the root cause may also require the assistance of other departments or staff members. For example, it may be necessary to ask the laboratory technician about the differences between methodologies of a particular lab test and an explanation of the type of testing that is performed within the office, and provide coders with the information necessary to assign the correct code based upon test methodology.

Develop Recommendations for a Corrective Action

The type of corrective action plan is totally dependent on the type of error. If a coding error, the simplest corrective action is education and the development of coding policies and procedures that are included in the practice's compliance manual.

Written standards, policies, and procedures are an essential component to correct coding and billing and ultimately appropriate reimbursement. Compliance policies should identify the services commonly ordered within the practice, as well as those that are at risk for inappropriate coding and billing, such as those that are found to have errors during an audit. The policies should include payer regulations and policies, as well as official coding guidelines. In some instances, medical record documentation should be addressed including examples of what is necessary to support code assignment. Compliance policies should also include issues such as medical necessity and coverage issues, proper use of modifiers, improper discounting, and unbundling issues.

The Office of Inspector General for Health and Human Services strongly recommends that physician practices develop compliance plans. The OIG believes that this is one initiative in preventing the submission of erroneous claims and in combating fraudulent conduct. The OIG recommends the following as components of a compliance plan:

- Conducting internal monitoring and auditing
- Implementing compliance and practice standards
- Designating a compliance officer or contact
- Conducting appropriate training and education
- Developing open lines of communication
- Enforcing disciplinary standards through well-publicized guidelines

The OIG published the OIG Compliance Program for Individual and Small Group Physician Practices in the October 5, 2000 *Federal Register,* which can be found at http://oig.hhs.gov/authorities/docs/physician.pdf.

Practices should also develop policies and procedures that include the proper steps for all major activities within the practice, including but not limited to such items as:

- Patient registration
- Collection of copayment
- Billing procedures
- Precertification
- Insurance validation
- Bad debt policies
- Collection of deductibles
- Financial hardship determinations
- Payment adjustments

The following is a sample of what a coding compliance policy could look like:

Facet Joint Injections

Coding Guidance
Facet joint injections should be reported using the appropriate codes from range 64490-64495. Correct code selection is dependent upon:

- Level of the spine injected
- Number of levels reported
- Whether the service was performed unilaterally or bilaterally

Single Level
A single level injection occurs when the physician administers one or more substances to a level using one or more needles. A physician may insert a needle and attach a small tube through which the first substance is administered via a syringe. The physician may then change out the syringe and administer a second substance. However, only one needle puncture is performed.

In another method, the physician inserts the needle, administers a substance, and then removes the needle and makes a second puncture with a new needle and syringe to administer an additional substance. Despite the fact that there are two puncture sites, only a single level is being treated.

In these scenarios, correct code selection is also contingent upon the specific area of the spine being treated. If the cervical or thoracic spine is treated, report 64490–64492; for the lumbar or sacral spine areas, report 64493–64495.

Multiple Levels
When the physician injects multiple levels of the spine, add-on codes 64491–64492 and 64494–64495, respectively, are reported.

Bilateral Injections
Modifier 50 should be appended when the documentation states that injections were made on the same level but on different sides. Add-on codes 64491–64492 or 64494–64495 should be reported twice when the documentation indicates that the injections were performed bilaterally. Do not report with modifier 50.

Anesthetic/Steroids
Report the name and dosage of the anesthetic agent and/or steroid agent administered with the appropriate HCPCS Level II code separately.

Modifier Guidelines
Append modifier 50 when documentation indicates that the injection was performed bilaterally.

According to the Medicare Physician Fee Schedule Database for 2020, the standard multiple procedure (modifier 51) and standard bilateral surgery adjustments apply to these codes.

Assistant at surgery (modifiers 80, 81, and 82) may be paid for these procedures. Cosurgery (modifier 62), and surgical team (modifier 66) concepts do not apply and therefore would not be paid separately.

Billing Guidelines
According to the National Correct Coding Initiative, this procedure may be billed when performed at the same time as another distinct service. Modifier 59

or an X{EPSU} modifier should be indicated on the claim to prevent denial. For more information on modifier 59 and the proper requirements for reporting, refer to modifier 59 in chapter 3.

Documentation

Medical record documentation should contain information regarding the preoperative evaluation leading to suspicion of the presence of facet joint pathology, as well as the provider's postoperative conclusions.

In addition, the anatomical area of the spine and the exact location of the injection site should be clearly notated, as well as the specific name and dosage of the anesthetic agent and/or steroid administered.

Local/National Coverage Issues

The following guidelines are contained in the local coverage determination effective January 8, 2019.

Indications and Limitations of Coverage and/or Medical Necessity

Medicare considers facet joint blocks to be reasonable and necessary for chronic pain (persistent pain for three (3) months or greater) suspected to originate from the facet joint. Facet joint block is one of the methods used to document/confirm suspicions of posterior element biomechanical pain of the spine. Hallmarks of posterior element biomechanical pain are as follows:

- The pain does not have a strong radicular component.
- There is no associated neurological deficit and the pain is aggravated by hyperextension, rotation, or lateral bending of the spine, depending on the orientation of the facet joint at that level.

A paravertebral facet joint represents the articulation of the posterior elements of one vertebra with its neighboring vertebrae. For purposes of this Local Coverage Determination (LCD), the facet joint is noted at a specific level by the vertebrae that form it (e.g., C4-5 or L2-3). It is further noted that there are two (2) facet joints at each level, left and right.

During a paravertebral facet joint block procedure, a needle is placed in the facet joint or along the medial branches that innervate the joints under fluoroscopic guidance and a local anesthetic and/or steroid is injected. After the injection(s) has been performed, the patient is asked to indulge in the activities that usually aggravate his/her pain and to record his/her impressions of the effect of the procedure. Temporary or prolonged abolition of the pain suggests that the facet joints are the source of the symptoms and appropriate treatment may be prescribed in the future. Some patients have long-lasting relief with local anesthetic and steroid; others require a denervation procedure for more permanent relief. Before proceeding to a denervation treatment, the patient should experience at least a 50 percent reduction in symptoms for the duration of the local anesthetic effect.

Diagnostic or therapeutic injections/nerve blocks may be required for the management of chronic pain. It may take multiple nerve blocks targeting different anatomic structures to establish the etiology of the chronic pain in a given patient. It is standard medical practice to use the modality most likely to establish the diagnosis or treat the presumptive diagnosis. If the first set of procedures fails to produce the desired effect or to rule out the diagnosis, the provider should proceed to the next logical test or treatment indicated. For the purpose of this paravertebral facet joint block LCD, an anatomic region is defined per the CPT® book as cervical/thoracic (64490, 64491, 64492) or lumbar/sacral (64493, 64494, 64495).

Limitations

Medicare does not expect that an epidural block or sympathetic block would be provided to a patient on the same day as facet joint injections. Multiple blocks on the same day can lead to an improper diagnosis or no diagnosis. Coverage will be extended for only one type of procedure during one day/session of treatment unless the patient has recently discontinued anticoagulant therapy for the purpose of interventional pain management.

Diagnostic Phase

- Procedures performed during the diagnostic phase should be limited to three (3) levels (whether unilateral or bilateral) for each anatomical region as defined in this LCD on any given date of service.

- A diagnostic block can be repeated once, at any given level, at least one week (preferably two weeks) after the first block. If repeated, strong consideration should be given to utilizing administration of an anesthetic of different duration of action. (This helps confirm the validity of the diagnostic facet block and may reduce the incidence of false positive responses due to placebo effect).

- Once a structure is proven to be negative as a pain generator, no repeat interventions should be directed at that structure unless there is a new clinical presentation with symptoms, signs, and diagnostic studies of known reliability and validity that implicate the structure.

Therapeutic Phase

- Other interventional pain management procedures done on the same day as paravertebral facet joint blocks should be rare. In certain circumstances a patient may present with both facet and sacroiliac problems. In this case, it is appropriate to perform both facet injections and SI injection at the same session assuming that these are therapeutic injections and that prior diagnostic injections (blocks) have demonstrated that both structures contribute to pain generation.

- The medical record must clearly support both procedures. It is recognized that this is not common, and the frequency with which these codes are combined will be monitored. Multiple procedure modifiers will apply to intra-articular sacroiliac injection.

Paravertebral blocks, facet joint injections, and medial branch blocks per Current Procedural Terminology (CPT) should be performed utilizing direct visualization with fluoroscopy and documented. Blocks performed without the use of fluoroscopy are considered not medically necessary. Per CPT, imaging guidance (fluoroscopy CT) and any injection of contrast are inclusive components of 64490-64495.

The CMS *Internet-Only Manual* (IOM) Pub.100-08, *Program Integrity Manual*, Chapter 13, Section 5.1, outlines that "reasonable and necessary" services are "ordered and/or furnished by qualified personnel." Services are considered medically reasonable and necessary only if performed by appropriately trained providers. A qualified physician for this service/procedure is defined as follows: 1) Physician is properly enrolled in Medicare. 2) Training and expertise must have been acquired within the framework of an accredited residency and/or fellowship program in the applicable specialty/subspecialty in the United States or must reflect equivalent education, training, and expertise endorsed by an academic institution in the United States and/or by the applicable specialty/subspecialty society in the United States.

ICD-10-CM Codes that Support Medical Necessity

Medicare is establishing the following limited coverage for CPT/HCPCS codes 64490, 64491, 64492, 64493, 64494, and 64495:

M25.50	Pain in unspecified joint
M47.14–M47.16	Other spondylosis with myelopathy, thoracic region—Other spondylosis with myelopathy, lumbar region
M47.21–M47.818	Other spondylosis with radiculopathy, occipito-atlanto-axial region—Spondylosis without myelopathy or radiculopathy, sacral and sacrococcygeal region
M47.891–M47.898	Other spondylosis, occipito-atlanto-axial region—Other spondylosis, sacral and sacrococcygeal region
M54.03–M54.09	Panniculitis affecting regions of neck and back, cervicothoracic region—Panniculitis affecting regions, neck and back, multiple sites in spine
M54.2	Cervicalgia
M54.5	Low back pain
M54.6	Pain in thoracic spine
M62.830	Muscle spasm of back
M96.1	Postlaminectomy syndrome, not elsewhere classified
Z79.01*	Long term (current) use of anticoagulants

* Use only as a supplemental code in addition to primary diagnosis, when anticoagulant therapy has been discontinued to facilitate therapeutic injections for pain management.

Documentation Requirements

Medical necessity for providing the service must be clearly documented in the patient's medical records.

Assessment of the outcome of this procedure depends on the patient's responses, therefore documentation should include:

- Whether the block was a diagnostic or therapeutic injection
- Pre- and postoperative evaluation of patient
- Patient education
- Subjective and objective responses from the patient regarding pain, including facet pain provocative maneuvers documented by pre-and postoperative measurement

According to ASIPP guidelines, a positive response to the paravertebral facet joint block is noted when a greater than 50 percent relief of pain is obtained.

Placement of the needle at the facet joint must be performed under the fluoroscopic guidance to ensure safety and accuracy of the injection procedure, and this must be documented in the patient's medical record.

Official Resources

CPT Assistant, August 2010, American Medical Association

Local Coverage Determination, L33930-Paravertebral Facet Joint Blocks, First Coast Service Options, Inc.

Local Coverage Determination, L34993-Facet Joint Injections, Medial Branch Blocks, and Facet Joint Radiofrequency Neurotomy, Noridian Healthcare Solutions, LLC

Medicare Payments for Facet Joint Injection Service, Office of Inspector General, OEI-05-07-00200, September 2008

Medicare Physician Fee Schedule Database, 2019

Medicare Transmittal 526, July 31, 2009, Centers for Medicare and Medicaid Services

National Correct Coding Initiative, Version 26.0

Audit and Monitoring

Last Review Date
01/01/2021

Reviewer
Mary Smith

Findings
An audit of 30 randomly selected facet joint injections was performed. The results revealed that for one claim the correct HCPCS Level II code for the steroid injection was not reported on the claim.

Corrective Action (Including Education)
None needed at this time.

Next Review Due
N/A

Implement Action Plan

Once an action plan is developed it should be reviewed by all parties involved. Any action plan should include steps that not only prevent problems from occurring, but most importantly, work well within the structure of the practice. If any action plan calls for the incorrect staff member to complete a task, it more than likely will not be performed. Likewise, staff may be able to identify areas where a step is too cumbersome and how to make it more manageable. If a process does not fit within the daily activities, it more than likely won't be performed.

When writing an action plan:

- **Determine who the plan is for.** If you are looking for a general plan to make sure the appropriate data is collected, the plan should identify the information needed but be broad enough to allow staff to identify esoteric objectives. However, if something is more specific such as precertification, a statement simply saying precertify procedures does not provide the necessary information the staff needs to determine which procedures need to be precertified and who should to perform it. Instead, provide a list of the procedures that should be precertified, identify who is responsible for precertifying the procedure, a form or template to use, and supply the contact information for the payers.

- **What are the costs?** If you suspect that the action plan will incur costs, try to identify where the costs lie and to predict how much the cost will be with estimate-based research. For example, if you know that a specific computer upgrade is necessary, call the vendor for an estimated cost of the software.

- **Stick to the point.** Write the action plan in a series of bullet-points, single-sentence actionable items. After each bullet, expand on the idea as much as possible and, if applicable, assign team members by name to each task based on their skills and abilities. Expanded points should include simple actionable steps, as well as broader directives. If unsure if an employee or coworker is up to a given task, be direct and ask if they think it is an appropriate fit for their position and if not, why.

Also, it is important to remember to keep action plans clear and concise. Try to make them short and to the point, while at the same time providing enough information so that the objectives and outcomes are clearly defined. Additional information, such as the individual steps to accomplish the goal, can be included in the policy and procedure manual or the compliance manual, or both.

Reevaluation

Once a corrective action has been put into place, a second review should be performed to determine whether the corrective action is having the desired effect.

Before performing the reevaluation, the appropriate time should have passed. Reevaluating too early means that there may not be enough records to determine if the corrective action is working. Reevaluating too late could mean that the corrective action is not working and the problem has only exacerbated.

© 2020 Optum360, LLC

For example, if a corrective action has been put in place for a coding issue, determine how frequently that procedure is performed before deciding when to reevaluate the effectiveness of the policy. If a procedure is performed 25 times a day, it can be reviewed much sooner than one that is performed 25 times a month.

Until such time as there are enough records to be reviewed, it is advisable to monitor the corrective action. Staff involved should be queried for the input and advice as to how the policies and procedures developed are working and what if any modifications are necessary. Also determine if there is any impact on other processes. Fixing one process could potentially "break" something somewhere else within the practice. Understanding the bigger picture and interacting with other departments helps to avoid potential problems.

Appendix 1. **Audit Worksheets**

Electronic Copies of Auditing Worksheets

This edition of the *Auditors' Desk Reference* includes access to Microsoft Word formatted copies of the auditing worksheets found in this manual. To access these worksheets go to this address:
www.optum360coding.com/2021AUDRWorksheets
Please use the following password to access updates: o360audr21

Customers are permitted to reproduce these worksheets for use within their own facility or medical practice. Wider licensing of this content is available. Other distribution is prohibited.

These audit worksheets can be used when auditing the different areas of CPT® codes.

Modifier Worksheet

The following worksheet may be used to collect the necessary data when auditing a medical record for modifier use.

Modifier Worksheet

Account/medical record number:

Date of service:

Date of review:

Reviewer:

Type of review:

Documentation						
	Supports Modifier Assignment		**Provides Necessary Detail**		**Authenticated**		**Comments**
	Yes	No	Yes	No	Yes	No	
Modifier							
Modifier							
Modifier							
Modifier							
Modifier							

Assignment

	Correct Modifier Assigned		Appended to Correct Code		Valid for Procedure		Guidelines Applied		No Code Describing Service		Comments
	Yes	No	Yes	No	Yes	No	Yes	No	Yes	No	
Modifier											
Modifier											
Modifier											
Modifier											

Reimbursement

	Fee Revisions Made		Comments
	Yes	No	
Modifier			
Modifier			
Modifier			
Modifier			

Payer Issues

	Modifier Processed		Payment Adjustment Made Correctly		Prevent Denial		Comments
	Yes	No	Yes	No	Yes	No	
Modifier							
Modifier							
Modifier							
Modifier							

Claim Issues

	Indicated on Claim Correctly		Claim Attachments Submitted			Payer Inquiries Responded To			Comments
	Yes	No	Yes	No	N/A	Yes	No	N/A	
Modifier									
Modifier									
Modifier									
Modifier									

Evaluation and Management Services Worksheets

Office and Other Outpatient Services Audit Worksheet
The following worksheet may be used to collect the necessary data when auditing a medical record for office and other outpatient services (99202–99205 and 99212–99215).

Record Number			DOS billed	
Attending		Signed Yes ❑ No ❑	DOS Rendered	

E/M Billed	E/M Documented	E/M Mod Bill		E/M Mod Doc	

Incident to:

When a yes is answered for **all** of the following, the service may be billed as incident to under Medicare guidelines.	Yes	No
Is the NPP an employee of the practice?	❑	❑
If this is a new patient, did the physician participate in the patient's care?	❑	❑
Was direct personal supervision by the physician provided for in-office encounters?	❑	❑
Does the physician have an active part in the ongoing care of the patient?	❑	❑

Shared Services:

For a service to be considered shared, **all** of the following questions must have an answer of yes.

	Yes	No
Are the NPP and physician employed by the same practice?	❑	❑
Are the clinically relevant portions of the E/M service documented by the physician?	❑	❑
Is there documentation from the physician for this encounter?	❑	❑
Is the physician documentation tied to the NPP's documentation?	❑	❑

History	Was a medically appropriate history documented? Yes ❑ No ❑
Examination	Was a medically appropriate exam documented? Yes ❑ No ❑

		Medical Decision Making		
Code	Level of MDM (Based on 2 out of 3 Elements of MDM)	Number and Complexity of Problems Addressed	Amount and/or Complexity of Data to be Reviewed and Analyzed *Each unique test, order, or document contributes to the combination of 2 or combination of 3 in Category 1 below.*	Risk of Complications and/or Morbidity or Mortality of Patient Management
99211 ❏	N/A	N/A	N/A	N/A
99202 ❏ 99212 ❏	Straight-forward	**Minimal** ❏ 1 self-limited or minor problem	❏ **Minimal or none**	❏ Minimal risk of morbidity from additional diagnostic testing or treatment
99203 ❏ 99213 ❏	Low	**Low** ❏ 2 or more self-limited or minor problems; or ❏ 1 stable chronic illness; or ❏ 1 acute, uncomplicated illness or injury	❏ **Limited** *(Must meet the requirements of at least 1 of the 2 categories)* ❏ **Category 1: Tests and documents** • **Any combination of 2 from the following:** • Review of prior external note(s) from each unique source* • Review of the result(s) of each unique test* • Ordering of each unique test* **or** ❏ **Category 2: Assessment requiring an independent historian(s)** *(For the categories of independent interpretation of tests and discussionof management or test interpretation, see moderate or high)*	❏ Low risk of morbidity from additional diagnostic testing or treatment
99204 ❏ 99214 ❏	Moderate	**Moderate** ❏ 1 or more chronic illnesses with exacerbation, progression, or side effects of treatment; or ❏ 2 or more stable chronic illnesses; or ❏ 1 undiagnosed new problem with uncertain prognosis; or ❏ 1 acute illness with systemic symptoms; or ❏ 1 acute complicated injury	❏ **Moderate** *(Must meet the requirements of at least 1 out of 3 categories)* ❏ **Category 1: Tests, documents, or independent historian(s)** • **Any combination of 3 from the following:** • Review of prior external note(s) from each unique source* • Review of the result(s) of each unique test* • Ordering of each unique test* • Assessment requiring an independent historian(s) **or** ❏ **Category 2: Independent interpretation of tests** • Independent interpretation of a test performed by another physician/other qualified health care professional (not separately reported) **or** ❏ **Category 3: Discussion of management or test interpretation** • Discussion of management or test interpretation with external physician/other qualified health care professional\appropriate source (not separately reported)	❏ Moderate risk of morbidity from additional diagnostic testing or treatment *Examples only:* • Prescription drug management • Decision regarding minor surgery with identified patient or procedure risk factors • Decision regarding elective major surgery without identified patient or procedure risk factors • Diagnosis or treatment significantly limited by social determinants of health

*   Note: Test panels such as 80047 are counted as a single laboratory test. The differentiation between single or multiple unique tests is defined in accordance with the CPT code set.

			Medical Decision Making	
Code	Level of MDM (Based on 2 out of 3 Elements of MDM)	Number and Complexity of Problems Addressed	Amount and/or Complexity of Data to be Reviewed and Analyzed *Each unique test, order, or document contributes to the combination of 2 or combination of 3 in Category 1 below.*	Risk of Complications and/or Morbidity or Mortality of Patient Management
99205 ❏ 99215 ❏	High	**High** ❏ 1 or more chronic illnesses with severe exacerbation, progression, or side effects of treatment; **or** ❏ 1 acute or chronic illness or injury that poses a threat to life or bodily function	**Extensive** *(Must meet the requirements of at least 2 out of 3 categories)* ❏ **Category 1: Tests, documents, or independent historian(s)** • **Any combination of 3 from the following:** • Review of prior external note(s) from each unique source*; • Review of the result(s) of each unique test*; • Ordering of each unique test*; • Assessment requiring an independent historian(s) **or** ❏ **Category 2: Independent interpretation of tests** • Independent interpretation of a test performed by another physician/other qualified health care professional (not separately reported) **or** ❏ **Category 3: Discussion of management or test interpretation** • Discussion of management or test interpretation with external physician/other qualified health care professional/appropriate source (not separately reported)	❏ **High risk of morbidity from additional diagnostic testing or treatment** *Examples only:* • Drug therapy requiring intensive monitoring for toxicity • Decision regarding elective major surgery with identified patient or procedure risk factors • Decision regarding emergency major surgery • Decision regarding hospitalization • Decision not to resuscitate or to de-escalate care because of poor prognosis

* Note: Test panels such as 80047 are counted as a single laboratory test. The differentiation between single or multiple unique tests is defined in accordance with the CPT code set.

Office and Other Outpatient Services Audit Worksheet – Time Only Reporting

Record Number			DOS billed	
Attending		Signed Yes ❏ No ❏	DOS Rendered	

History	Was a medically appropriate history documented? Yes ❏ No ❏
Examination	Was a medically appropriate exam documented? Yes ❏ No ❏

The table below shows the time required for each code.

Code	History & Exam	Medical Decision Making	Time in Minutes
99202	Medically appropriate	Straightforward	15–29
99203	Medically appropriate	Low level	30–44
99204	Medically appropriate	Moderate level	45–59
99205	Medically appropriate	High level	60–74
99211*	N/A	N/A	N/A
99212	Medically appropriate	Straightforward	10–19
99213	Medically appropriate	Low level	20–29
99214	Medically appropriate	Moderate level	30–39
99215	Medically appropriate	High level	40–54

*Physician presence is not required; presenting problems are minimal

The following activities are included in the provider's time when performed:
- ❏ Preparing to see the patient (e.g., review of tests)
- ❏ Performing a medically appropriate examination and/or evaluation
- ❏ Care coordination (not reported separately)
- ❏ Counseling and educating the patient/family/caregiver
- ❏ Documenting clinical information in the electronic or other health record
- ❏ Independently interpreting results (not reported separately) and communicating results to the patient/family/caregiver
- ❏ Obtaining and/or reviewing separately obtained history
- ❏ Ordering medications, tests, or procedures
- ❏ Referring and communicating with other health care professionals

Was code 99417 reported for prolonged services? Yes ❏ No ❏

The table below shows the time required to report each unit of 99417 in addition to 99205 or 99215.

New Patient	Code
60–74 minutes	99205
75–89 minutes	99205 x1 and 99417 x1
90–104 minutes	99205 x1 and 99417 x2
105 or more minutes	99205 x1 and 99417 x3 or more for each additional 15 minutes
Established Patient	**Code**
40–54 minutes	99215
55–69 minutes	99215 x1 and 99417 x1
70–84 minutes	99215 x1 and 99417 x2
85 or more minutes	99215 x1 and 99417 x3 or more for each additional 15 minutes

Code Assigned	Units	Code Documented	Units

Financial Impact			
Undercoding		Overcoding	
Code	Payment	Code	Payment
		Total Impact on Claim	

1995 Guidelines Audit Worksheet

The following worksheet may be used to collect the necessary data when auditing a medical record for evaluation and management services, excluding Office and Other Outpatient Services (99202–99205 and 99212–99215). For codes 99202–99205 and 99212–99215, see the audit worksheet on page 663.

Record Number				DOS billed	
Attending		Signed	Yes ❏ No ❏	DOS Rendered	

Incident to:

When a yes is answered for all of the following, the service may be billed as incident to under Medicare guidelines.

	Yes	No
Is the NPP an employee of the practice?	❏	❏
If this is a new patient, did the physician participate in the patient's care?	❏	❏
Was direct personal supervision by the physician provided for in-office encounters?	❏	❏
Does the physician have an active part in the ongoing care of the patient?	❏	❏

Shared Services:

For a service to be considered shared, the following questions must have a yes answer.

Was the service rendered at one of the sites identified below:	Yes	No
Inpatient	❏	❏
Outpatient	❏	❏
Emergency dept	❏	❏
Are the NPP and physician employed by the same practice?	❏	❏
Are the clinically relevant portions of the E/M service documented by the physician?	❏	❏
Is there documentation from the physician for this encounter?	❏	❏
Is the physician documentation tied to the NPP's documentation?	❏	❏

E/M Billed		E/M Doc		E/M Mod Bill		E/M Mod Doc			
History						Prob Foc	Exp Prob	Detailed	Compre-hensive
HPI—History of Present Illness Elements						Brief	Brief	Extend	Extend
Location		Severity		Timing		Modifying Factors	(1-3)	(1-3)	(4+)	(4+)
Quality		Duration		Context		Associated Signs and Symptoms				
ROS—Review of Systems Worksheet Signed ☐ Yes ☐ No Dated ☐ Yes ☐ No						None	Prob Pert (1)	Extend (2-9)	Comp (10+)
Constitu-tional	C/V		GU		Neuro	Endocrine				
Eyes	Respiratory		Musc		Psych	Allergy/Immun				
ENMT	GI		Integ		Heme/Lymph					
PFSH—Past medical, past family, social history						None	None	Pertinent (1)	Complete (2-3)
Past History—the patient's past experience with operations, illness, injuries and treatments									
Family History—a review of medical events in the patient's family, including diseases which may be hereditary or place the patient at risk									
Social History—an age appropriate review of past and current activities									

Exam Portion

Body Areas						Prob Foc	Exp Prob	Detailed	Compre-hensive
Head		Chest, breast, axilla	Abdomen		Back w/spine		1	(2-7)	(2-7)	8+
Neck			Genitalia		Each Extremity		Number			
Organ Systems									
Constitu-tional	ENMT		Respira-tory		Musculo	Psych				
Eyes	Cardio-vascular		GI		Skin	Heme Lymph Immuno				
			GU		Neuro					

Medical Decision Making

Diagnoses/ Management Options		Total	Amount/ Complexity of Data		MDM Grid				
Self limited/minor (2 max)	X1		Lab test (ordered or reviewed)	1	Dx/Mgt	0-1	2	3	4+
Est Prob/Stable	X1		X-ray (ordered or reviewed)	1	Data	0-1	2	3	4+
Est Prob/Worsening	X2		Medical proc (ordered or reviewed)	1	Risk	Min	Low	Mod	High
New Prob no workup (3 max)	X3		Discuss test w/perform phys	1	Final	Stfd	Low	Mod	High
New Prob additional workup	X4		Obtain old MR/hx other source	1					
Visit Time			Review/summarize old MR	2	Code Billed				
			Independent visualization	2	Code Documented				

Counseling Documented ❑ Yes ❑ No

Table of Risk Medical Decision Making

Level of Risk	Presenting Problem(s)	Diagnostic Procedure(s) Ordered	Management Options Selected
Minimal	One self-limited or minor problem (e.g., common cold, insect bite, tinea corporis)	• Laboratory test requiring venipuncture • Chest x-rays • EKG/EEG • Urinalysis • Ultrasound (e.g., echocardiography) • KOH prep	• Rest • Gargles • Elastic bandages • Superficial dressings
Low	• Two or more self-limited or minor problems • One stable chronic illness (e.g., well controlled hypertension, non-insulin-dependent diabetes, cataract, BPH) • Acute, uncomplicated illness or injury (e.g., cystitis, allergic rhinitis, simple sprain)	• Physiologic tests not under stress (e.g., pulmonary function tests) • Non-cardiovascular imaging studies with contrast (e.g., barium enema) • Superficial needle biopsies • Clinical laboratory tests requiring arterial puncture • Skin biopsies	• Over-the-counter drugs • Minor surgery with no identified risk factors • Physical therapy • Occupational therapy • IV fluids without additives

Level of Risk	Presenting Problem(s)	Diagnostic Procedure(s) Ordered	Management Options Selected
Moderate	• One or more chronic illnesses with mild exacerbation, progression or side effects of treatment • Two or more stable chronic illnesses • Undiagnosed new problem with uncertain prognosis (e.g., lump in breast) • Acute illness with systemic symptoms (e.g., pyelonephritis, pneumonitis, colitis) • Acute complicated injury (e.g., head injury with brief loss of consciousness)	• Physiologic tests under stress (e.g., cardiac stress test, fetal contraction stress test) • Diagnostic endoscopies with no identified risk factors • Deep needle or incisional biopsy • Cardiovascular imaging studies with contrast and no identified risk factors (e.g., arteriogram, cardiac catheterization) • Obtain fluid from body cavity (e.g., lumbar puncture, thoracentesis, culdocentesis)	• Minor surgery with identified risk factors • Elective major surgery (open, percutaneous or endoscopic) with no identified risk factors • Prescription drug management • Therapeutic nuclear medicine • IV fluids with additives • Closed treatment of fracture or dislocation without manipulation
High	• One or more chronic illnesses with severe exacerbation, progression or side effects of treatment • Acute or chronic illnesses or injuries that may pose a threat to life or bodily function (e.g., multiple trauma, acute MI, pulmonary embolus, severe respiratory distress, progressive severe rheumatoid arthritis, psychiatric illness with potential threat to self or others, peritonitis, acute renal failure) • An abrupt change in neurologic status (e.g., seizure, TIA, weakness, or sensory loss)	• Cardiovascular imaging studies with contrast with identified risk factors • Cardiac electrophysiological tests • Diagnostic endoscopies with identified risk factors • Discography	• Elective major surgery (open, percutaneous or endoscopic) with identified risk factors • Emergency major surgery (open, percutaneous, or endoscopic) • Parenteral controlled substances • Drug therapy requiring intensive monitoring for toxicity • Decision not to resuscitate or to de-escalate care because of poor prognosis

Procedures—Supplies			Procedure Modifiers			ICD-10-CM		
	Billed	Documented		Billed	Documented		Billed	Documented
1			1			1		
2			2			2		
3			3			3		
4			4			4		

1997 General Multisystem—Audit Worksheet

Record Number				DOS billed	
Attending		Signed	Yes ❑ No ❑	DOS Rendered	

Incident to:

When a yes is answered for all of the following, the service may be billed as incident to under Medicare guidelines.

	Yes	No
Is the NPP an employee of the practice?	❑	❑
If this is a new patient, did the physician participate in the patient's care?	❑	❑
Was direct personal supervision by the physician provided for in-office encounters?	❑	❑
Does the physician have an active part in the ongoing care of the patient?	❑	❑

Shared Services:

For a service to be considered shared, the following questions must have a yes answer.

Was the service rendered at one of the sites identified below:	Yes	No
Inpatient	❑	❑
Outpatient	❑	❑
Emergency dept	❑	❑
Are the NPP and physician employed by the same practice?	❑	❑
Are the clinically relevant portions of the E/M service documented by the physician?	❑	❑
Is there documentation from the physician for this encounter?	❑	❑
Is the physician documentation tied to the NPP's documentation?	❑	❑

E/M Billed		E/M Doc		E/M Mod Bill			E/M Mod Doc			
History							Prob Foc	Exp Prob	Detailed	Compre-hensive
HPI—History of Present Illness Elements							Brief (1-3)	Brief (1-3)	Extend (4+)	Extend (4+)
Location		Severity		Timing		Modifying Factors				
Quality		Duration		Context		Associated Signs and Symptoms				
ROS—Review of Systems Worksheet Signed ☐ Yes ☐ No Dated ☐ Yes ☐ No							None	Prob Pert (1)	Extend (2-9)	Comp (10+)
Constitu-tional		Cardio-vascular		GU	Neuro	Endocrine				
Eyes		Respiratory		Musc	Psych	Allergy/ Immun				
ENMT		GI		Integ	Heme/ Lymph					
PFSH—Past medical, past family, social history							None	None	Pertinent (1)	Complete (2-3)
Past History—the patients past experience with operations, illness, injuries and treatments										
Family History—a review of medical events in the patient's family, including diseases which may be hereditary or place the patient at risk										
Social History—an age appropriate review of past and current activities										

Exam Portion

Constitutional	Neck	Chest (breasts)	Skin	Problem Focused
• 3 + VS • Gen appearance	• Neck • Thyroid	• Inspection of breasts • Palpation breasts and axillae	• Inspect skin and subq tissue • Palpate skin and subq	1–5 elements
Eyes • Conjunctivae and lids • Pupils and irises • Ophthalmoscopic exam	Respiratory • Respiratory effort • Percussion chest • Palpation chest • Auscultation lungs	Lymphatic (2+ areas) • Neck • Groin • Axillae • Other	Genitourinary—MALE • Scrotal contents • Penis • Digital rectal exam	Expanded Problem Focused 6 or more elements
ENMT • Ears and nose • Otoscopic exam • Assess hearing • Mucosa, septum, and turbinates • Lips, teeth, and gums • Oropharynx	Cardiovascular • Palpate heart • Auscultation heart • Carotid arteries • Abdominal aorta • Femoral arteries • Pedal pulse • Extremity edema/varicosities	Gastrointestinal (Abdomen) • Abdomen—mass/tenderness • Liver and spleen • Hernia present/absent • Anus, perineum, and rectum • Stool sample when indicated	Genitourinary—FEMALE • External genitalia • Urethra • Bladder • Cervix • Uterus • Adnexa/parametria	Detailed 2 or more elements from at least 6 areas/systems OR 12 or more elements from at least two areas/systems

Musculoskeletal
• Gait and station
• Digits and nails
• Exam Areas (1+ areas)
  – Head and neck
  – Spine/rib/pelvis
  – Rt upper ext
  – Lt upper ext
  – Rt lower ext
  – Lt lower ext
• Exam elements:
  – Inspect and palpate
  – Range of motion
  – Stability
  – Muscle strength and tone
*Note any abnormalities
		Neurologic
		• Cranial nerves—deficits
		• Deep tendon reflex and pathologic
		• Sensation
			Psychiatric
			• Judgment and insight
			• Mental status
			  – Orientation
			  – Memory recent/remote
			  – Mood and affect
				Comprehensive
				All elements in at least 9 areas/systems and for each area document at least 2 elements from the 9 areas/systems

Medical Decision Making

Diagnoses/ Management Options		Total	Amount/ Complexity of Data		MDM Grid				
Self limited/minor (2 max)	X1		Lab test (ordered or reviewed)	1	Dx/Mgt	0-1	2	3	4+
Est Prob/Stable	X1		X-ray (ordered or reviewed)	1	Data	0-1	2	3	4+
Est Prob/Worsening	X2		Medical proc (ordered or reviewed)	1	Risk	Min	Low	Mod	High
New Prob no workup (3 max)	X3		Discuss test w/perform phys	1	Final	Stfd	Low	Mod	High
New Prob additional workup	X4		Obtain old MR/hx other source	1	See Table of Risk below				
Visit Time			Review/summarize old MR	2	Code Billed				
			Independent visualization	2	Code Documented				

Total points: Minimal = 1 Limited = 2 Multiple = 3 Extensive = 4 or more

Counseling Documented ❏ Yes ❏ No Nature and extent of counseling and/or coordination of care

Table of Risk Medical Decision Making

Level of Risk	Presenting Problem(s)	Diagnostic Procedure(s) Ordered	Management Options Selected
Minimal	One self-limited or minor problem (e.g., common cold, insect bite, tinea corporis)	• Laboratory test requiring venipuncture • Chest x-rays • EKG/EEG • Urinalysis • Ultrasound (e.g., echocardiography) • KOH prep	• Rest • Gargles • Elastic bandages • Superficial dressings
Low	• Two or more self-limited or minor problems • One stable chronic illness (e.g., well controlled hypertension, non-insulin-dependent diabetes, cataract, BPH) • Acute, uncomplicated illness or injury (e.g., cystitis, allergic rhinitis, simple sprain)	• Physiologic tests not under stress (e.g., pulmonary function tests) • Non-cardiovascular imaging studies with contrast (e.g., barium enema) • Superficial needle biopsies • Clinical laboratory tests requiring arterial puncture • Skin biopsies	• Over-the-counter drugs • Minor surgery with no identified risk factors • Physical therapy • Occupational therapy • IV fluids without additives

Level of Risk	Presenting Problem(s)	Diagnostic Procedure(s) Ordered	Management Options Selected
Moderate	• One or more chronic illnesses with mild exacerbation, progression or side effects of treatment • Two or more stable chronic illnesses • Undiagnosed new problem with uncertain prognosis (e.g., lump in breast) • Acute illness with systemic symptoms (e.g., pyelonephritis, pneumonitis, colitis) • Acute complicated injury (e.g., head injury with brief loss of consciousness)	• Physiologic tests under stress (e.g., cardiac stress test, fetal contraction stress test) • Diagnostic endoscopies with no identified risk factors • Deep needle or incisional biopsy • Cardiovascular imaging studies with contrast and no identified risk factors (e.g., arteriogram, cardiac catheterization) • Obtain fluid from body cavity (e.g., lumbar puncture, thoracentesis, culdocentesis)	• Minor surgery with identified risk factors • Elective major surgery (open, percutaneous or endoscopic) with no identified risk factors • Prescription drug management • Therapeutic nuclear medicine • IV fluids with additives • Closed treatment of fracture or dislocation without manipulation
High	• One or more chronic illnesses with severe exacerbation, progression or side effects of treatment • Acute or chronic illnesses or injuries that may pose a threat to life or bodily function (e.g., multiple trauma, acute MI, pulmonary embolus, severe respiratory distress, progressive severe rheumatoid arthritis, psychiatric illness with potential threat to self or others, peritonitis, acute renal failure) • An abrupt change in neurologic status (e.g., seizure, TIA, weakness, or sensory loss)	• Cardiovascular imaging studies with contrast with identified risk factors • Cardiac electrophysiological tests • Diagnostic endoscopies with identified risk factors • Discography	• Elective major surgery (open, percutaneous or endoscopic) with identified risk factors • Emergency major surgery (open, percutaneous, or endoscopic) • Parenteral controlled substances • Drug therapy requiring intensive monitoring for toxicity • Decision not to resuscitate or to de-escalate care because of poor prognosis

Procedures—Supplies			Procedure Modifiers			ICD-9-CM		
	Billed	Documented		Billed	Documented		Billed	Documented
1			1			1		
2			2			2		
3			3			3		
4			4			4		

1997 Evaluation and Management Worksheet

The following tool can be used when auditing evaluation and management services to determine the level of each key component.

History

Patient History	Elements of History	Total
Chief complaint—CC	Concise statement describing symptom, problem, condition, diagnosis, physician recommended return, reason for visit, usually in patient's own words. Required for all levels.	
History of present illness—HPI	Location, quality, severity, duration, timing, context, modifying factors, associated signs and symptoms	
Review of systems—ROS	Constitutional symptoms, eyes, ears, nose, mouth, throat, cardiovascular, respiratory, gastrointestinal, genitourinary, musculoskeletal, integumentary (skin and/or breast), neurological, psychiatric, endocrine, hematologic/lymphatic, allergic/immunologic	
Past, family, and/or social history—PFSH	Past medical (patient history), family history, social history	

The level of history can be determined using this table.

CC	Present	Present	Present	Present
HPI	>=1	>=1	>=4	>=4
ROS	0	>=1	>=2	>=10
PFSH	0	0	>=1	>=2
E/M level of service	Problem focused	Expanded problem focused	Detailed	Comprehensive

Note: All history elements must correspond to the table above; if not, decrease the E/M level by one.

Examination

The level of history can be determined using this table.

Level of Exam	Total organ system(s) or body area(s)examined
Problem Focused 1–5 elements identified by a bullet (•) in one or more organ system(s) or body area(s)	
Expanded Problem Focused 6 or more elements identified by a bullet (•) in one or more organ system(s) or body area(s)	

Detailed
    2 or more elements identified by a bullet (•) from at least 6 areas/systems
    OR 12 or more elements identified by a bullet (•) from at least two areas/systems	

Comprehensive All elements identified by a bullet (•) in at least 9 areas/systems and documentation of at least 2 elements from the 9 areas/systems	

Number of Diagnoses or Management Options	Amount and/or Complexity of Data to Be Reviewed	Risk of Complications and/or Morbidity or Mortality	Type of Decision Marking
Minimal	Minimal or none	Minimal	Straightforward
Limited	Limited	Low	Low
Multiple	Moderate	Moderate	Moderate
Extensive	Extensive	High	High

Documentation of Critical Care Time

Patient's Name: _____

Patient's Medical Record Number: _____

The services I provided to this patient were provided to treat _____

(State the condition the patient was treated for)

The services I provided required the highest level of my skills with direct and personal management of the patient's treatment. These services included:
- ❏ Medical record documentation
- ❏ Vital sign assessments
- ❏ Medication orders and management
- ❏ Reviewing all notes and previous visits
- ❏ Collaborating with other physicians on treatment options
- ❏ Care, transfer of care, and discharge plans
- ❏ Interpreting/reviewing all tests and studies
- ❏ Discussions with family or surrogate decision makers
- ❏ Other
- ❏ _____

The total critical care time was_____hours _____minutes. The total time does not include treating other patients, performing separately reportable procedures, or activities that were not directly related to the care of the patient.

Physician's signature:_____ Date:_____

Critical Care Audit Worksheet

Patient's name: _____

Patient's medical record number: _____

Date of service: _____

Date of review: _____

Reviewer: _____

Type of review: ❏ Prepayment   ❏ Postpayment

Reason for encounter: _____

Type of vital organ failure:

- ❏ Central nervous system failure
- ❏ Circulatory failure
- ❏ Shock
- ❏ Renal
- ❏ Hepatic
- ❏ Metabolic
- ❏ Respiratory

Were any additional services documented? (This time is included in the total critical care time.)

- ❏ 36000 Introduction of needle or intracatheter, vein
- ❏ 36410 Venipuncture, age 3 years or older, necessitating physician's skill or other qualified health care professional (separate procedure), for diagnostic or therapeutic purposes
- ❏ 36415 Collection of venous blood by venipuncture
- ❏ 36591 Collection of blood specimen from a completely implantable venous access device
- ❏ 36600 Arterial puncture, withdrawal of blood for diagnosis
- ❏ 43752 Naso- or oro-gastric tube placement, requiring physician's skill and fluoroscopic guidance
- ❏ 43753 Gastric intubation and aspiration(s) therapeutic, necessitating physician's skill (e.g., for gastrointestinal hemorrhage), including lavage if performed
- ❏ 71045 Radiologic examination, chest; single view
- ❏ 71046 Radiologic examination, chest; 2 views
- ❏ 92953 Temporary transcutaneous pacing
- ❏ 93561 Indicator dilution studies such as dye or thermodilution, including arterial and/or venous catheterization; with cardiac output measurements
- ❏ 93562 Indicator dilution studies such as dye or thermodilution, including arterial and/or venous catheterization; subsequent measurement of cardiac output
- ❏ 94002 Ventilation assist and management, initiation of pressure or volume preset ventilators for assisted or controlled breathing; hospital inpatient/observation, initial day
- ❏ 94003 Ventilation assist and management, initiation of pressure or volume preset ventilators for assisted or controlled breathing; hospital inpatient/observation, each subsequent day
- ❏ 94004 Ventilation assist and management, initiation of pressure or volume preset ventilators for assisted or controlled breathing; nursing facility, per day
- ❏ 94660 Continuous positive airway pressure ventilation (CPAP), initiation and management
- ❏ 94662 Continuous negative pressure ventilation (CNP), initiation and management
- ❏ 94760 Noninvasive ear or pulse oximetry for oxygen saturation; single determination
- ❏ 94761 Noninvasive ear or pulse oximetry for oxygen saturation; multiple determinations (e.g., during exercise)
- ❏ 94762 Noninvasive ear or pulse oximetry for oxygen saturation; by continuous overnight monitoring

Time spent in Critical Care	Start Time	End Time	Total Time	Was provider in constant attendance when critical care was provided?	
				Yes ❏ No ❏ If no, critical care codes should not be reported.	

Code Assigned	Units	Code Documented	Units		Comments
99291					
99292					

Additional Procedures (not included in bundled list)	Code Assigned	Code Documented	Modifier Assigned	Modifier Documented	

Financial Impact				
Undercoding		**Overcoding**		
Code	Payment	Code	Payment	
				Total Impact on Claim

Surgical Auditing Worksheet

Account/medical record number: _____

Date of service: _____

Date of review: _____

Reviewer: _____

Type of review: _____

CPT Code Assignment					
Procedure	Code Assigned	Code Documented	Modifier Assigned	Modifier Documented	Comments

Place of Service				Number of Units			
Indicated on Claim		Documented		Indicated on Claim		Documented	

Billable Supplies						Nonbillable Supplies					
Under Coding			Overcoding			Undercoding			Overcoding		
Code	Payment		Code	Payment		Code	Payment		Code	Payment	
			Total Impact on Claim								

Radiology Auditing Worksheet

The following worksheet may be used to collect the necessary data when auditing radiology services.

Account/medical record number: _____

Date of service: _____

Date of review: _____

Reviewer: _____

Type of review: _____

CPT Code Assignment					
Procedure	Code Assignment	Code Documented	Modifier Assigned	Modifier Documented	Comments

Place of Service			Number of Units		
	Indicated on Claim	Documented		Indicated on Claim	Documented

Billable Supplies		Nonbillable Supplies	
Provided		Provided	
Billed		Billed	

Financial Impact					
Undercoding			Overcoding		
	Code	Payment		Code	Payment
					Total Impact on Claim

Laboratory Auditing Worksheet

The following worksheet may be used when auditing laboratory services.

Account/medical record number: _____

Date of service: _____

Date of review: _____

Reviewer: _____

Type of review: _____

	Yes	No
Order for lab test in chart		
Result of lab test		

CPT Code				
CPT Code Assigned	Unbundled or Exploded?		Corrected CPT Code	
	Yes	No		

Modifier Assignment					
CPT Code	Modifier Assigned	Appended to correct code	Valid for Procedure	Guidelines Applied	Comments

Medical Necessity						
	Yes	No	Yes	No	Yes	No
Condition Documented						
ICD-10-CM Code Assigned Correctly						
Corrected ICD-10-CM Code						
Completed and signed ABN						

Units

Number of Units Performed	Number of Units Billed	Corrected Number of Units

Financial Impact	
Revised CPT Codes	
Revised Modifier Assignment	
Revised Units	
Total	

Medicine Auditing Worksheet

Account/medical record number:

Date of service:

Date of review:

Reviewer:

Type of review:

Immunizations/Vaccines/Toxoids CPT Code Assignment						
Substance	Code Assignment	Code Documented	Face-to-Face Counseling Documented	E/M Service Documented	E/M Service Billed	Comments

Therapeutic/Prophylactic Injections CPT Code Assignment						
Substance	Code Assignment	Code Documented	Face-to-Face Counseling Documented	E/M Service Documented	E/M Service Billed	HCPCS Level II Code Reported

Number of Units		
Billed	Documented	Comments

Other Medical Services CPT Code Assignment					
Procedure	Code Assignment	Code Documented	Modifier Assigned	Modifier Documented	Comments

Place of Service				Number of Units		
Indicated on Claim		Documented		Indicated on Claim		Documented

Billable Supplies						Nonbillable Supplies					
Undercoding			Overcoding			Undercoding			Overcoding		
Code	Payment		Code	Payment		Code	Payment		Code	Payment	
				Total Impact on Claim							

Non-Chemotherapy Injections and Infusion Auditing Worksheet

Account/medical record number: _____

Date of service: _____

Date of review: _____

Reviewer: _____

Type of review: _____

Diagnosis		
Documented	**ICD-10-CM**	**Reported Code**

Therapeutic, prophylactic or diagnostic injection		
❑ Subcutaneous (96372)	❑ Intramuscular (96372)	❑ Intra-arterial (96373)

Substance administered:	
HCPCS code:	HCPCS code reported:
The number of units documented:	Number of units billed:
Push/Drip 15 minutes or less	**Time if documented**
❑ Intra-arterial (96373)	
Substance administered:	
HCPCS code:	HCPCS code reported:
Number of units documented:	Number of units billed:
❑ IV Push, initial or single substance (96374)	
Substance administered:	
HCPCS code:	HCPCS code reported:
Number of units documented:	Number of units billed:
❑ Each additions push of **new** substance (96375)	
Substance administered:	
HCPCS code:	HCPCS code reported:
Number of units documented:	Number of units billed:
Substance administered:	
HCPCS code:	HCPCS code reported:
Number of units documented:	Number of units billed:
Substance administered:	

HCPCS code:	HCPCS code reported:
Number of units documented:	Number of units billed:

| **IV Infusion** ||

❑ Up to one hour (96365)

Substance administered:

HCPCS code:	HCPCS code reported:
Number of units documented:	Number of units billed:

❑ Each additional hour (96366)

Substance administered:

HCPCS code:	HCPCS code reported:
Number of units documented:	Number of units billed:

❑ Each new drug/substance (96367)

Substance administered:

HCPCS code:	HCPCS code reported:
Number of units documented:	Number of units billed:

❑ Concurrent infusion (96368)

Substance administered:

HCPCS code:	HCPCS code reported:
Number of units documented:	Number of units billed:

| **Subcutaneous infusion** ||

❑ Up to one hour (96369)

Substance administered:

HCPCS code:	HCPCS code reported:
Number of units documented:	Number of units billed:

❑ Each additional hour (96370)

Substance administered:

HCPCS code:	HCPCS code reported:
Number of units documented:	Number of units billed:

❑ Additional pump set-up (not to be reported with initial pump set-up) (93671)

Fracture Care Audit Worksheet

Date of service: _____

Date of review: _____

Reviewer: _____

Type of review: _____

Anatomical site: _____

Laterality: _____

Type of Fracture		
❏ Closed	❏ Open	
❏ Transverse	❏ Spiral	
❏ Comminuted	❏ Impacted	
❏ Greenstick	❏ Oblique	
❏ Displaced	❏ Nondisplaced	❏ Routine
❏ Delayed Healing	❏ Nonunion	❏ Malunion

How Injury Occurred		

❏ Fall
  ❏ From ladder
  ❏ From bike
	❏ Playing Sports	

❏ Auto Accident		
Sequela Documented	❏ Yes	❏ No

Treatment Type		
❏ Open Treatment	❏ Skin Traction	❏ Grafting
❏ Closed Treatment	❏ Internal Fixation	❏ Re-reduction
❏ Manipulation	❏ External Fixation	❏ Casting/Splinting
❏ Skeletal Traction	❏ Percutaneous Fixation	

Supplies			
Documented:	HCPCS Code:		
Code Reported:	Payer Allows Reporting	❏ Yes	❏ No

Diagnosis		
Documented	**ICD-10-CM**	**Reported Code**

 © 2020 Optum360, LLC

Procedure		
Documented	**CPT/HCPCS Code**	**Reported Code**

Note: See modifier worksheets to determine if CPT modifier is requited.

Wound Repair Audit Worksheet

Anatomical site (When multiple wounds are repaired, list each)

_____

_____

_____

_____

Size of wound (When multiple wounds are repaired, list each)

_____

_____

_____

Is the wound badly contaminated?	❑ Yes	❑ No

_____

_____

_____

How Injury Occurred

❑ Fall	From
❑ Auto Accident	
❑ Play Sports	Type of sport
❑ Additional Cutting	Indicate object

Closure:

❑ Single

❑ Layered

❑ Graft

❑ Flap

_____

_____

Any complicating factors?	❑ Yes	❑ No

If you answered yes above, please list factors:

_____

_____

_____

How closure was accomplished

❑ Glue

❑ Suture

❑ Layered closure

_____

Supplies

Documented	❑ Yes	❑ No
HCPCS Code:	Code Reported:	
Payer Allows Reporting	❑ Yes	❑ No

Diagnosis		
Documented	**ICD-10-CM**	**Reported Code**

Procedure		
Documented	**CPT/HCPCS Code**	**Reported Code**

Note: See modifier worksheets to determine if CPT modifier is required.

Lower Endoscopy Auditing Tool

Patient's Name: _____ Patient's Medical Record Number: _____

Date of Service: _____

Preoperative Diagnosis: _____

Procedure performed: _____

Findings:_____

Postoperative Diagnosis_____

Procedure performed:_____

❑ Diagnostic   ❑ Screening

Surgical with:

❑ Removal of foreign body-Location _____   Substance injected:_____

❑ With biopsy(ies)-Location _____   _____

❑ With directed submucosal injections-Location _____   _____

Were any of the following performed:

❑ With control of bleeding (unrelated to surgical procedures)

❑ With removal of foreign body-Location _____

❑ With decompression of volvulus-Location _____

❑ With ablation of lesions at-Location _____

❑ With removal of lesion by:

     ❑ Snare -Location _____

     ❑ Hot biopsy -Location _____

     ❑ Bipolar Location _____

❑ Dilation by balloon - Location _____ size of balloon _____mm

❑ Stent Placement -Location _____

❑ Endoscopic ultrasound -Location _____

❑ Ultrasound guided intramural or transmural FNA/Bx -Location _____

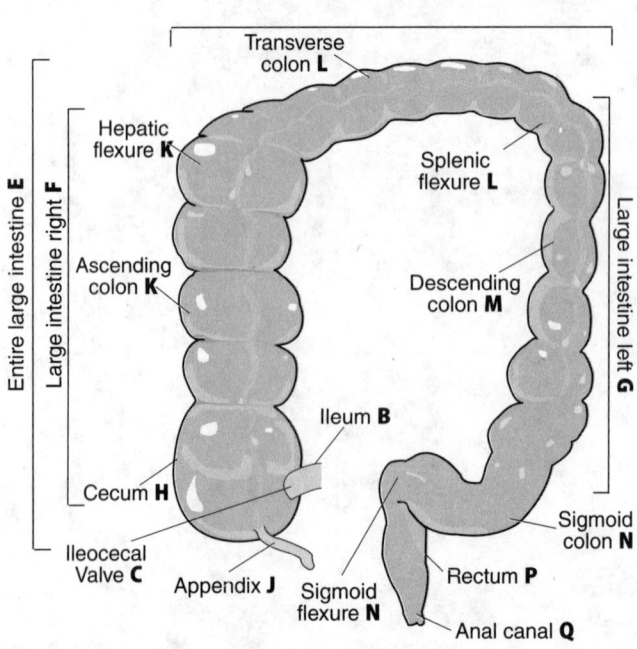

 © 2020 Optum360, LLC

Procedure	Code Assigned	Code Documented	Modifier Assigned	Modifier Documented	Comments

Number of Units		
Indicated on Claim	Documented	

Financial Impact			
Undercoding		Overcoding	
Code	Payment	Code	Payment
			Total Impact on Claim

Upper Endoscopy Auditing Tool

Patient's Name: _____ Patient's Medical Record Number: _____

Date of Service: _____

Preoperative Diagnosis: _____

Procedure performed: _____

Findings: _____

Postoperative Diagnosis _____

Procedure performed: _____

   ❏ Diagnostic   ❏ Screening

What kind of scope was the procedure performed with:

   ❏ Flexible, transnasal   ❏ Flexible, transoral   ❏ Rigid, transoral

Were any of the following performed:

   ❏ Biopsy(ies)-Location _____

   ❏ Ablation of lesions-Location _____

   ❏ Removal of lesion by: `

      ❏ Snare-Location _____

      ❏ Hot biopsy-Location _____

   ❏ Band ligation of esophageal varices-Location _____

   ❏ Control of bleeding (unrelated to surgical procedures)-Location _____

   ❏ Decompression of volvulus-Location _____

   ❏ Dilation by balloon-Location _____ size of balloon _____ mm

      ❏ Over a guidewire-Location _____

      ❏ Transendoscopic-Location _____

   ❏ Diverticulectomy of hypopharynx or cervical esophagus

   ❏ Removal of foreign body

   ❏ Injections   Substance injected: _____

      ❏ Directed submucosal injections-Location _____

      ❏ Injection of esophageal varices-Location _____

   ❏ Stent Placement -Location _____

   ❏ Endoscopic ultrasound -Location _____

   ❏ With optical endomicroscopy -Location _____

   ❏ Ultrasound guided intramural or transmural FNA/Bx -Location _____

Procedure	Code Assigned	Code Documented	Modifier Assigned	Modifier Documented	Comments

Number of Units		
Indicated on Claim	Documented	

Financial Impact

Undercoding		Overcoding	
Code	Payment	Code	Payment
		Total Impact on Claim	

Facet Joint Injection Audit Tool

Patient's Name: _____ Patient's Medical Record Number: _____

Date of Service: _____

Name of Provider: _____

Level injected:
- ☐ Level 1 Unilateral/Bilateral
- ☐ Level 2 Unilateral/Bilateral
- ☐ Level 3 Unilateral/Bilateral

Substance Administered: _____

Area:

- ☐ Lumbar   ☐ Thoracic   ☐ Cervical

Procedure	Code Assigned	Code Documented	Modifier Assigned	Modifier Documented	Comments

Number of Units	
Indicated on Claim	Documented

Billable Supplies				Nonbillable Supplies			
Undercoding		Overcoding		Undercoding		Overcoding	
Code	Payment	Code	Payment	Code	Payment	Code	Payment
					Total Impact on Claim		

Appendix 2. **Place-of-Service Codes**

Place-of-service (POS) codes indicate where services were rendered (e.g., in a hospital, clinic, laboratory or any facility other than the patient's home or physician's office). These codes should be reported on professional claims to specify the entity where services were rendered. Check with individual payers (e.g., Medicare, Medicaid, other private insurance) for reimbursement policies regarding these codes. POS codes are required in item 24b.

POS Code	Name	Description	Payment Rate Facility=F Nonfacility=NF
01	Pharmacy	A facility or location where drugs and other medically related items and services are sold, dispensed, or otherwise provided directly to patients	NF
02	Telehealth	The location where health services and health-related services are provided or received, through a telecommunication system. (Effective 1/1/17)	F
03	School	A facility whose primary purpose is education.	NF
04	Homeless Shelter	A facility or location whose primary purpose is to provide temporary housing to homeless individuals (e.g., emergency shelters, individual or family shelters).	NF
05	Indian Health Service Free-standing Facility	A facility or location, owned and operated by the Indian Health Service, which provides diagnostic, therapeutic (surgical and non-surgical), and rehabilitation services to American Indians and Alaska Natives who do not require hospitalization.	Not applicable for adjudication of Medicare claims; systems must recognize for HIPAA
06	Indian Health Service Provider-based Facility	A facility or location, owned and operated by the Indian Health Service, which provides diagnostic, therapeutic (surgical and non-surgical), and rehabilitation services rendered by, or under the supervision of, physicians to American Indians and Alaska Natives admitted as inpatients or outpatients.	Not applicable for adjudication of Medicare claims; systems must recognize for HIPAA
07	Tribal 638 Free-Standing Facility	A facility or location owned and operated by a federally recognized American Indian or Alaska Native tribe or tribal organization under a 638 agreement, which provides diagnostic, therapeutic (surgical and nonsurgical), and rehabilitation services to tribal members who do not require hospitalization.	Not applicable for adjudication of Medicare claims; systems must recognize for HIPAA
08	Tribal 638 Provider-Based Facility	A facility or location owned and operated by a federally recognized American Indian or Alaska Native tribe or tribal organization under a 638 agreement, which provides diagnostic, therapeutic (surgical and nonsurgical), and rehabilitation services to tribal members admitted as inpatients or outpatients.	Not applicable for adjudication of Medicare claims; systems must recognize for HIPAA
09	Prison-Correctional Facility	A prison, jail, reformatory, work farm, detention center, or any other similar facility maintained by either federal, state, or local authorities for the purpose of confinement or rehabilitation of adult or juvenile criminal offenders.	NF
10	Unassigned	N/A	

POS Code	Name	Description	Payment Rate Facility=F Nonfacility=NF
11	Office	Location, other than a hospital, skilled nursing facility (SNF), military treatment facility, community health center, State or local public health clinic, or intermediate care facility (ICF), where the health professional routinely provides health examinations, diagnosis, and treatment of illness or injury on an ambulatory basis.	NF
12	Home	Location, other than a hospital or other facility, where the patient receives care in a private residence.	NF
13	Assisted Living Facility	Congregate residential facility with self-contained living units providing assessment of each resident's needs and on-site support 24 hours a day, seven days a week, with the capacity to deliver or arrange for services including some health care and other services.	NF
14	Group Home	A residence, with shared living areas, where clients receive supervision and other services such as social and/or behavioral services, custodial service, and minimal services (e.g., medication administration).	NF
15	Mobile Unit	A facility unit that moves from place-to-place equipped to provide preventive, screening, diagnostic, and/or treatment services.	NF
16	Temporary Lodging	A short-term accommodation such as a hotel, campground, hostel, cruise ship, or resort where the patient receives care, and which is not identified by any other POS code.	NF
17	Walk-in Retail Health Clinic	A walk-in health clinic, other than an office, urgent care facility, pharmacy, or independent clinic and not described by any other Place of Service code, that is located within a retail operation and provides, on an ambulatory basis, preventive and primary care services.	Not applicable for adjudication of Medicare claims; systems must recognize for HIPAA
18	Place of Employment/ Worksite	A location, not described by any other POS code, owned or operated by a public or private entity where the patient is employed, and where a health professional provides ongoing or episodic occupational medical, therapeutic or rehabilitative services to the individual.	Not applicable for adjudication of Medicare claims; systems must recognize for HIPAA
19	Off Campus- Outpatient Hospital	A portion of an off-campus hospital provider based department which provides diagnostic, therapeutic (both surgical and nonsurgical), and rehabilitation services to sick or injured persons who do not require hospitalization or institutionalization.	F
20	Urgent Care Facility	Location, distinct from a hospital emergency room, an office, or a clinic, whose purpose is to diagnose and treat illness or injury for unscheduled, ambulatory patients seeking immediate medical attention.	NF
21	Inpatient Hospital	A facility, other than psychiatric, which primarily provides diagnostic, therapeutic (both surgical and nonsurgical), and rehabilitation services by, or under, the supervision of physicians to patients admitted for a variety of medical conditions.	F
22	On Campus- Outpatient Hospital	A portion of a hospital's main campus which provides diagnostic, therapeutic (both surgical and nonsurgical), and rehabilitation services to sick or injured persons who do not require hospitalization or institutionalization.	F
23	Emergency Room-Hospital	A portion of a hospital where emergency diagnosis and treatment of illness or injury is provided.	F

© 2020 Optum360, LLC

POS Code	Name	Description	Payment Rate Facility=F Nonfacility=NF
24	**Ambulatory Surgical Center**	A freestanding facility, other than a physician's office, where surgical and diagnostic services are provided on an ambulatory basis.	F
25	**Birthing Center**	A facility, other than a hospital's maternity facilities or a physician's office, which provides a setting for labor, delivery, and immediate postpartum care as well as immediate care of newborn infants.	NF
26	**Military Treatment Facility**	A medical facility operated by one or more of the Uniformed Services. Military treatment facility (MTF) also refers to certain former U.S. Public Health Service (USPHS) facilities now designated as Uniformed Service Treatment Facilities (USTF).	F
27-30	**Unassigned**	N/A	
31	**Skilled Nursing Facility**	A facility that primarily provides inpatient skilled nursing care and related services to patients who require medical, nursing, or rehabilitative services but does not provide the level of care or treatment available in a hospital.	F
32	**Nursing Facility**	A facility which primarily provides to residents skilled nursing care and related services for the rehabilitation of injured, disabled, or sick persons, or, on a regular basis, health-related care services above the level of custodial care to other than mentally retarded individuals.	NF
33	**Custodial Care Facility**	A facility which provides room, board and other personal assistance services, generally on a long-term basis, and which does not include a medical component.	NF
34	**Hospice**	A facility, other than a patient's home, in which palliative and supportive care for terminally ill patients and their families are provided.	F
35-40	**Unassigned**	N/A	
41	**Ambulance—Land**	A land vehicle specifically designed, equipped and staffed for lifesaving and transporting the sick or injured.	F
42	**Ambulance—Air or Water**	An air or water vehicle specifically designed, equipped and staffed for lifesaving and transporting the sick or injured.	F
43-48	**Unassigned**	N/A	
49	**Independent Clinic**	A location, not part of a hospital and not described by any other Place of Service code, that is organized and operated to provide preventive, diagnostic, therapeutic, rehabilitative, or palliative services to outpatients only.	NF
50	**Federally Qualified Health Center**	A facility located in a medically underserved area that provides Medicare beneficiaries preventive primary medical care under the general direction of a physician.	NF
51	**Inpatient Psychiatric Facility**	A facility that provides inpatient psychiatric services for the diagnosis and treatment of mental illness on a 24-hour basis, by or under the supervision of a physician.	F
52	**Psychiatric Facility-Partial Hospitalization**	A facility for the diagnosis and treatment of mental illness that provides a planned therapeutic program for patients who do not require full time hospitalization, but who need broader programs than are possible from outpatient visits to a hospital-based or hospital-affiliated facility.	F

POS Code	Name	Description	Payment Rate Facility=F Nonfacility=NF	
53	Community Mental Health Center	A facility that provides the following services: outpatient services, including specialized outpatient services for children, the elderly, individuals who are chronically ill, and residents of the CMHC's mental health services area who have been discharged from inpatient treatment at a mental health facility; 24 hour a day emergency care services; day treatment, other partial hospitalization services, or psychosocial rehabilitation services; screening for patients being considered for admission to State mental health facilities to determine the appropriateness of such admission; and consultation and education services.	F	
54	Intermediate Care Facility/Individuals with Intellectual Disabilities	A facility which primarily provides health-related care and services above the level of custodial care to mentally retarded individuals but does not provide the level of care or treatment available in a hospital or SNF.	NF	
55	Residential Substance Abuse Treatment Facility	A facility which provides treatment for substance (alcohol and drug) abuse to live-in residents who do not require acute medical care. Services include individual and group therapy and counseling, family counseling, laboratory tests, drugs and supplies, psychological testing, and room and board.	NF	
56	Psychiatric Residential Treatment Center	A facility or distinct part of a facility for psychiatric care which provides a total 24-hour therapeutically planned and professionally staffed group living and learning environment.	F	
57	Non-residential Substance Abuse Treatment Facility	A location that provides treatment for substance (alcohol and drug) abuse on an ambulatory basis. Services include individual and group therapy and counseling, family counseling, laboratory tests, drugs and supplies, and psychological testing.	NF	
58	Non-residential Opioid Treatment Facility	A location that provides treatment for opioid use disorder on an ambulatory basis. Services include methadone and other forms of Medication Assisted Treatment (MAT). (Effective January 1, 2020)		
59	Unassigned	N/A		
60	Mass Immunization Center	A location where providers administer pneumococcal pneumonia and influenza virus vaccinations and submit these services as electronic media claims, paper claims, or using the roster billing method. This generally takes place in a mass immunization setting, such as, a public health center, pharmacy, or mall but may include a physician office setting.	NF	
61	Comprehensive Inpatient Rehabilitation Facility	A facility that provides comprehensive rehabilitation services under the supervision of a physician to inpatients with physical disabilities. Services include physical therapy, occupational therapy, speech pathology, social or psychological services, and orthotics and prosthetics services.	F	
62	Comprehensive Outpatient Rehabilitation Facility	A facility that provides comprehensive rehabilitation services under the supervision of a physician to outpatients with physical disabilities. Services include physical therapy, occupational therapy, and speech pathology services.	NF	
63-64	Unassigned	N/A		
65	End-Stage Renal Disease Treatment Facility	A facility other than a hospital, which provides dialysis treatment, maintenance, and/or training to patients or caregivers on an ambulatory or home-care basis.	NF	
66-70	Unassigned	N/A		

POS Code	Name	Description	Payment Rate Facility=F Nonfacility=NF	
71	Public Health Clinic	A facility maintained by either State or local health departments that provides ambulatory primary medical care under the general direction of a physician.	NF	
72	Rural Health Clinic	A certified facility which is located in a rural medically underserved area that provides ambulatory primary medical care under the general direction of a physician.	NF	
73-80	Unassigned	N/A		
81	Independent Laboratory	A laboratory certified to perform diagnostic and or clinical tests independent of an institution or a physician's office.	NF	
82-98	Unassigned	N/A		
99	Other Place of Service	Other place of service not identified above	NF	